# A Case-Based Approach to PET/CT in Oncology

# A Case-Based Approach to PET/CT in Oncology

Edited by

**Victor H. Gerbaudo**
Brigham & Women's Hospital
Harvard Medical School

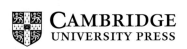
CAMBRIDGE
UNIVERSITY PRESS

CAMBRIDGE UNIVERSITY PRESS
Cambridge, New York, Melbourne, Madrid, Cape Town,
Singapore, São Paulo, Delhi, Mexico City

Cambridge University Press
The Edinburgh Building, Cambridge CB2 8RU, UK

Published in the United States of America
by Cambridge University Press, New York

www.cambridge.org
Information on this title: www.cambridge.org/9780521116831

First published 2012

Printed and Bound in the United Kingdom by the MPG Books Group

*A catalogue record for this publication is available from the
British Library*

*Library of Congress Cataloging-in-Publication data*

A case-based approach to PET/CT in oncology / edited by
Victor H. Gerbaudo.
    p. ; cm.
  Includes bibliographical references.
  ISBN 978-0-521-11683-1 (Hardback)
I. Gerbaudo, Victor H.
  [DNLM:  1.  Neoplasms–radionuclide imaging–Case Reports.
2.  Positron-Emission Tomography/Computed Tomography–Case
Reports.   QZ 241]
  616.99′407575–dc23

                                              2011048385

ISBN 978-0-521-11683-1 Hardback

Cambridge University Press has no responsibility for the persistence or
accuracy of URLs for external or third-party internet websites referred to
in this publication, and does not guarantee that any content on such
websites is, or will remain, accurate or appropriate.

Every effort has been made in preparing this book to provide accurate and
up-to-date information which is in accord with accepted standards and
practice at the time of publication. Although case histories are drawn
from actual cases, every effort has been made to disguise the identities of
the individuals involved. Nevertheless, the authors, editors and publishers
can make no warranties that the information contained herein is totally
free from error, not least because clinical standards are constantly
changing through research and regulation. The authors, editors and
publishers therefore disclaim all liability for direct or consequential
damages resulting from the use of material contained in this book.
Readers are strongly advised to pay careful attention to information
provided by the manufacturer of any drugs or equipment that they
plan to use.

DAMAGED

*To Fabiana, Sebastián and Sofía for understanding, patience and support during this demanding journey,*

*to my mother and father for believing in me,*

*to my teachers for wisdom, to my patients and students for inspiration, and last, but not least, to my colleagues who share the desire to conquer disease.*

*Y para vos Lolo, durante este emprendimiento entendí cuan grande es la verdad que una vez albergaron tus palabras, "no hay mejor pan que aquel horneado por uno mismo" y hoy lo comparto con vos...*

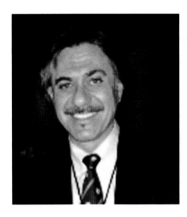

**Dr. Victor H. Gerbaudo** is the Director of the Nuclear Medicine and Molecular Imaging Program, and the Associate Director of Pulmonary Functional Imaging at the Brigham and Women's Hospital, Harvard Medical School, in Boston, Massachusetts, USA. He is a clinical Nuclear Oncology scientist with 20 years of experience in the field. His clinical, teaching and research efforts focus on the in-vivo qualitative and quantitative monitoring of tumor biology, imaging, and response to therapy with PET/CT. His teaching integrates the application of basic concepts of tumor pathophysiology and molecular pathology to oncologic imaging and to the interpretation and integration of imaging results into management decisions. Topics of interest include molecular imaging of tumor cell proliferation, perfusion, apoptosis and glycolytic metabolism. His research focuses on the assessment and characterization of tumor invasion and metastasis with positron imaging of thoracic malignancies (i.e., malignant pleural mesothelioma, lung cancer), as well as esophageal cancer, brain and gastrointestinal tumors. His work in this area has expanded the use of clinical PET/CT for metabolically guided tumor biopsy and ablation, and for metabolic grading and staging of human tumors, as it relates to histological grade, molecular pathology, surgical stage and survival. He has authored numerous original contributions, reviews, clinical communications and abstracts in the imaging and oncologic peer-reviewed literature, and has delivered more than 100 presentations on the role of PET in oncology around the world. Dr. Gerbaudo is a reviewer for numerous radiology and oncology journals, and serves in the Scientific Program Committee of the Society of Nuclear Medicine as subchairman of the Clinical Oncology track, and as the vice chairman of the education and research committee of the New England Chapter of Society of Nuclear Medicine. He is an active member of the Institute for Clinical PET of the Academy of Molecular Imaging, and of the International Mesothelioma Interest Group. Dr Gerbaudo also serves as an ad hoc expert lecturer on PET/CT in Oncology for the International Atomic Energy Agency.

# Contents

# Contributors

**Anthony P. Belanger, PhD**
Division of Nuclear Medicine and Molecular Imaging,
Department of Radiology, Brigham and Women's Hospital
and Harvard Medical School,
Boston, MA, USA

**Ronald Boellaard, PhD**
Department of Nuclear Medicine and PET Research VU
University Medical Center, Amsterdam, the Netherlands

**Scott Britz-Cunningham, MD, PhD**
Division of Nuclear Medicine and Molecular Imaging,
Department of Radiology, Brigham and Women's Hospital
and Harvard Medical School, Boston, MA, USA

**Muhammad A. Chaudhry, MD**
Division of Nuclear Medicine, Department of Radiology
and Radiological Sciences, Johns Hopkins University Hospital,
Baltimore, MD, USA

**Wei Chen, MD, PhD**
Department of Molecular and Medical Pharmacology,
Ahmanson Biological Imaging, David Geffen School of
Medicine at UCLA, Los Angeles, CA, USA

**Hubert H. Chuang, MD**
Department of Nuclear Medicine, MD Anderson Cancer
Center, Houston, TX, USA

**Timothy R. DeGrado, PhD**
Division of Nuclear Medicine,
Department of Radiology,
Mayo Clinic, Rochester, MN, USA

**Dominique Delbeke, MD, PhD**
Department of Radiology and Radiological Sciences,
Vanderbilt University School of Medicine,
Nashville, TN, USA

**Laura A. Drubach, MD**
Division of Nuclear Medicine and Molecular Imaging,
Department of Radiology, Children's Hospital of Boston
and Harvard Medical School, Boston, MA, USA

**Einat Even-Sapir, MD, PhD**
Department of Nuclear Medicine, Tel Aviv Sourasky Medical
Center, Tel Aviv, Israel

**Kent P. Friedman, MD**
Department of Radiology, NYU School of Medicine,
New York, NY, USA

**Victor H. Gerbaudo, PhD**
Division of Nuclear Medicine and Molecular Imaging,
Department of Radiology, Brigham and Women's Hospital
and Harvard Medical School, Boston, MA, USA

**Ritu R. Gill, MBBS**
Division of Thoracic Radiology, Department of Radiology,
Brigham and Women's Hospital and Harvard Medical School,
Boston, MA, USA

**Denis J. Gradinscak, MBB, FRANZCR**
Department of Nuclear Medicine, Westmead Hospital,
Sydney, Australia

**Frederick D. Grant, MD**
Division of Nuclear Medicine and Molecular Imaging,
Department of Radiology, Children's Hospital of Boston
and Harvard Medical School, Boston, MA, USA

**Ravinder Grewal, MD**
Division of Nuclear Medicine, Department of Radiology,
Memorial Sloan-Kettering Cancer Center, New York, NY, USA

**Jon M. Hainer, BS**
Division of Nuclear Medicine and Molecular Imaging,
Department of Radiology, Brigham and Women's Hospital,
Boston, MA, USA

**Otto S. Hoekstra, MD, PhD**
Department of Nuclear Medicine and PET Research, VU
University Medical Center, Amsterdam, the Netherlands

**Laura L. Horky, MD, PhD**
Division of Nuclear Medicine and Molecular Imaging,
Department of Radiology, Brigham and Women's Hospital
and Harvard Medical School, Boston, MA, USA

**Ora Israel, MD**
Department of Nuclear Medicine, Rambam Health Care Center, Haifa, Israel

**Aaron C. Jessop, MD, PhD**
Department of Nuclear Medicine, MD Anderson Cancer Center, Houston, TX, USA

**Chun K. Kim, MD**
Division of Nuclear Medicine and Molecular Imaging, Department of Radiology, Brigham and Women's Hospital and Harvard Medical School, Boston, MA, USA

**Lale Kostakoglu, MD, MPH**
Division of Nuclear Medicine, Department of Radiology, Mount Sinai School of Medicine, New York, USA

**Homer A. Macapinlac, MD**
Department of Nuclear Medicine, MD Anderson Cancer Center, Houston, TX, USA

**Stephen C. Moore, PhD**
Division of Nuclear Medicine and Molecular Imaging, Department of Radiology, Brigham and Women's Hospital and Harvard Medical School, Boston, MA, USA

**Mi-Ae Park, PhD**
Division of Nuclear Medicine and Molecular Imaging, Department of Radiology, Brigham and Women's Hospital and Harvard Medical School, Boston, MA, USA

**Stephan Probst, MD**
Department of Radiology, NYU School of Medicine, New York, NY, USA

**Saiyada N. F. Rizvi**
Dept. of Nuclear Medicine and PET Research, VU University Medical Center, Amsterdam, the Netherlands

**Christiaan Schiepers, MD, PhD**
Department of Molecular and Medical Pharmacology, David Geffen School of Medicine at UCLA, Los Angeles, CA, USA

**Heiko Schöder, MD**
Division of Nuclear Medicine, Department of Radiology, Memorial Sloan-Kettering Cancer Center, New York, NY, USA

**Stuart Silverman, MD**
Abdominal Imaging and Intervention, Department of Radiology, Brigham and Women's Hospital and Harvard Medical School, Boston, MA, USA

**Sigrid Stroobants**
Department of Nuclear Medicine, Antwerp University Hospital, Edegem, Belgium

**Servet Tatli, MD**
Abdominal Imaging and Intervention, Department of Radiology, Brigham and Women's Hospital and Harvard Medical School, Boston, MA, USA

**S. Ted Treves, MD**
Division of Nuclear Medicine and Molecular Imaging, Department of Radiology, Children's Hospital of Boston and Harvard Medical School, Boston, MA, USA

**Richard L. Wahl, MD**
Division of Nuclear Medicine, Department of Radiology and Radiological Sciences, Johns Hopkins University Hospital, Baltimore, MD, USA

**Katherine A. Zukotynski, MD**
Department of Imaging, Dana Farber Cancer Institute and Harvard Medical School, Boston, MA, USA

# Foreword

Who could have predicted that the discoveries by Roentgen of X-rays, by Becquerel of radioactivity, by Warburg of the aerobic glycolysis of tumors, and the solution of the Radon problem by Cormack would lead to one of the most powerful medical technologies in the care of cancer patients? But it did and this (not so slim) volume organized by Victor Gerbaudo shows the result.

The development of PET/CT for cancer was mostly a case of technology first – application second. This is in contrast to those technologies where there is a clear need and a technology developed to meet it. Originally concerned in applications to brain imaging, all parts (PET, CT, DG) were adapted to oncology once it was remembered that tumors as well as the brain use glucose as a fuel. After a slow but rapidly progressing start over the past fifteen years, inhibited, in part, by gatekeeping agencies' inability to realize its potential, PET/CT has become central to diagnosis, staging, assessing response to therapy and in the planning of radiation therapy for a host of cancers. This compendium demonstrates how far it has come and points to some uses, such as in image-guided therapy, for the future.

This book should be read by both imagers and oncologists; it should appeal to expert and novice alike. The first part, concerning the sciences and technology basic to PET/CT, not only reviews traditional physics, instrumentation, and radiopharmaceutical chemistry but adds material on information systems and functional anatomy as well. The second part provides a general background for each organ system followed by case-based exemplars. The expert-authors bring to each chapter a broad experience.

The power of mixing functional imaging with anatomical detail has only begun to be realized. As the systematic variation of genetic components in disease are translated into metabolic/biochemical manifestations and as appropriate radio-labeled agents are developed to reflect them, we can expect new insights into patho-physiology as well as new approaches to nosology and to the planning and monitoring of treatments. Today's FDG-PET/CT in cancer will be the founding example.

*S. James Adelstein*
Harvard Medical School
Boston, Massachusetts

# Preface

Clinical Positron Emission Tomography (PET) with the glucose analog $^{18}$F-fluorodeoxyglucose (FDG) has already gained its place as a routine clinical imaging test in today's clinical and surgical practice of oncology. Its inherent ability to interrogate the biologic behavior of neoplastic molecular pathways in one whole-body scan has made it a very important and in some cases indispensable, diagnostic and staging tool for cancer patients. The end result has been its significant impact in the medical management of these patients.

*A Case-Based Approach to PET/CT in Oncology* applies PET basic and clinical science concepts to the detailed analysis of well-illustrated cases of daily clinical practice. It shows imaging practitioners and clinical and surgical oncologists the important role that PET imaging plays in the care of cancer patients, as it influences management and outcomes.

Part I starts with the physics and instrumentation of PET imaging, followed by a chapter on PET probes that stresses the potential of FDG and other tracers which hopefully soon will be reaching the clinic. A chapter describing the role of information systems in medical imaging and PET/CT in particular introduces the reader to the foundations of the electronic media, so as to be able to recognize the possible pitfalls and to the extent possible, adjust for them to minimize misinterpretation and error. Part I concludes with a chapter describing the basic biodistribution and image patterns observed in the normal FDG-PET image.

Part II is devoted to the oncologic applications of PET imaging. The cancer types discussed per organ system are those in which the published data support good clinical accuracy of the technique. Each chapter starts with an introduction to the general concepts and epidemiology, staging and treatment overview of the cancer type being addressed. This is followed by a thorough description of the role of PET/CT in the diagnosis, initial staging, restaging and monitoring response to therapy; concepts that are applied and exemplified by the cases that follow.

Each case starts with a clinical history, followed by a detailed description of the PET/CT technique employed. The image findings are described as they should appear in the clinical imaging report. The latter unfolds in a detailed discussion of the pathophysiology of the disease, including when appropriate or when known, the molecular basis of radiotracer uptake in the lesion being described. Teaching points highlight the role of FDG and other radiotracers when applicable, in cancer diagnosis, staging, restaging, and monitoring response to treatment, together with its reported accuracy. The additional information provided by fusion imaging is discussed, as it increases confidence during image interpretation for optimal clinical decision making. In addition, the authors elaborate on the PET-driven changes in management, and on the take-home message from each case. A chapter on the methodological aspects of monitoring response to cancer therapy discusses, and exemplifies with everyday cases, the advantages of using tumor metabolic changes as the early predictors of therapeutic sensitivity. The last chapter describes our experience and the complementary role of functional imaging to guide interventional procedures, such as biopsies and ablations. We report on the advantages and limitations of the technique while attempting to minimize sampling errors from cancerous lesions in which metabolic disease precedes morphologic changes.

All chapters, including those on the basic sciences, are clinically oriented, and demonstrate an important clinical application for the practicing radiologist, the nuclear medicine physician, and Residents and Fellows in training. This text attempts to balance practical aspects of anatomo-functional imaging while answering clinical oncology questions, therefore clinical and surgical oncologists and their trainees should also find this book to be a reliable resource for their daily practice.

*Victor H. Gerbaudo*
Boston, Massachusetts

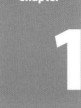

**Chapter**

# PET and PET/CT physics, instrumentation, and artifacts

Stephen C. Moore and Mi-Ae Park

This chapter provides background material essential for understanding the scientific and technical underpinnings of the image-formation process in positron emission tomography (PET). X-ray computed tomography (CT) will also be briefly discussed, though in much less detail. Instead, we will emphasize, later in this chapter, the ways in which the CT acquisition and resulting images influence reconstructed PET images. Because the terminology used to describe the most important nuclear physics and PET instrumentation concepts may be unfamiliar to some readers, we have highlighted certain key words and expressions in bold font when these terms are first introduced. For more advanced treatments of selected topics related to PET instrumentation and imaging, readers are referred to physics texts, such as those by Cherry *et al.* (1) and Wernick and Aarsvold (2).

## Radioactive decay: positron emission, annihilation, and detection

In this section, we discuss the basic nuclear physics concepts on which PET imaging is based. We begin by presenting some information and terminology related to the decay of radioactive atoms, in general, as well as more detailed and specific descriptions of positron decay. Along the way, we will discuss several key characteristics of radioactive nuclei that emit positrons; these will later be shown to influence the quality of PET images.

## Radioactive decay

There are many different types of radioactive elements, called **radionuclides**. While all such elements possess **unstable** nuclei, different categories of radioactive elements have been defined according to the manner in which they transform themselves to allow the constituents of the nucleus, i.e., protons and neutrons, to assume a more stable arrangement. When such a transformation occurs, we say that the nucleus has **decayed** from a higher energy, unstable state to a lower energy, more stable state, or often to a fully stable **ground**

state. The total mass-energy of the resulting ground-state atom is less than that of the initial radionuclide. The energy lost by the radioactive nucleus during its decay is normally transferred to one or more particles that are emitted from the atom; thus, it is often possible to determine quite precisely the moment when an unstable nucleus decays, by detecting the emitted radiation using one of several types of radiation detectors. Depending on the **decay mode**, the emitted radiation can consist of charged particles which have mass (e.g., an electron, or a positively charged electron called a **positron**), or particles with zero mass and zero charge (e.g., a **photon**, which is the fundamental particle or "carrier" of electromagnetic radiation). Very commonly, both massive and massless particles are emitted during the decay of a single radioactive atom. The type and number of particles emitted in any given nuclear decay are characteristic properties of the decay mode. Some radioactive elements can decay by more than one possible mode.

Each nucleus can be uniquely characterized by an **atomic number, Z**, and a **mass number, A**, where Z is the number of protons in the nucleus, and A is the sum of the number of protons and neutrons in the nucleus. Stable nuclei generally have approximately the same number of protons and neutrons (or somewhat more neutrons than protons), whereas unstable nuclei usually have an excess number of protons or neutrons. Two or more radionuclides which have the same number of protons, but a different number of neutrons within their nuclei are called **radioisotopes** of the same element. For example, iodine-123, iodine-125, and iodine-131 are all radioisotopes. There are several unique properties of every radionuclide; these include the nuclide's decay mode (or combination of modes), its decay **transition energy** (which is divided among the resulting decay particles), and its **half-life**, which is the time required for half of the initial number of radioactive nuclei in a sample to decay. While we can never predict the exact moment in time when a given nucleus will decay, or – for multiple, or complex decay modes – the exact decay mode or the exact energy of each of the possible emitted particles, we do know these properties quite well in a statistical sense. In fact,

*A Case-Based Approach to PET/CT in Oncology*, ed. Victor H. Gerbaudo. Published by Cambridge University Press.
© Cambridge University Press 2012.

the phenomenon of radioactive decay can be described as a so-called Poisson statistical process and, for any given radionuclide, we can state with a high degree of certainty the *average* time required for a large number of such radioactive nuclei to be reduced by one-half (i.e., the radionuclide's half-life). Similarly, we can reliably predict the average number of emitted particles of any given type, as well as the distribution of their energies.

## Positron decay

Unstable nuclei possessing an excess number of protons often become more stable by undergoing **positron decay**. (This is also sometimes referred to as positive **beta decay**, because positrons or electrons emitted from a nucleus during a radioactive decay are commonly called positive or negative **beta particles**.) During positron decay, a positively charged proton in the nucleus ($p^+$) appears to change into a neutral (zero-charge) neutron ($n^0$) while, simultaneously, a positron ($\beta^+$) is emitted from the nucleus, along with a zero-mass, neutral particle called a neutrino ($\nu^0$). Because a proton, essentially, turns into a neutron during the decay, the initial element is transformed into another element whose atomic number, Z, is reduced by one, but whose mass number, A, remains unchanged. Sometimes, following positron decay, the nucleus will end up with an appropriate ratio of protons to neutrons to be stable; however, the combined properties of all of the nuclear constituents may still not result in a fully stable state, in which case the nucleus is said to be in a **metastable state**. When this occurs, the metastable nucleus generally decays further to the ground state by rearranging its nuclear constituents and emitting one or more photons in the process. (When photons are emitted from a nucleus, they are referred to as **gamma** radiation.) Positron or $\beta^+$ decay (including, for some radionuclides, one or more possible neutral gamma photons, $\gamma^0$) can thus be summarized symbolically by the formula:

$$p^+ \rightarrow n^0 + \beta^+ + \nu^0 \ (+\gamma^0{}_1 + \gamma^0{}_2 + \cdots).$$

Note that the total electrical charge is conserved in this decay process, as it must be. The left-hand side of the equation shows a proton with a single positive charge (+1), and the sum of the charges of all particles on the right-hand side is also +1.

## Positron emitters used in biomedical imaging

It can be seen from this formula that the transition energy associated with a *pure* positron decay (with no accompanying gamma photons) is shared among three particles: a neutron which remains bound within the nucleus, a positron, and a neutrino. Because there are three decay particles which share the nuclear transition energy, the kinetic energy of the emitted positron is not restricted to a single value but, instead, is characterized by a continuous **energy spectrum**, ranging from zero up to some maximum value, $E_{\beta,max}$, which is different for each different radionuclide. The average positron energy is, typically, about one-third of $E_{\beta,max}$.

Most positron emitters used for biomedical imaging applications have relatively short half-lives, ranging from seconds to minutes, although there are exceptions. Examples of commonly used radioactive elements which decay by positron emission (and their half-lives) include fluorine-18 ($^{18}$F; $T_{1/2} = 110$ min.), carbon-11 ($^{11}$C; $T_{1/2} = 20$ min.), nitrogen-13 ($^{13}$N; $T_{1/2} = 10$ min.), oxygen-15 ($^{15}$O; $T_{1/2} = 122$ s), and rubidium-82 ($^{82}$Rb; $T_{1/2} = 75$ s). Some of these positron emitters, e.g., $^{11}$C, $^{13}$N, $^{15}$O, are radioisotopes of corresponding stable elements ($^{12}$C, $^{14}$N, $^{16}$O) that are ubiquitous throughout all biologic systems. This affords the opportunity to radiolabel many different bio-molecules of interest simply by replacing a stable element in the molecule with the corresponding positron-emitting isotope. The stable isotopes corresponding to other positron emitters, such as $^{18}$F and $^{82}$Rb are found less commonly in living systems; however, some of these radionuclides can still be used to label various analogs of bio-molecules, e.g., the glucose analog, $^{18}$F-fluorodeoxyglucose (FDG), while others can be used in the form of radioactive salts, e.g., $^{82}$Rb-chloride, which behaves as a potassium analog in vivo.

## Electron capture

It is important to note that not all positron emitters decay solely by $\beta^+$ decay; some unstable radionuclides characterized by an excess number of protons can also decay by a competing process, known as **electron capture**, in which an inner-shell atomic electron is captured by the nucleus, where it combines with a proton and, effectively, changes into a neutron. Just as for $\beta^+$-decay, a neutrino is produced during electron capture, although no positron results from this decay mode:

$$p^+ + e^- \rightarrow n^0 + \nu^0.$$

Carbon-11 is an example of a radionuclide which decays either by positron emission (in 97% of decays), or by electron capture (in 3% of decays). Clearly, if a positron emitter decays much more frequently by electron capture, then this radionuclide would probably not be very useful for PET imaging, since its positron yield per nuclear decay would be very low.

## Positron annihilation

In positron emission tomography, the positrons themselves are not directly detected to form images. This is because positrons have a short range in tissue (less than a few millimeters), which means that almost none of them will escape the patient's body to be detected. After an emitted positron loses most of its kinetic energy, by scattering off of multiple electrons along its path, it combines with a nearby electron to form an atomic-like species known as **positronium**. This extremely short-lived state promptly results in the annihilation of the positron and electron to produce two photons which are emitted back-to-back in opposite directions. (See Figure 1.1.) Both of the **annihilation photons** have the same energy – 511 thousand (kilo) electron volts (keV) – which is the rest-mass energy of the electron and the positron from which the photons originated. To be used for PET image formation, both of these photons must escape the patient and then be detected simultaneously in two of the many thousands of PET detectors which encircle the patient in a modern PET scanner. It should be mentioned that the neutrino emitted during $\beta^+$ decay is almost impossible to detect because neutrinos only interact in matter with extremely low probability. Although they do not play a direct role in the PET image-formation process, neutrinos do influence the energy spectrum and range of the positrons with which they share the energy made available in the decay process.

## The PET measurement process

A schematic view of a PET detector ring is shown in Figure 1.2A, along with an illustration of a single positron-annihilation event occurring within a patient's body, and the resulting two 511-keV annihilation photons being detected in coincidence in two opposing detectors. The path along which the back-to-back annihilation photons travel is defined by the two detectors in

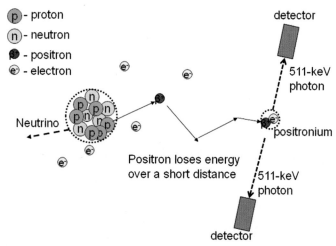

**Figure 1.1** Positron decay and annihilation. The emitted positron travels a distance of up to several millimeters, depending on its initial energy (Table 1.1). After losing energy by multiple scatter interactions, the positron and an electron annihilate to form two 511-keV photons, emitted in opposite directions.

which the photons are detected. This path is often called a PET **line-of-response**, or **LOR**. Because all of the detectors are electronically placed in coincidence with all other detectors within an arc on the other side of the patient, it is easy to see there are a great many possible LORs in a PET scanner. As each coincidence-pair event is detected in the PET scanner, the system electronics computes the unique LOR associated with the two detectors which "fired." Each LOR is mapped to a unique location in a computer memory, which is incremented every time an event is detected along the corresponding LOR.

Figure 1.2B shows only those LORs which connect a single detector to all the detectors on the other side of the patient. During the acquisition of PET data, certain LORs will record more decay events, while others will record fewer events, depending on the distribution of radioactivity within the patient's body. At the end of the PET acquisition, each LOR will have recorded a total number of counts proportional to the *integral* of the radioactivity concentration along that LOR. It is clear from Figure 1.2B that the pattern of all LORs involving a single detector resembles a "fan" of LORs across the patient. In fact, we often refer to this data format as **fan-beam projection data**. All of the other detectors around the ring will also have their own coincidence fans of data. Given a complete set of such angular projection data, which includes fan-beam projections from all angles around the PET detector ring, it is possible to reconstruct an image corresponding to the concentration of the positron-emitting radionuclide within a transaxial "slice" through the patient's body. For those readers who are already knowledgeable about X-ray CT, the fan-beam projection concept should be quite familiar. In CT, the scanner records fan-beam projections connecting each X-ray source position, i.e., during the rotation of an X-ray tube, to all opposing detectors. In CT, each projection-ray is a measurement of the integral of the so-called **linear attenuation coefficient** along the line, whereas in PET, each projection ray is proportional to the integral of the radiotracer's activity concentration along the LOR. Therefore, the image intensity (brightness) in a given region of a reconstructed CT image is proportional to the region's linear attenuation coefficient (related to the region's density and the effective atomic

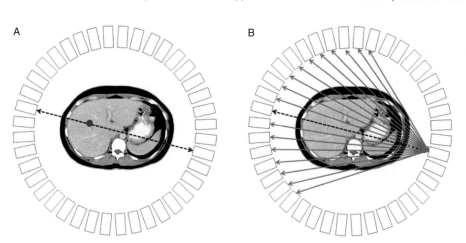

**Figure 1.2** (A) A single coincidence line-of-response (LOR) defined by two detector elements; (B) a fan-beam projection of coincidence LORs, shown superimposed on a X-ray CT transaxial section through the abdomen.

number of the material), whereas the local image intensity in reconstructed PET images is proportional to the concentration of radioactivity in the region in units of decays per second per mL (Bq/mL), or μCi/mL (where 1 μCi = 37 kBq).

The earliest PET tomographs consisted of a single ring of detectors; these systems acquired and reconstructed data from a single transaxial section of the patient at one time. To image additional "slices" required stepping the patient table through the PET scanner, and acquiring another set of coincidence projections at each additional desired axial slice location. Modern PET scanners have many more rings of detectors surrounding the patient, which permit more slices within a larger axial range (typically 15–20 cm) to be imaged simultaneously.

## Spatial resolution of PET images

The spatial resolution of an imaging system determines our ability to resolve two distinct features that are close together in the patient being imaged. A system with good spatial resolution will allow us to visually discriminate the two features when they are very close together, whereas a system with poor resolution will only permit us to resolve the features when they are farther apart. Spatial resolution is often described by a single number representing the **full-width-at-half-maximum (FWHM)** of the so-called **point-spread function (PSF)**. If a very tiny point-source of radioactivity is imaged in a PET scanner, then the PSF is just the blurred image of this source. The FWHM of the PSF is simply a measure of the extent or width of the blurred PSF at the location corresponding to half of the maximum image brightness within the point. The FWHM is also a convenient measure because it also provides an indication of the distance of separation between two point sources at which they would blur together, and no longer be resolvable as two separate sources. In PET imaging, the spatial resolution is primarily affected by the following factors: detector size, positron range, photon non-colinearity, and image reconstruction. These factors will now be discussed, one by one.

## Detector size

The effective width of the lines-of-response connecting any pair of detectors is obviously affected by the size of the detectors themselves; the use of smaller detectors implies that the LOR connecting them will be "narrower," i.e., its width will be known more precisely, whereas wider detectors will lead to a greater uncertainty in our ability to localize annihilation events, with a concomitant deterioration of spatial resolution. As shown in Figure 1.3, the FWHM of the LOR is not constant everywhere; since two detectors must simultaneously detect both coincident photons, the detector resolution varies along the LOR. It turns out that the detector PSF is approximately triangular in shape at the mid-point between the two detectors, where the detector resolution, R, is best and the FWHM is equal to half the detector size, d. The detector PSF becomes increasingly wider for annihilation events located closer to

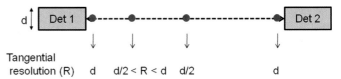

**Figure 1.3** Detector resolution, R, depends on the width of a detector element, d, perpendicular to the LOR, and varies with the source location along the LOR. The detector element size, d, is typically several millimeters in most PET scanners.

either of the two detectors; the worst detector resolution is found immediately adjacent to a detector, where the PSF shape is approximately rectangular with a FWHM of the detector PSF equal to the detector size.

These considerations imply that a large number of very small detectors should be used in PET scanners; however, there are other important factors which must be considered when designing a PET system. Importantly, the detectors are often the most expensive components in the scanner, so a large increase in the number of detectors may not be possible. Another consideration is that there is always a small gap between detector elements. This implies that a system containing a larger number of smaller detectors will have a greater percentage of "dead-space" between detectors, which decreases the overall detection efficiency of the scanner. Finally, when more detector elements are used in a system, it becomes more difficult to identify accurately the exact detector element in which a photon interaction occurred.

## Positron range

Ideally, we would like each positron-decay event to be located along a well-defined LOR in the PET scanner. Unfortunately, however, as shown in Figure 1.1, the positron can sometimes travel through a distance up to several millimeters away from its point of origin, before annihilating with an electron to produce the back-to-back photons which define the LOR associated with the event. Because the positron's path through the surrounding materials can be quite tortuous, owing to multiple scattering, this means that, in some cases, a positron might end up back near its origin before it loses enough energy to annihilate. In this case, there would be very little loss of spatial information because the annihilation would occur close to the point of nuclear decay. However, on average, most positrons are located somewhat farther from their point-of-origin when they annihilate. The maximum possible energy of the emitted positrons, their average energy, and the root-mean-square (rms) position deviation from the location of the positron decays are listed in Table 1.1 for a variety of common positron emitters. (Beta-particle energy values are shown in units of millions of electron volts, MeV.)

## Photon non-colinearity

The positron and electron which comprise the short-lived positronium "atom" both have some (generally small) kinetic energy and momentum before they annihilate to produce

**Table 1.1** Properties of some positron emitters.

| Radionuclide | $E_{max}$ (MeV) | $E_{ave}$ (MeV) | RMS position deviation in water (mm) |
|---|---|---|---|
| $^{11}$C | 0.96 | 0.38 | 0.42 |
| $^{13}$N | 1.19 | 0.49 | 0.57 |
| $^{15}$O | 1.72 | 0.73 | 1.02 |
| $^{18}$F | 0.64 | 0.24 | 0.23 |
| $^{82}$Rb | 3.35 | 1.52 | 2.60 |

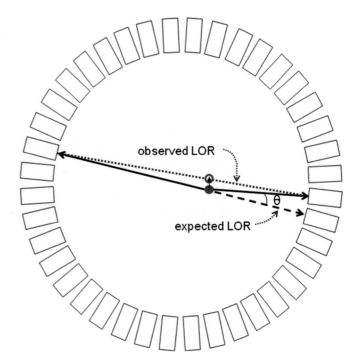

**Figure 1.4** Resolution degradation arising from non-colinearity in the directions of the two 511-keV annihilation photons.

back-to-back photons. If their combined momentum before the annihilation had a significant component in a direction perpendicular to the direction along which the annihilation photons are emitted, then, because each vector component of momentum must be conserved, it turns out that the angle between the annihilation photons will not always be exactly 180 degrees but, instead, will deviate slightly from 180 degrees from event to event. Since the LOR is defined by the straight line connecting the two detectors which sense the annihilation photons, it can be seen from Figure 1.4 that any non-colinearity in the directions of the two annihilation photons will introduce an additional uncertainty in the determination of the event location. Because this effect produces an *angular* deviation, the magnitude of the position uncertainty arising from photon non-colinearity increases with the diameter of the PET scanner's detector ring. The resolution attributable to photon non-colinearity has been shown (3) to be well approximated by the following empirical function of ring diameter, in centimeters:

$$FWHM_{non-col}(cm) \sim 0.0022 \times ring\ diameter\ (cm).$$

Thus, for a whole-body PET scanner with a ring-diameter of 90 cm, the FWHM resolution attributable to non-colinearity is approximately 2 mm.

## System resolution and reconstructed resolution

The FWHM of the overall system resolution can be approximated fairly well as the quadrature sum (i.e., the square-root of the sum of squares) of the various contributing factors:

$$FWHM_{sys} = \sqrt{FWHM_{det}^2 + rms_{range}^2 + FWHM_{non-col}^2}.$$

For a PET system with 4.2-mm wide detectors and a ring-diameter of 90 cm, the resolution near the center of the scanner is thus expected to be ~ 2.9 mm when imaging F-18, whereas if the same system is used to image Rb-82, the system resolution is ~ 3.9 mm.

So far, we have only discussed those factors contributing to the overall system resolution which are limited by the fundamental physics of positron decay and annihilation, as well as by the "hardware" design of the PET tomograph. It is important to realize, however, that the resolution of the final

PET images will also be influenced by the type of tomographic reconstruction algorithm (e.g., filtered-backprojection, iterative maximum-likelihood, etc.), as well as by the user's choice of reconstruction parameters, which generally affect the "tradeoff" between reconstructed image resolution and image noise. Because the choice of reconstruction method and parameters often depends strongly on the type of PET study being performed, there is a rather wide range of reconstructed resolution values utilized in clinical practice.

## Detector depth-of-interaction effect on spatial resolution

As seen in Figure 1.5, when considering the detector spatial resolution perpendicular to LORs located at larger radial distances from the center of the PET scanner, there is an additional degrading factor which can be attributed to a lack of knowledge about the depth within each detector where the photon interaction occurred. For LORs near the center of the PET scanner, we also have no knowledge of the **depth-of-interaction (DOI)** in the detectors; however, the DOI effect only degrades spatial resolution significantly for LORs at large radial offsets, where the DOI uncertainty, essentially, makes the detectors appear to be wider than they actually are. The worse resolution attributable to this effect could be improved by using thinner detectors; however, this can be counter-productive because thinner detectors will significantly reduce the scanner's detection efficiency. Another (expensive) approach to reduce the influence of the detector DOI effect is to utilize two layers of independent detector elements, without reducing the total thickness of the detectors. For this method to work, the system must be able to determine which of the two detector layers detected the photon interaction; there are various ways of doing this (4), but these are beyond the scope of this chapter.

## PET detectors and system geometry; 2-D and 3-D imaging modes; random- and scatter-coincidence events

## PET detectors

The detectors used in most PET scanners are made from high-density inorganic scintillation crystals, coupled to photomultiplier tubes. The purpose of the photomultiplier tubes is to detect a pulse

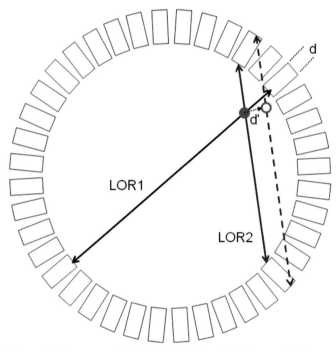

**Figure 1.5** The apparent width, d', of LOR 2 – located at a large radial distance from the center of the scanner – is increased by uncertainty in the detector depth-of-interaction (DOI), whereas the width, d, of the more centrally located LOR 1 is relatively unaffected by DOI uncertainty.

of light created in one or more scintillation crystals when an incident annihilation photon undergoes an interaction. As discussed above, to obtain good spatial resolution, the individual detector crystals should be very small in cross-section (e.g., 4.2 × 6.3 mm), but they must be thick enough (e.g., 20 to 30 mm deep) to stop most of the 511-keV photons entering the crystal. In most PET scanners, the individual crystal elements are organized into **detector blocks** (Figure 1.6), viewed by a 2×2 array of photomultiplier tubes (5). The blocks are usually fabricated from a single large rectangular crystal, into which relatively deep grooves are cut to segment the block into individual crystal elements. Regardless of whether grooved blocks or individual discrete elements are used, however, each element should be optically isolated to some extent from its neighboring crystal elements, to reduce the light cross-talk from one crystal element to others within the block. This is often accomplished by coating the surfaces of each element with an opaque, light-reflecting layer. In actuality, as described below, a small amount of light spreading within the block is necessary for determining the exact crystal in which an incident annihilation photon interacted.

When a photon from a positron–electron annihilation interacts in a scintillation crystal, a flash of visible light photons is created within a very small region surrounding the interaction point. The intensity or brightness of this flash, i.e., the number of light photons generated, is linearly proportional to the total energy deposited in the crystal during the annihilation photon's interaction. The number of light photons emitted per unit time after the initial interaction can generally be described by a rapid exponential or bi-exponential decay. Most of the time, one of two types of interactions will occur in the crystal: either photoelectric absorption or Compton scattering of the incident photon. If a 511-keV photon's energy is fully absorbed, e.g., by a photoelectric interaction in the scintillation crystal, then the number of visible light photons created in the crystal will be greater than the number of light photons generated by an annihilation photon undergoing a Compton-scatter interaction in the crystal, since the scattered photon carries some of the energy away from the initial interaction point. The scattered photon might then interact again in either the same or a different detector element, or it could escape the detector material altogether. Clearly,

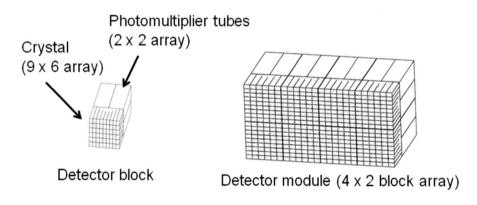

**Figure 1.6** Illustration of a PET detector block (left) and module (right). Crystal element dimensions typically range from 4 to 6 mm in cross-section, and 20 to 30 mm in depth.

photoelectric interactions are preferable because more energy is deposited at the first interaction point and more scintillation light is produced in comparison to a Compton interaction.

Because the grooves in the crystal block are cut less deep in the center of the block than near the edges, the light from an interaction in the central crystal elements will spread out more over the four photomultiplier tubes, in comparison with the light from an interaction in one of the corner crystals. The crystal where the interaction took place can usually be identified quite accurately by calculating (in the detector block's electronics) two appropriate linear combinations of the photomultiplier tube signals, one for the crystal's horizontal location and the other for its vertical location (e.g., Figure 1.6), and dividing by the total energy deposited in this event, which is, essentially, the sum of the light signals from all four photomultiplier tubes.

Based on the considerations described above, we are now in a position to summarize the most important physical attributes of scintillation-detector materials used for PET imaging. The best scintillators clearly need to be fast and bright, but they should also have a high stopping power (linear attenuation coefficient), and a high **photofraction** (percentage of photoelectric, as opposed to Compton or other interactions). In addition, the wavelength of the visible light produced in the scintillator should be reasonably well matched to the spectral sensitivity of the photomultiplier tubes used to detect the light. **Fast scintillators** are those in which the light flash takes place almost immediately after the annihilation-photon interacts in the crystal, so that the system can determine if a coincident photon was detected at almost the same time in some other detector on the other side of the PET scanner. A **coincidence timing window** width ranging from somewhere between 6 and 12 nanoseconds is used to define coincidence events in most PET systems today. An equally important consideration, however, is that the light pulse must decay very rapidly, so that the detector block will be ready to accept and process the next event as soon as possible.

**Bright scintillators** produce enough light with each interaction to permit unambiguous identification of the crystal in which the interaction took place; if too few light photons are available for the event position calculation, then there could be a large uncertainty in determining the crystal of interaction, which degrades spatial resolution. Furthermore, the total energy of the detected photon would also not be known with good precision if too few light photons are produced per event. The energy information is useful for reducing the number of detected photons which have scattered too many times in either the patient or the detector, or both. This is accomplished electronically by using a **pulse-height discriminator** to reject events producing light signals that are either too low (too few light photons) or too high (too many light photons). Events detected with too much energy occasionally occur when two or more photons from two different decays are detected in the same detector block at almost the same time.

**Table 1.2** Some properties of scintillation crystals.

| Property | NaI(Tl) | BGO | LSO | LaBr$_3$ |
|---|---|---|---|---|
| Density (g/mL) | 3.67 | 7.1 | 7.4 | 5.3 |
| Effective Z | 51 | 75 | 66 | 47 |
| Attenuation length at 511 keV (cm) | 2.91 | 1.04 | 1.14 | 2.13 |
| Decay time (ns) | 230 | 300 | 40 | 35 |
| Light photons/MeV | 41 000 | 9000 | 26 000 | 61 000 |

Good scintillator materials for PET should also have a high **stopping power** at 511 keV. The stopping power is directly related to the linear attenuation coefficient, which implies that the detectors should have a high effective atomic number, as well as a high physical density. In this case, the detector material's attenuation length – which is the inverse of its linear attenuation coefficient at 511-keV – would be short enough that most annihilation photons would interact within a 2- to 3-cm-thick crystal. Furthermore, the photofraction should also be as high as possible, since more energy is deposited in the crystal during photoelectric interactions, in comparison with Compton-scatter interactions. Finally, if a 511-keV photon scatters in one crystal element, but then deposits most of its energy in some other crystal in the same detector block, this could also introduce an error in the LOR associated with the event.

The properties of a few standard scintillators used in nuclear medicine applications are shown in Table 1.2. (For additional properties, the reader is referred to reference (6).) It can be seen that thallium-doped sodium-iodide, NaI(Tl), which is used in most gamma cameras for lower energy single-photon nuclear medicine imaging, has a significantly lower effective atomic number and density than those of bismuth germanate (BGO) and lutetium oxyorthosilicate (LSO), which are used in most PET scanners today. Because of its low stopping power or, equivalently, its longer attenuation length at 511 keV, NaI(Tl) is not often used for PET imaging, despite its reasonably fast light decay time and relatively high total photon yield per MeV of energy deposited during the interaction of the annihilation photon. Among the more commonly used PET scintillators, BGO has better stopping power than LSO; however, LSO is significantly faster and brighter than BGO. Lanthanum bromide, (LaBr$_3$) despite its longer attenuation length than LSO, is faster and brighter than LSO; for this reason, lanthanum bromide may be better suited than LSO for use in specialized **time-of-flight** PET systems (7), in which the location of the point where the positron annihilated is estimated using the photon arrival-time difference of the two detectors which define the LOR.

## PET scanner geometry and acquisition modes

There are two different ways of acquiring data in detector-ring-based PET systems. In the so-called two-dimensional

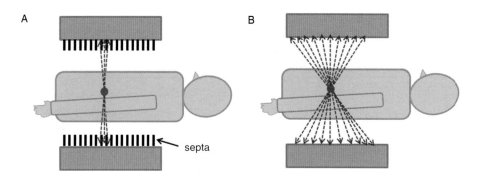

Figure 1.7 PET data acquisition modes: (A) 2-D; (B) 3-D.

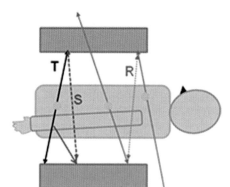

Figure 1.8 Three coincidence-event topologies: (black) a true coincidence, (red) a scattered coincidence, and (blue) a random coincidence. Dashed (dotted) lines represent incorrectly assigned LORs for scattered (random) coincidence events.

(2-D) mode, LORs are acquired in a slice-by-slice manner; in other words, coincidence events are only allowed between detector crystals located within the same axial ring of detectors or, in some cases, among detectors in two or three adjacent detector rings. In this mode, potential coincidence events between detectors located farther apart in the axial direction are limited further through the use of annular septa, made from tungsten or lead, which physically restrict the axial acceptance angle for possible coincidence events by attenuating photons traveling towards the detector ring at larger angles of incidence (e.g., Figure 1.7A). In three-dimensional (3-D) data-acquisition mode, the axial collimator septa are removed from the scanner, and coincidence events between detectors located in more widely separated detector rings are also included as valid events (Figure 1.7B). Obviously, 3-D mode allows many more valid coincidence LORs than 2-D mode, so a PET scanner's count sensitivity is typically about 6–10 times higher in 3-D mode than in 2-D mode. In recent years, there has been a clear increase in the use of 3-D-mode scanning (8), for reasons described below.

Some PET systems are still manufactured with both 2-D and 3-D mode data-acquisition capability; such scanners have retractable annular septa which are positioned appropriately within the scanner for 2-D-mode scanning, but can be quickly and automatically moved out of the scanner for 3-D-mode acquisitions. Other manufacturers are now selling PET scanners which can only acquire data in 3-D mode. Because the photon flux hitting the detector crystals is much higher in 3-D than in 2-D mode when the axial collimators are present, PET scanners based on fast scintillator crystals, such as LSO, may be somewhat more useful for 3-D-mode scanning than systems with slower crystals. Nevertheless, very good-quality 3-D scans are also being routinely acquired today with slower BGO-based scanners. While the detectors in each ring could, in principle, be placed in coincidence with detectors in all other axial rings, in practice, the manufacturers often specify some **maximum acceptable ring difference** which is less than the total number of detector rings in the system.

For 3-D-mode imaging, the PET system's sensitivity for detecting positron-annihilation events occurring near the middle of the scanner in the axial direction is significantly higher than its sensitivity for detecting annihilations located near either end of the scanner. This is because many more detector rings are

available for recording coincidences between back-to-back annihilation photons in the middle of the scanner than near its ends. In fact, at the extreme edges of the scanner's axial field-of-view (FOV), only one detector ring can acquire valid coincidence events. For event positions in between the center and the ends, the system coincidence sensitivity decreases linearly from its maximum value in the center to its lowest value at the end rings. On the other hand, in 2-D-mode imaging, the PET scanner's sensitivity is more constant along the axial direction. One important implication of the falloff in 3-D count sensitivity near the axial ends of the PET gantry is that a larger overlap between adjacent axial bed positions must be used for 3-D-mode imaging over multiple bed positions, in comparison with 2-D-mode PET, in order to better equalize the count sensitivity over the entire axial region being scanned. In practice, this means that if, for example, five 15-cm axial bed positions are sufficient to cover the torso region in a 2-D-mode whole-body scan, then seven bed positions might be required to achieve the same axial coverage in 3-D mode. Fortunately, however, because of the greater overall count sensitivity in 3-D mode, less acquisition time is needed for each bed position in 3-D than in 2-D, so a whole-body PET scan can still often be acquired in the same time, or even more rapidly, in 3-D mode than in 2-D mode.

## Types of coincidence events; corrections for randoms and scatter

PET scanners acquire three different types of coincidence events, as illustrated in Figure 1.8. The most desirable event topology is a **true-coincidence** event, in which both photons from one positron–electron annihilation are detected back-to-back along the correct LOR. Sometimes, however, one or both of the annihilation photons undergo Compton scattering in the patient before being detected. In this case, the **scatter-coincidence** event will appear to originate along an incorrect LOR. Finally, it is often possible for two annihilation photons originating from two *different* nuclear decays to be detected by chance within the coincidence time window, which will also lead to an incorrectly specified LOR; this type of event is called a **random coincidence**. Ideally, we would like to preserve all of the true-coincidence events, while rejecting all scatter- and random-coincidence events before reconstructing images; however, it is not possible to reject all of the "bad events" with current PET technology. By using detectors with improved performance characteristics, it is possible to reduce the number of detected scatter and random coincidences, but not to eliminate them completely. Fortunately, however, techniques have been developed to compensate for these sources of error while reconstructing PET images.

One can reduce the number of detected random-coincidence events by simply using a narrower coincidence time window; however, this approach will also reject more true-coincidence events because the timing resolution of the detectors is not perfect. By using fast scintillators, like some of those shown in Table 1.2, PET instrument designers are able to set narrower coincidence time windows in order to reduce the contribution of randoms to the PET coincidence data; however, the percentage of randoms in most whole-body PET studies is still, typically, 10–15% in 2-D mode, and 30–35% in 3-D mode, so correction for the random events is still required. One correction method is known as **delayed-window randoms subtraction**. With this approach, the PET scanner records two different types of coincidences. One type consists of all of the events described above which fall within the usual **prompt-coincidence** window; however, the scanner additionally can search for events detected in a **delayed window**; these consist of events in which the second photon is detected within a different time window that is set to be much later than the time when the first photon was detected. The time delay between the two detected photon events is chosen to be large enough so that a true- or scatter-coincidence event could never be detected in the delayed window; however, the LOR distribution of random coincidences in a delayed window is, statistically, the same as that observed in the prompt window. Although the delayed-window randoms approach provides accurate estimates of the rate of random coincidences along each LOR, these estimates are "noisy," i.e., there can be a large variability of the estimates of the random-coincidence contribution to each LOR. For this reason, lower noise approaches have been devised; in one such method, the random-coincidence count-rate is computed from the so-called **single-event** count-rate on each detector (9). To use this **randoms-from-singles** method, the scanner's electronics must be able to keep track of the total number of photons detected per second, which is the singles count-rate, in all of the

detector elements. For a coincidence time window width, $\tau$, it can be shown that a good estimate of the expected random-coincidence count-rate, R, along any given LOR is then simply given by:

$$R = 2\,\tau\,S_1\,S_2,$$

where $S_1$ and $S_2$ are the singles count-rates recorded for the two detector elements defining the LOR.

Turning our attention now to the scatter-coincidence events, one way to reduce the number of these less desirable events would be, in principle, to use detectors with improved energy resolution. Because photons which undergo Compton scattering in the patient lose some energy in the process, if the detectors could measure a scattered photon's energy with great accuracy, we should be able to reject more scattered events. However, even when using the brightest scintillation detectors shown in Table 1.2, the energy resolution of the detectors is not great, so a wide energy window must still be used in order to include most of the desirable true-coincidence events. The fraction of scattered photons detected within the scanner's energy window is then still rather large, i.e., approximately 20–30% in 2-D mode, and 40–60% in 3-D mode.

Two general approaches have been developed to estimate the scattered-photon contribution to the projection data. One simple method, most often used for 2-D PET imaging, assumes that the scattered photon contribution can be estimated (after subtraction of random coincidences) by mathematically smoothing the coincidence-projection data using blurring functions which are measured using sources located at several different radial positions in a cylindrical phantom (10). Estimating the scatter data in 3-D-mode imaging is more challenging (11, 12); this is generally accomplished by starting from an initial estimate of the PET image, along with an attenuation map (e.g., obtained from CT), and then using these to compute the expected distribution of scatter-coincidence events; this calculation is based on the Klein–Nishina formula, which describes the angular distribution of Compton-scattered photons. Once the scattered-photon contribution to the raw data has been estimated, it can be used to refine the PET emission-image estimate, and the process could then be repeated in an iterative fashion until the estimated scatter contribution to the projection data no longer changes significantly.

Finally, we point out that there are two different general approaches to correcting for random and scatter coincidences. In one approach, the estimates of these "bad-coincidence" contributions are first subtracted from the measured projection data. Then, the remaining coincidence data, which would ideally represent only true-coincidence events at this point, can be reconstructed by one of several different tomographic reconstruction algorithms. There are a couple of possible problems with data-subtraction techniques. First, the subtracted projections could contain some negative values, for example, if the random or scatter contributions were overestimated, or if the projection data simply had too many statistical

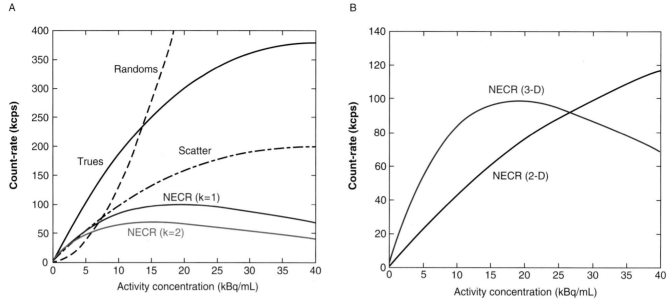

**Figure 1.9** (A) Count-rates in 3-D mode vs. activity concentration; (B) noise-equivalent count-rate (NECR) curves for 3-D and 2-D mode scanning.

noise variations. While negative projection LOR values do not adversely affect some reconstruction algorithms, such as **filtered backprojection** methods, they can, however, cause serious problems for certain types of **iterative reconstruction algorithms**, which require that both the projection data and the reconstructed image be positive. Second, whenever one noisy data set is subtracted from another noisy data set, the relative statistical variability of the resulting data is significantly increased in comparison with the noise in the original data. Therefore, even if the subtraction approach is, on average, *unbiased*, or accurate, the subtraction technique is known to produce an amplification of the reconstructed PET image noise, which adversely affects overall image quality.

The other approach is to include the estimates of random and scatter coincidences *additively* when estimating the total projection data within an iterative reconstruction algorithm. In the popular **maximum-likelihood image reconstruction** methods (13) this approach provides an important advantage, because such methods rely on the assumption that the total projection data can be described by a joint Poisson statistical model of the counting noise in all of the detector elements. If the scatter and random coincidences are subtracted from the data, this assumption is violated, whereas if these "bad-coincidence" contributions are included additively, then the Poisson-statistics assumption can be preserved, which mitigates problems with excessive noise amplification during image reconstruction.

## Noise-equivalent count-rate (NECR)

A useful approximate metric for assessing the deleterious effect of random and scatter coincidences on overall PET image quality is the so-called noise-equivalent count-rate (NECR) (14). NECR is the count-rate recorded by an *ideal* PET scanner

(i.e., a scanner that could perfectly reject all random and scatter coincidences) which would yield PET images with a noise level the same as that obtained from a *real* PET scanner after correcting for randoms and scatter. For a PET scanner recording true-coincidence rate, T, scatter-coincidence rate, S, and random-coincidence rate, R, the NECR is given by:

$$NECR = \frac{T^2}{(T + S + kR)}.$$

In this formula, the multiplier "k" in the denominator is 2 when the delayed-window randoms subtraction method is used, or 1 when a very low-noise randoms estimate, e.g., the randoms-from-singles approach, is used.

3-D-mode count-rate curves are shown in Figure 1.9A as a function of the activity concentration within a phantom; these curves were measured for a modern PET scanner equipped with LYSO detector modules. (LYSO is similar to LSO, in terms of the basic properties listed in Table 1.2.) It can be seen that the true-coincidence count-rate initially increases linearly with activity concentration, until the system begins to lose events at high count-rates because of increasing detector "dead-time." The scatter-coincidence count-rate is approximately half of the trues count-rate; the shapes of these curves are the same because a loss of counts at high rates due to detector dead-time influences the trues and scatters in the same way. The random-coincidence count-rate is initially much less than that of the true- and scatter-coincidences; however, the randoms rate increases rapidly, i.e., as the *square* of activity concentration, which causes the noise-equivalent count-rate (NECR) to increase to a maximum value (in this case, at an activity concentration of about 16–19 kBq/mL) and then to decrease with further increases in activity concentration. The maximum NECR for this scanner in 3-D mode occurs at approximately 19 kBq/mL when estimating randoms from singles (k = 1), and near 16 kBq/mL when using delayed-window randoms (k = 2).

In Figure 1.9B, we compare, for the same scanner, the NECR measured in 3-D mode with that measured in 2-D mode. In the low activity-concentration range, i.e., less than about 20 kBq/mL, 3-D mode appears to offer a significant advantage over 2-D mode. It is important to point out, however, that the phantom used for measuring these NECR curves is different from real patients in several respects. Most importantly, the fraction of detected scatter events is often higher in patient 3-D-mode imaging than in phantom imaging, especially for large patients. A higher scatter-fraction has the effect of reducing the activity concentration yielding the maximum NECR. For this reason, it is usually recommended that less activity be injected for whole-body FDG patient imaging in 3-D mode, i.e., to make sure that the count-rate values do not lead to a NECR value beyond the peak of the curve. An injection of ~12 mCi (~450 MBq), followed by an one-hour delay before imaging leads to a typical patient soft-tissue activity-concentration value of less than ~5 kBq/mL, which should be safely below the NECR peak, even for quite large patients. For 2-D-mode imaging, on the other hand, a higher activity injection is generally used to increase the 2-D NECR enough to achieve image quality comparable to that seen in 3-D mode. As shown in Figure 1.9B, the 2-D NECR curve has not yet reached its peak even by 40 kBq/mL. (In fact, this scanner's peak NECR was found at ~76 kBq/mL in 2-D mode.) In most clinics, patient dosimetry conditions limit the injected dose to ~20 mCi (740 MBq), which implies that we are always operating far below the peak NECR in 2-D mode.

Figure 1.10 shows two different transaxial slices through the same torso phantom, scanned in both 2-D mode and 3-D mode. Even though the acquisition time and activity concentration were both less in 3-D mode, compared with 2-D mode, the overall level of image noise is clearly better in the 3-D images than in the 2-D images, for the same degree of lesion contrast.

## Attenuation compensation

### The attenuation problem in PET

We have so far addressed three topologies of PET events which arise from true, random, and scatter coincidences. There are,

however, many additional positron decays which never yield a detected coincidence event, even when the two annihilation photons are directed perfectly along one of the many valid LORs defined by the detector geometry of the PET scanner. Frequently, these events are lost because one or both of the annihilation photons are **attenuated** by the patient's body before reaching the detectors. Events which are "lost" to attenuation consist of two types: first, those events in which one or both photons are absorbed photoelectrically within the patient and, second, those in which one of the photons scatters, but is not detected (or both photons scatter and are not detected). If only one of the two annihilation photons is detected, this will contribute to the singles count-rate of the system and, possibly, to the random-coincidence count-rate, but not to the useful coincidence count-rate.

The problem with attenuation in PET imaging is that it introduces a fundamental ambiguity into the measurement process. This ambiguity is illustrated in Figure 1.11, where it can be seen that the same number of valid coincidence events could be detected along a given LOR either by imaging

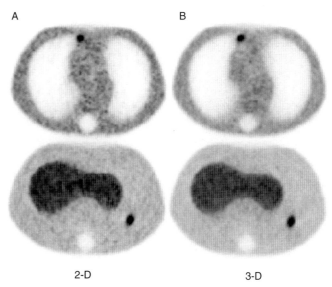

2-D          3-D

**Figure 1.10** FDG-PET images of two different transaxial slices of a torso phantom, acquired (A) in 2-D mode and (B) in 3-D mode.

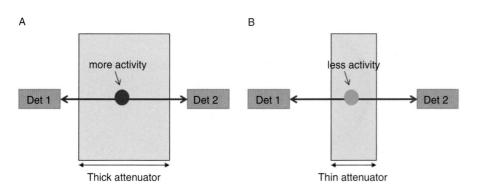

**Figure 1.11** Illustration of a fundamental ambiguity in FDG-PET imaging: the same coincidence count-rate can be observed from (A) a high activity source, embedded in a thick attenuator, as from (B) a lower activity source inside a thinner attenuator.

a high-activity source attenuated by a thick attenuator, or by imaging a lower activity source, attenuated by a thinner attenuator. Ideally, the reconstructed PET images should reflect solely the local concentration of radioactivity in the patient's body, and should not be influenced by the distribution of attenuating material within the patient. Therefore, in order to resolve the basic measurement ambiguity inherent in PET imaging, we need to correct as well as possible for the loss of photons by attenuation.

Figure 1.12 shows images from a patient whole-body PET study, reconstructed with and without attenuation correction.

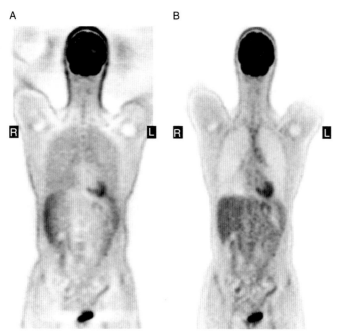

**Figure 1.12** Whole-body coronal FDG-PET images following reconstruction (A) without and (B) with attenuation correction.

When compensation for attenuation is not included in the reconstruction, there appear to be dark-line artifacts, erroneously indicating higher activity concentration around the periphery of the patient images and the outside of abdominal organs, such as the liver. In addition, even though the lung activity concentration is less than that of the soft tissue, the lungs appear to be "hotter" than the soft tissue in images not corrected for attenuation. These artifacts in uncorrected images are a natural consequence of inconsistencies between the expected projection images and the actual measured projections. Figure 1.13 shows that, for two concentric circular regions, even though the "lung" activity concentration is less than that of the "soft tissue," nevertheless, since the lung is less attenuating, its activity in the attenuated projection profile appears incorrectly to be higher than that of the soft tissue; this effect is what causes reconstructed lung images with apparently higher activity concentration (Figure 1.13C).

## Attenuation correction in stand-alone PET scanners

To correct for photon attenuation in PET, it is necessary to measure or estimate reliably the integral of the attenuation "map" along every LOR which traverses the patient. Before the advent of PET/CT scanners, this was generally accomplished by using from one to three radioactive sources which rotated around the patient to perform a **transmission scan**. Most stand-alone PET scanners utilize "pin sources" of the positron-emitter $^{68}$Ge for this purpose (15); this radionuclide has a half-life of 271 days, so the rotating $^{68}$Ge sources only need to be replaced every 6–12 months or so. Because the flux of 511-keV annihilation photons being emitted from the $^{68}$Ge pins is substantially higher than that from the PET radionuclide in the patient, most of the counts detected in coincidence during the transmission scan, in fact, arise from events in which one of the two coincidence photons is transmitted

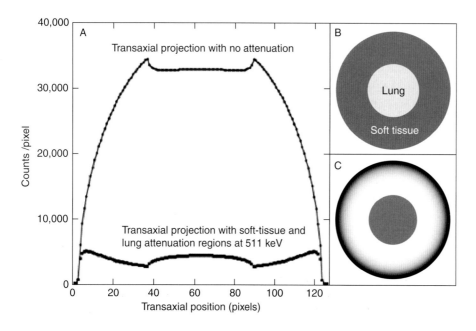

**Figure 1.13** Demonstration of the effects of a non-uniform distribution of soft tissue and lung attenuation. (A) Projection profiles with and without attenuation, and ideal transverse slices reconstructions (B) with and (C) without attenuation correction, illustrating the apparent increase of activity around the periphery of the phantom, as well as in the lower activity "lung" region.

from a $^{68}$Ge pin through the patient and detected on the other side of the patient. If the intensity of $^{68}$Ge annihilation photons emitted from the source along a given direction (defined by one of the PET scanner's LORs) is given by $I_0$, then the intensity transmitted through the patient along the same LOR is given by:

$$I = I_0 \exp\left\{ -\int_{LOR} \mu_{511}(\mathbf{x})\mathbf{dx} \right\},$$

where $\mu_{511}(\mathbf{x})$ is the linear attenuation coefficient for 511-keV photons at location, x, along the LOR. $I_0$ can be measured simply by acquiring a $^{68}$Ge transmission scan with no patient in the scanner, and I is the same measurement when the patient is present. By taking the natural log of both sides of the equation, and rearranging the result, it can be seen that the desired integral of the attenuation along the LOR is given by:

$$\int_{LOR} \mu(\mathbf{x})\mathbf{dx} = \ln(\mathbf{I}_0) - \ln(\mathbf{I}).$$

If this quantity is measured separately for every LOR, which is accomplished during the rotation of the $^{68}$Ge pin sources, it is possible not only to correct the emission data for the integrated attenuation along the LOR – e.g., by dividing the emission LORs by the integral expression above – but also to reconstruct an image representing the measured attenuation value at every location within the patient. This image is quite similar to that obtained with a CT scanner, with some exceptions, as we shall see. Most importantly, the spatial resolution of a transmission image measured using a radionuclide source in a stand-alone PET scanner is significantly degraded in comparison with the exquisite (often sub-millimeter) spatial resolution that can be obtained with a modern CT scanner.

It should also be mentioned that some stand-alone scanners utilize a gamma-photon emitter, such as $^{137}$Cs, rather than a positron emitter, to measure the attenuation correction factors and attenuation map (16). This is possible because the system knows where the sources are at all times during their rotation; therefore, each LOR is simply defined by the line connecting a given source location to the appropriate detector on the other side of the patient. Cs-137 has a long half life ($\sim$30 years), so this source does not need to be replaced within the life-time of most PET systems; however, its principal gamma photon energy used for this measurement is 662 keV, so with $^{137}$Cs, we are actually measuring the attenuation at this energy, rather than at 511 keV, the energy necessary for PET attenuation correction. Nevertheless, as we shall see, it is possible to scale the attenuation maps measured at one energy in order to estimate those that would be measured at another energy, with fairly good accuracy.

## Attenuation correction in PET/CT scanners

In modern, hybrid PET/CT scanners, the CT scanner, itself, provides the attenuation map used to correct the PET data for photon attenuation by the patient. This means that the radionuclide sources used for attenuation correction in stand-alone PET systems do not need to be present in a hybrid PET/CT system, although most systems still utilize one such source for PET detector-gain calibration, for coincidence-timing calibration, and/or for measuring detector efficiencies.

Hybrid PET/CT systems (17) consist, essentially, of a PET scanner and a CT scanner, with a single shared patient table which moves sequentially through both scanners. If the patient does not move during or between the PET and CT scans, then, in principle, the PET and CT images can be spatially aligned, or **registered** perfectly to each other. To accomplish this, it has proven necessary to develop new patient-support approaches, such as that shown in Figure 1.14. Instead of simply moving the table top through the gantry over a fixed support-base (which is the method used most often in stand-alone scanners), if the PET/CT scanner can move the base along with its table top, then Figure 1.14 demonstrates that the end of the table supporting the patient will bend or flex by the same amount when the patient is scanned in the PET system as when he or she was scanned in the CT scanner.

The basic principle of CT imaging is quite similar to that described above for the transmission image obtained in a stand-alone PET scanner. In a modern CT scanner, however, the radionuclide source is replaced by an X-ray tube which rotates continuously at high speeds, e.g., as fast as one-third of a second per rotation. The X-ray tube emits a very high flux of X-ray photons, with a broad distribution of energies characterized by a maximum energy of 120 keV or 140 keV, depending on the high-voltage applied to the tube. The CT scanner's detectors are also different from those used for PET. Because of the high photon flux impinging on the CT detectors, it is generally not possible to count individual photons in each detector element; instead, the solid-state CT detectors are only used to measure the *integrated* photon flux density hitting each detector.

Early generations of CT scanners used a single ring of detectors in the axial direction, and volumetric CT scanning was accomplished by scanning a single slice at a time, then moving the patient couch one "step" in the axial direction, then scanning again, and so on until the desired patient volume was covered. This scan mode is referred to as "step-and-shoot" mode. More modern CT scanners, on the other hand, are now equipped with multiple rows of detectors which can cover a wide range in the axial direction of the scanner. Many PET/CT scanners installed in the USA are currently using 16-detector-row CT systems, and many centers have CT scanners equipped with 64 or even more detector rows. Figure 1.15 shows that these systems do not need to acquire data in step-and-shoot mode. Although this is still possible, faster scanning can now be accomplished by moving the patient table continuously through the gantry while also rotating the X-ray tube continuously, and simultaneously acquiring integrated X-ray flux measurements from all of the detector elements. For reasons evident in Figure 1.15, this type of scan is referred to as a **helical scan**. If the width of the detector array in the axial direction is exactly equal to the distance traveled by

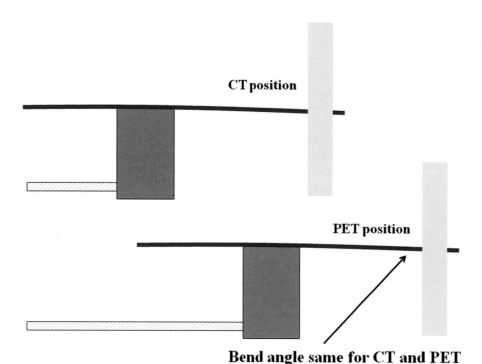

**Figure 1.14** If the FDG-PET-CT patient table support moves along with the table, the table will bend the same amount in both the PET and CT scanners.

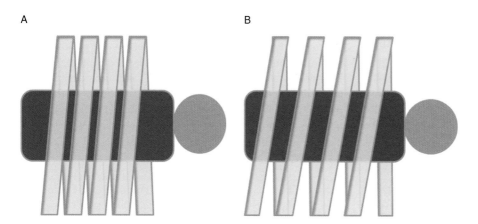

**Figure 1.15** Helical CT orbits acquired with (A) low and (B) high values of pitch.

the table during one rotation of the X-ray tube, the scan is being acquired with a value of **pitch** of 1.0. Even faster volumetric scanning can be accomplished using higher values of pitch; for example, a pitch of 2.0 means that the table travels a distance equal to twice the axial width of the detector array during each rotation of the X-ray tube. Although high values of pitch can provide fast volumetric scanning, unfortunately, because of more limited data sampling, interpolation errors and artifacts can often be seen, particularly if the patient moves during the acquisition. The increasing number of detector rows being used in modern CT scanners permits rapid scanning over organs like the lungs or the heart without the need to use a high value of pitch. This has proved to be advantageous for PET/CT imaging because high pitch can lead to CT image artifacts, which are then reflected in the corresponding PET images when the CT scan is used for attenuation correction.

## Conversion of CT attenuation values to linear attenuation coefficients at 511 keV

The X-ray tube in a PET/CT scanner is generally operated at a peak voltage of 120 to 140 kV$_p$. Because the mean effective beam energy of the emitted X-ray spectrum is typically about one-third of its maximum energy, this implies that the resulting attenuation maps, expressed in **CT numbers** (also called **Hounsfield units**), are appropriate for photons with an average energy of approximately 40–50 keV. In order to correct PET measurements for attenuation, it is necessary to transform the CT numbers to linear attenuation coefficients at 511 keV (18). Figure 1.16 shows that a simple **bilinear transformation** can be used to accomplish this conversion quite accurately for most tissue types found in the body (19). One linear conversion is used for CT numbers in the range

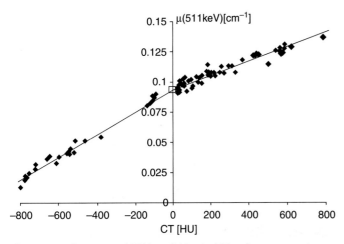

**Figure 1.16** Conversion of CT Hounsfield units (HU) to linear attenuation-coefficient values appropriate for FDG-PET imaging at 511 keV. (With kind permission from Springer Science+Business Media: *European Journal of Nuclear Medicine*, C Burger, G Goerres, S Schoenes, A Buck, AHR Lonn, GK von Schulthess, "PET attenuation coefficients from CT images: experimental evaluation of the transformation of CT into FDG-PET 500-keV attenuation coefficients." 2002;**29**:922–7, Fig. 2b.)

from −1000 (air) up to 0 (water, or some soft tissues), while another linear conversion is used to cover the range of attenuation from that of soft tissue up to that of bone.

## Artifacts and inaccuracies in PET/CT
### Effect of metallic implants

When a high-Z material, e.g., an implant made from tungsten, stainless steel, or some other metal, is present in the patient, the attenuation coefficient resulting from the transformation shown in Figure 1.16 can be quite inaccurate. Generally, the attenuation coefficient at 511 keV obtained with this transformation will be overestimated. The effect of an artifactually increased attenuation coefficient on the corrected PET image is to *increase* the apparent local reconstructed activity; and, conversely, an artifactually decreased attenuation coefficient leads to an apparently *decreased* PET activity. Figure 1.17B shows a "hot spot" in the attenuation-corrected FDG PET image which could be mistaken for a hypermetabolic lymph node, for example. However, the corresponding CT image indicates that the patient had a pacemaker in the same location. Because the pacemaker's

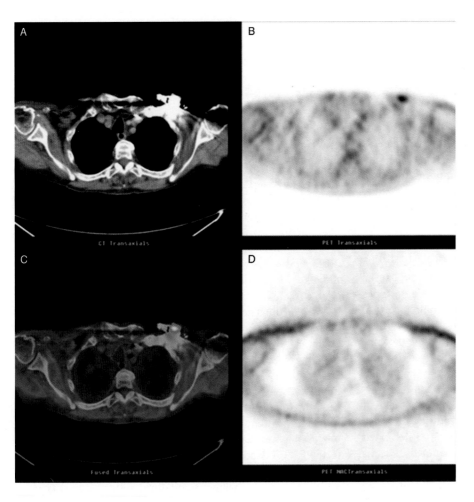

**Figure 1.17** Artifact from a high Z material (pacemaker). (A) CT; (B) FDG-PET image, corrected using the CT-derived attenuation map; (C) fused CT and corrected FDG-PET images; (D) FDG-PET image reconstructed with no attenuation correction. (With kind permission from CD Rajadhyaksha, JA Parker, L Barbaras, VH Gerbaudo, *Joint Program in Nuclear Medicine* Teaching File: "Normal and Benign Pathologic Findings in 18FDG-PET and PET/CT: an Interactive Web-Based Image Atlas" (http://www.jpnm.org/petctatlas.html).)

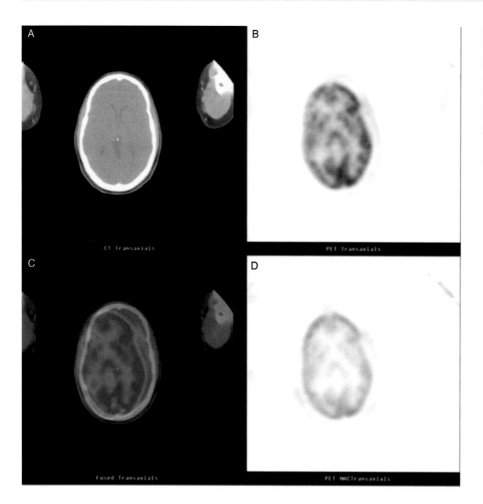

**Figure 1.18** Left–right brain asymmetry artifact from patient motion between the CT and FDG-PET acquisitions: (A) CT; (B) FDG-PET corrected using the CT-derived attenuation map; (C) fused CT and corrected FDG-PET images; (D) FDG-PET image reconstructed without attenuation correction. (With kind permission from CD Rajadhyaksha, JA Parker, L Barbaras, VH Gerbaudo, *Joint Program in Nuclear Medicine* Teaching File: "Normal and Benign Pathologic Findings in 18FDG-PET and PET/CT: an Interactive Web-Based Image Atlas" (http://www.jpnm.org/petctatlas.html).)

attenuation coefficient at 511 keV was overestimated by the transformation in Figure 1.16, this led to an artifactual increase in the reconstructed PET counts in the same region. One useful way of confirming this observation is by examining the same PET images reconstructed with *no* attenuation compensation. As seen in Figure 1.17D, the apparent hot spot is no longer visible when attenuation compensation is not performed.

## Effect of patient motion or PET/CT misregistration

Figure 1.18 shows a brain PET/CT imaging study in which the attenuation-corrected PET image (Figure 1.18B) demonstrates an apparent left–right asymmetry especially in the cortical uptake of the tracer, FDG. By examining the alignment of the PET and CT images, however, it can be seen that the patient's head clearly moved between the CT and the PET acquisitions. This means that the left side of the patient's brain, which appears to be deeper inside the patient's head, has been over-corrected for attenuation. On the other hand, the right side of the brain, which has apparently been rotated outside the head, has been undercorrected for attenuation, leading to decreased image intensity, and the resulting left–right asymmetry. Just as we saw in the previous section, when the PET reconstruction is performed without attenuation correction (Figure 1.18D), the apparent asymmetry is no longer observed.

## Effects of CT motion artifacts

Figure 1.19A shows an artifact or possible lesion in the patient's right lower-lung region. The CT scan used for the attenuation correction of this study (not shown) was acquired while the patient was breathing, using a scanner with a high value of pitch for the helical scan. This led to a "detached liver" artifact in which the dome of the liver appeared to be located within the right lung on the CT scan. When this artifactual CT scan was used for attenuation correction of the PET study, the activity in this region of the lung was overcorrected, thereby causing the observed PET artifact. As before, reconstruction of the PET data without attenuation correction (Figure 1.19B) eliminated the detached liver-dome artifact.

Figure 1.20 illustrates the opposite situation, in which the CT scan was acquired at or near full end-inspiration, while the PET data were acquired during normal respiration. In this case, the top of the liver appears artifactually to be located in a region of lower density lung attenuation, resulting in the observed photopenic region immediately above the liver. In fact, PET/CT studies like the one shown here have led most practitioners to recommend that the CT scan should be acquired during shallow respiration, rather than during a breath-hold at full-inspiration. When using a modern multidetector CT system equipped with 16 or more detector rows, and acquiring helical scans with a reasonable value of pitch (e.g., near 1.0), not only are liver–lung mismatches seldom observed, but in addition, helical scan artifacts, such as the detached liver dome shown in Figure 1.19, are also almost never seen.

## Inaccuracies in measured standardized uptake values (SUV)

If all of the corrections described earlier in this chapter have been implemented correctly, PET images have the potential to be quantitatively accurate, i.e., the image pixel values can

reliably be converted to absolute values of local activity concentration, measured in µCi/mL (or Bq/mL) in tissue. This has led clinical practitioners to search for meaningful approaches to compare image voxel values from patient to patient, as well as across different states of health and disease, in normal as well as in cancerous or inflamed tissues. The quantitative capabilities of PET imaging have also led naturally to the concept of the **standardized uptake value (SUV)** for assessment of various findings on PET images. The basic idea behind SUV can be described easily by imagining the unlikely situation in which all of the activity administered to a patient ends up being distributed uniformly throughout the patient's body. This condition is then used to define the value of activity concentration which corresponds to a SUV value of 1.0. For example, if 10 mCi (370 MBq) of FDG were administered to a patient weighing 100 kg, then after correcting for all physics effects described earlier, as well as for the decay of the radioactivity between injection and imaging, a tissue activity concentration of 0.1 µCi/g would be used to set the SUV scale. In other words, a local concentration of 0.1 µCi/g would, in this case, correspond to SUV = 1.0, while a concentration of 0.5 µCi/g, for example, would represent SUV = 5.0. The higher the measured activity concentration in a tissue, the higher its SUV and, therefore, the higher its apparent rate of FDG metabolism.

Several different factors can lead to inaccurate SUVs. It is clear from the basic SUV concept described above that the patient's weight and injected dose must be known quite accurately, along with the time of injection and the time of the scan, for decay correcting the image data. In addition, if any of the factors described in the previous sections of this chapter leads to inaccuracies in the absolute tracer activity concentration within the PET images, this will also adversely affect the calculation of local SUVs. Finally, a particularly serious factor

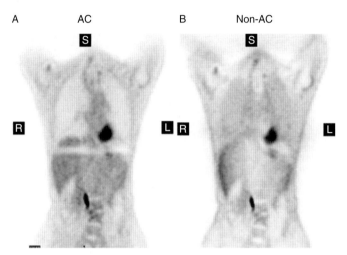

**Figure 1.19** Attenuation artifact resulting from apparent separation of the liver dome in a CT image (not shown) acquired with a high value of pitch. (A) FDG-PET coronal image reconstructed using artifactual CT image for attenuation correction, (B) same coronal section reconstructed with no attenuation correction.

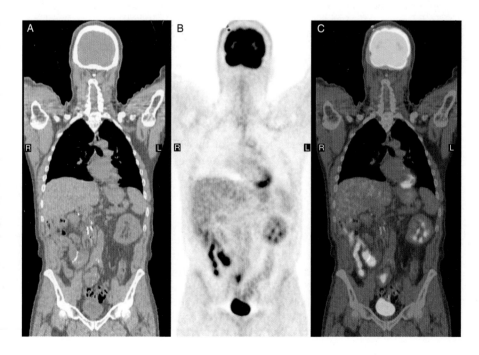

**Figure 1.20** (A) CT image acquired during breath-hold near end-inspiration; (B) corresponding FDG-PET image acquired during continuous normal breathing, demonstrating a curvilinear "cold" artifact immediately above the liver; (C) fused CT and FDG-PET images.

affecting SUV measurements is the size of the lesion whose SUV we would like to measure. Because small lesions (e.g., tumors or lymph nodes) can be significantly blurred by the spatial resolution of the PET system, this can cause image counts to be moved from inside the lesion boundary to outside the lesion, thereby decreasing the lesion's average SUV (**SUV-ave**). Because of this count **spill-out** phenomenon – which is often somewhat erroneously referred to as the **partial-volume effect** – many clinicians prefer to utilize the so-called **SUV-max** metric, which is defined as the maximum SUV observed in any voxel within the lesion of interest. SUV-max is influenced somewhat less than SUV-ave by count spill-out, although the relative precision (reproducibility) of SUV-max measurements is worse than that of SUV-ave, because SUV-max is based solely on a single voxel value.

## Summary

We have seen that there are many fundamental physics factors and technical details which can significantly impact the accuracy and the precision of PET and PET/CT images presented to the radiologist for interpretation. A good understanding of the various sources of error is essential for performing optimal PET/CT patient-imaging studies, as well as for discriminating between true clinical findings and artifacts in the reconstructed images.

## References

1. Cherry SR, Sorenson J, Phelps ME. *Physics in Nuclear Medicine*. Philadelphia, PA: Saunders Medical, 2003.

2. Wernick MN, Aarsvold JN, eds. *Emission Tomography: The Fundamentals of PET and SPECT*. San Diego, CA: Elsevier Academic Press, 2004.

3. Moses WW, Derenzo SE. Empirical observation of resolution degradation in positron emission tomographs utilzing block detectors. *J Nucl Med* 1993;**34**:101P.

4. Saoudi A, Pepin CM, Dion F et al. Investigation of depth-of-interaction by pulse-shape discrimination in multicrystal detectors read out by avalanche photodiodes. *IEEE Trans Nucl Sci* 1999;**46**:462–7.

5. Casey M, Nutt R. A multicrystal two-dimensional BGO detector system for positron emission tomography. *IEEE Trans Nucl Sci* 1986;**33**:460–3.

6. van Eijk CWE. Inorganic scintillators in medical imaging. *Phys Med Biol* 2002; **47**:R85–R106

7. Kuhn A, Surti S, Karp JS et al. Design of a lanthanum bromide detector for time-of-flight PET. *IEEE Trans Nucl Sci* 2004;**51**:2550–7.

8. Bendriem B, Townsend DW. *The Theory and Practice of 3D PET*. Dordrecht: Kluwer,1998.

9. Cooke BE, Evans AC, Fanthome EO, Alarie R, Sendyk AM. Performance figure and images from the Therascan 3128 positron emission tomograph. *IEEE Trans Nucl Sci* 1984;**31**:640–4.

10. Bergstrom M, Eriksson L, Bohm C, Blomqvist G, Litton J. Correction for scatter radiation in a ring detector positron camera by integral transformation of the projections. *J Comput Assist Tomogr* 1983; **10**:845–50.

11. Ollinger JM. Model-based scatter correction for fully 3D PET. *Phys Med Biol* 1996;**41**:153–76.

12. Watson CC, Newport D, Casey ME. A single-scatter simulation technique for scatter correction in 3D PET. In P Grangeat, JL Amans (Eds.), *Fully Three-Dimensional Image Reconstruction in Radiology and Nuclear Medicine*. Dordrecht: Kluwer Academic,1996, pp.255–68.

13. Shepp LA, Vardi Y. Maximum likelihood reconstruction in positron emission tomography, *IEEE Trans Med Imag* 1982;**1**:113–22.

14. Strother SC, Casey ME, Hoffman EJ. Measuring PET scanner sensitivity: relating count rates to image signal-to-noise ratios using noise equivalent counts. *IEEE Trans Nucl Sci* 1990;**37**:783–8.

15. Watson CC, Eriksson L, Casey ME et al. Design and performance of collimated coincidence point sources for simultaneous transmission measurements in 3-D PET. *IEEE Trans Nucl Sci* 2001;**48**:673–9.

16. Karp JS, Muehllehner G, Qu H, Yan XH. Singles transmission in volume imaging PET with a Cs-137 source. *Phys Med Biol* 1995;**40**:929–44.

17. Beyer T, Townsend DW, Brun T et al. A combined PET/CT scanner for clinical oncology. *J Nucl Med* 2000;**41**:1369–79.

18. Kinahan PE, Townsend DW, Beyer T, Sashin D. Attenuation correction for a combined 3D PET/CT scanner. *Med Phys* 1998;**25**:2046–53.

19. Burger C, Goerres G, Schoenes S et al. PET attenuation coefficients from CT images: experimental evaluation of the transformation of CT into PET 500-keV attenuation coefficients. *Eur J Nucl Med* 2002;**29**:922–7.

# PET probes for oncology

Anthony P. Belanger and Timothy R. DeGrado

## Introduction

Although current clinical PET imaging of cancer predominantly utilizes the glycolysis probe, [18]F-fluorodeoxyglucose (FDG), a large effort is being made to discover, develop and clinically implement novel PET probes to evaluate other aspects of the tumor microenvironment and cancer cell biology. In this chapter, we discuss the major areas of novel PET probe development with emphasis on those probes that have been implemented in clinical studies and may be in routine use in some PET imaging centers. We have structured each section with an introduction to the significance of the targeted biological process, a brief description of the synthesis of the probe, and a summary of the reported clinical applications. It is shown that PET probes represent a growing armamentarium for use in diagnosing and monitoring treatment of human tumors.

## Glycolysis
## Significance

D-glucose is metabolized in normal living cells via glycolysis, a 10-step process ultimately forming two molecules each of pyruvate, NADH, ATP, H$^+$, and water. In normal tissue, pyruvate is generally oxidized to $CO_2$ in the mitochondria to form an additional 34 molecules of ATP. Tumors exhibit enhanced glycolysis and conversion of pyruvate to lactate even in the presence of oxygen. This phenomenon was first noted by Warburg (1) and recently linked to expression of the M2 splice isoform of pyruvate kinase (2). As a consequence of decreased ATP production, glucose uptake is increased to meet the energy requirements of rapid cell division. The upregulation of glucose uptake in tumor tissue relative to normal tissue provides an effective means for differentiating a variety of cancers including lymphoma (Hodgkin's and non-Hodgkin's), colorectal, head and neck, breast, lung, and melanoma. Largely due to their biochemical association with tumor viability, glucose-derived PET probes have been studied for over 30 years and represent one of the most clinically utilized classes of radiopharmaceuticals.

## [18]F-fluorodeoxyglucose

Employed in over 90% of all clinical PET studies, [18]F-fluorodeoxyglucose ([[18]F]FDG, referred to in this volume as FDG) is by far the most widely used PET tracer for oncological evaluation. FDG behaves analogously to D-glucose with regards to initial uptake and phosphorylation, but unlike glucose, it cannot be further metabolized within the decay time of the [18]F radioisotope. Unable to exit the cell, phosphorylated FDG accumulates in high concentrations in tissue with elevated glucose uptake. This has aided in the grading of cancers, as benign tumors show lower rates of glycolysis than malignant tumors. However, not all tissues with elevated rates of glycolysis are indicative of malignancy. Adenomas, fibroids, inflammatory tissue, and normal tissue are all susceptible to false positive interpretation as malignant tumors depending on the individual patient and the conditions under which the study is being performed (3). In response to this drawback, numerous studies have shown that modifying patient diet can significantly reduce erroneous diagnosis across a variety of tumor types (4).

### Synthesis

FDG is now commonly synthesized using automated synthesis modules. The method currently used in routine clinical production is derived from the Hamacher synthesis, using nucleophilic [[18]F]F$^-$ (5). A precursor solution of mannose triflate (1,3,4,6-tetra-O-acetyl-2-trifluoromethanesulfonyl-β-D-mannopyranose) in acetonitrile is reacted with [[18]F]F$^-$ at reflux for 5 minutes to incorporate the [18]F atom into the sugar moiety. The protective acyl groups are then hydrolyzed under acidic or basic conditions (see Figure 2.1). Radiopharmaceutical production facilities are able to efficiently and reproducibly synthesize FDG with high radiochemical yields (50–80%) and specific activity using this method.

### Applications

PET imaging of FDG is typically performed 45–60 minutes post-injection (tumor accumulation reaching a maximum 2 hours post-injection) with a dose of ~15mCi for an average

*A Case-Based Approach to PET/CT in Oncology*, ed. Victor H. Gerbaudo. Published by Cambridge University Press.

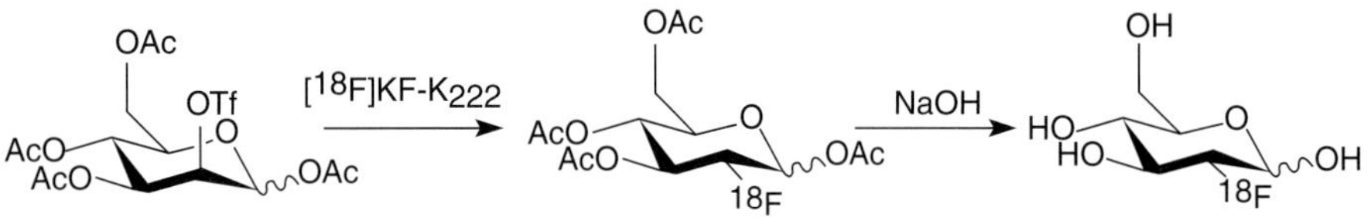

**Figure 2.1** Synthesis of $^{18}$F-FDG.

adult patient. FDG-PET provides metabolic information that complements CT and MRI (which provide mainly anatomical information) for staging and monitoring of treatment of a large variety of cancer types (3).

FDG-PET and PET/CT have proven highly effective in characterizing solitary pulmonary nodules as compared with CT alone, ultimately decreasing the number of unnecessary biopsies that result in benign findings (6). For staging and restaging of lymphoma, FDG-PET/CT has been shown in several studies to have significantly higher specificity without loss of sensitivity as compared with CT (7). Use of FDG-PET/CT has also been shown to provide increased detection of lymphoma bone involvement as compared with CT alone or in combination with bone marrow biopsy (8).

While FDG is successful in imaging many cancers, its uptake properties are suboptimal in certain types such as bone and prostate. Renal clearance of FDG leads to accumulation in the bladder, interfering with the ability to image the nearby prostate, while lower rates of glycolysis seem to be responsible for difficulties in imaging certain types of metastatic bone cancer. Inflammation can also be problematic in FDG-PET imaging due to increased glycolytic activity. Inflammatory effects of radiation therapy may muddle FDG assessment of treatment effectiveness (9).

## Amino acid transport

### Significance

Similar to the rationale of the glucose-derived radiotracer FDG, amino acid-based radiotracers allow for detection and imaging of various cancer types based upon their enhanced uptake as compared with normal tissue. Amino acid radiotracers can offer advantages over FDG in certain conditions due to higher tumor-to-background contrast and lower uptake in benign pathologies. FDG limitations in brain imaging include: low sensitivity for low-grade gliomas, non-specific FDG uptake in inflammatory lesions, and poor tumor boundary delineation due to high uptake in gray matter (see reference (10) for further discussion of amino acid metabolism and imaging).

## [methyl-$^{11}$C]Methionine (MET)

The investigation of [methyl-$^{11}$C]methionine (MET) as an imaging agent was reported as early as 1976 (11, 12). The short half-life of carbon-11 permits higher injectable doses ($\sim$20 mCi), allowing for detailed MET studies of tumor metabolism in brain.

### Synthesis

While many versions of L-[methyl-$^{11}$C]methionine synthesis have arisen over the years (11–15), all utilize $^{11}$C-methylation

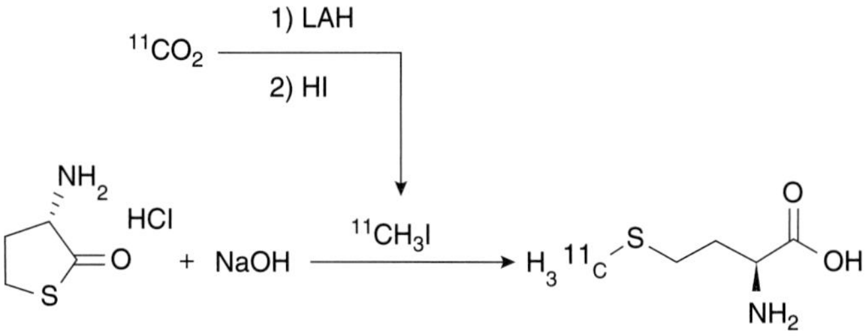

**Figure 2.2** Synthesis of $^{11}$C-methionine.

of the precursor L-homocysteine thiolactone hydrochloride (see Figure 2.2). Notable advances in the synthetic approach include on-Sep-Pak methylation which avoids time-consuming HPLC purification (14), and development of a fast in-loop (HPLC loop), room temperature $^{11}$C methylation reaction, which is capable of a 38% radiochemical yield in a production time of just 12 minutes (15).

### Applications

Although primarily utilized for imaging cerebral gliomas (10), MET has also shown great potential in imaging head and neck cancers (16), melanoma (17), non-Hodgkin's lymphoma (18), metastatic prostate cancer (19), and assessing breast cancer therapy response (20). The distinction between enhanced amino acid transport and increase energy uptake allows MET–PET to accurately diagnose and assess treatment where an FDG-PET study may be inadequate due to increased glucose uptake in inflammatory tissue, lower tumor to blood ratio, or general contrast enhancement in surrounding normal tissue.

## $^{18}$F-F-DOPA

The short half-life associated with [$^{11}$C]methionine (20.4 minutes) has spurred the development of $^{18}$F-labeled amino acids in order to eliminate the need for an in-house cyclotron. One such tracer, 3,4-dihydroxy-6–$^{18}$F-fluoro-L-phenylalanine (F-DOPA), is an analog of the natural biological precursor of dopamine, L-dopa. Since dopamine itself is unable to cross the blood–brain barrier, F-DOPA is synthesized and transported across the blood–brain barrier with kinetics similar to those of unlabeled L-dopa and subsequently decarboxylated in vivo to give the desired $^{18}$F-labeled dopamine (21). Initially investigated as an imaging tracer for diseases directly related to dopamine presence and metabolism such as Parkinson's and schizophrenia, F-DOPA has steadily worked its way into oncology imaging.

### Synthesis

The most common approach to synthesizing F-DOPA involves electrophilic fluorination ([$^{18}$F]F$_2$) of an organo-tin precursor

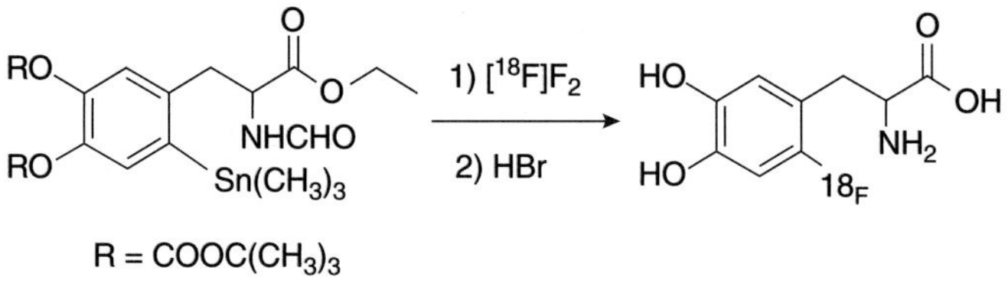

Figure 2.3 Synthesis of 6-$^{18}$F-fluoro-L-dopa.

as shown in Figure 2.3, giving the product in 25% radiochemical yield in 60 minutes (22), however, low specific activity and low regioselectivity often hinder [$^{18}$F]F$_2$ radiosyntheses. Alternative nucleophilic syntheses of F-DOPA have been reported which attempt to circumvent these problems, however radiochemical yields tend to be low, and synthesis of the precursors can be quite complicated (23).

### Applications

Aside from its use to assess dopamine levels and metabolism, FDOPA has been reported as a good surrogate for [$^{11}$C] methionine for imaging brain tumors (24). An 81-patient study reported that "[$^{18}$F]-F-DOPA PET was more accurate than [$^{18}$F]-FDG PET for imaging of low-grade tumors and evaluating recurrent tumors" (25). It has also shown great promise in diagnosis and localization of a variety of neuroendocrine tumors with high sensitivity and specificity (26).

## O-(2-[$^{18}$F]fluoroethyl)-L-tyrosine (FET)

Another commonly used artificial amino acid is O-(2-[$^{18}$F] fluoroethyl)-L-tyrosine, or FET (27). Initial studies reported that of 28 different amino acids investigated, [$^{14}$C]tyrosine displayed the third-highest brain uptake, feeding interest in developing a $^{18}$F-labeled tyrosine imaging agent (28). Also contributing to it's promise as a useful imaging agent, FET is synthesized in reasonable radiochemical yields as compared with other potential $^{18}$F amino acid targets displaying high brain uptake.

### Synthesis

The synthesis of FET utilizes no-carrier-added $^{18}$F-fluoride, producing the desired radiotracer in 40% radiochemical yield in 50 min (27). The approach involves mono-fluorination of ethylene glycol-1,2-ditosylate which is then added to the tyrosine salt precursor.

Although the synthetic route depicted in Figure 2.4 is currently the method commonly used in clinical production,

a new synthesis of FET has recently been reported using 2-bromoethyl triflate which offers simplified purification methods, abbreviated synthesis time (35 minutes) and a 45% radiochemical yield (29).

### Applications

Based on differential tracer uptake kinetics, FET is capable of detection and distinction of low- and high-grade gliomas (30). When combined with MRI, the tracer provides enhanced prognostic value in cases of untreated low-grade gliomas (31) and significantly improves the identification of cellular glioma tissue and allows definite histological tumor diagnosis (32). Similar to other amino acid radiotracers, FET can differentiate tumors from radiation-induced contrast enhancement in the brain (33), but remains inferior to FDG as a peripheral tumor-diagnostic PET tracer (34).

## New agents
### [$^{18}$F]1-amino-3-fluorocyclobutane 1-carboxylic acid (FACBC)

The $^{18}$F-labeled unnatural amino acid [$^{18}$F]1-amino-3-fluoro-cyclobutane 1-carboxylic acid, or FACBC, has recently been evaluated as a brain tumor-imaging probe. Tumor to brain ratios of 6.6 were observed at 20 minutes post-injection (35). Other preliminary FACBC studies have shown utility in imaging prostate carcinoma (36) and guiding prostate radio-therapy (37).

## Cellular proliferation and apoptosis
## Significance

Uncontrolled cellular proliferation is a characteristic hallmark of cancer. The imbalance between cell division and cell death underlies tumor growth, microenvironmental changes, and ultimately tumor progression to metastasis and mortality. Accordingly, many anticancer therapies are aimed specifically at inhibiting cellular proliferation or stimulation of apoptosis, and their success is dependent on the functioning of the tumor cell cycle. Thus, the assessment of rates of proliferation and apoptosis in tumors has both prognostic and therapeutic value. In vitro assays for proliferation are typically performed by an immunoassay against the protein Ki-67 which is expressed only in the nuclei of cells that are actively dividing. Prior to the use of Ki-67, the most common assay for cellular proliferation was the estimation of DNA synthesis rate by quantitation of the incorporation of $^3$H- or $^{14}$C-labeled

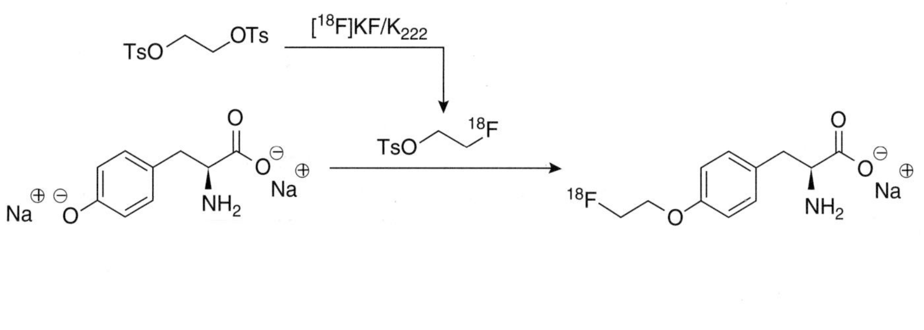

Figure 2.4 Synthesis of $^{18}$F-FET.

thymidine into tissue DNA. This method measures the fraction of cells in the S-phase of the cell cycle, which has been shown to be a very good prognostic for various cancers (38). The activity of thymidine kinase (TK), the enzyme family that catalyzes the phosphorylation of thymidine, correlates with the DNA synthesis rate.

Apoptosis (programmed cell death) and necrosis (uncontrolled cell death) are distinct processes of cell death. Apoptosis has come to be defined as one of a number of active forms of cell death that involve induction of certain "death receptors" (TNFR, FasR) and signaling pathways (caspases), modification of the nuclear matrix, release of endonucleases, and changes in DNA condensation. Necrosis results from physiochemical damage from outside the cell, resulting in sudden metabolic failure. Necrosis is characterized by cell swelling and rupture, leading to a local inflammatory reaction. Apoptosis can lead to necrosis in the event of ATP depletion.

## 3'-deoxy-3'-$^{18}$F-fluorothymidine (FLT)

As a PET radiotracer of cellular proliferation, [$^{11}$C]thymidine was developed and utilized to non-invasively and quantitatively evaluate thymidine kinetics in various human tumors (reviewed in (39)). Since the short half-life of carbon-11 limits the use of this radiotracer to a few academic PET centers, a number of $^{18}$F-labeled analogs have been investigated. The most extensively studied $^{18}$F-labeled thymidine analog is 3'-deoxy-3'-$^{18}$F-fluorothymidine (FLT). The development and biological characterization of FLT has been previously reviewed (38). FLT is transported into the cell and phosphorylated by TK1, but is not incorporated into DNA. Its kinetics in tissue are therefore analogous to those for FDG. For FLT, the rate-limiting step is the phosphorylation step, which in most conditions tracks with DNA synthesis rate.

### Synthesis

The first synthesis of FLT employed an $O^2,O^3$-anhydro precursor that gave modest radiochemical yields (40). Yield was improved by use of an N-BOC, protected nosylate precursor shown in Figure 2.5 (41). Nucleophilic [$^{18}$F] fluorination was followed by deprotection in acid, HPLC purification and sterile filtration. The synthesis has been fully automated, and gives typical radiochemical yields approaching 50%.

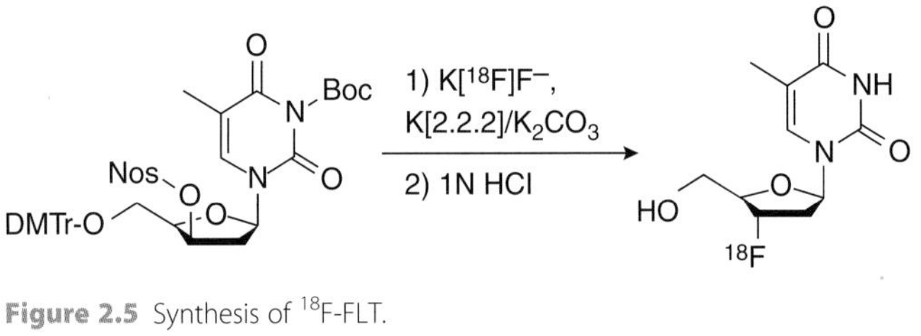

**Figure 2.5** Synthesis of $^{18}$F-FLT.

### Applications

FLT uptake has been shown to correlate with Ki-67 levels in resected tumors in patients with lung cancer (42), malignant lymphoma (43), brain gliomas (44) and breast cancer (45). However, FLT uptake was not found to correlate with Ki-67 levels in gastric cancer (46). FLT uptake has been shown in animal tumor models to be sensitive to monitor early biochemical changes in response to therapies (47, 48), but the effectiveness of FLT-PET to monitor response to therapy in patient trials has yet to be defined.

## New agents

The 2'-fluoropyrimidine, $^{18}$F-FMAU, is under investigation as a proliferation probe that is phosphorylated by TK1 and incorporated into DNA (49). It shows high uptake in the normal heart, kidneys, and liver, in part because of the role of mitochondrial thymidine kinase 2. Sigma-2 receptor binding ligands are under preclinical investigation as proliferation probes (50).

Although a number of PET probes for apoptosis are in preclinical development, none has reached widespread use. $^{99m}$Tc-labeled Annexin-V was developed as a SPECT tracer having high affinity to bind to phosphatidyl serine residues that are exposed on the surface of cells undergoing apoptosis and necrosis (51). Although this tracer was able to predict outcome in treated cancer patients (52), clinical trials were discontinued due to poor biodistribution and signal : noise properties. Annexin-V has been labeled with Fluorine-18 and shows feasibility as a probe for apoptosis in preclinical models (53). A malonic acid derivative, $^{18}$F-ML-10 (ApoSense), has shown accumulation in a cerebral artery occlusion model that correlated with histologic evidence of cell death (54).

## Choline transport and phosphorylation
## Significance

Choline (trimethylethanolamine) is a primary component of membrane phospholipids. The first step toward its metabolism to phospholipids is phosphorylation by choline kinase. Choline kinase is over-expressed in a broad array of tumor types, including prostate (55), breast (56), lung (57), sarcoma (58), ovarian (59), hepatocellular carcinoma (60), and brain tumors (61). Enhanced choline phosphorylation in tumor cells results in elevated levels of phosphocholine (PC). Proton magnetic resonance spectroscopic imaging (MRSI) of human tumors in vivo has demonstrated increased PC levels (55–57), as well as decreased PC levels in response to chemotherapies (60, 62). PET imaging after intravenous administration of PET choline analogs provides assessment of rates of transport and metabolic trapping. Thus, choline-PET data are reflective of perfusion-dependent delivery, transport and choline kinase-mediated phosphorylation of circulating choline (63–66). On the other hand, the MRSI-measured pool size of choline-containing metabolites is influenced by rates of synthesis and degradation of each entity, and the intracellular choline pool may be replenished by both endogenous and exogenous sources. The development of [11]C- and [18]F-labeled choline analogs as PET probes for choline uptake and metabolism are presently reviewed.

# [11]C-choline

## Synthesis

[11]C-choline is synthesized in high radiochemical yield by reaction of [11]C-methyl iodide or [11]C-methyl triflate with dimethylethanolamine (Figure 2.6) (63). A cation-exchange solid-phase extraction (SPE) cartridge was employed to purify the product. An automated synthesis of [11]C-choline was first reported by Hara et al. (67), for which radiochemical yields of 45% (uncorrected) were obtained. Radiochemical yield was improved to 60% by use of a "loop" reaction method (68).

## Applications

Hara et al. (63) were the first to demonstrate the potential of choline-PET imaging in oncology. High uptake of [11]C-choline was shown in patients with brain tumors. Low normal uptake in brain allowed excellent delineation of malignant regions. In 1998, Hara et al. (64) showed excellent potential of [11]C-choline as a prostate cancer probe. This seminal work stimulated many other groups to investigate [11]C-choline in prostate cancer (69–70), esophageal (71), lung (72), and other tumor types (73). Although its short half-life (20 m) limits its use to PET imaging facilities that have cyclotrons, [11]C-choline has found clinical utility in staging (71–75) and evaluation of recurrent disease (70, 75). Pelvic imaging of gynecologic, prostate and bladder cancers is benefitted by the very low urinary excretion of [11]C-choline. Significant promise has been shown for its use in monitoring of therapeutic response (70, 76). It is important to note that [11]C-choline uptake reflects active transport of choline by malignant tissue, but the relationship of choline uptake and cellular proliferation has not been clarified. A study that compared [11]C-choline uptake in primary prostate cancer before prostatectomy with post-surgical histopathology showed that choline uptake did not correlate with cellular proliferation rate as determined by Ki-67 staining (77). On the other hand, other studies in transformed human cell lines (78) and human cancer cell lines (79) have demonstrated a strong correlation between choline kinase-α activity and S-phase fraction (proliferation). To properly interpret imaging data with choline analogs, the observer must consider that the accumulation of radioactivity in tissue is not only dependent on choline kinase activity, but also tumor perfusion and choline transport (65). The rapid blood clearance of choline-based radiotracers renders them highly dependent on

perfusion. Furthermore, tissue hypoxia, a feature of poorly perfused tumors, modulates choline kinase activity (80).

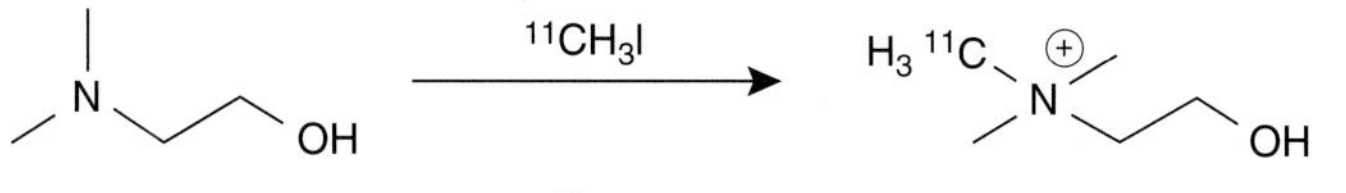

# [18]F-FCH/[18]F-FECH

## Synthesis

[18]F-labeled analogs of choline were developed to provide longer-lived radiotracers of choline uptake and metabolism. The fluoromethyl analog, [18]F-FCH (FCH), was developed by DeGrado and co-workers (65), while the fluoroethyl analog, [18]F-FECH (FECH), was investigated by Hara et al. (66). The syntheses of FCH and FECH employed [[18]F]fluoroalkylations of dimethylethanolamine (Figure 2.7). The [[18]F]fluoroalkylating synthon for FCH may be [[18]F]fluoromethyl bromide (65) or [[18]F]fluoromethyl triflate (81). For FECH, [[18]F]fluoroethyl tosylate is employed. Radiochemical yields for both FCH and FECH were in the 30–50% range (corrected) (65, 66). Recent improvements on automation and radiochemical yields have been reported for FCH (82) and FECH (83).

## Applications

The clinical applications of [18]F-labeled choline analogs in oncologic PET imaging are the same as those of [11]C-choline (recently reviewed in (84)). The longer half-life of [18]F provides for more practical clinical scheduling, and longer and more flexible scanning protocols. Two-phase and 3-phase imaging protocols have been employed to help differentiate cancer from normal tissues on the basis of differences of tracer kinetic properties. Although a head-to-head comparison of imaging characteristics of FCH and FECH has yet to be reported, the separate literature on these two agents suggest similar biodistribution, tumor uptake, and pharmacokinetics. This is not surprising since structure-activity studies of cholines for low-affinity choline transport (85) and choline kinase (86) show tolerance for replacement of one of the N-methyl groups of choline with an ethyl moiety. A potential drawback for imaging of pelvic tumors is that the urinary excretion for both fluorinated analogs is significantly higher than for [11]C-choline. However, the rapid blood clearance and tumor accumulation of the choline analogs allows for delineation of tumor uptake before radioactivity enters the ureters or bladder (65). Alternatively, the urinary contribution in later images can be ameliorated by hydration and voiding prior to PET scanning as is commonly employed in FDG imaging.

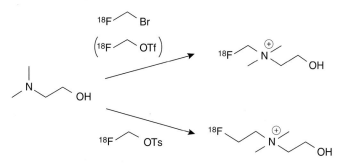

**Figure 2.6** Synthesis of methyl-[11]C-choline.

**Figure 2.7** Synthesis of [18]F-FCH and [18]F-FECH.

## Angiogenesis

### Significance

Continued growth of a solid tumor requires adequate perfusion. Upregulation of a family of cell surface receptors known as integrins has been implicated in aiding tumor growth by facilitating angiogenesis, potentially leading to tumor metastasis. By exploiting the integrin recognition (specifically integrin $\alpha_v\beta_3$) of the tri-peptide sequence argentine-glycine-aspartic acid (RGD), angiogenesis probes have been successfully developed (87).

### $^{18}$F-Galacto-RGD

Initial studies of cyclic RGD peptides using $^{125}$I showed liver and intestinal activity retention (88). By linking the cyclic peptide fragment to a sugar moiety, liver uptake was decreased and $^{18}$F-labeling could easily be achieved. The resultant $^{18}$F-Galacto-RGD displays low tracer concentration in organs and stable accumulation in $\alpha_v\beta_3$-expressing tumors, giving a high signal to noise ratio up to 2 hours p.i. (87).

#### Synthesis

The multistep synthesis of $^{18}$F-Galacto-RGD (Figure 2.8) involves first synthesizing and cyclizing the peptidic fragment. This peptide is then linked to the sugar and subsequently $^{18}$F-labeled using 4-nitrophenyl-2-[$^{18}$F]fluoropropionate (this is synthesized from [$^{18}$F]F$^-$). The reader is directed to reference (89) for further details.

#### Applications

While $^{18}$F-Galacto-RGD is relatively new, it has already successfully imaged $\alpha_v\beta_3$ expression in a variety of cancers including glioblastoma multiforme (90), breast (91), squamous cell carcinoma of the head and neck (92) and non-small cell lung cancer (93). In comparing FDG-PET to $^{18}$F-Galacto-RGD-PET, initial findings indicate that FDG is more sensitive for tumor staging, while $^{18}$F-Galacto-RGD-PET is useful in imaging angiogenesis and planning and assessing $\alpha_v\beta_3$ targeted therapies (92, 93).

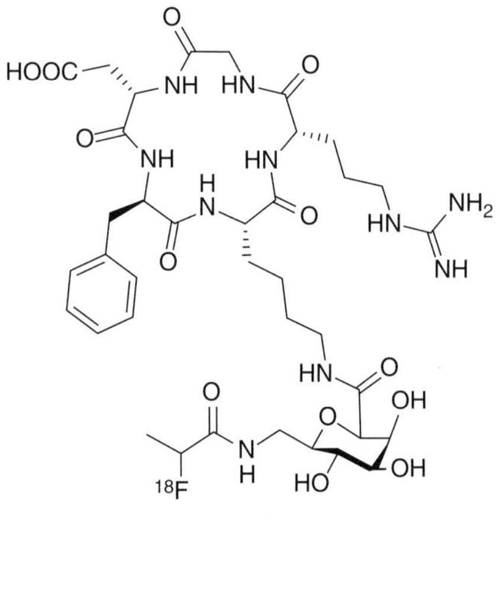

Figure 2.8 Structure of $^{18}$F-Galacto-RGD.

## New agents

Recently, research groups have labeled RGD peptides with radiometals such as $^{64}$Cu, however, these new probes have yet to be used in the clinic (94).

## Hypoxia

### Significance

Tumor hypoxia arises when the oxygen supply does not match the metabolic demand. Hypoxia can result from limitations in tumor perfusion (oxygen delivery) and/or increased diffusive distance from nutritive blood vessels. Hypoxia induces both proteomic and genomic changes in tumor cells leading to a large number of changes in functional status. Whereas in normal tissues, sustained hypoxia will lead to apoptosis, cancer cells respond through HIF-1$\alpha$-dependent mechanisms to arrest the cell-cycle, reduce energy-consuming processes, and render the cell in a dormant (quiescent) state. Meanwhile, the proteomic changes result in upregulation of processes involved with tumor invasiveness, metastasis and malignant phenotype (95). The downregulation of the cell cycle in response to hypoxia renders the cells less responsive to radiation therapy and certain chemotherapies. It has been clearly established through invasive tissue oxygenation measurements and non-invasive imaging studies with hypoxic probes that tumor hypoxia is predictive of poor survival in cervical cancer and head and neck tumors. Given the clinical relevance of an imaging method to assess tumor hypoxia, a considerable amount of attention has been given over the last 20 years to the development of PET probes for hypoxia, and several agents are currently undergoing clinical trials.

### FMISO

[$^{18}$F]fluoromisonidazole (1-(2-nitroimidazolyl)-2-hydroxy-3-fluoropropane) (FMISO), is the most widely used PET probe for non-invasive assessment of regional tissue hypoxia. FMISO is one of a large number of radiolabeled 2-nitroimidazoles that are under evaluation as hypoxia imaging agents (96). The mechanism by which 2-nitroimidazoles are retained in hypoxic tissues is now reasonably well understood. After diffusive transport into cells, the 2-nitro group accepts an electron to form an $NO_2^-$ radical anion. In the presence of oxygen, the nitro radical is readily oxidized, returning the nitroimidazole radiopharmaceutical to its parent state. However, in low oxygen concentrations, a competing reaction becomes significant: the nitro radical may react with nitroreductase enzymes to form a 2-electron reduction product that cannot be reoxidized by oxygen. The labeled nitroimidazole goes on to form an alkylating agent that reacts indiscriminately with intracellular macromolecules to be irreversibly trapped within the cell. Since the octanol/water partition coefficients of many of these agents are near 1, they are freely diffusible and homogenously distributed in the body within an hour after injection, maintaining a volume of distribution essentially equal to that of total body

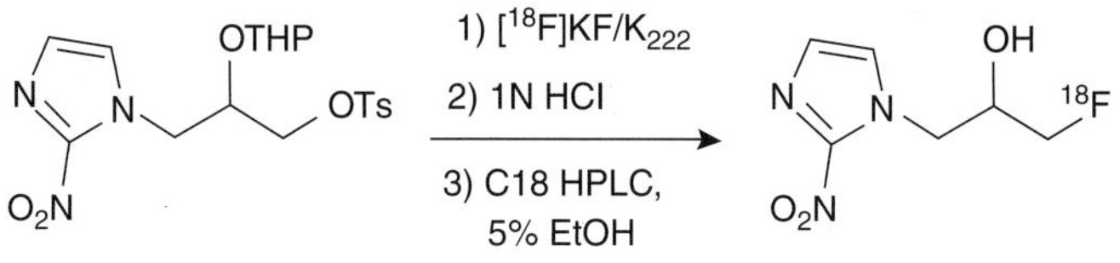

Figure 2.9 Synthesis of [18]F-FMISO.

water. Thus, the kinetics of FMISO and other nitroimidazoles are near ideal to indicate hypoxia from the ratio of concentration of radioactivity measured in tumor tissue to normal tissue (e.g., muscle). Furthermore, the stable whole-body distribution minimizes the potential of a confounding influence of tissue perfusion. Because FMISO only accumulates in hypoxic cells with functional nitroreductase enzymes, there is no accumulation in necrotic cells.

## Synthesis

FMISO is commonly synthesized in a 2-step procedure analogous to the synthesis procedure for FDG (Figure 2.9) (97). The synthesis is accomplished in about 35 min. Typical radiochemical yields are 25–30%. The product is racemic at the alcohol group, but has been shown to have the same biodistribution characteristics as the pure enantiomer (96).

## Applications

Selective retention of FMISO is observed in hypoxic tissue by 1 h after injection and persists for 2.5 h. The optimal imaging time for quantitation of the tumor/plasma and tumor/normal tissue concentration ratios is 2 h post-injection (98). Good correlation was found between FMISO tumor:muscle ratio and intraoperative $pO_2$ measurements in head and neck cancer (99), but not in soft tissue sarcomas (100). FMISO imaging has shown feasibility to assess hypoxia in brain tumors (101), head and neck cancer (99), renal tumors (102), and non-small cell lung cancer (103). Hypoxia on FMISO-PET predicts adverse prognosis in head and neck cancer (104), and decrease of FMISO uptake after chemotherapy or chemoradiotherapy was associated with favorable treatment response (103, 104).

## New agents

Several second-generation nitroimidazoles are under investigation as hypoxia imaging probes. [18]F]fluoroazomycin arabinofuranoside (FAZA) was found to have higher tumor: background ratios relative to FMISO in EMT6 tumor-bearing BALB/c mice (105) and initial studies in patients with head and neck cancer appear encouraging (105). Other [18]F]fluorinated nitroimidazoles in development include [18]F]fluoroerythronitroimidazole (FETNIM) (106), [18]F]fluoroetanidazole (FETA) (107), and EF5 (108). The radiocopper metal complex agent, diacetyl-bis-(N4-methylthiosemicarbazone) (ATSM) was developed as a longer-lived hypoxia imaging agent (109), although a mechanistic understanding of tissue retention related to hypoxia has not been completely clarified. In an initial study in patients with non-small cell cancer, [60]Cu-ATSM uptake

predicted response to chemotherapy and radiochemotherapy. In patients with cancer of the uterine cervix, hypoxia as indicated by [60]Cu-ATSM-PET was a significant independent predictor of tumor recurrence (110).

## Osseous tumors and metastases
### Significance

[18]F-fluoride was one of the earliest used PET radiotracers, having been introduced in the early 1960s as an excellent skeletal scintigraphy imaging agent (111). The availability of [99m]Tc generators and the thick NaI(Tl) crystals required for imaging the 511-KeV photons given off by [18]F annihilation events precluded widespread use of [18]F-fluoride as a bone imaging agent. The introduction of high-sensitivity PET scanners and the explosion of interest in producing large quantities of FDG led to facilities which could easily produce [18]F-fluoride and perform whole-body bone scans with higher spatial resolution than scintigraphy or SPECT would permit.

## [18]F-Fluoride
### Synthesis

[18]F-fluoride is produced from the nuclear reaction of [[18]O] $H_2O$ in the cyclotron target. The irradiated water is then flushed from the target through an ion-exchange resin. The [18]F-fluoride is eluted from the resin with saline and passed through a sterilizing filter, before administration to human subjects.

### Applications

The use of [18]F-fluoride-PET has provided clinicians with a powerful tool for imaging skeletal metastases of a variety of cancers with 13% higher sensitivity than projection images (112). Compared to widely used [99m]Tc scintigraphy, [18]F-fluoride-PET has significantly higher sensitivity in detecting skeletal lesions (113). Dual-modality [18]F-fluoride-PET/CT has been shown to accurately detect and differentiate malignant from benign lesions using a low-dose CT scan, minimizing the need for separate studies (114). Pilot studies have recently been performed using a comprehensive imaging cocktail of FDG and [18]F-fluoride in a single PET/CT scan for efficient whole-body cancer screening (115).

## Estrogen receptor
### Significance

The estrogen receptor is associated with malignancy of certain breast cancers (116). This has led to the development of antiestrogen therapies which block the division of estrogen dependent tumor cells (117). The estrogen receptor ERα displays increased expression in estrogen dependent tumors (ER+ tumors) and has been shown to have prognostic value and aid in predicting the effectiveness of hormone therapy for a given patient (118). This increased expression of ERα can be imaged using estrogen-based radiotracers which bind to the target in a high ratio relative to surrounding normal tissue and ER– tumor tissue (119).

## $^{18}$F-fluoroestradiol (FES)

Presently, the most successful estrogen based ER imaging agent is the tracer $^{18}$F-fluoroestradiol (FES). While a variety of other agents such as betaFMOX have shown comparable and even enhanced ER binding in vitro and in small animal studies, FES remains the best tracer for human studies most likely due to species specific estrogen delivery and metabolism associated with sex hormone binding globulin (SHBG) which is present in primates but lacking in rats (120). In primates, SHBG aids in biodistributing FES within the timeframe of $^{18}$F imaging and protects FES from metabolism (121).

### Synthesis

The synthesis of FES was first reported by Kiesewetter *et al.* in 1984 (122). In addition to stability issues associated with the precursor, this synthesis was complicated by a LiAlH$_4$ ketone reduction and triflate removal. Several years later a synthesis was reported by Tewson *et al.* using a more stable precursor and simplified synthesis (123) (Figure 2.10). This synthesis was then incorporated into an automated module giving radiochemical yields in the 50% range and allowing for several doses to be synthesized at once (124).

A recent advance allows for the production of FES using a disposable cassette system and the GE TracerLab MX module (typically used for FDG synthesis) giving the radiotracer in 45% radiochemical yield (125).

### Applications

FES-PET studies primarily focus on breast cancer imaging. After initially demonstrating success at imaging primary breast tumors (126), FES-PET imaging performed on patients with metastatic breast cancer resulted in 93% sensitivity in one study and 88% agreement with ER assay in another, allowing for unprecedented non-invasive assessment of ER+ expression in breast cancer (127, 128). FES uptake in ER+ tumors may have predictive value in determining the success rate of various therapies such as tamoxifen (129) and aromatase inhibitor therapy (130), however, more studies need to be performed before any clear conclusions can be drawn. Aside from imaging breast cancer, preliminary combined FDG/FES-PET studies have demonstrated potential value in differential diagnosis of uterine tumors (131).

## New agents

Preliminary in vitro studies performed on structural variants of FES have shown some potential for new estrogen-based tracers with enhancing uptake in ER+ tumors (132). Other ER ligand classes such as cyclofenils are in early stages of investigation as potential radiotracers for imaging ER+ tumors (133).

## Androgen receptor

### Significance

Early stage prostate neoplasms often overexpress the androgen receptor (AR). Most of these tumors eventually become hormone independent, complicating treatment (134). Unlike ER+ tumors in breast tissue, there has been poor correlation between AR expression and hormone therapy response (135). This has been attributed to the cellular heterogeneity of AR expression in poor responders to hormone therapy, making immunohistochemical tumor analysis less reliable than expected. The ability to image the tumor using PET with an appropriate AR binding ligand could provide a better representation of AR expression and perhaps provide predictive value for hormone therapy response.

## 16β-[$^{18}$F]fluoro-5α-dihydrotestosterone (FDHT)

Of three AR ligands initially investigated in male baboons, 16β-[$^{18}$F]fluoro-5α-dihydrotestosterone (FDHT) showed the highest absolute uptake and highest tumor to soft tissue ratio (134). These properties combined with the tracer's simple synthesis made it a choice candidate for evaluation in human subjects.

### Synthesis

The synthesis of FDHT (Figure 2.11) is similar to the early syntheses of FES and consists of [$^{18}$F] nucleophilic fluorination of a triflate precursor followed by ketone reduction and ketal deprotection to give the desired product in 30% radiochemical yield (136).

### Applications

So far, very few clinical PET studies have been performed using FDHT. The initial human study found that FDHT was

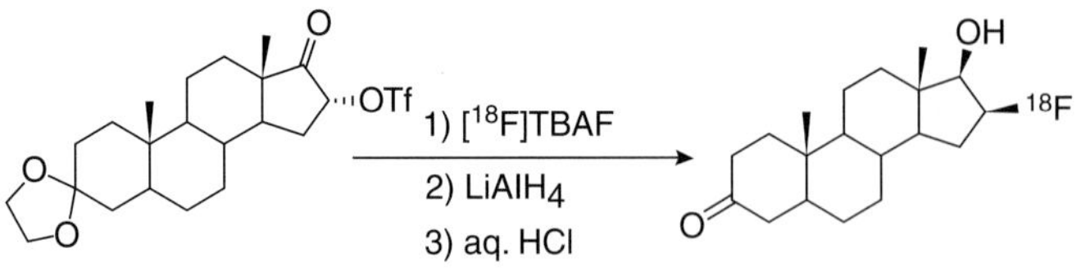

**Figure 2.11** Synthesis of $^{18}$F-FDHT.

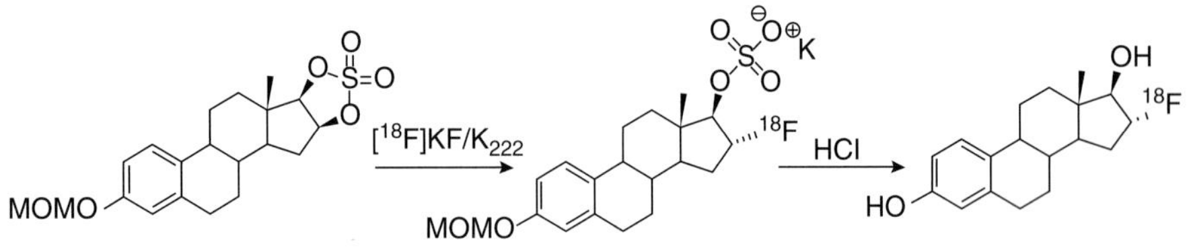

**Figure 2.10** Synthesis of $^{18}$F-FES.

effective at detecting metastatic lesions of prostate cancer (137). The high binding observed for FDHT to prostate cancer relative to normal tissue supports the observation that AR over-expression is present in androgen-independent tumors. While a follow-up study involving 19 men with advanced prostate cancer revealed FDHT-PET sensitivity of 63%, the tracer detected 17 unsuspected lesions in five patients. The report also showed a decrease in FDHT uptake in tumors after administration of the anti-androgen drug flutamide, further supporting that tracer uptake is a receptor-mediated process (138). Thus, FDHT can provide valuable insight into cancer pharmacology for use in treatment determination and assessment of therapy response.

## New agents

The new tracer $^{18}$F-FMDHT has shown high AR specificity and sensitivity in rat studies, however human studies have yet to be performed (139). Non-steroidal AR antagonists such as 3-F-NNDI and (+/−)-3-[$^{76}$Br]bromo-hydroxyflutamide have recently been investigated but have shown little success due to poor target tissue distribution properties (140, 141).

## Somatostatin receptor

### Significance

The somatostatin receptor is expressed in a variety of tissues and cancers. It is highly expressed in pancreatic cancer and neuroendocrine tumors, particularly carcinoid tumors and the gastroenteropancreatic tumors. Early work in imaging of neuroendocrine tumors identified $^{111}$In- and $^{123}$I-labeled analogs of the therapeutic peptide, octreotide, as useful probes of the somatostatin receptor in tumors (142, 143). It was recognized that a positive scan may predict the ability of octreotide therapy to control symptoms of hormonal hypersecretion in neuroendocrine tumors (144). The reported sensitivity for tumor detection with $^{111}$In-DTPA-octreotide ranges from 60% to 90% and the specificity ranges from 85% to 98% (145). The SPECT imaging technique is limited by long acquisition periods (24–48 h), administration of laxatives to avoid significant accumulation of bowel activity, high physiologic uptake in the liver and kidneys, and rather low spatial resolution and high statistical noise. Radiolabeling with PET isotopes was developed to address these limitations.

## $^{68}$Ga-labeled octreotide analogs

Although $^{18}$F-labeled octreotide analogs were the first PET analogs of octreotide to be developed, $^{68}$Ga-labeled somatostatin analogs have received significantly more clinical interest, particularly in the European Union (146–148). The radiometal $^{68}$Ga has a physical half-life of 68 min and requires a chelator for attachment to the octreotide peptide. Several $^{68}$Ga-labeled somatostatin analogs have been investigated, including 1,4,7,10-tetraazacyclododecane-N,N$'$, N$''$,N$'''$-tetraacetic-acid-D-Phe1-Tyr3-octreotide (DOTATOC) (147), (1-(1-carboxy-3-carbo-tert-butoxypropyl)-4,7-(carbo-tert-butoxymethyl)-1,4,7-triazacyclononane-[Tyr3]-octreotide (NODAGATOC) (148), and DOTA-NOC (146).

### Synthesis

$^{68}$Ga-labeled octreotides are labeled by complexation of $^{68}$Ga to the conjugated chelate. $^{68}$Ga is obtained from a $^{68}$Ge/$^{68}$Ga generator by elution in dilute HCl. To this eluate carrier Ga$^{3+}$ is added, followed by evaporation to dryness and redissolution in acetate buffer pH 4.8. $^{68}$Ga-DOTATOC is thus prepared by adding to such a solution 14 mL 1 mmol/L aqueous DOTA-TOC solution and heating the mixture for 15 min at 95 °C (147). Subsequently, the pH is adjusted to 7.0 and uncomplexed $^{68}$Ga is retained on a reverse-phase cartridge (SepPAK C18; Waters Corp., Milford, MA), whereas $^{68}$Ga-DOTATOC is eluted with ethanol. After evaporation of the organic solvent, the compound is redissolved in 5.0 mL 0.01 mol/L phosphate-buffered saline pH 7.4. Specific activities obtained were 15–18 MBq $^{68}$Ga/nmol of ligand.

### Applications

$^{68}$Ga-labeled octreotides have been shown to be effective imaging agents for somatostatin receptor positive tumors. At 10 min after injection, about 80% of the $^{68}$Ga-DOTATOC is rapidly cleared from blood with a half-life of 3.5 min, leading to high tumor : background ratios as early as 15 min post-injection (147). The enhanced spatial resolution of PET allows detection and visualization of smaller tumors. Clinical applications include imaging of meningiomas (147), neuroendocrine tumors (146), gastroenteropancreatic neuroendocrine tumors (149), bronchial carcinoid (150), and hepatocellular carcinoma (151).

## Other agents

A glycosylated analog, N(alpha)-(1-deoxy-D-fructosyl)-N (epsilon)-(2-[$^{18}$F]fluoropropionyl)-Lys(0)-Tyr(3)-octreotate (Gluc-Lys([$^{18}$F]FP)-TOCA) showed lower liver uptake due to lower lipophilicity (152). The $^{18}$F-labeled analogs have received less attention because of the relative ease of production of the $^{68}$Ga-labeled analogs.

## Fatty acid synthesis

### Significance

The fatty acid synthesis pathway provides long-chain fatty acids necessary for membrane lipid synthesis. It also has an important role in regulation of lipid signaling pathways that regulate tumor cell survival. The precursor for fatty acid synthesis is malonyl-CoA produced by action of acetyl-CoA carboxylase (ACC) on cytosolic acetyl-CoA. Cytosolic acetyl-CoA can arise from cytosolic citrate via ATP citrate lyase (ACL) activity or, to a lesser extent, activation of exogenous acetate by cytosolic acetyl-CoA synthetase (ACSS2) (153). Fatty acid synthase (FAS) is a key enzyme in the fatty acid synthesis pathway, and is over-expressed in a wide variety of tumors. FAS levels correlate with tumor grade and invasiveness (154). The tumorigenic properties of FAS over-expression appear to be independent of its role in fatty acid synthesis, but instead mediated through regulation of the signaling pathways (155). Targeted inhibition of FAS slows tumor growth and induces apoptosis in cultured cells (156). Thus, imaging of the fatty acid synthesis pathway using $^{11}$C-acetate as a metabolic substrate may allow assessment of this important process in human tumors (157).

# $^{11}$C-Acetate

## Synthesis

The radiochemical synthesis of $^{11}$C-acetate has undergone only minor variations since its initial publication in 1943 (158). Advances have been made in synthesis automation (159, 160). The common approach is to react $^{11}$CO$_2$ with a methyl Grignard reagent, followed by treatment with an aqueous acid such as HCl (Figure 2.12). Typical decay-corrected radiochemical yields fall in the range of 60–70% and optimized synthesis times are approximately 20 min.

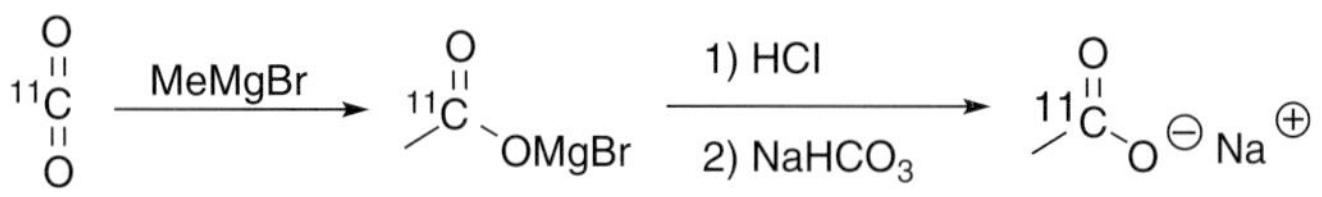

**Figure 2.12** Synthesis of $^{11}$C-acetate.

## Applications

$^{11}$C-Acetate was first evaluated as an oncologic tracer in renal cell carcinoma by Shreve *et al.* (157) who reported accumulation of tracer in tumors as opposed to metabolic clearance in normal renal cortex. Subsequent studies showed utility for imaging of prostate cancer (161), hepatocellular carcinoma (162), brain tumors (163), lung cancer (164), head and neck cancer (165), and thymoma (166). High clinical interest has been given in evaluation of recurrent prostate cancer (161, 167) and the use of $^{11}$C-acetate-PET images to guide radiation treatment to the primary prostatic tumor (168).

# Other agents

$^{18}$F-Fluoroacetate (FAc) is under investigation as a longer-lived analog of $^{11}$C-acetate. Preliminary imaging studies in a patient with prostate cancer showed accumulation of FAc in metastases, although higher urinary excretion of radioactivity was seen in rats and baboons (169).

# References

1. Warburg O. On the origin of cancer cells. *Science* 1956;**123**:309–314.

2. Christofk HR, Vander Heiden MG, Harris MH *et al.* The M2 splice isoform of pyruvate kinase is important for cancer metabolism and tumour growth. *Nature* 2008;**452**:230–3.

3. Phelps M. *PET: Molecular Imaging and its Biological Applications.* New York: Springer, 2004, p. 621.

4. Williams G, Kolodny GM. Suppression of myocardial 18F-FDG uptake by preparing patients with a high-fat, low-carbohydrate diet. *Am J Roentgenol* 2008;**190**:W151–6.

5. Hamacher K, Coenen HH, Stocklin G. Efficient stereospecific synthesis of no-carrier-added 2-[18F]-fluoro-2-deoxy-D-glucose using aminopolyether supported nucleophilic substitution. *J Nucl Med* 1986;**27**:235–8.

6. Jeong SY, Lee KS, Shin KM *et al.* Efficacy of PET/CT in the characterization of solid or partly solid solitary pulmonary nodules. *Lung Cancer* 2008;**61**:186–94.

7. Stumpe KD, Urbinelli M, Steinert HC *et al.* Whole-body positron emission tomography using fluorodeoxyglucose for staging of lymphoma: effectiveness and comparison with computed tomography. *Eur J Nucl Med* 1998;**25**:721–8.

8. Moog F, Kotzerke J, Reske SN. FDG PET can replace bone scintigraphy in primary staging of malignant lymphoma. *J Nucl Med* 1999;**40**:1407–13.

9. Haberkorn U, Strauss LG, Dimitrakopoulou A *et al.* PET studies of fluorodeoxyglucose metabolism in patients with recurrent colorectal tumors receiving radiotherapy. *J Nucl Med* 1991;**32**:1485–90.

10. Singhal T, Narayanan TK, Jain V, Mukherjee J, Mantil J. 11C-L-methionine positron emission tomography in the clinical management of cerebral gliomas. *Mol Imaging Biol* 2008;**10**:1–18.

11. Langstrom B, Lundqvist H. The preparation of 11C-methyl iodide and its use in the synthesis of 11C-methyl-L-methionine. *Int J Appl Radiat Isot* 1976;**27**:357–63.

12. Comar D, Cartron J, Maziere M, Marazano C. Labelling and metabolism of methionine-methyl-11 C. *Eur J Nucl Med* 1976;**1**:11–14.

13. Davis J, Yano Y, Cahoon J, Budinger TF. Preparation of 11C-methyl iodide and L-[S-methyl-11C]methionine by an automated continuous flow process. *Int J Appl Radiat Isot* 1982;**33**:363–9.

14. Pascali C, Bogni A, Iwata R *et al.* High efficiency preparation of L-[S-methyl-11C]methionine by on-column [11C]methylation on C18 Sep-Pak. *J Label Comp Radiopharm* 1999;**42**:715–24.

15. Gomez V, Gispert JD, Amador V, Llop J. New method for routine production of L-[methyl-11C] methionine: in loop synthesis. *J Label Comp Radiopharm* 2008;**51**:83–6.

16. Leskinen-Kallio S, Lindholm P, Lapela M, Joensuu H, Nordman E. Imaging of head and neck tumors with positron emission tomography and [11C]methionine. *Int J Radiat Oncol Biol Phys* 1994;**30**:1195–9.

17. Lindholm P, Leskinen S, Någren K *et al.* Carbon-11-methionine PET imaging of malignant melanoma. *J Nucl Med* 1995;**36**:1806–10.

18. Leskinen-Kallio S, Ruotsalainen U, Någren K, Teräs M, Joensuu H. Uptake of carbon-11-methionine and fluorodeoxyglucose in non-Hodgkin's lymphoma: a PET study. *J Nucl Med* 1991;**32**:1211–18.

19. Macapinlac HA, Humm JL, Akhurst T Differential metabolism and pharmacokinetics of L-[1-(11C)]-methionine and 2-[(18)F] fluoro-2-deoxy-D-glucose (FDG) in androgen

independent prostate cancer. *Clin Positron Imaging* 1999;**2**:173–81.

20. Lindholm P, Lapela M, Någren K *et al.* Preliminary study of carbon-11 methionine PET in the evaluation of early response to therapy in advanced breast cancer. *Nucl Med Commun* 2009;**30**:30–6.

21. Firnau G, Garnett ES, Sourkes TL, Missala K. (18F) Fluoro-Dopa: a unique gamma emitting substrate for Dopa decarboxylase. *Experientia* 1975;**31**:1254–5.

22. Namavari M, Bishop A, Satyamurthy N, Bida G, Barrio JR. Regioselective radiofluorodestannylation with [18F]F2 and [18F]CH3COOF: a high yield synthesis of 6-[18F]Fluoro-L-dopa. *Int J Rad Appl Instrum A* 1992;**43**:989–96.

23. Lemaire C, Damhaut P, Plenevaux A, Comar D. Enantioselective synthesis of 6-[fluorine-18]-fluoro-L-dopa from no-carrier-added fluorine-18-fluoride. *J Nucl Med* 1994;**35**:1996–2002.

24. Becherer A, Karanikas G, Szabó M *et al.* Brain tumour imaging with PET: a comparison between [18F]fluorodopa and [11C]methionine. *Eur J Nucl Med Mol Imaging* 2003;**30**:1561–7.

25. Chen W, Silverman DH, Delaloye S *et al.* 18F-FDOPA PET imaging of brain tumors: comparison study with 18F-FDG PET and evaluation of diagnostic accuracy. *J Nucl Med* 2006;**47**:904–11.

26. Becherer A, Szabó M, Karanikas G *et al.* Imaging of advanced neuroendocrine tumors with (18)F-FDOPA PET. *J Nucl Med* 2004;**45**:1161–7.

27. Wester HJ, Herz M, Weber W *et al.* Synthesis and radiopharmacology of O-(2-[18F]fluoroethyl)-L-tyrosine for tumor imaging. *J Nucl Med* 1999;**40**:205–12.

28. Oldendorf WH. Brain uptake of radiolabeled amino acids, amines, and hexoses after arterial injection. *Am J Physiol* 1971;**221**:1629–1639.

29. Zuhayra M, Alfteimi A, Forstner CV *et al.* New approach for the synthesis of [18F]fluoroethyltyrosine for cancer imaging: simple, fast, and high yielding automated synthesis. *Bioorg Med Chem* 2009;**17**:7441–8.

30. Pöpperl G, Kreth FW, Herms J *et al.* Analysis of 18F-FET PET for grading of recurrent gliomas: is evaluation of uptake kinetics superior to standard methods? *J Nucl Med* 2006;**47**:393–403.

31. Floeth FW, Pauleit D, Sabel M *et al.* Prognostic value of O-(2–18F-fluoroethyl)-L-tyrosine PET and MRI in low-grade glioma. *J Nucl Med* 2007;**48**:519–27.

32. Pauleit D, Floeth F, Hamacher K *et al.* O-(2-[18F]fluoroethyl)-L-tyrosine PET combined with MRI improves the diagnostic assessment of cerebral gliomas. *Brain* 2005;**128**(Pt 3):678–87.

33. Pöpperl G, Götz C, Rachinger W *et al.* Value of O-(2-[18F]fluoroethyl)-L-tyrosine PET for the diagnosis of recurrent glioma. *Eur J Nucl Med Mol Imaging* 2004;**31**:1464–70.

34. Pauleit D, Stoffels G, Schaden W *et al.* PET with O-(2–18F-Fluoroethyl)-L-Tyrosine in peripheral tumors: first clinical results. *J Nucl Med* 2005;**46**:411–16.

35. Shoup TM, Olson J, Hoffman JM *et al.* Synthesis and evaluation of [18F] 1-amino-3-fluorocyclobutane-1-carboxylic acid to image brain tumors. *J Nucl Med* 1999;**40**:331–8.

36. Schuster DM, Votaw JR, Nieh PT *et al.* Initial experience with the radiotracer anti-1-amino-3-18F-fluorocyclobutane-1-carboxylic acid with PET/CT in prostate carcinoma. *J Nucl Med* 2007;**48**:56–63.

37. Jani AB, Fox TH, Whitaker D, Schuster DM. Case study of anti-1-amino-3-F-18 fluorocyclobutane-1-carboxylic acid (anti-[F-18] FACBC) to guide prostate cancer radiotherapy target design. *Clin Nucl Med* 2009;**34**:279–84.

38. Bading JR, Shields AF. Imaging of cell proliferation: status and prospects. *J Nucl Med* 2008;**49** Suppl **2**:64S–80S.

39. Mankoff DA, Shields AF, Krohn KA. PET imaging of cellular proliferation. *Radiol Clin North Am* 2005;**43**:153–67.

40. Grierson JR, Shields AF. Radiosynthesis of 3′-deoxy-3′-[(18)F]fluorothymidine: [(18)F]FLT for imaging of cellular proliferation in vivo. *Nucl Med Biol* 2000;**27**:143–56.

41. Martin SJ, Eisenbarth JA, Wagner-Utermann U *et al.* A new precursor for the radiosynthesis of [18F]FLT. *Nucl Med Biol* 2002;**29**:263–73.

42. Buck AK, Halter G, Schirrmeister H *et al.* Imaging proliferation in lung tumors with PET: 18F-FLT versus 18F-FDG. *J Nucl Med* 2003;**44**:1426–1431.

43. Buck AK, Bommer M, Stilgenbauer S *et al.* Molecular imaging of proliferation in malignant lymphoma. *Cancer Res* 2006;**66**:11055–61.

44. Choi SJ, Kim JS, Kim JH *et al.* [18F]3′-deoxy-3′-fluorothymidine PET for the diagnosis and grading of brain tumors. *Eur J Nucl Med Mol Imaging* 2005;**32**:653–9.

45. Kenny LM, Vigushin DM, Al-Nahhas A *et al.* Quantification of cellular proliferation in tumor and normal tissues of patients with breast cancer by [18F]fluorothymidine-positron emission tomography imaging: evaluation of analytical methods. *Cancer Res* 2005;**65**:10104–12.

46. Kameyama R, Yamamoto Y, Izuishi K *et al.* Detection of gastric cancer using 18F-FLT PET: comparison with 18F-FDG PET. *Eur J Nucl Med Mol Imaging* 2009;**36**:382–8.

47. Sugiyama M, Sakahara H, Sato K *et al.* Evaluation of 3′-deoxy-3′-18F-fluorothymidine for monitoring tumor response to radiotherapy and photodynamic therapy in mice. *J Nucl Med* 2004;**45**:1754–8.

48. Waldherr C, Mellinghoff IK, Tran C *et al.* Monitoring antiproliferative responses to kinase inhibitor therapy in mice with 3′-deoxy-3′-18F-fluorothymidine PET. *J Nucl Med* 2005;**46**:114–20.

49. Sun H, Sloan A, Mangner TJ *et al.* Imaging DNA synthesis with [18F] FMAU and positron emission tomography in patients with cancer. *Eur J Nucl Med Mol Imaging* 2005;**32**:15–22.

50. Tu Z, Xu J, Jones LA *et al.* Fluorine-18-labeled benzamide analogues for imaging the sigma2 receptor status of solid tumors with positron emission tomography. *J Med Chem* 2007;**50**:3194–204.

51. Hayes MJ, Moss SE. Annexins and disease. *Biochem Biophys Res Commun* 2004;**322**:1166–70.

52. Belhocine T, Steinmetz N, Hustinx R *et al.* Increased uptake of the apoptosis-imaging agent (99m)Tc recombinant human Annexin V in human tumors after one course of chemotherapy as a predictor of tumor response and patient prognosis. *Clin Cancer Res* 2002;**8**:2766–74.

53. Murakami Y, Takamatsu H, Taki J *et al.* 18F-labelled annexin V: a PET tracer for apoptosis imaging. *Eur J Nucl Med Mol Imaging* 2004;**31**:469–74.

54. Reshef A, Shirvan A, Waterhouse RN et al. Molecular imaging of neurovascular cell death in experimental cerebral stroke by PET. *J Nucl Med* 2008;**49**:1520–8.

55. Kurhanewicz J, Vigneron DB, Hricak H et al. Three-dimensional H-1 MR spectroscopic imaging of the in situ human prostate with high (0.24–0.7-cm3) spatial resolution. *Radiology* 1996;**198**:795–805.

56. Ronen SM, Rushkin E, Degani H. Lipid metabolism in T47D human breast cancer cells: 31P and 13C-NMR studies of choline and ethanolamine uptake. *Biochim Biophys Acta* 1991;**1095**:5–16.

57. Onodera K, Okubo A, Yasumoto K et al. 31P nuclear magnetic resonance analysis of lung cancer: the perchloric acid extract spectrum. *Jpn J Cancer Res* 1986;**77**:1201–6.

58. Yanagawa T, Watanabe H, Inoue T et al. Carbon-11 choline positron emission tomography in musculoskeletal tumors: comparison with fluorine-18 fluorodeoxyglucose positron emission tomography. *J Comput Assist Tomogr* 2003;**27**:175–82.

59. Torizuka T, Kanno T, Futatsubashi M et al. Imaging of gynecologic tumors: comparison of (11)C-choline PET with (18)F-FDG PET. *J Nucl Med* 2003;**44**:1051–6.

60. Kuo YT, Li CW, Chen CY et al. In vivo proton magnetic resonance spectroscopy of large focal hepatic lesions and metabolite change of hepatocellular carcinoma before and after transcatheter arterial chemoembolization using 3.0-T MR scanner. *J Magn Reson Imaging* 2004;**19**:598–604.

61. Alger JR, Frank JA, Bizzi A et al. Metabolism of human gliomas: assessment with H-1 MR spectroscopy and F-18 fluorodeoxyglucose PET. *Radiology* 1990;**177**:633–41.

62. Glunde K, Serkova NJ. Therapeutic targets and biomarkers identified in cancer choline phospholipid metabolism. *Pharmacogenomics* 2006;**7**:1109–23.

63. Hara T, Kosaka N, Shinoura N, Kondo T. PET imaging of brain tumor with [methyl-11C]choline. *J Nucl Med* 1997;**38**:842–7.

64. Hara T, Kosaka N, Kishi H. PET imaging of prostate cancer using carbon-11-choline. *J Nucl Med* 1998;**39**:990–5.

65. DeGrado TR, Coleman RE, Wang S et al. Synthesis and evaluation of 18F-labeled choline as an oncologic tracer for positron emission tomography: initial findings in prostate cancer. *Cancer Res* 2001;**61**:110–117.

66. Hara T, Kosaka N, Kishi H. Development of (18)F-fluoroethylcholine for cancer imaging with PET: synthesis, biochemistry, and prostate cancer imaging. *J Nucl Med* 2002;**43**:187–99.

67. Hara T, Yuasa M. Automated synthesis of [11C]choline, a positron-emitting tracer for tumor imaging. *Appl Radiat Isot* 1999;**50**:531–3.

68. Reischl G, Bieg C, Schmiedl O, Solbach C, Machulla HJ. Highly efficient automated synthesis of [(11)C] choline for multi dose utilization. *Appl Radiat Isot* 2004;**60**:835–8.

69. Kotzerke J, Gschwend JE, Neumaier B. PET for prostate cancer imaging: still a quandary or the ultimate solution? *J Nucl Med* 2002;**43**:200–2.

70. de Jong IJ, Pruim J, Elsinga PH, Vaalburg W, Mensink HJ. 11C-choline positron emission tomography for the evaluation after treatment of localized prostate cancer. *Eur Urol* 2003;**44**:32–8; discussion 38–9.

71. Jager PL, Que TH, Vaalburg W et al. Carbon-11 choline or FDG-PET for staging of oesophageal cancer? *Eur J Nucl Med* 2001;**28**:1845–9.

72. Pieterman RM, Que TH, Elsinga PH et al. Comparison of (11)C-choline and (18)F-FDG PET in primary diagnosis and staging of patients with thoracic cancer. *J Nucl Med* 2002;**43**:167–72.

73. Khan N, Oriuchi N, Ninomiya H et al. Positron emission tomographic imaging with 11C-choline in differential diagnosis of head and neck tumors: comparison with 18F-FDG PET. *Ann Nucl Med* 2004;**18**:409–17.

74. Kobori O, Kirihara Y, Kosaka N, Hara T. Positron emission tomography of esophageal carcinoma using (11)C-choline and (18)F-fluorodeoxyglucose: a novel method of preoperative lymph node staging. *Cancer* 1999;**86**:1638–48.

75. Tuncel M, Souvatzoglou M, Herrmann K et al. [(11)C]Choline positron emission tomography/computed tomography for staging and restaging of patients with advanced prostate cancer. *Nucl Med Biol* 2008;**35**:689–95.

76. Liu D, Hutchinson OC, Osman S et al. Use of radiolabelled choline as a pharmacodynamic marker for the signal transduction inhibitor geldanamycin. *Br J Cancer* 2002;**87**:783–9.

77. Breeuwsma AJ, Pruim J, Jongen MM et al. In vivo uptake of [11C]choline does not correlate with cell proliferation in human prostate cancer. *Eur J Nucl Med Mol Imaging* 2005;**32**:668–73.

78. Ramirez de Molina A, Gallego-Ortega D, Sarmentero-Estrada J et al. Choline kinase as a link connecting phospholipid metabolism and cell cycle regulation: implications in cancer therapy. *Int J Biochem Cell Biol* 2008;**40**:1753–63.

79. Nimmagadda S, Glunde K, Pomper MG, Bhujwalla ZM. Pharmacodynamic markers for choline kinase down-regulation in breast cancer cells. *Neoplasia* 2009;**11**:477–84.

80. Bansal A, Shuyan W, Hara T, Harris RA, Degrado TR. Biodisposition and metabolism of [(18)F]fluorocholine in 9L glioma cells and 9L glioma-bearing fisher rats. *Eur J Nucl Med Mol Imaging* 2008;**35**:1192–203.

81. Iwata R, Pascali C, Bogni A et al. [18F] fluoromethyl triflate, a novel and reactive [18F]fluoromethylating agent: preparation and application to the on-column preparation of [18F] fluorocholine. *Appl Radiat Isot* 2002;**57**:347–52.

82. Kryza D, Tadino V, Filannino MA, Villeret G, Lemoucheux L. Fully automated [18F]fluorocholine synthesis in the TracerLab MX FDG Coincidence synthesizer. *Nucl Med Biol* 2008;**35**:255–60.

83. Pascali G, D'Antonio L, Bovone P, Gerundini P, August T. Optimization of automated large-scale production of [(18)F]fluoroethylcholine for PET prostate cancer imaging. *Nucl Med Biol* 2009;**36**:569–74.

84. Bauman G, Belhocine T, Kovacs M et al. (18)F-fluorocholine for prostate cancer imaging: a systematic review of the literature. *Prostate Cancer Prostatic Dis* Advance online publ. 16 August 2011; doi: 10.1038/pcan.2011.35.

85. Wright SH, Wunz TM, Wunz TP. A choline transporter in renal brush-border membrane vesicles: energetics

and structural specificity. *J Membr Biol* 1992;**126**:51–65.

86. Clary GL, Tsai CF, Guynn RW. Substrate specificity of choline kinase. *Arch Biochem Biophys* 1987;**254**:214–21.

87. Haubner R, Wester HJ, Weber WA *et al.* Noninvasive imaging of alpha(v) beta3 integrin expression using 18F-labeled RGD-containing glycopeptide and positron emission tomography. *Cancer Res* 2001;**61**:1781–5.

88. Haubner R, Wester HJ, Reuning U *et al.* Radiolabeled alpha(v)beta3 integrin antagonists: a new class of tracers for tumor targeting. *J Nucl Med* 1999;**40**:1061–71.

89. Haubner R, Kuhnast B, Mang C *et al.* [18F]Galacto-RGD: synthesis, radiolabeling, metabolic stability, and radiation dose estimates. *Bioconjug Chem* 2004;**15**:61–9.

90. Schnell O, Krebs B, Carlsen J *et al.* Imaging of integrin alpha(v)beta(3) expression in patients with malignant glioma by [18F] Galacto-RGD positron emission tomography. *Neuro Oncol* 2009;**11**:861–70.

91. Beer AJ, Niemeyer M, Carlsen J *et al.* Patterns of alphavbeta3 expression in primary and metastatic human breast cancer as shown by 18F-Galacto-RGD PET. *J Nucl Med* 2008;**49**:255–9.

92. Beer AJ, Grosu AL, Carlsen J *et al.* [18F] galacto-RGD positron emission tomography for imaging of alphavbeta3 expression on the neovasculature in patients with squamous cell carcinoma of the head and neck. *Clin Cancer Res* 2007;**13**(22 Pt 1):6610–16.

93. Beer AJ, Lorenzen S, Metz S *et al.* Comparison of integrin alphaVbeta3 expression and glucose metabolism in primary and metastatic lesions in cancer patients: a PET study using 18F-galacto-RGD and 18F-FDG. *J Nucl Med* 2008;**49**:22–9.

94. Chen X, Park R, Tohme M *et al.* MicroPET and autoradiographic imaging of breast cancer alpha v-integrin expression using 18F- and 64Cu-labeled RGD peptide. *Bioconjug Chem* 2004;**15**:41–9.

95. Vaupel P, Mayer A. Hypoxia in cancer: significance and impact on clinical outcome. *Cancer Metastasis Rev* 2007;**26**:225–39.

96. Krohn KA, Link JM, Mason RP. Molecular imaging of hypoxia. *J Nucl Med* 2008;**49** Suppl **2**:129S–48S.

97. Lim JL, Berridge MS. An efficient radiosynthesis of [18F] fluoromisonidazole. *Appl Radiat Isot* 1993;**44**:1085–91.

98. Lee ST, Scott AM. Hypoxia positron emission tomography imaging with 18f-fluoromisonidazole. *Semin Nucl Med* 2007;**37**:451–61.

99. Gagel B, Reinartz P, Dimartino E *et al.* pO(2) Polarography versus positron emission tomography ([(18)F] fluoromisonidazole, [(18)F]-2-fluoro-2′-deoxyglucose). An appraisal of radiotherapeutically relevant hypoxia. *Strahlenther Onkol* 2004;**180**:616–22.

100. Bentzen L, Keiding S, Nordsmark M *et al.* Tumour oxygenation assessed by 18F-fluoromisonidazole PET and polarographic needle electrodes in human soft tissue tumours. *Radiother Oncol* 2003;**67**:339–44.

101. Valk PE, Mathis CA, Prados MD, Gilbert JC, Budinger TF. Hypoxia in human gliomas: demonstration by PET with fluorine-18-fluoromisonidazole. *J Nucl Med* 1992;**33**:2133–7.

102. Lawrentschuk N, Poon AM, Foo SS *et al.* Assessing regional hypoxia in human renal tumours using 18F-fluoromisonidazole positron emission tomography. *BJU Int* 2005;**96**:540–6.

103. Gagel B, Reinartz P, Demirel C *et al.* [18F] fluoromisonidazole and [18F] fluorodeoxyglucose positron emission tomography in response evaluation after chemo-/radiotherapy of non-small-cell lung cancer: a feasibility study. *BMC Cancer* 2006;**6**:51.

104. Hicks RJ, Rischin D, Fisher R *et al.* Utility of FMISO PET in advanced head and neck cancer treated with chemoradiation incorporating a hypoxia-targeting chemotherapy agent. *Eur J Nucl Med Mol Imaging* 2005;**32**:1384–91.

105. Grosu AL, Souvatzoglou M, Roper B *et al.* Hypoxia imaging with FAZA-PET and theoretical considerations with regard to dose painting for individualization of radiotherapy in patients with head and neck cancer. *Int J Radiat Oncol Biol Phys* 2007;**69**:541–51.

106. Lehtio K, Oikonen V, Nyman S *et al.* Quantifying tumour hypoxia with fluorine-18 fluoroerythronitroimidazole ([18F]FETNIM) and PET using the tumour to plasma ratio. *Eur J Nucl Med Mol Imaging* 2003;**30**:101–8.

107. Rasey JS, Hofstrand PD, Chin LK, Tewson TJ. Characterization of [18F]fluoroetanidazole, a new radiopharmaceutical for detecting tumor hypoxia. *J Nucl Med* 1999;**40**:1072–9.

108. Ziemer LS, Evans SM, Kachur AV *et al.* Noninvasive imaging of tumor hypoxia in rats using the 2-nitroimidazole 18F-EF5. *Eur J Nucl Med Mol Imaging* 2003;**30**:259–66.

109. Fujibayashi Y, Taniuchi H, Yonekura Y *et al.* Copper-62-ATSM: a new hypoxia imaging agent with high membrane permeability and low redox potential. *J Nucl Med* 1997;**38**:1155–60.

110. Dehdashti F, Grigsby PW, Mintun MA *et al.* Assessing tumor hypoxia in cervical cancer by positron emission tomography with 60Cu-ATSM: relationship to therapeutic response – a preliminary report. *Int J Radiat Oncol Biol Phys* 2003;**55**:1233–8.

111. Blau M, Nagler W, Bender MA. Fluorine-18: a new isotope for bone scanning. *J Nucl Med* 1962;**3**:332–4.

112. Petren-Mallmin M, Andreasson I, Ljunggren O *et al.* Skeletal metastases from breast cancer: uptake of 18F-fluoride measured with positron emission tomography in correlation with CT. *Skeletal Radiol* 1998;**27**:72–6.

113. Langsteger W, Heinisch M, Fogelman I. The role of fluorodeoxyglucose, 18F-dihydroxyphenylalanine, 18F-choline, and 18F-fluoride in bone imaging with emphasis on prostate and breast. *Semin Nucl Med* 2006;**36**:73–92.

114. Even-Sapir E, Metser U, Flusser G *et al.* Assessment of malignant skeletal disease: initial experience with 18F-fluoride PET/CT and comparison between 18F-fluoride PET and 18F-fluoride PET/CT. *J Nucl Med* 2004;**45**:272–8.

115. Iagaru A, Mittra E, Yaghoubi SS *et al.* Novel strategy for a cocktail 18F-fluoride and 18F-FDG PET/CT scan for evaluation of malignancy: results of the pilot-phase study. *J Nucl Med* 2009;**50**:501–5.

116. Lippman M, Bolan G, Huff K. The effects of estrogens and antiestrogens on hormone-responsive human breast cancer in long-term tissue culture. *Cancer Res* 1976;**36**:4595–601.

117. Locker GY. Hormonal therapy of breast cancer. *Cancer Treat Rev* 1998;**24**:221–40.

118. Donegan WL. Prognostic factors. Stage and receptor status in breast cancer. *Cancer* 1992;**70**(6 Suppl):1755–64.

119. Kumar R. Targeted functional imaging in breast cancer. *Eur J Nucl Med Mol Imaging* 2007;**34**:346–53.

120. Jonson SD, Welch MJ. PET imaging of breast cancer with fluorine-18 radiolabeled estrogens and progestins. *Q J Nucl Med* 1998;**42**:8–17.

121. Jonson SD, Bonasera TA, Dehdashti F *et al.* Comparative breast tumor imaging and comparative in vitro metabolism of 16alpha-[18F]fluoroestradiol-17beta and 16beta-[18F]fluoromoxestrol in isolated hepatocytes. *Nucl Med Biol* 1999;**26**:123–30.

122. Kiesewetter DO, Kilbourn MR, Landvatter SW *et al.* Preparation of four fluorine-18-labeled estrogens and their selective uptakes in target tissues of immature rats. *J Nucl Med* 1984;**25**:1212–21.

123. Lim JL, Berridge MS, Tewson TJ. Preparation of [18F]16a-fluoro-17b-estradiol by selective nucleophilic substitution. *10th International Symposium on Radiopharmaceutical Chemistry, Kyoto, Japan, October 1993,* 1993.

124. Römer J, Füchtner F, Steinbach J, Johannsen B. Automated production of 16alpha-[18F]fluoroestradiol for breast cancer imaging. *Nucl Med Biol* 1999;**26**:473–9.

125. Oh SJ, Chi DY, Mosdzianowski C *et al.* The automatic production of 16alpha-[18F]fluoroestradiol using a conventional [18F]FDG module with a disposable cassette system. *Appl Radiat Isot* 2007;**65**:676–81.

126. Mintun MA, Welch MJ, Siegel BA *et al.* Breast cancer: PET imaging of estrogen receptors. *Radiology* 1988;**169**:45–8.

127. Dehdashti F, Mortimer JE, Siegel BA *et al.* Positron tomographic assessment of estrogen receptors in breast cancer: comparison with FDG-PET and in vitro receptor assays. *J Nucl Med* 1995;**36**:1766–74.

128. Mortimer JE, Dehdashti F, Siegel BA *et al.* Positron emission tomography with 2-[18F]Fluoro-2-deoxy-D-glucose and 16alpha-[18F]fluoro-17beta-estradiol in breast cancer: correlation with estrogen receptor status and response to systemic therapy. *Clin Cancer Res* 1996;**2**:933–9.

129. Mortimer JE, Dehdashti F, Siegel BA *et al.* Metabolic flare: indicator of hormone responsiveness in advanced breast cancer. *J Clin Oncol* 2001;**19**:2797–803.

130. Linden HM, Stekhova SA, Link JM *et al.* Quantitative fluoroestradiol positron emission tomography imaging predicts response to endocrine treatment in breast cancer. *J Clin Oncol* 2006;**24**:2793–9.

131. Tsujikawa T, Yoshida Y, Kudo T *et al.* Functional images reflect aggressiveness of endometrial carcinoma: estrogen receptor expression combined with 18F-FDG PET. *J Nucl Med* 2009;**50**:1598–604.

132. Seimbille Y, Rousseau J, Bénard F *et al.* 18F-labeled difluoroestradiols: preparation and preclinical evaluation as estrogen receptor-binding radiopharmaceuticals. *Steroids* 2002;**67**:765–75.

133. Seo JW, Comninos JS, Chi DY *et al.* Fluorine-substituted cyclofenil derivatives as estrogen receptor ligands: synthesis and structure-affinity relationship study of potential positron emission tomography agents for imaging estrogen receptors in breast cancer. *J Med Chem* 2006;**49**:2496–511.

134. Bonasera TA, O'Neil JP, Xu M *et al.* Preclinical evaluation of fluorine-18-labeled androgen receptor ligands in baboons. *J Nucl Med* 1996;**37**:1009–15.

135. Barrack ER, Tindall DJ. A critical evaluation of the use of androgen receptor assays to predict the androgen responsiveness of prostatic cancer. *Prog Clin Biol Res* 1987;**239**:155–87.

136. Liu A, Dence CS, Welch MJ, Katzenellenbogen JA. Fluorine-18-labeled androgens: radiochemical synthesis and tissue distribution studies on six fluorine-substituted androgens, potential imaging agents for prostatic cancer. *J Nucl Med* 1992;**33**:724–34.

137. Larson SM, Morris M, Gunther I *et al.* Tumor localization of 16beta-18F-fluoro-5alpha-dihydrotestosterone versus 18F-FDG in patients with progressive, metastatic prostate cancer. *J Nucl Med* 2004;**45**:366–73.

138. Dehdashti F, Picus J, Michalski JM *et al.* Positron tomographic assessment of androgen receptors in prostatic carcinoma. *Eur J Nucl Med Mol Imaging* 2005;**32**:344–50.

139. Garg S, Doke A, Black KW, Garg PK. In vivo biodistribution of an androgen receptor avid PET imaging agent 7-alpha-fluoro-17 alpha-methyl-5-alpha-dihydrotestosterone ([(18)F]FMDHT) in rats pretreated with cetrorelix, a GnRH antagonist. *Eur J Nucl Med Mol Imaging* 2008;**35**:379–85.

140. Parent EE, Dence CS, Sharp TL, Welch MJ, Katzenellenbogen JA. Synthesis and biological evaluation of a fluorine-18-labeled nonsteroidal androgen receptor antagonist, N-(3-[18F]fluoro-4-nitronaphthyl)-cis-5-norbornene-endo-2,3-dicarboxylic imide. *Nucl Med Biol* 2006;**33**:615–24.

141. Parent EE, Jenks C, Sharp T, Welch MJ, Katzenellenbogen JA. Synthesis and biological evaluation of a nonsteroidal bromine-76-labeled androgen receptor ligand 3-[76Br]bromo-hydroxyflutamide. *Nucl Med Biol* 2006;**33**:705–13.

142. Bakker WH, Krenning EP, Breeman WA *et al.* Receptor scintigraphy with a radioiodinated somatostatin analogue: radiolabeling, purification, biologic activity, and in vivo application in animals. *J Nucl Med* 1990;**31**:1501–9.

143. Lamberts SW, Bakker WH, Reubi JC, Krenning EP. Somatostatin-receptor imaging in the localization of endocrine tumors. *N Engl J Med* 1990;**323**:1246–9.

144. Bakker WH, Albert R, Bruns C *et al.* [111In-DTPA-D-Phe1]-octreotide, a potential radiopharmaceutical for imaging of somatostatin receptor-positive tumors: synthesis, radiolabeling and in vitro validation. *Life Sci* 1991;**49**:1583–91.

145. Schmidt M, Fischer E, Dietlein M. Clinical value of somatostatin receptor imaging in patients with suspected head and neck paragangliomas. *Eur J Nucl Med Mol Imaging* 2002;**29**:1571–80.

146. Wild D, Macke HR, Waser B *et al.* 68Ga-DOTANOC: a first compound for PET imaging with high affinity for somatostatin receptor subtypes 2 and 5. *Eur J Nucl Med Mol Imaging* 2005;**32**:724.

147. Henze M, Schuhmacher J, Hipp P *et al.* PET imaging of somatostatin receptors using [68GA]DOTA-D-Phe1-Tyr3-octreotide: first results in patients with meningiomas. *J Nucl Med* 2001;**42**:1053–6.

148. Eisenwiener KP, Prata MI, Buschmann I et al. NODAGATOC, a new chelator-coupled somatostatin analogue labeled with [67/68Ga] and [111In] for SPECT, PET, and targeted therapeutic applications of somatostatin receptor (hsst2) expressing tumors. Bioconjug Chem 2002;13:530–541.

149. Junik R, Drobik P, Malkowski B, Kobus-Blachnio K. The role of positron emission tomography (PET) in diagnostics of gastroenteropancreatic neuroendocrine tumours (GEP NET). Adv Med Sci 2006;51:66–8.

150. Ambrosini V, Castellucci P, Rubello D et al. 68Ga-DOTA-NOC: a new PET tracer for evaluating patients with bronchial carcinoid. Nucl Med Commun 2009;30:281–6.

151. Freesmeyer M, Schulz S, Knosel T, Settmacher U. Imaging of somatostatin receptor subtype 2 in advanced hepatocellular carcinoma by 68Ga-DOTATOC PET. Nuklearmedizin 2009;48:N17–18.

152. Wieder H, Beer AJ, Poethko T et al. PET/CT with Gluc-Lys-([(18)F]FP)-TOCA: correlation between uptake, size and arterial perfusion in somatostatin receptor positive lesions. Eur J Nucl Med Mol Imaging 2008;35:264–71.

153. Yoshii Y, Furukawa T, Yoshii H et al. Cytosolic acetyl-CoA synthetase affected tumor cell survival under hypoxia: the possible function in tumor acetyl-CoA/acetate metabolism. Cancer Sci 2009;100:821–7.

154. Swinnen JV, Roskams T, Joniau S et al. Overexpression of fatty acid synthase is an early and common event in the development of prostate cancer. Int J Cancer 2002;98:19–22.

155. Knowles LM, Yang C, Osterman A, Smith JW. Inhibition of fatty-acid synthase induces caspase-8-mediated tumor cell apoptosis by up-regulating DDIT4. J Biol Chem 2008;283:31378–84.

156. Pizer ES, Chrest FJ, DiGiuseppe JA, Han WF. Pharmacological inhibitors of mammalian fatty acid synthase suppress DNA replication and induce apoptosis in tumor cell lines. Cancer Res 1998;58:4611–15.

157. Shreve P, Chiao PC, Humes HD, Schwaiger M, Gross MD. Carbon-11-acetate PET imaging in renal disease. J Nucl Med 1995;36:1595–601.

158. Buchanan, JM, Hastings AB, Nesbett FB. The role of carboxyl-labeled acetic, propionic, and butyric acids in liver glycogen formation. J Biol Chem 1943;150:413–25.

159. Pike VW, Horlock PL, Brown C, Clark JC. The remotely-controlled preparation of a 11C-labelled radiopharmaceutical-[1–11C]acetate. Int J Appl Radiat Isot 1984;35:623–7.

160. Iwata R, Ido T, Tada M. Column extraction method for rapid preparation of [11C]acetic and [11C]palmitic acids. Appl Rad Isot 1995;46:117–21.

161. Oyama N, Akino H, Kanamaru H et al. 11C-acetate PET imaging of prostate cancer. J Nucl Med 2002;43:181–6.

162. Delbeke D, Pinson CW. 11C-acetate: a new tracer for the evaluation of hepatocellular carcinoma. J Nucl Med 2003;44:222–3.

163. Spence AM, Mankoff DA, Muzi M. Positron emission tomography imaging of brain tumors. Neuroimaging Clin N Am 2003;13:717–39.

164. Higashi K, Ueda Y, Matsunari I et al. 11C-acetate PET imaging of lung cancer: comparison with 18F-FDG PET and 99mTc-MIBI SPET. Eur J Nucl Med Mol Imaging 2004;31:13–21.

165. Sun A, Sörensen J, Karlsson M et al. 1-[11C]-acetate PET imaging in head and neck cancer – a comparison with 18F-FDG-PET: implications for staging and radiotherapy planning. Eur J Nucl Med Mol Imaging 2007;34:651–7.

166. Sakurai H, Kaji M, Suemasu K. Thymoma of the middle mediastinum: 11C-acetate positron emission tomography imaging. Ann Thorac Surg 2009;87:1271–4.

167. Kotzerke J, Volkmer BG, Neumaier B et al. Carbon-11 acetate positron emission tomography can detect local recurrence of prostate cancer Eur J Nucl Med Mol Imaging 2002;29:1380–4.

168. Seppälä J, Seppänen M, Arponen E, Lindholm P, Minn H. Carbon-11 acetate PET/CT based dose escalated IMRT in prostate cancer. Radiother Oncol 2009;93:234–40.

169. Ponde DE, Dence CS, Oyama N et al. 18F-fluoroacetate: a potential acetate analog for prostate tumor imaging – in vivo evaluation of 18F-fluoroacetate versus 11C-acetate. J Nucl Med 2007;48:420–8.

**Chapter**

# 3

# PET/CT information systems

Jon M. Hainer

While radiology was founded when X-rays spoiled a piece of photographic film, modern medical imaging has evolved to become primarily electronic. Computers, electromagnetic storage systems, and information networks are rapidly replacing photographic film as the means of viewing, storing, and distributing radiologic images. As with any media, however, these electronic systems have idiosyncrasies that can lead to misinterpretation and error. It is therefore vital for radiologists to understand the foundations of the electronic media, so as to be able to recognize these pitfalls and, to the extent possible, adjust for them.

Using some interesting images as starting points, we will discuss how modern systems store and display two-dimensional (2-D) and three-dimensional (3-D) images, as well as describe the additional text data necessary to provide the proper context for the imaging.

## Two-dimensional radiologic imaging

In Figure 3.1, we have four identical images. Well, at least the images are identical in terms of how they are stored on a computer. On the screen, they are clearly very different. While the basic structures of the images generally appear similar, color and intensity have been varied to emphasize different aspects of the images. Given that the images were created from identical datasets, what could account for these differences? To understand this better, let us delve into how radiology images are stored and displayed using computer systems. We will start by examining the foundations of 2-D radiologic images, and explore how they relate to the pictures that actually appear on a computer monitor.

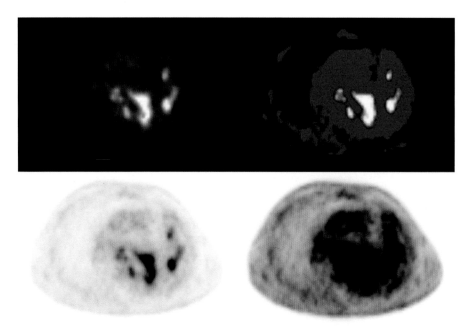

**Figure 3.1** Four equivalent FDG-PET images.

**Figure 3.2** Overview of binary numbers.

In a base 10 (decimal) counting system, the following 10 digits are used:

0, 1, 2, 3, 4, 5, 6, 7, 8, 9

When creating multi-digit numbers, each digit in the decimal number represents that digit multiplied by a power of 10:

| 4305 (decimal) | = | $(4 \times 10^3) + (3 \times 10^2) + (0 \times 10^1) + (5 \times 10^0)$ |
|---|---|---|
| | = | 4000 + 300 + 0 + 5 |
| | = | 4305 (decimal) |

In a base 2 (binary) counting system, the following 2 digits are used:

0, 1

When creating multi-digit numbers, each digit in the binary number represents that digit multiplied by a power of 2:

| 11001 (binary) | = | $(1 \times 2^4) + (1 \times 2^3) + (0 \times 2^2) + (0 \times 2^1) + (1 \times 2^0)$ |
|---|---|---|
| | = | 16 + 8 + 0 + 0 + 1 |
| | = | 25 (decimal) |

# Foundations of computerized imaging

Before we get too deep into the radiology aspect of this discussion, however, it's good to have a very basic understanding of how computers store any type of data. Computer systems use electric circuits, magnetic disks, optical disks, and other media to store and process information. What these media have in common is that they are all composed of millions of distinct data-storing units, called **bits**, and each of these bits can only exist in one of two states. If we use an electric circuit to store a bit, for example, the circuit can either have electricity coursing through it or it can be devoid of electricity. Bits on an optical disc, like a CD-ROM, can either reflect light or scatter light being projected from a laser. When computer programmers deal with these two discrete states, they represent the bits using the numbers 1 and 0. For example, 1 means that this circuit carries an electric charge, while 0 means that it does not. Since we have now given these bits a numeric value, by stringing several of them together in series, we can count. We are not counting in our normal base-10 system of 1,2,3,4 …, however. We are counting in a base-2 numeric system called the binary system. In binary, all numbers are represented by 1s and 0s, as shown Figure 3.2. Computers store everything as binary numbers.

That being said, images by nature are not numbers. How would someone go about converting an image into a series of numbers that can be stored on a computer? Let us start with an image, like the one in Figure 3.3. If we take this picture of blossoms and put a piece of graph paper with very small boxes over it, then we've created a grid, or matrix, of smaller pictures. Each box in this matrix is called a **pixel**. For each of these pixels, we will identify the predominant color and replace the entire area of the pixel with that color. Perhaps a given pixel in the image of the flower is more purple than anything else. We then break that purple color down into its three basic **component colors** – red, green, and blue – and give each of these component colors a value from 0 to 255 based on that color's intensity (255 is the highest value that can be stored by 8 bits. It is the number 11111111 in binary.) Figure 3.3 shows this process for one specific pixel.

We then apply this numeric conversion to every pixel in the original image matrix, starting at the left and going to the right, then restarting at the left on the next line of the image, and so on, to create a series of numbers representing the color of each pixel in the matrix grid. If you feed this series of color intensities to a computer monitor with the dimensions of the matrix, it will perform the operation in reverse and display a rather decent facsimile of the original image. We have thus changed a picture into numbers, which can be stored on a computer and displayed on a computer monitor.

Before we continue with radiology images, let us discuss a couple more things about photographic imaging. The first thing to note is that if you make the pixels in your matrix physically smaller and use a lot more of them, then the image will look smoother and less "blocky." The number of the pixels in the image is sometimes called the "image resolution" (although the reader should be aware that this usage of the term is somewhat different than that discussed in Chapter 1, in which the number of pixels determined the image **sampling**, whereas **resolution** was determined primarily by the underlying image-acquisition hardware). On the other hand, for computer programmers and image processors, image resolution or sampling is conventionally denoted by the number of pixels from left to right in a given image, followed by a multiplication sign, and then followed by the number of rows

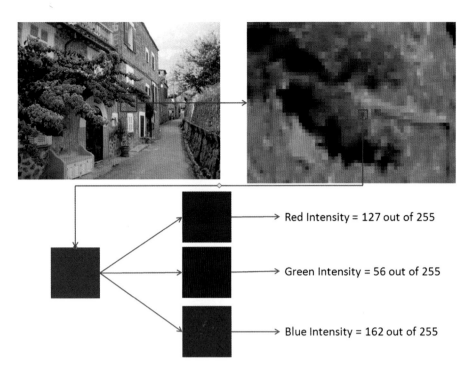

**Figure 3.3** Pixelizing a photograph and decomposing one pixel into its component colors.

Red Intensity = 127 out of 255

Green Intensity = 56 out of 255

Blue Intensity = 162 out of 255

The Numeric Value of the Selected Pixel is 127, 56, 162.

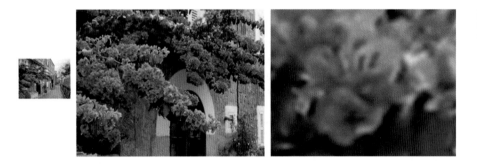

**Figure 3.4** Shrunken images lose detail; images close to their original resolution look sharpest, while enlarged images appear blurry.

of pixels from the top to the bottom of the image. When you hear that your computer monitor has a resolution of 1,280 × 1,024, this is an indication that you have 1,280 pixels going across the screen from left to right, and 1,024 pixels going down the screen from top to bottom, which provides a matrix with a total of 1,310,720 pixels over the entire screen. While an image may be stored at one resolution, a direct pixel-to-pixel translation to the monitor may not be appropriate, as it may make the image too large or too small to be useful. The computer will frequently use some complex calculations to expand images to larger resolutions or compress them to smaller resolutions, depending on how large you want them to appear on the screen. In this way, radiologic imaging software generally allows users to modify image sizes as necessary. It is important to note that as you enlarge a picture to a higher resolution, it can become grainier and more blocky in appearance, as seen in the inset of Figure 3.3. When images are enlarged using automated procedures on our radiology workstations, however, these programs often utilize a smoothing

procedure (called "interpolation") to reduce this blocky appearance; in this case, the image just appears blurrier. By contrast, as you shrink an image, it may look sharper, but details can blend together. Examples of expanding and compressing image resolutions can be seen in Figure 3.4.

## Two-dimensional imaging

Now that we have a basic understanding of how photographic images are stored and displayed on a computer, let us compare this process to radiologic imaging. A radiologic image is very similar to a visual image in that it is a matrix of numbers that is interpreted by a computer to display a visual image on the screen. Is it really the case that the numeric values in the pixels of radiologic images represent colors? What color is an X-ray or gamma ray? How would a photon know the color of an organ inside the body? Of course, radiology pictures are not photographs, and they have no intrinsic color information. Instead, each pixel in a radiologic image is a numerical

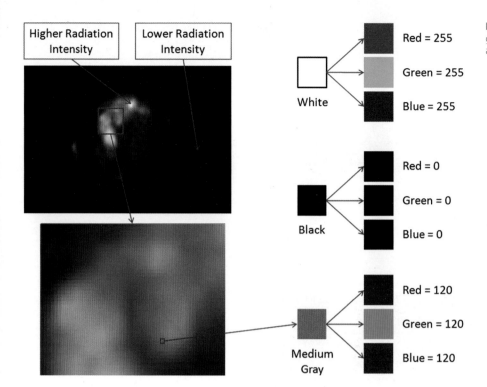

**Figure 3.5** Component color intensities in grayscale are equal, and values of 0 always display as black.

representation of the number of X-ray or gamma photons that has either passed through or originated from the point in the body represented by the pixel. In general, the pixel value is between 0 and 65,535 (a 16-bit number), and, for nuclear medicine images, is measured in Becquerel/milliliter (Bq/mL).

While radiologic images consist of a matrix of pixels that represent intensity of radiation, rather than color, they clearly must be displayed using some sort of color on a color monitor. How is that color determined? One simple way is to set the intensity of all three of the component colors to the relative intensity of the pixel. When the red, green, and blue intensities on the screen are all the same, this combination will yield varying shades of gray. When red, green, and blue all have values of 0, for instance, the color black will be displayed on a monitor. If we set red, green, and blue all to 255 (the highest intensity value on many color monitors), the pixel will be white. If red, green, and blue all have values of 128, we'll see medium gray. In other words, using this approach of equal mixtures of red, green, and blue, the image will always be displayed in "grayscale," with darker pixels indicating areas of low radiation intensity or radiotracer uptake, and lighter pixels indicating areas of high radiation intensity or uptake, as shown in Figure 3.5.

## Color look-up tables

While this is a very simple way to display the images, it is certainly not the only way. In reality, all that we have done here is simply to assign grayscale pixel color values to the radiation intensities. There is no reason, however, that we couldn't

assign any pixel color values to the intensity of uptake. If we want the highest intensities to be red, we can just assign to the higher-intensity pixels the component color values for shades of red. If we want lower intensities to be blue, we can assign to the lower-intensity pixels screen-color numeric values that will be displayed as blue. Doing this, we may end up with a colorful image on the screen that highlights areas of higher uptake and diminishes areas of lower intensity. The color-mapping scheme that is used to assign colors to radiation intensities is called a **look-up table** (or **LUT**) (1). Color look-up tables are frequently used to view PET images, especially when those images are fused to CT. CT images, however, are traditionally viewed with the standard grayscale. Figure 3.6 displays the same PET image using several different color look-up tables. Remember, the radiation intensities of the individual pixels do not change – only the colors with which those intensities are displayed change.

While it is aesthetically pleasing to see images in color, this property, alone, does not seem like a good enough reason to view radiologic images in color. What is the real purpose of color look-up tables? To answer that, note the difference in the way that the lesion appears in the four different images in Figure 3.6. The contrast of the grayscale images is not nearly as sharp as the contrast of the color images. The reds and whites of the color images seem to "jump out" in comparison with their grayscale counterparts. This can be useful for quickly identifying areas of disease, especially those that are small. That same high contrast that initially captures a viewer's eye, however, may also tend to make that viewer assign too much importance to the area. As a radiologist uses color look-up

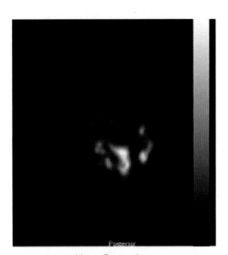

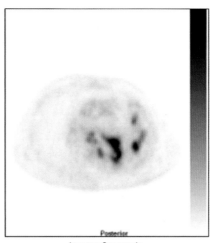

**Figure 3.6** Four common look-up tables (LUT).

Linear Grayscale
Intensity Colors (Low to High):
Black, Dark Gray, Medium Gray, Light Gray, White

Inverse Grayscale
Intensity Colors (Low to High):
White, Light Gray, Medium Gray, Dark Gray, Black

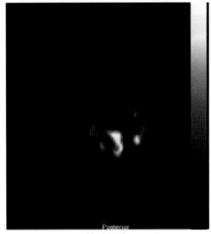

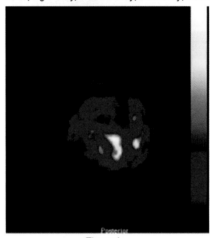

Hot Metal
Intensity Colors (Low to High):
Black, Red, Orange, Yellow, White

Thermal
Intensity Colors (Low to High):
Black, Blue, Red, Yellow, White

tables, it is of vital importance to understand the idiosyncrasies of the tables that are being used. Clearly, certain look-up tables are better for identifying subtle findings, while others are better for accurately assessing relative radiotracer uptake in different regions of an image.

## Image contrast (window-leveling)

Now that we understand that radiology images are a matrix of radiologic intensities that are converted to color to be displayed on a computer monitor, let us pause for a minute and consider our original images in Figure 3.1. Could color conversion and look-up tables be responsible for the radically different patterns that we see? Clearly, it has something to do with it. The top-left image is a standard grayscale image, while the top-right image uses a color look-up table with a variety of colors to display the image. The two bottom images, however, both use an inverse grayscale look-up table, but for some reason still look very different.

In addition to assigning a look-up table to be used for displaying radiologic images, a radiologist may also manually adjust the contrast of those images. This process of adjusting the contrast of a radiologic image is frequently called **window-leveling**. How does window-leveling work? Consider an image containing a range of pixel intensity values between 0 and 65,535, where the majority of the pixels of interest fall between the values of 5,000 and 10,000. That is a relatively tight range out of the entire available range from 0 to 65,535, so if we use a grayscale look-up table with values of 0 being black and values of 65,535 being white, then all of these pixels are going to be similar shades of gray. This does not provide very much contrast, and we may not be able to differentiate the structures in the image using this scale. However, the look-up table can be scaled. In most viewing programs, the grayscale can be changed so that instead of 0 being the lower bound of the scale, it becomes whatever we want it to be, for example 5,000. Any pixels with a value of 5,000 or below will now be black.

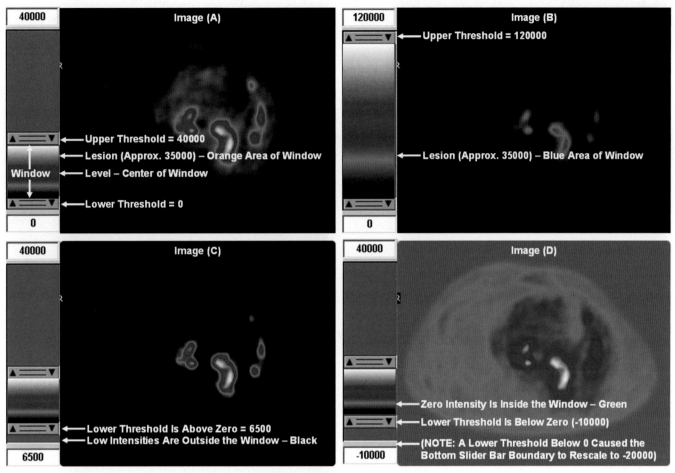

**Image (A) – A PET image with an appropriate window / level.**
**Image (B) – Increasing the window size causes high intensity areas to fall lower on the color scale.**
**Image (C) – Moving the lower threshold above 0 causes low intensity areas to display as black.**
**Image (D) – Moving the lower threshold below 0 causes zero intensity pixels to map to the green area of the color scale.**

**Figure 3.7** Adjusting contrast with window-leveling.

Similarly we may change the upper bound of the scale from 65,535 to 10,000. Now, every pixel with a value of 10,000 or greater will be white. Every pixel in-between those values will be assigned a new color value. Those closest to 5,000 will now be nearly black, while those near 10,000 will be nearly white. By re-applying the look-up table over a smaller **window** at a certain **level** of the intensity spectrum, we have modified our image on the screen to have appropriate contrast. Note that this works for color look-up tables, just as well as it does for grayscale tables. Everything at or below the lower bound of the window becomes the lower-bound color, while everything at or above the upper bound becomes the upper-bound color. Everything in-between is readjusted to fit the new contrast window accordingly.

It is also important to note that the upper and lower bounds of the window frequently expand beyond the range of the actual pixel intensities of the image. For example, suppose that the lowest pixel intensity is 5,000. Setting the lower bound of the window of a grayscale look-up table to 5,000 will make that pixel black – invisible against the background. If we

set that lower bound to 1,000, however, the pixel will likely appear dark gray and thus become visible against the background of 0-value pixels.

Figure 3.7 displays four PET images. These images are all displayed using a color look-up table where the colors progress through black, green, blue, purple, red, orange, yellow, and finally white, as the intensity of the pixels increases. In Image (A), the upper and lower bounds of the contrast window are set appropriately with an upper bound of 40,000 and a lower bound of 0, showing a properly window-leveled PET image. The intensities of the lesions fall on the orange range of the look-up table's color spectrum. In Image (B), the upper threshold has been increased from 40,000 to 120,000. Expanding the window in this way has stretched the color spectrum so that the lesion intensity is now in the bluish-green range. In Image (C), the upper bound has been brought back down to 40,000, but the lower bound has been raised from 0 to 6,500. Here we see that the lower-intensity pixels inside the patient's body now have values below the lower bound of the look-up table and thus display as black, the color at the bottom of the look-up table. Finally, in Image (D), we have changed the lower bound to −10,000. Stretching the window below the zero-intensity level has put the zero intensity into the green area of the color spectrum. All of the zero-intensity pixels in the background outside of the patient's body now appear as the zero-intensity shade of green.

While an extremely wide display window may cover the entire spectrum of intensities (e.g., from 0 to 65,535), such a window is rarely useful. Many PET viewing programs will attempt to generate appropriate window-leveling settings automatically. Through a process called normalization (2), these programs will examine the values of all of the pixel data and attempt to estimate the initial upper and lower bounds for the PET display. If this estimation is calculated incorrectly, the user may have to manually adjust the window and/or level to yield the appropriate image brightness and contrast. Similarly, CT viewing programs often have pre-set intensity windows designed for specific organs or areas of the body. If these settings are inadequate for a given image or are assigned incorrectly, they may also be changed by hand for better viewing.

Through our discussion of window-leveling for contrast control, we have just solved the second part of our initial imaging mystery. A combination of color look-up tables and changes in contrast via window-leveling account for the drastic differences in the appearance of identical radiologic images. So, now that we understand the basics of how a radiologic image appears on the screen, let us ask a more basic question:

If you just walked up to a computer monitor and saw this picture on the screen, how would you know whose image is being displayed?

## Radiology information systems and data processing

Note the PET image in Figure 3.8. What do we notice about this image that was missing in our discussion in the previous section? Clearly, this image is presented with some very important text information describing the patient, the study being performed, the date of the study, and other descriptors. Simple things like knowing the name of the patient in question is so second nature that we rarely stop to wonder how this information consistently appears on the screen. These data are vitally important, however, to ensure the integrity of the diagnostic process in radiology. They cannot at any point be separated from the actual images. Having a picture with no name is equally as useless as having a name with no picture.

All radiologic images are stored along with data relevant to patient demographics, as well as with study information and additional information specific to how a given image relates to other images in the same study. Furthermore, vital data that describe how an image must be displayed, e.g., its resolution, must be stored with the pixel data, as well. Before we can continue on to discuss three-dimensional and multi-modality imaging, we must briefly discuss the systems that will be

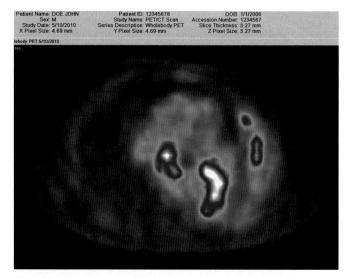

**Figure 3.8** A radiologic image presented with patient demographic information.

displaying these images and how these systems store and retrieve the essential, associated text and numeric data.

## Stand-alone workstations versus PACS

Unlike photographic images, radiologic images are rarely viewed with simple software like an unenhanced web browser. Generally, they are displayed on high-end computer systems with impressive graphical capabilities. Many of these computer systems are self-contained, meaning that the program for viewing the images, the image pixel data, and the text data related to the image, are all stored on a single **stand-alone workstation**. A radiologic scanner (e.g., a CT or PET scanner) is a prime example of a stand-alone system. Once the image-collection process of the scanner has been completed, all patient data – the patient name, study data, pixel data, etc. – are stored locally on a computer system sitting in the scanner's control room. At this point, it cannot be viewed anywhere else in the hospital. This image acquisition workstation then transmits all of the image and associated data, usually over a computer network, to a different computer where a radiologist can look at it. Sometimes the radiologist's viewing workstation is stand-alone, as well, but more frequently, the data are sent to a much more complex, multi-computer system called a **PACS**.

PACS is the acronym for **Picture Archiving and Communications System** (3). A PACS system stores all imaging and related text data in large data repositories called **PACS servers** that are accessible over a computer network to many different imaging workstations called **PACS clients** or **PACS workstations**. PACS servers are rarely in the same room as their clients. Usually, these servers reside in rooms specifically designed to be computer warehouses; rows and rows of computers lined up for easy access and maintenance by PACS administrators. PACS servers are designed to receive new data from imaging equipment over the network, store the data in a very organized manner, archive them for many years and quickly retrieve the data via the network to PACS clients that request it.

PACS clients, on the other hand, are the systems that radiologists usually use for viewing radiologic images. They are usually located in offices and reading rooms convenient to the doctors that will be using them. They are used to query the PACS server for a list of all radiology studies that a patient may have had at a given institution, to view any of the images from those studies, and frequently to create and retrieve text reports from previously acquired imaging procedures.

Stand-alone and PACS systems have one thing in common, which is that image data and text data are both stored in a highly organized way in a database.

## Storage of radiologic data – databases

As with most information, the most efficient way to store and retrieve radiologic data on a computer system is with a program specifically designed for that purpose, called a **database program**. A database program is simply specialized software that has been designed to store a wide variety of information in a very organized manner. This highly structured organization allows huge stores of data to be searched very quickly for specific subsets. In addition, the use of highly structured data ensures that the information stored in the database meets certain minimal levels of quality control for completeness and accuracy. For example, a radiology system database program may require a technologist to enter a patient's family name to be associated with that person's images. This ensures that we can always identify the patient to whom the images belong. The database may also require that a date of birth is actually a real date, rather than a bunch of random characters. These data rules help to guarantee the integrity of the data in the database, although they clearly do not prevent all errors.

Stand-alone workstations and PACS servers always use some type of database to store and retrieve the data associated with their images. Frequently, the actual pixel values of the images are stored in the database as well. That being said, there are many different companies that make database tools, and once the vendor has the tools, the variety of data structures that they can create with those tools is infinite. This complexity creates a huge problem. Given the incredibly diverse possibilities of creating radiologic data structures and the lack of compatibility between many of the database toolsets, how can we be certain that each vendor is collecting adequate information for their image sets, and how can we ensure that images created on one vendor's cameras may be transferred and moved to another vendor's viewing station?

## Transferring imaging and data between systems – DICOM

To solve the problems associated with moving images between disparate radiology systems, the medical community has developed a single, standard protocol for temporarily storing and transferring radiologic images. This protocol is called **Digital Imaging and Communications in Medicine**, and is generally referred to as **DICOM** (4). When transferring information between DICOM-compliant systems, vendors extract all of the important demographic, study, and image data from their proprietary databases and store those data in so-called "flat files," which are similar to a word-processing or spreadsheet file. These DICOM files may be moved in some way, usually over the network or via CD-ROM, to another vendor's imaging system. Since the DICOM files are strongly formatted, and more importantly, always formatted in a very similar way, the receiving vendor's database may very quickly identify the data and import them to the corresponding storage locations within its own database structure. Without a standard such as DICOM, large PACS systems that accept images from multiple vendors could not exist.

Beyond simply allowing interoperability between systems, DICOM has had a very important side-effect that has greatly simplified the discussion of how text and image data are stored on a system. Since vendors are now required, for all intents and purposes, to provide DICOM interoperability, they have begun designing their system databases with that in mind. As a result, the DICOM data structure is virtually mirrored in the database design of most modern radiology systems. If we understand how images are stored in the DICOM format, we will have a pretty good understanding of the way that those images are stored in the databases underlying most imaging software. In addition, since radiology software user interfaces frequently mirror the data structures in the database, understanding the DICOM format goes a long way towards helping us use different vendors' software, as well.

## DICOM basics – data modules contain patient, study, series, and instance data

The first thing to understand about DICOM is that all information that is pertinent to any specific image is stored in every single flat file. While multiple files may be combined to create a 3-D volume (more on this later) or a dynamic image, each and every file in the group will have common information. This ensures that if one file in a group is separated from the other files in the group, we still have every piece of information necessary to display that image, to identify the patient to whom it belongs, and to know when and under what conditions the image was acquired.

With so much information in each file, the data must be stored in a structured way to be easily recoverable. Every piece of information is tagged and identified internally within the DICOM file in two ways. First, each piece of data is assigned a **group number** associating it with a **data module**. A data module is simply a group of related data. For example, patient demographic information is all grouped in the same data module by assigning to it a data module number of 0010. When a radiology information system attempts to read these

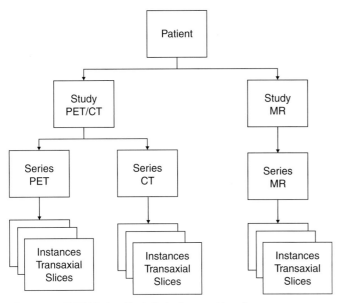

**Figure 3.9** DICOM Patient/Study/Series/Instance hierarchy.

data, it knows that if the data-module number is 0010, then the data relate to patient demographics. In addition to the data module, each piece of data is also assigned a second so-called "tag," called the **element number**. The element number specifically identifies the purpose of a piece of data within the data module. Standard data modules and element numbers are defined by a consortium of electrical equipment vendors called the **National Electrical Manufacturers Association**, or **NEMA** (5). At the time of this writing, the DICOM standard that defines all data modules and element numbers (along with everything else related to DICOM) could be found using a web browser at ftp://medical.nema.org/medical/dicom/2011/.

Many data modules and element numbers are specifically assigned in the DICOM standard. Frequently, however, vendors may create their own vendor-specific data modules and element numbers to store data that are important for their software, but may not be included in the standard. These extensible, proprietary fields are generally ignored by competing vendors. That being said, it is important that vendors create their DICOM files as close as possible to the standard, so as to avoid problems when other vendors try to import their files.

Each DICOM file has many data modules and elements, and many of them are modality dependent. PET images would not have certain data modules that are necessary for CT imaging, and vice-versa. There are four data modules that are extremely important, however, and are included in every DICOM file. These data modules form the foundation for identifying patients, describing distinct radiology studies, and creating separate image sets. These vital data modules are described below (Figure 3.9):

- The **Patient data module** includes elements describing patient demographics. This includes such elements as patient ID number, patient name, patient date of birth, patient gender, patient age, etc. If the patient data-module

fields are identical between two separate DICOM files, then a radiology information system will assume that the image sets refer to the same patient and store them accordingly.

- The **Study data module** includes information that is pertinent to a single scheduled study within a radiology department. If a study has multiple acquisitions, for example a PET acquisition and a CT acquisition, then the PET and the CT DICOM files will have common information in the Study data module. The study data include elements like a unique study identification number, description, date, accession number used for scheduling and billing, the referring physician's name, etc. When a radiology information system sees DICOM files with important study information in common, it will assume that the image sets were acquired during the same study and stores them accordingly.

- The **Series data module** includes information that is pertinent to a single image acquisition. It is called a series, because many acquisitions actually yield a group of images, rather than a single image, and so these may be stored in a group of DICOM files. For example, a PET acquisition results in a group of many individual 2-D images, rather than a single 3-D volume. (We will describe how 3-D images are created a bit later in the chapter.) These individual images are grouped together as a series of images. Using our PET/CT example from the Study data module description, although our PET and CT scans have identical Study data, they have separate Series data. Series data include a unique series identification number, a series description, the date and the time that the series was created, etc. When a radiology information system sees DICOM files, which have important series information in common, it assumes that the image sets are from the same acquisition and stores them accordingly.

- The **Instance data module** has information pertinent to an individual image contained in a DICOM file. For example, instance data would describe a single 2-D slice of a multi-slice PET series. Instance data include a unique instance identification number, an instance time and date, and a few other entries describing the single piece of radiology images. The instance is the smallest unit of radiologic imaging data.

It is important to note that the patient, study, series, and instance data are related to each other in a hierarchical structure, as shown in Figure 3.9. As mentioned previously, groups of DICOM files with certain DICOM elements that are identical will be related to each other. For example, in most radiology software, if the patient ID and patient name are identical in a group of DICOM files, the system will assume that the files describe the same patient. Similarly, if the unique study identification number is identical in certain files, then DICOM software will assume that the images were acquired as part of the same study. If the patient information is identical, but the study unique identifier is different, however, DICOM software

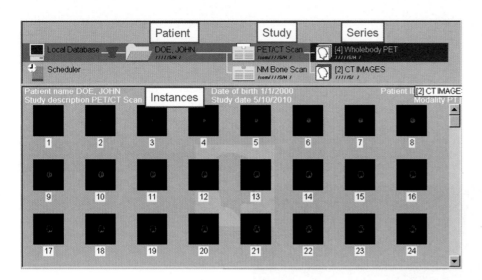

**Figure 3.10** An example of DICOM hierarchy from a common user interface.

will assume that the images belong to the same patient, but were acquired as different studies. Along those same lines, if the series-identification numbers are identical, then the DICOM files will be assumed to be part of the same acquisition. Note, however, that instance-identification numbers should never be identical. If they are, then DICOM systems will assume that the DICOM files are identical copies of each other and frequently ignore one of the files as a duplicate.

As mentioned previously, most vendors are now mirroring this same DICOM patient/series/study/instance hierarchy in their own software and user interfaces. Figure 3.10 shows the patient browser from a common imaging vendor. In this example, the hierarchy is clearly indicated in the display.

The reader will find it useful to keep the DICOM hierarchical Patient/Study/Series/Instance model in mind when viewing radiologic imaging text data. It goes a long way towards explaining inconsistencies in imaging displays. In addition to those data, some other vital data are also stored in databases and DICOM files. As we work with 3-D images, it is important to know that some data specific to changing 2-D images to 3-D images has to be stored somewhere.

## Image relationship data

As mentioned before, the very same databases and DICOM files that contain our Patient, Study, Series, and Instance information, also contain some other data that are vital to creating 3-D images as well. As we shall see, 3-D images are generally built from a series of 2-D images. These 2-D images have a variety of data that describe how they relate to each other and to the real world. Data items such as image size, scanner table position, image "depth" (bits per pixel), and others, are used by the computer to arrange the 2-D images into a 3-D image. The details about how that occurs will be discussed in the next section. In the meantime, however, it suffices simply to remember where this text and numerical data are stored – in databases while on a PACS server or a stand-alone workstation, and in DICOM files while in transit between them.

By now, we already have a reasonable understanding of how text data are stored in imaging software databases and DICOM transfer files. When we see patient demographic information and study information displayed over an image on the screen, it should be clear that it is not a trivial matter to make the data appear there. By using highly organized databases, radiology PACS servers or stand-alone workstations collect, store, and quickly retrieve required information, as well as a plethora of other data related to specific radiologic images. Using the DICOM protocol, these images can be transferred between workstations created by different vendors. Since the different vendors are now all using DICOM to transmit their images, they frequently use the DICOM Patient/Study/Series/Instance hierarchy in their data structures and user interfaces. And most importantly for 3-D images, these data structures allow for the storage of image-relationship data that can be used for creating the 3-D images. So, without further delay, let us discuss the creation of 3-D images.

## Three-dimensional radiologic imaging

Note the images in Figure 3.11. In general, the PET and CT scans acquired with a hybrid PET/CT system tend to encompass the same portions of the patient's body. If the CT scan starts at the head and goes to the thighs, the PET scan normally covers head to thigh, as well. In the case above, the study appears to be missing PET image data from the chest down. You might think, perhaps, that the technologist did not acquire data from the entire PET image volume, but a quick phone call to the technologists would confirm that the entire PET image was acquired, and that the images look correct on the PET/CT acquisition console. Something clearly failed during the transmission of the images, but what is it about 3-D radiologic images that would permit only half of the image to be displayed? We will answer this question in a few pages, but first, to understand the cause of this problem, it will be useful to know how 3-D images are stored and transferred among various radiology workstations.

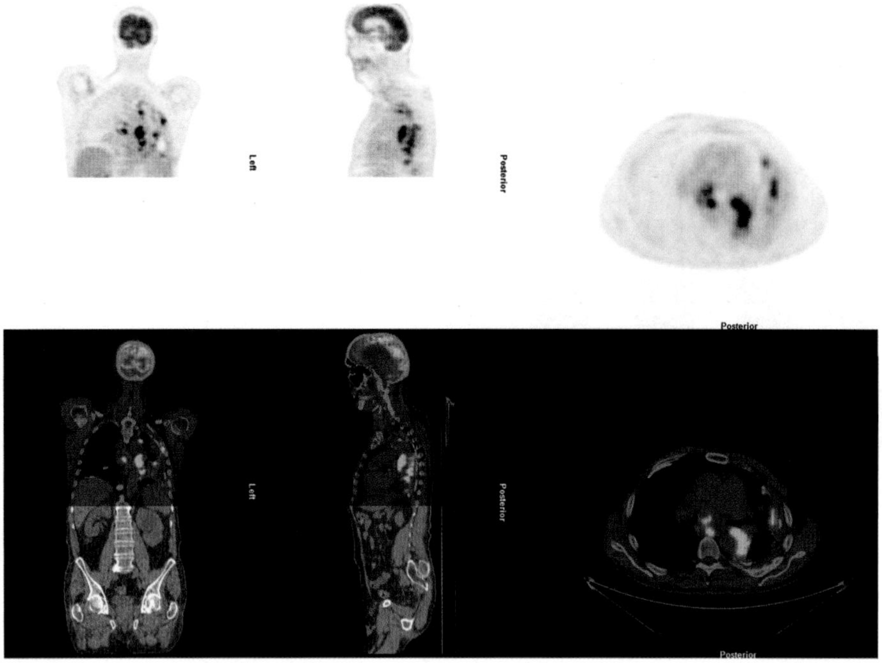

**Figure 3.11** Half of a FDG-PET image.

## Creating a 3-D matrix from a series of 2-D matrices

To start this discussion, let us first review what we know about 2-D imaging. Two-dimensional images consist of a matrix of pixels representing intensities, and there are associated text data representing such things as patient, study, series, and instance information. As mentioned previously, however, those text data also contain many other important things, as well. In the **DICOM Image-Presentation Data Module**, for example, there exists a substantial amount of information about how the stream of pixel data should be displayed. The image-presentation module contains, among other things, data entries for the image resolution. Since the pixel data are stored as a single line of intensities, knowing the resolution is crucial for understanding how many pixels should be included along each line of the image displayed on the screen. Another entry in the image presentation is the **pixel spacing**; this describes the distance in millimeters horizontally and vertically between the centers of adjacent pixels. Using this information, the computer can calculate the real-world size of objects, e.g., tumors or organs, within the images, using ruler tools included with most radiology imaging software. Data that describe the contextual basis for other data are frequently called **meta-data**. When meta-data describe not only the context of the immediate image but also its relationship to other images in the same series, we can use multiple 2-D images to create 3-D images.

Consider, for example, the images in Figure 3.12. This figure displays a series of PET transaxial slices. Most imaging systems store a series of 2-D PET or CT transaxial images, which may be used to synthesize the 3-D-image volume. As we look through the transaxial images in Figure 3.12, we realize that each one was acquired at a position slightly above the image on its left and slightly below the image on its right; thus, the images have an order associated with them. They are not randomly arranged on the screen. Additionally, "slightly above" and "slightly below" are not random either. Each 2-D image is precisely a known distance above the one prior to it, and it is precisely the same distance below the image following it. This distance between the images is known as the **slice thickness**. One can perceptually synthesize a 3-D image from this series of 2-D images by mentally stacking them on top of each other, while leaving a space equivalent to the slice thickness between them. We have now created a 3-D volume of stacked images that represents the patient's body (Figure 3.13).

A PET or CT 3-D DICOM volume consists of a series of 2-D images of transaxial slices "stacked" on top of each other in this way. These slices are identified and ordered by their distance in millimeters from the origin of the scan using a DICOM/Database field called **slice location**. Once stacked, each pixel in a given 2-D image has corresponding pixels from the preceding slice below it and the succeeding slice above it (unless, of course, it is in the top or bottom plane). Our 2-D matrix is now a 3-D matrix and the points in our matrix are no longer called pixels (a 2-D term), but instead are referred to as **voxels** (a 3-D term). It is vitally important to remember, however, that the distances between points in our 3-D matrix are not necessarily equal. While the pixel spacing along the x-axis and y-axis of the transaxial slices is frequently (but not necessarily) the same, the slice thickness along the volume's z-axis is commonly not the same as the pixel spacing. The result is a 3-D matrix with different distances between neighboring points in the transaxial vs. axial directions.

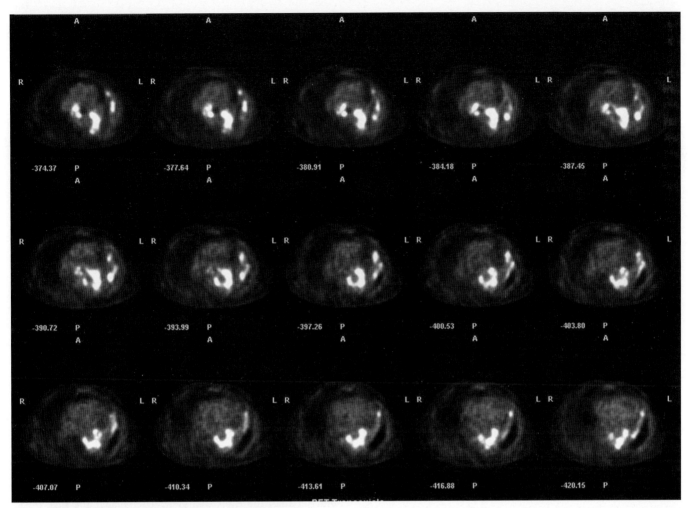

**Figure 3.12** A series of 2-D transaxial images.

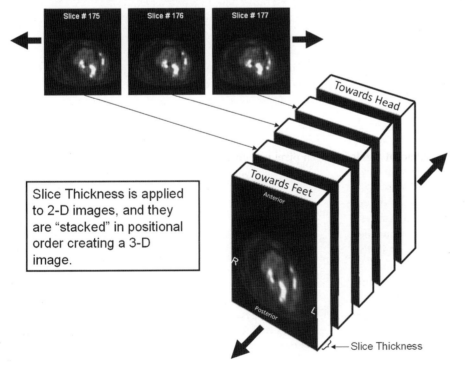

**Figure 3.13** Stacking 2-D images to create a 3-D volume.

Slice Thickness is applied to 2-D images, and they are "stacked" in positional order creating a 3-D image.

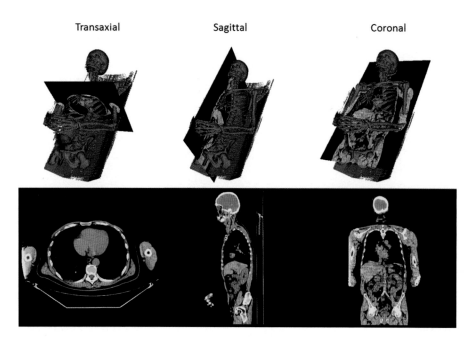

Transaxial          Sagittal          Coronal

**Figure 3.14** Transaxial, sagittal, and coronal images.

## PET/CT 3-D triangulation mode – transaxial, coronal and sagittal views

Once a 3-D matrix exists, the computer can perform complex calculations on the data to rotate the matrix. Instead of viewing a set of transaxial images, for example, the image volume can be rotated to show a set of coronal sections through the image volume. The **coronal view** of the 3-D matrix shows a stack of images with the patient's head at the top, the feet at the bottom, and with both shoulders visible, i.e., frontal views. Once rotated, the image volume is "re-sliced" so as to obtain a new series of images containing all of the coronal slices of the body starting from the anterior surface and increasing towards the posterior surface.

Similarly, this coronal 3-D matrix can be rotated 90 degrees about a different axis to display a **sagittal view**. The sagittal view of the 3-D matrix shows a series of images with the patient's head at the top and feet on the bottom, with the anterior surface on the left and the posterior on the right, i.e., a set of views from the left side of the patient (Figure 3.14).

The calculations required to perform these re-orientations and re-slicings are relatively complex and outside of the scope of this chapter. One important aspect of the process to note, however, is that the pixel data become less accurate when each transformation occurs. We have already discussed the difference between pixel spacing, the distance in millimeters between the pixels along the x-axis and y-axis in a transaxial image, and slice thickness, the distance between pixels in the z-axis of the 3-D matrix. Since the x-axis and y-axis values of the pixel spacing are generally the same, they correspond extremely well to a computer monitor where imaging pixels are also equal distances apart on both axes. When we begin "stacking" 2-D images to create a 3-D matrix, however, the distance between levels on the stack (the z-axis) is frequently

quite different than the others. This means that as the images are rotated, we cannot simply rotate the matrix without compensating for the different pixel spacing along different axes. We must perform additional calculations using the slice thickness to convert the z-axis distances to be identical to the x-axis and y-axis. If the distance between pixels is smaller than the slice thickness (as is almost always the case) then the data must be interpolated in order to fill in the missing pixels. This data interpolation can cause the coronal and sagittal views to look blurrier than the transaxial view. The smaller the slice thickness, however, the less the data interpolation, and the sharper the coronal and sagittal images will appear.

On clinical workstations, transaxial, coronal, and sagittal slices are frequently displayed on the screen simultaneously with a cross hair showing the point at which the three planes intersect. This view is called a **3-D triangulation viewing mode**. The user may scroll forward or backward through the slices in any of the three views. Frequently, the clinical software allows the user to click the mouse pointer on a specific voxel on one view, and the two adjacent views will immediately change to the corresponding slices containing that same voxel. Figure 3.15 shows a sample PET triangulation view. Note the cross-hairs indicating the point at which the three planes intersect.

The triangulation mode is the workhorse of PET/CT imaging today, and is included in every modern PET/CT viewing stand-alone and PACS workstation. The ability to rapidly examine different planes of the body in orientations that are immediately familiar to most viewers is vital. It is important to note, however, that some other useful 3-D tools exist, as well.

## Oblique views

One useful tool which is increasingly available on many workstations allows the user to create non-standard oblique views.

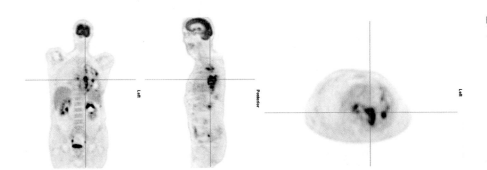

**Figure 3.15** FDG-PET triangulation mode.

An **oblique view** simply results from rotating the 3-D matrix to a position other than the standard transaxial, coronal, or sagittal views. The rotation does not even have to be a 90° increment of the original transaxial view. Many modern systems simply allow the user to "grab" the image with the computer's mouse and "drag" the point clicked to a different point on the screen. The image will rotate along the axis defined by the mouse movement to the new orientation. The computer will then re-sample the matrix in the new orientation and re-slice the image along this new orientation allowing the user to scroll through the volume in a non-standard way. This can be exceptionally useful for orienting an organ that may not normally correspond to the standard transaxial, sagittal, and coronal orientations. For example, quite often, a patient may be scanned with their head and neck at a non-standard angle; in this case, all planes of the image volume can be rotated to position the head in the conventional manner used for viewing and interpretation.

### Maximum intensity projection (MIP)

One frequently used viewing application that is based on a set of oblique views is called the **maximum intensity projection**, or **MIP** (6). In a MIP ciné view, the image is rotated, usually around the axial direction of the patient. For any given rotation angle, each voxel perpendicular to the current 2-D plane of projection at that position is scanned, and the pixel with the highest intensity is displayed. For any given point in the rotation, this creates an image more similar to a 2-D X-ray, where the body is "flattened," and the most intense areas within it appear on the screen. While cycling through the various rotation angles, an illusion is created in which the body appears to spin in 3-D with areas of intensity close to the outside of the body appearing to make wide arcs around the axis, while areas of intensity closer to the central axis seem to follow narrower arcs. Since the MIP view requires that the image rotate in order to perceive the 3-D effect, it is very difficult to display a MIP adequately on a book page, but Figure 3.16 attempts to show several views of a MIP image as it rotates around. In many workstations, the rotating MIP is displayed on the screen at the same time as the three images which form the triangulation view. The user may frequently use the mouse to click on findings seen on the MIP, and then the triangulation view will change accordingly to the corresponding views of the selected voxel in the three primary planes.

## 3-D imaging and DICOM

As we discuss the creation of 3-D images as "stacks" of 2-D slices, let us now backtrack a bit and review how that relates to the DICOM transport files. As mentioned previously, DICOM frequently uses a series of files containing 2-D images that are related to each other by the encapsulated contextual data to create more complex images. In this way, a group of many DICOM files – each containing a 2-D transaxial image – can be grouped together to form a 3-D PET or CT image. For example, if 250 transaxial image files belonging to the same DICOM series are transmitted to a DICOM-compliant imaging workstation, that workstation will combine the 2-D instances together to form a coherent 3-D volume.

Now let us think back on our example in Figure 3.11. That figure showed a full-size whole-body CT image, but only half of the total image volume was displayed for the PET study. Knowing what we know now, what could have happened to cause the image to be displayed in this way? Imaging workstations automatically generate 3-D volumes from a series of DICOM files. Each and every DICOM image file contains all of the contextual information necessary to place it appropriately at the correct location in the 3-D stack. And we know that the 2-D image files used to create 3-D images are generally stored in order of increasing the transaxial planes. Could it be that only a subset of the transaxial DICOM files had arrived at the workstation, yet the workstation had all of the data necessary to create a partial 3-D volume? That is, indeed, what happened in this case.

Many imaging workstations do not require the entire DICOM series to be present to display 3-D volumes. The workstations import the DICOM files on a file-by-file basis. From each and every DICOM file, all of the data necessary to create even a partial 3-D volume is imported into the appropriate fields of the workstation's database. In many cases, if a user attempts to open a partial DICOM series, the system will successfully recreate the 3-D volume based on the images that it has. More than likely, the PET image in Figure 3.11 was the result of a DICOM file transfer that failed to complete. Perhaps the transmitting station was shut down during the transfer, perhaps the network failed during the transfer, or perhaps the user simply tried to open the image set before the transfer was complete. The result is

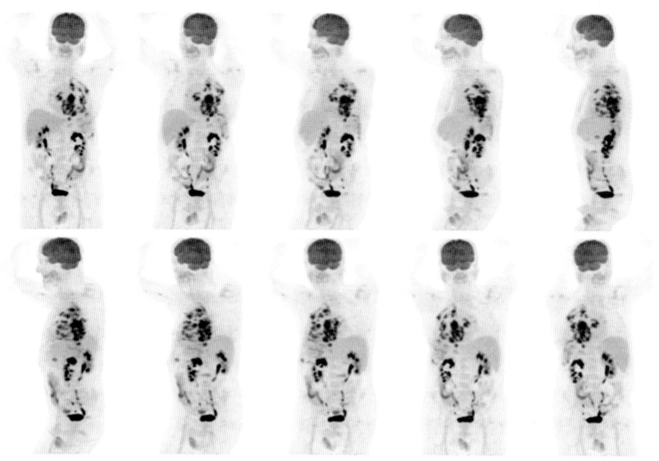

**Figure 3.16** Maximum intensity projections (MIP).

the same for all three possibilities. Instead of a complete whole-body image, the system had enough information to do the best that it could – namely create a partial 3-D volume. The solution to fixing this problem is most likely as simple as requesting that the technologist who performed the study should resend the complete image set to the viewing workstation. Once the complete image sets arrives, we should be ready to view the correct images – perhaps displaying the PET and CT images together. This brings us to our next topic: image registration and fusion.

## Image registration and fusion

One of the biggest strengths of modern PET/CT imaging workstations is the ability to view both PET and CT images together as a cohesive whole. By using synchronized displays and fusion imaging, metabolic findings can be very precisely localized to specific anatomic structures. As Figure 3.17 shows, PET and CT images can be tightly integrated into displays that synchronize images in separate display panels and even show both images superimposed in the same frame. How is this possible? What is going on to make this functionality available?

To answer these questions, we must have a brief discussion about image registration and fusion. Before delving too deeply

into these topics, however, let us clear up one point of common confusion. Frequently in the clinical laboratory setting, the terms "registration" and "fusion" are used interchangeably. Common parlance tends to indicate that either term can be used to describe images that show two modalities superimposed and displayed on a single panel of a workstation. This is not the case, however. The two terms describe two separate, but related processes. **Image registration** is the process of "morphing" two or more separate images of a patient's body into "matching" 2-D or 3-D coordinate spaces. Using image registration, images with drastically different resolution, pixel spacings and slice-thickness values, as well as with drastically different patient positions and orientations, can be modified so that all of those variables become approximately equal for the two registered image sets. **Image fusion**, on the other hand, takes these already pre-registered image volumes and superimposes them as one or more images displayed on a computer monitor. With an understanding of that distinction, let us go forward and discuss these processes in more detail.

### Image registration

As mentioned previously, image registration is the process of taking two or more disparate medical images and modifying them so that they are spatially aligned within the same coordinate system. Usually this is accomplished by selecting one of the images as the **target image**, an image which will not change during the course of the image manipulation. The remaining

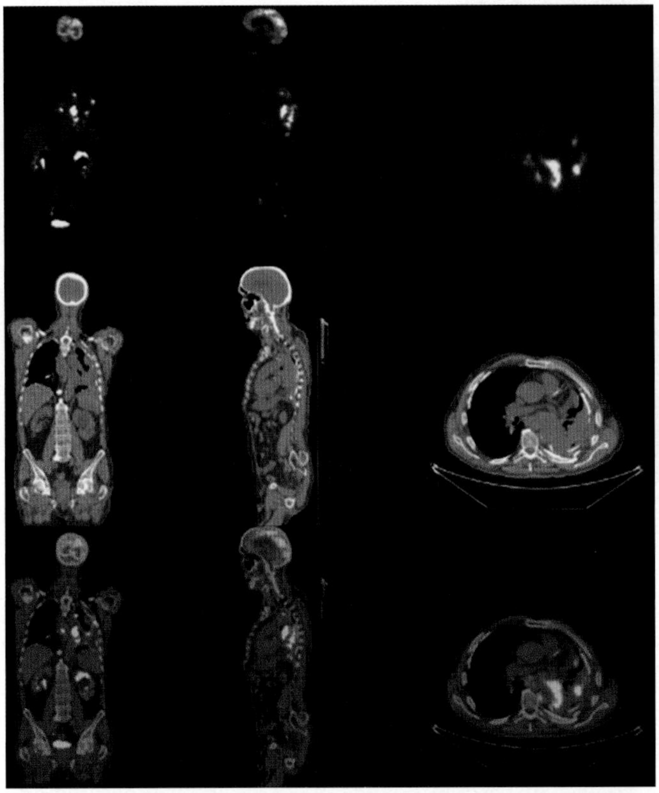

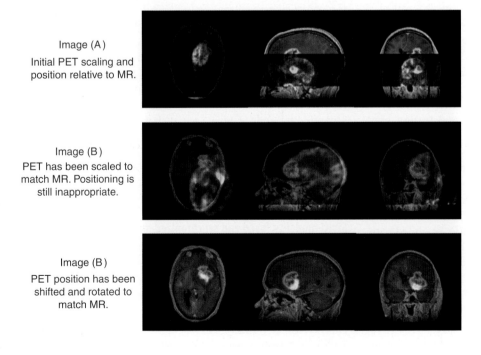

**Figure 3.17** Image fusion display.

image or images are known as **object images**. An object image will be modified to closely resemble the target image in certain ways, depending on the so-called "objective function" used during the registration process. For the purposes of our discussion, we will use an example of a brain scan acquired with an MR image as the target image volume and a PET image as the object image volume, as shown in Image (A) of Figure 3.18.

For our example our MR image has a resolution of $256 \times 256$, a pixel spacing of 1.106 mm, a slice thickness of 0.9 mm, and a total of 208 2-D transaxial images which make up the 3-D volume. Our PET image, on the other hand, has a resolution of $128 \times 128$, a pixel spacing of 3.406 mm, a slice thickness of 3.27 mm, and a total of 47 2-D transaxial images which make up the 3-D volume. From Figure 3.18, you can see that the MR images of the brain are positioned drastically differently than those from the PET. In order to make these images "match" for fusion, the following steps must take place. Since the PET image is the object image, it will be modified to match the coordinate space and positioning of the MR image. The MR image will not change. Using complex calculations that are outside of the scope of this discussion, the 3-D matrix which holds the PET image volume will be changed from its original $128 \times 128$ resolution, 3.406 mm pixel spacing, 3.27 mm slice thickness, and 47 number of transaxial slices to match the MRI image volume's $256 \times 256$ resolution, 1.106 mm pixel spacing, 0.9 mm slice thickness, and 208 number of slices. Once this scaling is done, as shown in Image (B) of Figure 3.18, the PET 3-D matrix will be rotated, reformatted and compared with the original MRI to see if the image is closer or farther away to the correct positioning. If the image positioning is

**Figure 3.18** Rigid registration of brain MR and FDG-PET images.

Image (A)
Initial PET scaling and position relative to MR.

Image (B)
PET has been scaled to match MR. Positioning is still inappropriate.

Image (B)
PET position has been shifted and rotated to match MR.

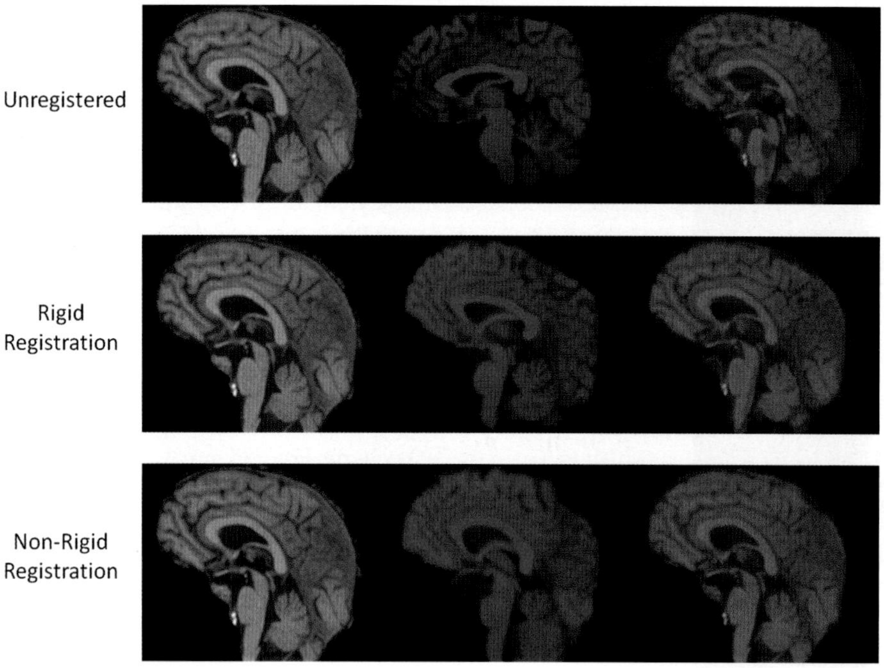

**Figure 3.19** Rigid vs. non-rigid registration of FDG-PET and CT brain imaging.

worse, then the computer will use the previous position and try a slightly different position change. If the positioning is better, the new position will be kept and used as the basis for another position change. This trial and error method of position changes is repeated many times, a process called **iteration**, until the object-image volume's positioning is very close to that of the target-image volume.

At this point, the registration process will frequently stop, and the object-image's 3-D matrix will be saved as new 3-D matrix or DICOM-like series of 2-D slices in the workstation's database. When the process stops at this point, it is called a **rigid registration**. As described, a rigid registration only scales (resizes), shifts (moves), and/or rotates the volume. It never "warps" or changes the volume in any other way. Image (C) in Figure 3.18 shows the final results of the rigid registration of the MR and PET images.

In cases where a rigid registration is not deemed to be adequate, the additional step of **non-rigid registration** may be applied. Non-rigid registration generally starts from the results of the rigid-registration procedure and attempts to stretch, or compress, features within the object image to match similar features in the target image. This occurs in a non-linear fashion, so that certain volumes of the image may be modified more or less than others. For example, if a CT is acquired during a breath-hold, the lungs will be greatly expanded with air. If a corresponding PET is acquired in a condition of continuous shallow breathing by the patient, the image of the lungs will be considerably smaller. Non-linear registration will attempt to alter the 3-D matrix to have the PET lung area more closely match the expanded CT lung area. Areas outside the lungs may be compacted to make up the difference. If the same images include an area representing the head, the PET image

in that area may not be affected much at all. Figure 3.19 shows fused images illustrating the difference between a rigid and a non-rigid brain registration procedure.

It is vitally important to note that complex registration processes can drastically change the imaging results. The more an image is resized, placed into a matrix of different dimensions, shifted, rotated, and warped, the less accurate it becomes. Shapes and boundaries of lesions will become distorted and blurred. Quantitative values will also lose their accuracy. While the registration process is incredibly useful for comparing results of tests from different modalities, the results should be interpreted more cautiously as the changes required to create them become more drastic. To solve this issue, PET and CT images are now commonly obtained on the same hybrid imaging system during the same session, in principle with no patient motion between the PET and CT studies. The PET-CT scanner's software is designed to save the separate PET and CT image sets such that the changes required for registration are minimal, preserving the integrity and accuracy of the original images. Once accurately registered images sets have been created and saved, they may be used by imaging workstations for synchronized displays and fusion imaging.

### Multi-modality fused and synchronized imaging

Once PET and CT images have been properly registered, either through an automated computerized registration process, or through a semi-automated process (in which the user interacts with the registration program), or by being acquired in such a way as to be closely registered without the need for advanced processing, the images can be viewed in more cohesive ways. One of the most useful views is the one that shows the PET

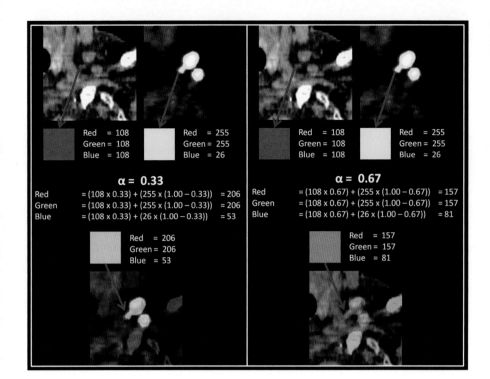

**Figure 3.20** A FDG-PET/CT fusion image with the degree of alpha-blending set to two different levels.

image superimposed over the CT. This combination of PET and CT imaging is called **image fusion**. Image fusion can be accomplished in several ways, but the most common is through a process called **alpha-blending** (7). Alpha-blending takes two pre-registered images and, on a pixel-by-pixel basis, separates each pixel into its three component color intensities. The two base color intensities are merged into a new intensity that is a blend, or mixture of the two values. The blending is based on the following equation where $\alpha$ is a value between 0 and 1:

$$Intensity_{New} = Intensity_1(\alpha) + Intensity_2(1 - \alpha)$$

As alpha increases, the color intensities represented by Intensity$_1$ will have more of an emphasis on the final color of the pixel. As alpha decreases, the color intensities represented by Intensity$_2$ will have more emphasis. Thus, if Pixel$_1$ is medium gray and Pixel$_2$ is yellow, a higher alpha value will result in a pixel that is mostly gray with a slight tinge of yellow. In the same example, a lower alpha value will result in a pixel that is mostly yellow with a tinge of gray. Figure 3.20 illustrates alpha-blending at two levels for alpha.

One thing to note about image fusion is the number of user-controllable variables that influence the displayed images. The user can change the look-up table and window-leveling settings for the primary image, the look-up table and window-leveling for the secondary image and the alpha value. All of these changes will have drastic effects on the final fused image. For example, if the user selects two grayscale images, there will usually not be enough color or contrast differences between the original images to be useful. Additionally, if the window-leveling is set such that large portions of an original image are at maximum intensity, this tends to over-power the other image unless the fused image is created with an alpha value that highly emphasizes the less intense image.

Along with fusion, another feature common to most imaging workstations is **synchronized 3-D image triangulation**. This feature provides a display layout that is similar to that used for standard, single-modality 3-D image triangulation, but now the PET, CT, and fused images are all displayed on the screen simultaneously. Because these images are pre-registered, it is very easy for the software to update all three displays whenever one of them is changed. For example, if a user were to click on a voxel on the PET transaxial image, not only would the corresponding coronal and sagittal images on the PET change, but so would the images on both the CT and the fused displays. All of the views on each of the PET, CT, and fused displays would continuously show the same portions of the patient's anatomy.

## Take-home message

- Two-dimensional matrices contain numeric pixel values which represent relative radiation intensity at various points in the subject's body.
- Given a sequential series of these 2-D matrices, along with information about the relative pixel spacing and slice thickness, one can create a 3-D matrix that a computer can rotate and re-slice to show in a variety of orientations.
- Three primary orientations – the transaxial, coronal, and sagittal views – show these images in orientations at right-angles to the natural axes of the body.

- Computer systems store these data numerically in a database and can transmit the data to other very different computer systems using the DICOM radiologic imaging standard.
- By using specialized acquisition techniques and complex calculations, 3-D matrices from different acquisitions can be registered, and the resulting images can then be combined to display fused images.

Clearly this is just the beginning. As the field of radiology advances, the data gathered from images will be used in more and more useful ways. Dynamic PET and CT images, which show volumes changing over time to adjust for bodily functions like breathing and movement, are rapidly becoming a reality. By understanding the relationship of computers and imaging today, we prepare ourselves for the challenges of tomorrow.

## Acknowledgement

The editor and the author acknowledge the valuable suggestions from Dr. Stephen Moore, Director of Nuclear Medicine Physics at Brigham and Women's Hospital.

## References

1. Oberholzer M, Ostreicher M, Christen H, Brühlmann M. Methods in quantitative image analysis. *Histochem Cell Biol* 1996;**105**(5):333–55.

2. Acton PD, Zhuang H, Alavi A. Quantification in PET. *Radiol Clin North Am* 2004;**42**(6):1055–62, viii.

3. Huang HK, Mankovich NJ, Taira RK *et al.* Picture archiving and communication systems (PACS) for radiological images: state of the art. *Crit Rev Diagn Imaging* 1988;**28**(4):383–442.

4. Bidgood WD Jr, Horii SC. Introduction to the ACR-NEMA DICOM standard. *Radiographics* 1992;**12**(2):345–55.

5. Busemann-Sokole E, Cradduck TD. National Electrical Manufacturers Association. *J Nucl Med* 1983;**24**(10):973–4.

6. Fujiwara T, Miyake M, Watanuki S *et al.* Easy detection of tumor in oncologic whole-body PET by projection reconstruction images with maximum intensity projection algorithm. *Ann Nucl Med* 1999;**13**(3):199–203.

7. Bican J, Janeba D, Táborská K, Veselý J. Image overlay using alpha-blending technique. *Nucl Med Rev Cent East Eur* 2002;**5**(1):53.

# Functional anatomy of the FDG image

Scott Britz-Cunningham and Victor H. Gerbaudo

## The physiologic basis of FDG uptake

[18]F-fluorodeoxyglucose (FDG) is an index molecule for glucose metabolism, a highly complex physiologic process. It is practically a truism that malignant cells proliferate rapidly, and thus tend to have a high metabolic rate (1, 2). However, this statement conceals as much as it reveals. The "metabolism" depicted by a PET scan image cannot be treated as a simple continuum, with benign and inert tissues at the low end (white = "good"), and rampant malignancies at the high end (black = "bad"). There are many kinds of metabolism, and glucose is not the only metabolic currency. Nor is glucose metabolism uniform; it has many competing pathways, often within the same cell. These include both catabolic (energy-producing) or anabolic (energy-consuming) processes, such as the pentose phosphate pathway.

FDG uptake does not directly correspond to the presence or activity of any single molecular target. Every count in every pixel on an ordinary PET scan is a summation of numerous factors, including delivery of tracer molecules to the tissues (plasma input function) and the microscopic and macroscopic architecture of the tissue itself. These are not academic trivia; intimate understanding of these factors is essential for accurate interpretation of PET images. Oversimplification is the most common and perhaps the most dangerous error in reading PET scans.

## Glucose transporters

The cell membrane is impermeable to sugars. Although glucose and other six-carbon sugars lie at the very root of metabolism and of life itself, they can only enter the cell by permission, through highly restricted portals. Foremost among these is the GLUT family of transporters (also known as SLC2, or solute carrier family 2), 13 isoforms of which are presently known (3, 4). Each GLUT isoform consists of 12 transmembrane helices. The binding of a molecule of sugar on the outer side of the membrane induces a conformational change in the transporter molecule, which translocates the sugar and releases it on the inner side. Since this is not an energy-dependent

process, another sugar molecule can be picked up just as easily inside the cell, and transported back out again (3). The net result is facilitated diffusion of sugar in *either* direction, from the side of higher concentration to the lower, whichever it may be.

The various GLUT isoforms differ in their specificity (fructose, for example, is the sole substrate for GLUT-5), and in their tissue expression. Some, like GLUT-1, tend to be constitutively active. Others, such as GLUT-4, are synthesized ahead of need, but remain sequestered in vesicles until insulin stimulation recruits them to the plasma membrane. From the standpoint of PET/CT imaging with FDG, the crucial point is that the synthetic molecule fluorodeoxyglucose is also a substrate for these transporters, with transport kinetics very similar to glucose itself. Some idea of the variety of this gene family can be gained from Table 4.1, which summarizes the pattern of expression of each of the isoforms.

In addition to facilitated diffusion, glucose can be imported into the cell by energy-dependent active transport. This is particularly important in the absorptive epithelia of the small intestine and proximal renal tubule, which need to transport glucose against a concentration gradient. These tissues rely upon Na+/glucose symporters SGLT-1 and SGLT-2 (5). The SGLT family (also known as SLC5A, or solute carrier family 5A) contains at least seven homologous sequences. Although FDG is also a substrate, its affinity for these transporters is less than glucose. In the kidney, this means that reabsorption of FDG is less efficient than that of glucose, which is a primary reason for the intense accumulation of FDG in the renal collecting systems and bladder on PET/CT scans (6).

## Hexokinase

GLUT transporters tend only to equalize the concentration of glucose (and FDG) on either side of the cell membrane. They are not capable of concentrating their substrates within the cell. Were GLUT the end of the story, target tissues, including tumors, would gradually reach an equilibrium activity on PET/CT equal to that of the blood pool, and would then stop. FDG imaging is only possible because of the action of a

*A Case-Based Approach to PET/CT in Oncology*, ed. Victor H. Gerbaudo. Published by Cambridge University Press.
© Cambridge University Press 2012.

**Table 4.1** Glucose transporter family.

| Transporter | Class | Location | Features |
|---|---|---|---|
| GLUT-1 | I | Widely expressed | Key to basal metabolism<br>Upregulated in many tumors<br>Deficiency: seizure disorder |
| GLUT-2 | I | Hepatocytes; pancreatic beta cells; basolateral intestinal/renal epithelium | Deficiency: Fanconi–Bickel syndrome |
| GLUT-3 | I | Neurons | |
| GLUT-4 | I | Fat and muscle; cerebellum | Preformed enzyme is translocated from storage vesicle to cell membrane by insulin or exercise |
| GLUT-5 | II | Spermatozoa; intestinal apical membrane | Fructose transporter |
| GLUT-6 | III | Leukocytes; brain; spleen | |
| GLUT-7 | II | Apical membrane of small intestine, colon; liver; endoplasmic reticulum | High affinity for glucose, fructose |
| GLUT-8 | III | Testis; blastocyst; brain; muscle; fat; placenta | |
| GLUT-9 | II | Liver; kidney; spleen | |
| GLUT-10 | III | Liver; pancreas | |
| GLUT-11 | II | Heart; skeletal muscle | |
| GLUT-12 | III | Muscle; fat; breast; small intestine; prostate | Insulin-responsive |
| GLUT-13 | III | Glia, neurons | Proton-coupled myoinositol transporter |

critical enzyme, **hexokinase** – the "unsung hero" of PET/CT technology.

Hexokinase is a "gatekeeper" – the first enzyme encountered in both the glycolytic and oxidative pathways of glucose metabolism. It is single-handedly responsible for tissue localization of FDG, since phosphorylated FDG is no longer a substrate for the GLUT transporter, and is therefore trapped in place. Hexokinase activity is promoted by insulin and hypoxia, and is allosterically inhibited by its product, glucose-6-phosphate. Several isoforms of hexokinase have been identified in humans (7, 8). Types I and II are activated by binding to the mitochondrial membrane through a voltage-dependent anion channel, in which location they are well positioned to integrate glycolysis with oxidative metabolism. Type II also has an anti-apoptotic action through its effect upon protein kinase B (PKB/Akt), and is upregulated in cancer cells. Type III is a perinuclear form, which does not bind mitochondria. Type IV, also known as glucokinase, is constitutively active in the liver and pancreas. In liver tumors, there is often a shift in expression from Type IV to Type II or Type I.

## Phosphatases

The glucose-6-phosphatases (three isoforms known) are enzymes involved in the final processing and release of glucose in gluconeogenesis and glycogenolysis. They act as the reverse of hexokinase, converting glucose-6-phosphate back into glucose (or FDG-6-phosphate back into FDG). These products, of course, are perfect substrates for reverse transport via GLUT

back out of the cell. Hence, where phosphatase activity is high, FDG-6-phosphate will fail to concentrate, and the target tissue will be poorly visualized on PET imaging.

Phosphatase activity is high in liver, kidney, intestine, and resting skeletal muscle. Well-differentiated tumors arising from these tissues may retain some of this activity, and may thus show lower resultant levels of FDG uptake than would be expected from their proliferative or metabolic rate. In particular, hepatocellular carcinoma has been shown to have high phosphatase activity, which contributes to the difficulty of distinguishing this tumor from normal hepatic background (9).

## Rate limitation and control

Depending on the physiologic context, any of these processes may be rate-limiting for the uptake of glucose (and thus of FDG). In most tissues, GLUT is active at low, constitutive levels of expression. When glucose is abundant, the transporters are easily saturated, and GLUT expression itself limits the rate of uptake. This is why tumors, which express GLUT at higher levels than normal tissue, are able to concentrate FDG activity much more intensely than background. However, when GLUT is functioning at very high levels (e.g., after insulin stimulation of GLUT-4), the choke point may pass to hexokinase. In starvation and acute ischemia, it is delivery of blood-borne glucose to the tissue that is rate limiting. In such cases, the PET/CT image may show a suboptimal tumor-to-background ratio.

# Quantifying FDG uptake

Forming a PET/CT image is a quantitative process. The images viewed on screen are simply cross-sections of a 3-D map of activity throughout the body, rendered on a light–dark scale which is intuitively interpreted by the reader's eye. To supplement what the eye perceives, all current PET/CT display systems provide a quantitative measure of activity, the standardized uptake value (SUV). This represents the ratio of activity within a pixel or volume of interest to the average activity everywhere else in the body. The SUV is not new information; it simply assigns a number to what the eye estimates instinctively. However, it can be useful to eliminate perceptual bias (to keep the eye "honest"), or to compare foci of uptake that are physically remote from each other.

Behind the concept of SUV is an assumption that "more" and "less" are significant. Back to our truism, again: tumoral uptake is high; normal tissue uptake is low. But, as we have seen, the FDG activity at any point integrates complex interactions of glucose transporters, hexokinase, phosphatase, as well as other physiologic factors such as perfusion rates, competition with sugar substrates, and so forth. These, in turn, are not static, but are in constant change in response to the metabolic conditions of the target tissue and the body as a whole. Table 4.2 lists a few of the most relevant factors. Note should be made, however, that few of the entries on the list exist in isolation; most of them have secondary effects upon each other.

Tumors have their own set of uptake-modifying factors (Table 4.3). To begin with, they are not made up of uniform solid balls of cells. They tend to be heterogeneous, often because of features, like necrosis, desmoplasia, or an infiltrative pattern of spread, that are individually characteristic of each histologic subtype. A squamous cell carcinoma of the lung does not look like carcinoid under the microscope; nor does it on an FDG image. The clinically experienced PET/CT reader will be aware of these characteristics, and will read each scan with one eye on the biopsy report, judging the significance of any findings in light of the expected pattern and intensity of uptake. Conversely, when evaluating a still-unbiopsied lesion, the FDG uptake may help to define the set of possible tumor types to be considered. The object of many of the following chapters of this book will be to acquaint the reader with these special patterns of tumoral uptake.

A PET/CT scanner is, obviously, a mechanical device, and as such it imposes a number of technical and geometric factors that can also affect the measurement and display of FDG activity (Table 4.4). While some of these can be minimized by good technique, their impact will be all too familiar to any experienced PET/CT interpreter. When identified by hindsight on a completed scan, it may be difficult to estimate the extent to which they affect uptake of any specific lesion. However, the first rule of dealing with artifacts is to recognize that they exist.

The upshot of all this is that the PET/CT image, or the SUV derived from it, represents at best an approximation – a kind

**Table 4.2** General biological factors affecting $^{18}$F-fluorodeoxyglucose (FDG) uptake.

Total body volume of distribution (affected by body composition)

Perfusion

Cellularity

Metabolic rate of tissue
- Constitutive/housekeeping functions
- Proliferation
- Specialized activity

Need for carbon skeletons for anabolic pathways (e.g., pentose phosphate pathway)

Dominant metabolic pathway: glycolysis vs. aerobic oxidation

Hypoxia

Serum glucose levels

Serum insulin levels

Expression of glucose transporters (at least 12 isoforms are presently known, with varying $K_M$ for glucose)

Expression and activity of hexokinase

Expression and activity of glucose-6-phosphatase

Availability of alternative fuel molecules (fatty acids, ketones, etc.)

Organ activity
- Skeletal muscle: movement or isometric tension
- Brain
    - Sensory stimulation (e.g., light)
    - Intellectual activity
    - Wakefulness
- Glands: secretory activity
    - Salivation
    - Lactating breast

Smooth muscle: bowel peristalsis, gastric contractions

Temperature response:
- Shivering
- Hypermetabolic fat

Fever (affects basal metabolic rate)

Renal excretion of radiotracer, affected by:
- Hydration
- Diuresis
- Age

Local attenuating factors: bowel contents, edema

of Gordian knot of metabolic, tumoral, and technical complexities which the busy clinician can never expect to unravel. There will always remain two crucial but fundamentally irreducible uncertainties: *How accurate is the uptake information I am observing?* And, assuming that the uptake is accurate, *what tumors or physiologic and pathologic processes are included or excluded by it?*

Table 4.3 Tumor-specific factors.

Angiogenesis

Chemotherapy/radiotherapy

Hormonal stimulation

Location (bone, soft tissue, lung)

Presence of mucin or other acellular elements

Chronic inflammatory infiltrate within tumor. (Many tumors undergo necrosis, or immune response stimulated by specific tumor antigens)

Total tumor burden. (Where a large amount of tumor is present, the FDG pool is divided among all of it, and the measured SUV will decrease, as will the SUV of tissues such as brain and liver)

FDG, [18]F-fluorodeoxyglucose; SUV, standardized uptake value.

Table 4.4. Technical factors.

Dose infiltration

Retention of radiotracer in ports/catheters

Time of imaging after injection (may have differing effects upon different tissues, due to varying uptake rates)

Recovery coefficient/partial volume effects (especially for small or irregular structures)

Camera resolution

Reconstruction filter

Method of attenuation correction

Placement of region of interest (ROI)

Some confidence can be gained by comparing the uptake in a lesion of interest with some sort of internal control – typically, background activity in the organ where the lesion is found. This may help to cancel out some of the grossest factors that are likely to perturb FDG uptake measurements. However, the adjoining tissue may not always be the ideal standard for comparison. The metabolism of aerated lung, for example, is very different from that of a pulmonary adenocarcinoma. For that reason, it has been long-established practice at our institution to compare lesion activity, not to adjoining tissue, but to basal ganglia or to cerebral cortex. Like most tumors, the brain has a high rate of metabolism, which is dependent wholly upon glucose as an energy source. Furthermore, in both cases GLUT-1 is the dominant glucose transporter. The comparative activity ratio (CAR) between these two tissues is simple to calculate, and it can help to distinguish malignant from benign lesions, as well as to facilitate comparisons between serial studies (10).

## Standard whole-body distribution of FDG uptake

Table 4.5 shows the range of uptake seen in normal tissues in 105 scans performed at the Brigham and Women's Hospital. Table 4.6 shows the same data, normalized to activity in the brain (comparative activity ratios). From these data, it can easily be seen that FDG uptake varies widely between tissue types, with some normal tissues (brain, kidney, stomach, rectum) having physiologic uptake as intense as that of malignant tumors (Figure 4.1). Furthermore, even a single tissue type can show wide variation (stomach, bowel) within the normal physiologic range of activity. Although much of this variability can be rationalized by invoking the modifying factors discussed in the previous section, in practice it is essential to become familiar with the natural range for each tissue before abnormal findings can be recognized and assessed.

The following is a brief overview of uptake characteristics in various sites of the body.[1]

**Brain and spinal cord.** Brain uptake in the cortical ribbon and basal ganglia is intense, reflecting high neuronal metabolic rates and a preference for glucose as an energy source (Figures 4.2 and 4.3). This can make it difficult to identify small cortical or subcortical tumors, for which MRI is a more sensitive modality. White matter uptake is very low. Cerebellar uptake is slightly less than cerebral cortex (opposite to the pattern seen on SPECT imaging with HMPAO or ECD). Focally increased uptake is normal in the midline cerebellum (vermis). In the spine, mild to moderate uptake can usually be seen in the cervical and lumbar ganglia, which should not be confused with true lesions.

**Lymphoid tissue.** Intense uptake due to chronic reactive changes is commonly seen in the tonsils and adenoids (the latter particularly in children). While usually symmetric, this can be unilateral, a very problematic finding in patients with lymphoma or primary head and neck cancer. When there are no clear-cut CT findings to correlate with asymmetric FDG uptake, the only diagnostic recourse may be direct examination by an otolaryngologist, or a follow-up PET/CT study to assess stability.

Mild chronic reactive uptake is frequently seen in cervical, axillary, mediastinal, and inguinal nodes. Typically these will have benign morphology (reniform shape, fatty hilum) on CT. A **grossly enlarged** lymph node with only mild uptake is unlikely to represent metastasis from an intensely FDG-avid primary malignant tumor. However, **small** nodes with mild uptake may represent micrometastases, and should be identified for inclusion in any staging biopsy or mediastinoscopy, if feasible.

Lymphatic metastases tend to spread station-by-station, along pathways that have been anatomically characterized for many tumor types (discussed in the following chapters). Thus, for example, in a patient with limited-stage lung cancer, an FDG-avid inguinal lymph node is unlikely to be metastatic. However, in abdominal and pelvic cancers, nodes from the upper paraaortic stations may drain directly to a left supraclavicular node (Virchow's node). Furthermore, skip metastases are not uncommon in patients who have previously undergone

**Table 4.5** Reference ranges for standardized uptake value (SUV) of $^{18}$F-fluorodeoxyglucose (FDG) in normal tissues and benign and iatrogenic lesions on PET/CT.

| Site | Number | Range | Mean | Std. dev. | Coeff. of variation |
|---|---|---|---|---|---|
| Bladder | 96 | 3.1–167.0 | 32.5 | 25.9 | 0.8 |
| Renal pelvis | 99 | 3.0–119.4 | 30.5 | 23.9 | 0.8 |
| Basal ganglia | 105 | 5.0–24.7 | 11.8 | 3.8 | 0.3 |
| Cerebral cortex | 105 | 5.0–24.4 | 11.7 | 4 | 0.3 |
| Cerebellum | 105 | 4.7–18.0 | 9.6 | 2.5 | 0.3 |
| Ureter | 77 | 1.2–39.4 | 8.9 | 8.1 | 0.9 |
| Bowel | 99 | 2.2–15.8 | 5 | 2.5 | 0.5 |
| Stomach | 100 | 1.4–9.4 | 4.1 | 1.2 | 0.3 |
| Tongue base | 100 | 1.3–9.9 | 3.8 | 1.5 | 0.4 |
| Oropharynx | 99 | 1.1–8.0 | 3.6 | 1.4 | 0.4 |
| Vertebral body | 101 | 2.0–9.6 | 3.6 | 1.2 | 0.3 |
| Rectum | 94 | 1.2–13.0 | 3.4 | 1.7 | 0.5 |
| Spleen | 99 | 1.7–7.8 | 3.2 | 0.9 | 0.3 |
| Esophagus | 100 | 1.6–5.7 | 2.9 | 0.7 | 0.3 |
| Muscle | 102 | 1.2–7.1 | 2.7 | 1.2 | 0.5 |
| Parotid | 103 | 1.2–6.3 | 2.6 | 0.8 | 0.3 |
| Vertebral facet | 92 | 1.5–5.7 | 2.6 | 0.7 | 0.3 |
| Benign pulmonary hilum | 102 | 1.0–3.7 | 2.4 | 0.6 | 0.2 |
| Aortic blood pool | 102 | 1.4–3.9 | 2.4 | 0.4 | 0.2 |
| Liver | 100 | 1.5–3.6 | 2.4 | 0.4 | 0.2 |
| Acromioclavicular joint | 102 | 0.2–4.3 | 1.9 | 0.7 | 0.4 |
| Thyroid (non-focal) | 76 | 0.8–4.9 | 1.7 | 0.6 | 0.3 |
| Normal breast | 102 | 0.5–2.8 | 1.3 | 0.5 | 0.4 |
| Fat | 101 | 0.4–4.9 | 0.9 | 0.6 | 0.7 |
| Lung | 102 | 0.3–1.9 | 0.6 | 0.2 | 0.4 |
| Fracture | 19 | 0.8–5.5 | 2.7 | 1.2 | 0.5 |
| Uterine fibroid | 7 | 1.7–2.7 | 2.2 | 0.3 | 0.1 |
| Thyroid (focal) | 21 | 1.9–12.3 | 1.7 | 0.6 | 0.3 |
| Pulmonary atelectasis | 14 | 0.9–2.5 | 1.6 | 0.4 | 0.3 |
| Pleural effusion | 12 | 0.7–2.1 | 1.4 | 0.4 | 0.3 |
| Gastrojejunal tube | 2 | 4.1–5.8 | 5 | 1.2 | 0.2 |
| Ileostomy | 3 | 1.5–5.4 | 3.3 | 2 | 0.6 |
| Bowel anastomosis | 8 | 1.7–7.4 | 3.3 | 1.9 | 0.6 |
| Incision | 17 | 1.2–4.3 | 2.6 | 0.9 | 0.4 |
| Breast biopsy site | 2 | 1.3–2.0 | 2.2 | 1.2 | 0.6 |

All values are maximum standardized uptake value (SUV), except for bladder, lung, pleural effusion, liver and non-focal thyroid, which are averaged over the entire organ or derived from the average of multiple measurements.

**Table 4.6** Reference ranges for standardized uptake value (SUV) of [18]F-fluorodeoxyglucose (FDG) in normal tissues and benign and iatrogenic lesions on PET/CT.

| Site | Number | Range | Mean | Std. dev. | Ratio of std. dev./mean |
|---|---|---|---|---|---|
| Bladder | 96 | 3.1–167.0 | 32.5 | 25.9 | 0.8 |
| Renal pelvis | 99 | 3.0–119.4 | 30.5 | 23.9 | 0.8 |
| Basal ganglia | 105 | 5.0–24.7 | 11.8 | 3.8 | 0.3 |
| Cerebral cortex | 105 | 5.0–24.4 | 11.7 | 4 | 0.3 |
| Cerebellum | 105 | 4.7–18.0 | 10.6 | 11.2 | 1.1 |
| Ureter | 77 | 1.2–39.4 | 8.9 | 8.1 | 0.9 |
| Bowel | 99 | 2.2–15.8 | 5 | 2.5 | 0.5 |
| Stomach | 100 | 1.4–9.4 | 4.1 | 1.2 | 0.3 |
| Tongue base | 100 | 1.3–9.9 | 3.8 | 1.5 | 0.4 |
| Oropharynx | 99 | 1.1–8.0 | 3.6 | 1.4 | 0.4 |
| Vertebral body | 101 | 2.0–9.6 | 3.6 | 1.2 | 0.3 |
| Rectum | 94 | 1.2–13.0 | 3.4 | 1.7 | 0.5 |
| Spleen | 99 | 1.7–7.8 | 3.2 | 0.9 | 0.3 |
| Esophagus | 100 | 1.6–5.7 | 2.9 | 0.7 | 0.3 |
| Muscle | 102 | 1.2–7.1 | 2.7 | 1.2 | 0.5 |
| Parotid | 103 | 1.2–6.3 | 2.6 | 0.8 | 0.3 |
| Vertebral facet | 92 | 1.5–5.7 | 2.6 | 0.7 | 0.3 |
| Benign pulmonary hilum | 102 | 1.0–3.7 | 2.4 | 0.6 | 0.2 |
| Aortic blood pool | 102 | 1.4–3.9 | 2.4 | 0.4 | 0.2 |
| Liver | 100 | 1.5–3.6 | 2.4 | 0.4 | 0.2 |
| Acromioclavicular joint | 102 | 0.2–4.3 | 1.9 | 0.7 | 0.4 |
| Thyroid (non-focal) | 76 | 0.8–4.9 | 1.7 | 0.6 | 0.3 |
| Normal breast | 102 | 0.5–2.8 | 1.3 | 0.5 | 0.4 |
| Fat | 101 | 0.4–4.9 | 0.9 | 0.6 | 0.7 |
| Lung | 102 | 0.3–1.9 | 0.6 | 0.2 | 0.4 |
| Fracture | 19 | 0.8–5.5 | 2.7 | 1.2 | 0.5 |
| Uterine fibroid | 7 | 1.7–2.7 | 2.2 | 0.3 | 0.1 |
| Thyroid (focal) | 21 | 1.9–12.3 | 1.7 | 0.6 | 0.3 |
| Pulmonary atelectasis | 14 | 0.9–2.5 | 1.6 | 0.4 | 0.3 |
| Pleural effusion | 12 | 0.7–2.1 | 1.4 | 0.4 | 0.3 |
| Gastrojejunal tube | 2 | 4.1–5.8 | 5 | 1.2 | 0.2 |
| Ileostomy | 3 | 1.5–5.4 | 3.3 | 2 | 0.6 |
| Bowel anastomosis | 8 | 1.7–7.4 | 3.3 | 1.9 | 0.6 |
| Incision | 17 | 1.2–4.3 | 2.6 | 0.9 | 0.4 |
| Breast biopsy site | 2 | 1.3–2.0 | 2.2 | 1.2 | 0.6 |

All values are maximum SUV, except for bladder, which is averaged over the entire bladder.

radiation, chemotherapy, or sentinel node resection, which can interrupt the normal pattern of lymphatic drainage. In such cases, an FDG-avid node in any plausible drainage pathway is best presumed "guilty, until proven innocent."

**Salivary glands**. A symmetric pattern of mild to moderate uptake is typically seen in the parotid and submandibular glands. Asymmetric activity can reflect sialadenitis (on the hotter side), or atrophy, ductal obstruction, or radiation-induced changes

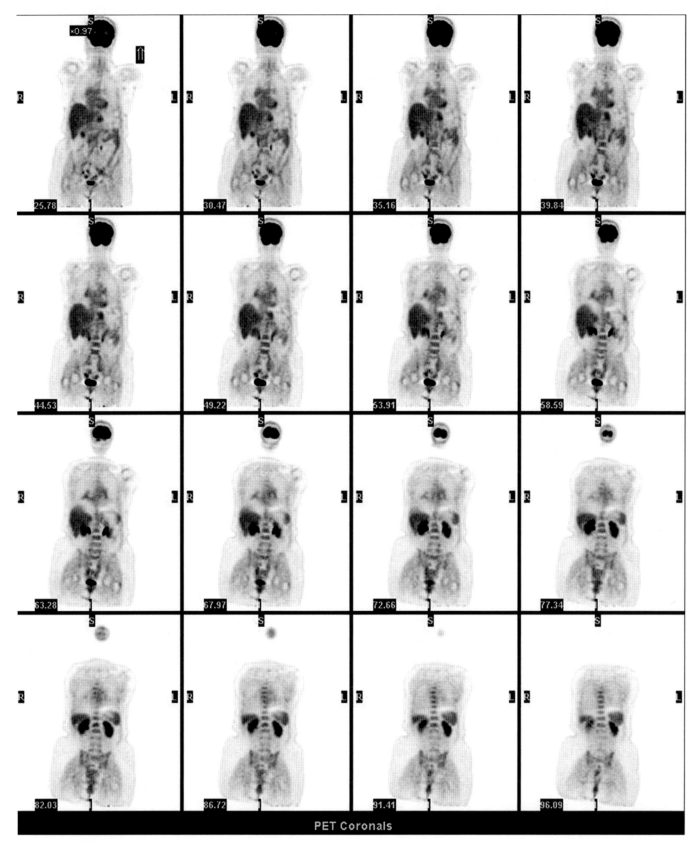

**Figure 4.1** Normal FDG biodistribution.

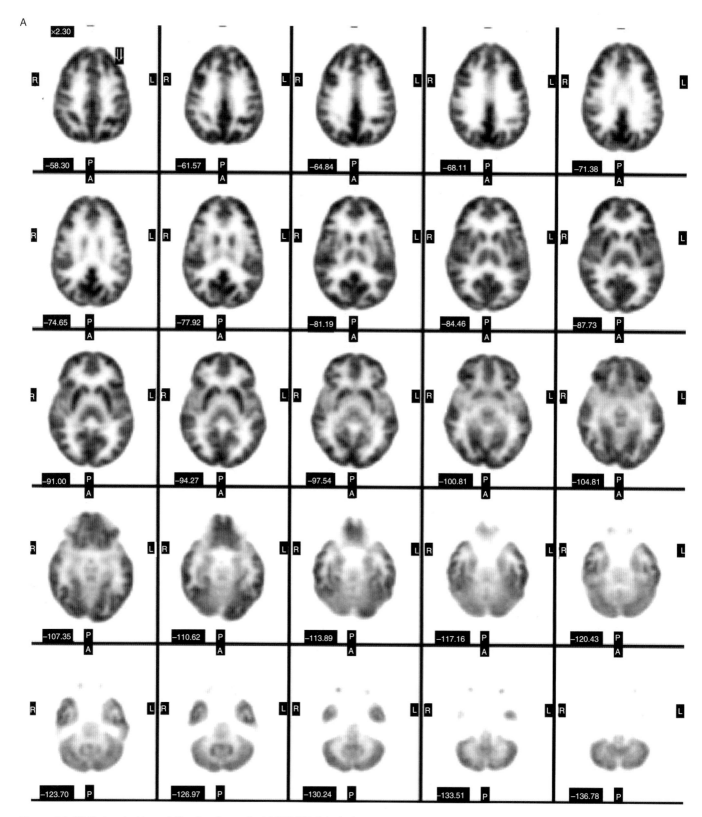

**Figure 4.2** (A) Black and white and (B) color of normal axial FDG-PET of the brain.

B

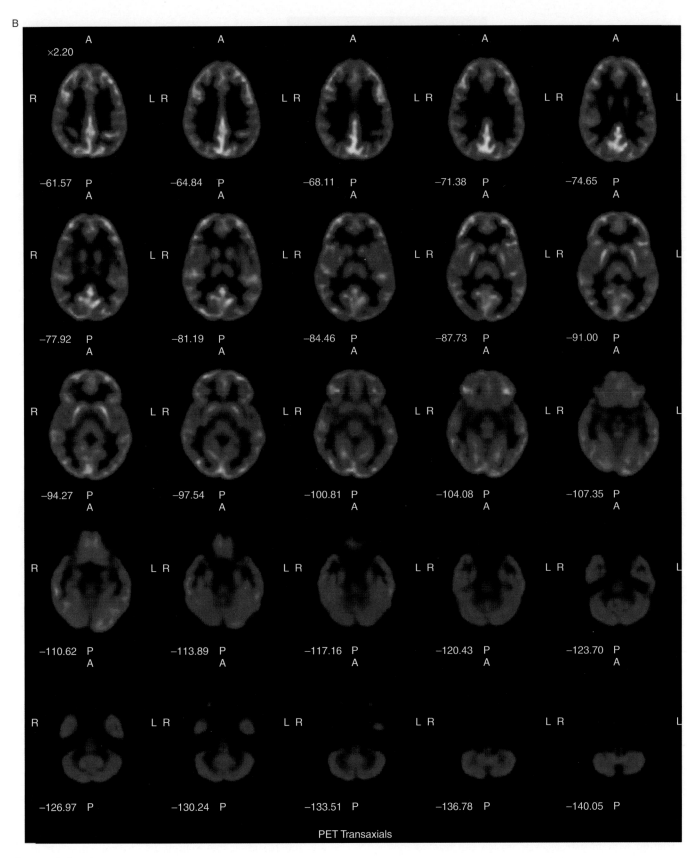

Figure 4.2 (cont.)

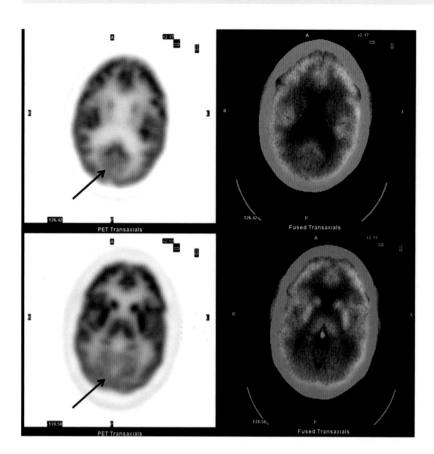

**Figure 4.3** A 45-year-old female with epilepsy. History of blindness secondary to Stevens Johnson syndrome. FDG activity is decreased in the bilateral occipital poles and medial occipital cortex (arrows) adjacent to the caudal half of the calcarine fissure consistent with known blindness. There is no hypometabolic focus to suggest the presence of an interictal seizure focus.

(on the colder side). Focally increased activity in a parotid gland may represent an intraparotid lymph node (normal or diseased) or a true parotid neoplasm.

**Tongue and vocal cords.** Intense uptake is commonly seen at the insertion of the genioglossus and geniohyoid muscles at the midline of the mandible, and at times in the body of the tongue itself (Figure 4.4). This is often exacerbated by streak artifact on the CT, due to metal dental fillings. Although sometimes unavoidable, it can be minimized by keeping the patient from speaking, drinking, or eating during the uptake period after injection.

**Thyroid.** Diffuse uptake can be physiologic or may reflect non-specific thyroiditis (including subacute thyroiditis, Graves' disease, or Hashimoto's thyroiditis) (11, 12). Focal uptake has a significant chance of reflecting thyroid cancer, and should be followed up with thyroid ultrasound in all cases (13, 14).

**Thymus.** Uptake in the involuted thymus is normally indistinguishable from connective tissue background. However, mildly increased uptake can be seen in younger patients and in adults as a rebound effect after chemotherapy (Figure 4.5). Uptake that is significantly greater than this is unlikely to be physiologic, and should raise concern for thymoma, thymic carcinoma, or lymphoma.

**Breast.** Mild subareolar uptake is normal. There is mild variation with menstrual cycle, which can lead to moderate uptake in the post-ovulatory phase. Moderate or even intense uptake can be seen with lactation (Figure 4.6). In males,

gynecomastia is usually associated with mild to moderate uptake. Fat necrosis after lumpectomy can have persistent uptake in the mild-to-moderate range, due to the presence of macrophage-derived giant cells.

**Lung.** On attenuation-corrected images, aerated lungs will show minimal uptake relative to soft-tissue or blood-pool background (Figure 4.1). Blood vessels and bronchi at the lobar or segmental level will show uptake greater than aerated lung, and must be distinguished from tumors of low avidity. Atelectasis is often accompanied by mild uptake (15); above a CAR of 30% or an SUV of 3.0, aspiration pneumonia should be considered. Pulmonary emboli and infarcts can have mild-to-moderate uptake in the acute or subacute phase, and must be carefully distinguished from tumors (16, 17) (Figure 4.7).

**Heart.** Cardiac uptake is extremely variable, and can range from minimal to intense, depending on the levels of glucose, insulin and free fatty acids in blood (17, 18). When FDG imaging is performed for tumor targeting, a long fasting state is recommended. This will minimize blood glucose levels and in the majority of the cases, cardiac FDG uptake, as myocytes shift their metabolism from glucose to free fatty acids. At our institution, cancer imaging is performed after a long fasting period of 6–12 hours. Cardiac FDG activity can also be minimized by a fatty meal protocol at breakfast on the day of the study, and at supper the evening before. Note, however, that, even with the best protocol, patches of residual uptake can often be seen (Figure 4.8). Focal uptake is commonly seen in

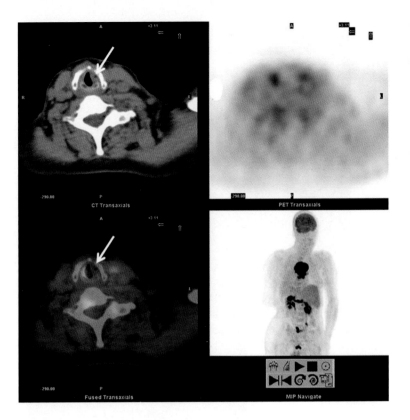

**Figure 4.4** Vocal cord paralysis: FDG accumulation in the right internal laryngeal muscles, with contralateral laryngeal nerve palsy with no radiotracer uptake (arrows) caused by compression of the recurrent laryngeal nerve by the highly FDG-avid mediastinal mass.

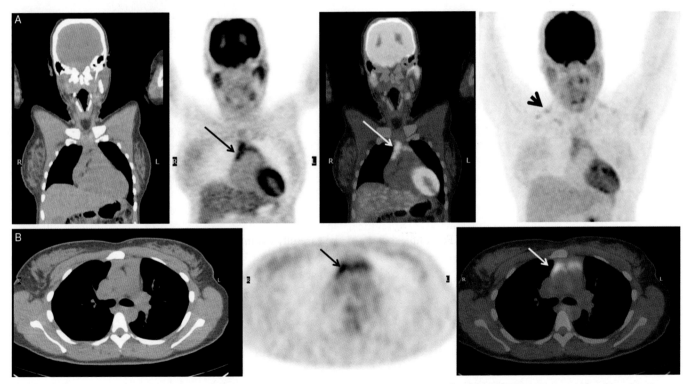

**Figure 4.5** Thymic rebound. (A) coronal CT, FDG-PET, fused FDG-PET/CT, and MIP; (B) axial CT, FDG-PET, fused FDG-PET/CT. A 33-year-old female undergoing FDG-PET/CT imaging for restaging of her invasive ductal breast cancer, status post-chemotherapy for 6 months. There is mild non-specific FDG activity in the nasopharyngeal lymphoid tissues, submandibular glands and the parotid glands. In the anterior mediastinum there is a soft tissue density just deep to the sternum with a location and configuration consistent with thymic tissue with mild-to-moderate FDG activity representing thymic rebound post-chemotherapy (arrows). There is minimal FDG activity in both right and left breasts, with activity in the right breast slightly greater than the left breast, consistent with prior therapy to the right breast. In the supraclavicular regions there are small foci of mild FDG activity secondary to brown fat (arrowhead on MIP image).

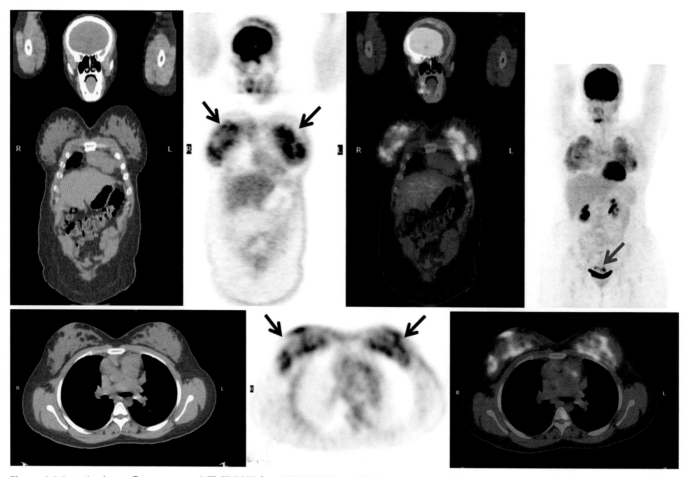

**Figure 4.6** Lactating breast: Top row: coronal CT, FDG-PET, fused FDG-PET/CT, and MIP; Bottom row: axial CT, FDG-PET, fused FDG-PET/CT. A 26-year-old female with anterior mediastinal mass (not shown). FDG-PET/CT was obtained to evaluate for thymic hyperplasia, thymoma, or lymphoma. There is heterogeneous intense FDG uptake in the breasts bilaterally consistent with lactation (arrows). Linear and focal area of FDG uptake immediately superior to the bladder in the anterior midline uterus is noted on the MIP image (red arrow), likely representing healing surgical scar from recent cesarean section.

the papillary muscles. A more problematic finding is intense uptake in an atrial appendage. Only by careful correlation with the CT can a mediastinal node or mass be excluded.

**Blood pool.** Relative activity in the blood pool decreases slightly over time, as tracer is taken up by target tissues or cleared in the urinary tract. A consistent interval between injection and imaging will minimize any diagnostic difficulty; however in patients with renal failure, clearance may be delayed. Small foci of moderate activity are often seen in medium- or large-sized vessels, often near bifurcations. Where there is no corresponding CT abnormality, these may be attributable to slight motion-induced or attenuation-correction related artifacts. However, where calcifications or vessel-wall thickening is present, or where the abnormality is extensive, ulcerated plaques or vasculitis should be considered in the differential.

**Liver.** The liver shows a characteristic nutmeg pattern of background heterogeneity within the mild-to-moderate range, reflecting both metabolic versatility and the presence of a finely interspersed blood pool in the form of venules and sinusoids (Figure 4.1). While intensely avid large metastases

can still be reliably detected, small lesions may be difficult to evaluate against this background. Particularly troublesome are tiny foci of uptake in the high-to-moderate range, without CT correlates, which could represent either metastases or simple background noise. One useful rule is to examine the focus in question on each of the three principal imaging axes. If increased activity is seen on two or more adjacent slices on each axis, then background noise is less likely, and follow-up with MRI or a repeat PET/CT scan may be recommended to further study the possibility of metastasis.

Liver uptake is usually slightly higher than spleen. However, it may be decreased in fatty infiltration, and selectively preserved where there is focal sparing. Uptake may also be decreased in hepatic cirrhosis. Cysts are typically seen as photopenic "holes" on the PET images, although cysts under 1 cm in size may be averaged into the surrounding background, and may thus be undetectable. Cavernous hemangiomas tend to have uptake similar to the liver itself, and are rarely appreciable.

**Spleen.** Splenic uptake is usually homogeneous, in the mild-to-moderate range, and slightly less than liver (Figure 4.1).

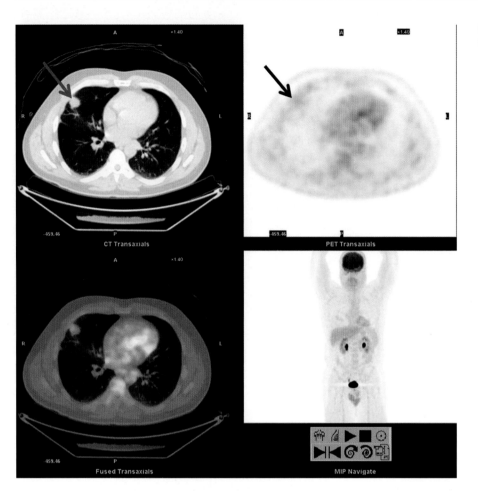

**Figure 4.7** Pulmonary infarct with mild FDG uptake.

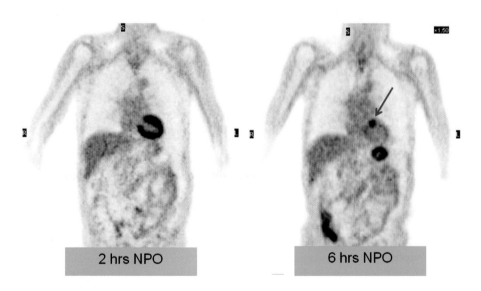

**Figure 4.8** Left: FDG-PET coronal image obtained after a 2-hour fasting period. Notice intense FDG uptake throughout the heart. Right: same patient imaged after fasting for 6 hours, showing that the base of the heart (arrow) is the last myocardial segment to switch from glycolytic to fatty-acid metabolism.

It can be increased in portal hypertension. Diffusely increased uptake in the moderate range can also reflect increased hematopoiesis in anemia or after chemotherapy and/or stimulation with GCSF (Figure 4.14). This should be distinguished from the diffuse pattern of intense uptake, often heterogeneous, which is characteristic of sepsis or infiltrative involvement by lymphoma or leukemia.

**Gastrointestinal tract.** Gastrointestinal uptake can be variable to a troublesome degree. Intense uptake can often be seen in the stomach and colon, particularly the cecum/ascending

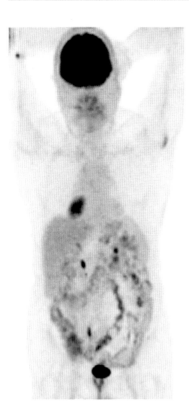

Figure 4.9 Normal GI tract FDG uptake.

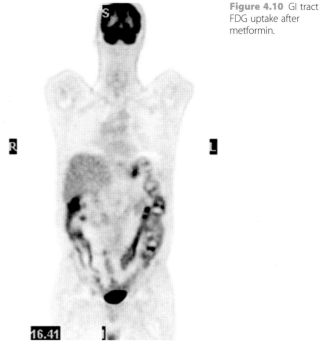

Figure 4.10 GI tract FDG uptake after metformin.

colon and rectosigmoid (Figure 4.9). In the cecum, this has been attributed to a concentration of lymphoid tissue in Peyer's patches. Elsewhere, it may be due to peristalsis, or to factors not yet appreciated. Moderate focal uptake at the gastroesophageal junction is common. This may be either purely physiologic, or may reflect chronic esophagitis due to gastroesophageal reflux. Intense uptake involving long segments of intestine (most frequently the colon) is often seen in diabetics on Metformin therapy (19) (Figure 4.10), and may be reduced after discontinuing the medication for at least 2 or 3 days (20, 21). Segmental uptake may reflect colitis, or, in the distal ileum, active Crohn's disease. Focal areas of intense activity in the colon should always be scrutinized; while these are commonly physiologic or artifactual, adenoma or adenocarcinoma can be difficult to exclude, even with an unremarkable CT. Follow-up with colonoscopy should be considered, particularly where a similar focus is seen on serial PET/CT studies.

**Adrenal glands.** Focal uptake in the adrenals can be quite problematic, since the adrenals are a common site of metastasis, and also of benign nodules/adenomas (see Chapter 7). The "benign range" has been reported to extend to an SUV of 3.5 (equivalent to a brain CAR of 35%). A large nodule with uptake no higher than this is unlikely to represent a metastasis from a primary that has intense uptake. However, for smaller nodules, or where the primary tumor has only mild or moderate uptake, metastasis cannot be excluded with certainty, and dedicated CT or MR adrenal protocols are required.

**Urinary tract.** Urinary activity is invariably intense except in cases of renal failure, precluding definitive evaluation of the kidneys or bladder for urinary tract cancer (although metastases can usually be assessed without difficulty). Most often, the urinary activity is considerably higher than all but the most extremely intense tumors (Figure 4.1). The renal parenchyma is better evaluated on the CT portion of the exam. Renal cysts are acellular structures and should be completely photopenic on PET; even mild activity should raise suspicion for renal cell carcinoma.

Focal uptake associated with ureteral peristalsis is common, but can be difficult to distinguish from metastatic lymph nodes in the pelvis or retroperitoneum. Where such activity is present, the ureters must be carefully traced on the CT from their origin in the renal pelvis to the site of uptake.

**Skeletal muscle.** Uptake is usually low, but can be increased after activity. Athletes who work out can have significant uptake the following day, so rigorous physical activity should be avoided the day before a scan. Uptake in sternocleidomastoid or neck muscles is common, and can be asymmetric. So can uptake in muscles of mastication (temporalis, masseter, and medial and lateral pterygoids) (Figure 4.11). The conformity to the expected muscle belly will usually prevent confusion with true lesions; however, uptake can be focal (frequently in the suboccipital muscles), and may need to be carefully differentiated from misregistered uptake in a vertebra or lymph node. Diffuse muscular uptake usually reflects increased serum insulin levels, either in diabetics with chronic insulin resistance, or in normal patients who have eaten sugary or starchy foods within four hours prior to the exam (Figure 4.12). Focally intense uptake can be seen at sites of recent muscle trauma, or after cardioversion (Figure 4.13).

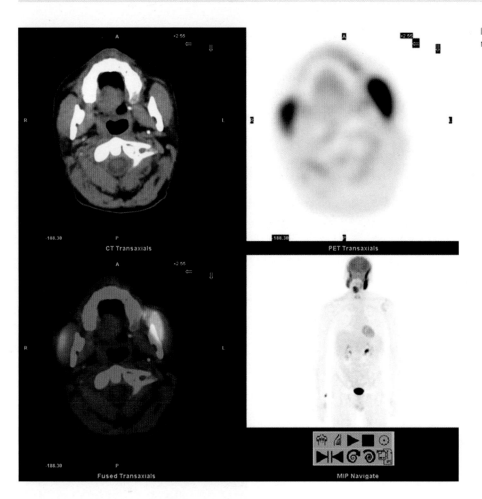

Figure 4.11 FDG uptake in muscles of mastication.

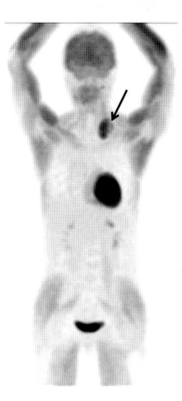

Figure 4.12 A 42-year-old male with recently diagnosed lung adenocarcinoma underwent FDG-PET imaging for initial staging. Note diffuse, moderately intense muscular uptake due hyperinsulinemia. Arrow points to patient's FDG-avid tumor.

**Bone**. Most skeletal uptake is mild and reflects bone marrow activity. In younger patients, marrow activity is quite uniform, however, with aging there is a piecemeal replacement of red marrow with fatty tissue, leading to heterogeneity of uptake, particularly in the spine and sacroiliac region. This can be so irregular that sometimes it may be difficult to exclude metastases. In such cases, a negative CT may not be conclusive, since small or permeative metastases may be inapparent. The only recourse may be MRI, or, failing that, reevaluation of the most suspicious sites on a follow-up PET/CT. Bone marrow uptake can be diffusely increased in anemia or chronic inflammation, and very markedly so after chemotherapy (Figure 4.14). Treated/extinct metastases are usually photopenic on PET and may have a sclerotic appearance on CT. Hemangiomas in the spine are also photopenic on PET, with a "corduroy" pattern of thickened trabeculae on CT. Slightly more prominent uptake is normally seen in articular portions of mobile joints. This can increase to moderate-to-intense levels if active arthritis is present, or at tendinous insertions in cases of enthesopathy.

**Ovary/uterus**. Moderate uptake in the uterine cavity can be seen during mid-cycle (around the time of ovulation) and during the period of menstrual flow (22), as well as in the

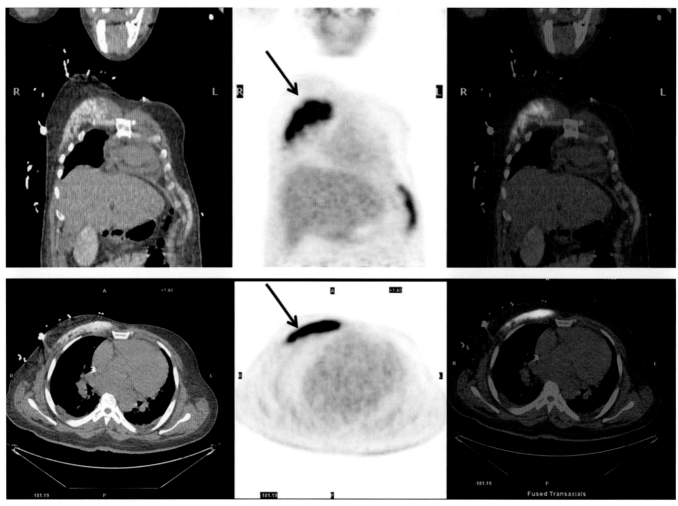

Figure 4.13 Intense chest wall muscle FDG uptake (arrows) after cardioversion.

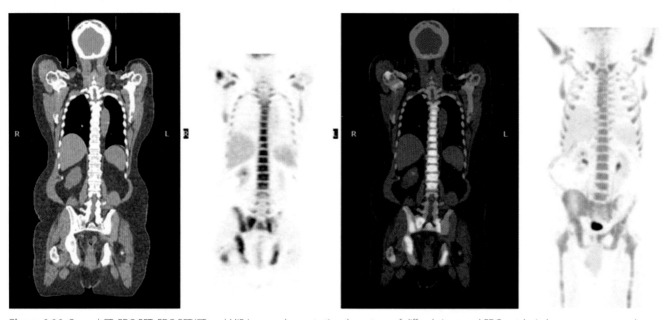

Figure 4.14 Coronal CT, FDG-PET, FDG-PET/CT, and MIP images, demonstrating the pattern of diffusely increased FDG uptake in bone marrow expansion after granulocyte colony-stimulating factor (GCSF) therapy.

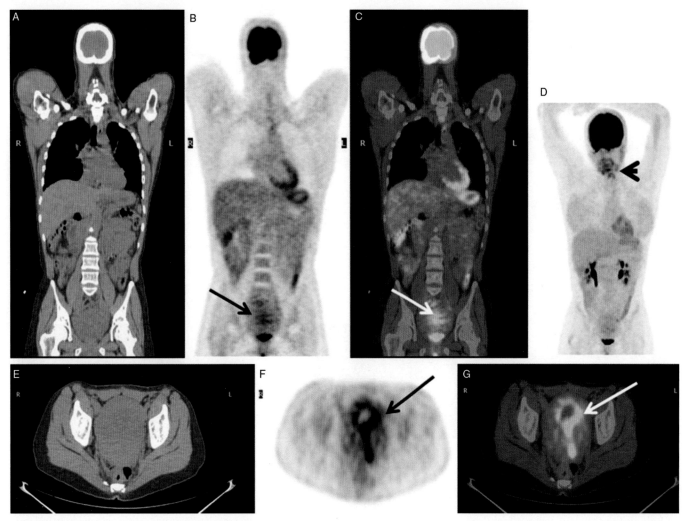

**Figure 4.15** Post-partum endometritis: 36-year-old female with a history of mediastinal lymphoma undergoing FDG-PET/CT for restaging. There is symmetric mild increased FDG uptake in the oropharynx (D: arrowhead), which likely represents benign lymphoid activity. Focus of high uptake within the endometrial cavity of a post-partum uterus (arrows in B, C, F, and G) representing endometritis.

post-partum uterus (Figure 4.15). Endometritis can have a similar appearance, and needs to be excluded by history. Endometrial uptake in a post-menopausal female is always abnormal, and raises concern for endometrial hyperplasia or carcinoma. It should be followed by gynecologic consult in all cases. In an ovulating female, focal ovarian uptake can be seen in ruptured follicles or corpora lutea. An ovarian malignancy can have a similar appearance; if a differential diagnosis is essential, a repeated PET/CT scan after two or more weeks will usually show decrease or resolution of benign uptake (Chapter 12).

**Testis and scrotum.** Baseline uptake is usually in the moderate range, but should be symmetric. Asymmetric uptake could reflect tumor on the hotter side, or torsion or infarct on the colder side. Epididymitis can be seen as a small focus of increased uptake lying directly atop the testis, however this may be difficult to distinguish from tumor and physical exam and ultrasound follow-up is usually indicated. Hydroceles are common, and can be easily spotted as well-circumscribed photopenic areas with fluid density on CT. Inguinal hernias have low uptake if only fat-containing, unless there is chronic inflammation. Herniated bowel will show variable uptake, usually physiologic; however, intense uptake could indicate inflammation or impending strangulation. Rarely, hernias will contain bladder, with very intense urinary uptake.

**Prostate.** Uptake is usually mild, and similar to muscle or soft-tissue background, even in cases of benign prostatic hypertrophy. Very intense focal uptake centrally is occasionally seen due to urethral urinary excretion; this can be very prominent after transurethral resection of the prostate (TURP). Focal uptake that is not centrally located may represent prostatitis or prostatic carcinoma. Note, however, that many prostate cancers are not FDG avid, and the absence of abnormal uptake in a patient with known or suspected prostate cancer is not diagnostically probative.

**Brown fat.** White fat has very low uptake, similar to lung. However, thermogenic brown adipose tissue (BAT) can show moderate to intense uptake, typically in a symmetrical

A

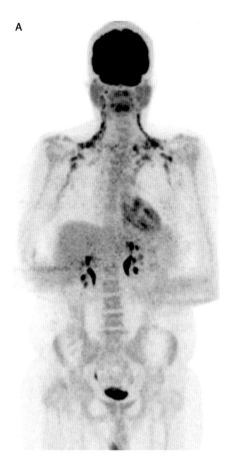

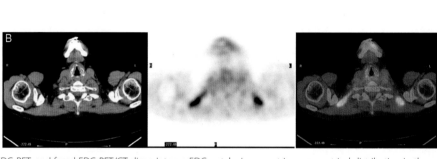

B

**Figure 4.16** Brown fat uptake: (A) MIP; (B) axial CT, FDG-PET, and fused FDG-PET/CT slices. Intense FDG uptake is present in a symmetrical distribution in the neck and supraclavicular regions (A and B). The foci of uptake colocalize with areas of fat density permitting its unequivocal identification (B).

distribution in the lower neck and supraclavicular regions and along the thoracic costovertebral junctions (Figures 4.16 and 4.17). Brown fat uptake may also be found below the diaphragm, as diffuse or even focal extraperitoneal-parahepatic and/or perirenal uptake. Most frequent in children, it may also be seen in adults, particularly women, in the winter months. On PET/CT, the foci of uptake colocalize with areas of fat density, which usually permits unequivocal identification. However, where uptake is very extensive, or where there is significant misregistration between the PET and CT images, cervical or supraclavicular lymphadenopathy may be difficult to exclude. In such cases, a repeat PET/CT may be useful. Ensuring that the patient is kept in an adequately heated environment during the uptake period may help to minimize BAT uptake. Other reported methods include pre-treatment with propranolol or other beta blockers (23), or with a fatty-meal protocol (24).

**Post-surgical changes.** Granulation tissue related to surgical incisions or biopsy tracts will show moderate uptake that gradually resolves, typically within 3–6 months. Intense or persistent uptake raises concern for wound infection. Tumoral seeding of the incision should also be considered if focally intense uptake is accompanied by a distinct mass on CT, or uptake increases in extent on serial studies. Surgical clips,

sutures, mesh, ostomies, tracheotomies, and other foreign bodies often show moderate uptake that can persist indefinitely, due to the aggregation of macrophage-derived giant cells, which are highly FDG-avid. This non-progressive, focal uptake is not accompanied by a distinct mass on CT, and should not be confused with true tumor recurrence at the resection margin. Injection granulomas also feature a giant-cell reaction, and can show uptake in the mild-to-moderate range for a year or more after injection (Figure 4.17).

If mediastinoscopy is performed prior to PET/CT in a patient with lung cancer, typical biopsy-tract changes usually occasion no difficulty (Figure 4.18). However, reactive changes in unsampled lymph nodes can lead to a mild-to-moderate increase in uptake. These changes are non-specific, and can be very difficult to distinguish from nodal metastases. Where such uncertainty exists, it is best acknowledged, although if the mediastinoscopy itself is negative, the surgeon may choose to consider these nodes as "innocent, until proven guilty."

**Chemotherapy.** The immediate effect of chemotherapy is to decrease uptake in bone marrow, although this is rarely seen unless follow-up imaging is performed very early. Once the nadir of myelosuppression has been passed, there is a physiologic rebound of hematopoiesis, which is often

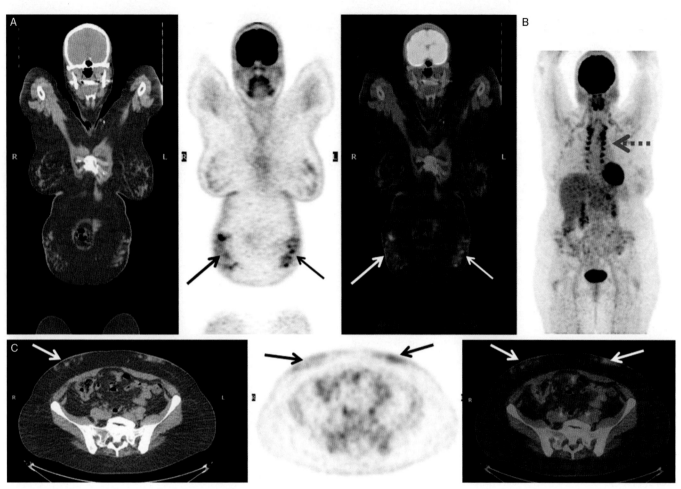

**Figure 4.17** Injection granulomas: (A) coronal CT, FDG-PET, and fused FDG-PET/CT slices; (B) MIP; (C) axial CT, FDG-PET, and fused FDG-PET/CT slices. A 49-year-old female with a history of breast cancer. FDG-PET/CT was obtained for restaging. Images show increased uptake in the paravertebral fat (B: dotted arrow). In addition, there is mild FDG uptake associated with soft tissue nodules in the anterior abdominal wall due to heparin injection granulomas (arrows).

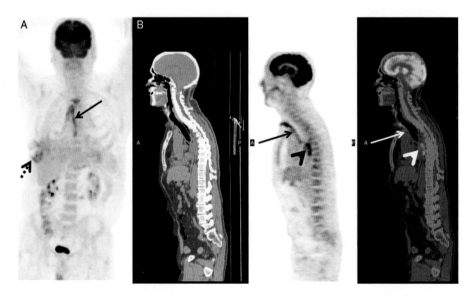

**Figure 4.18** Mediastinoscopy: (A) MIP; (B) sagittal CT, FDG-PET, and fused FDG-PET/CT slices. A 70-year-old female with a history of right epithelial subtype pleural mesothelioma undergoing FDG-PET/CT imaging for restaging. There is abnormal linear FDG activity in the anterior neck extending into the chest, compatible with a post-operative inflammatory reaction from a recent cervical mediastinoscopy (arrows). Abnormal FDG activity is also present in the posterior mediastinum, which may be related to nodal disease (arrowhead), but cannot be differentiated from the FDG activity secondary to mediastinoscopy. Moderate FDG activity in the inferior right chest wall corresponding to recent surgery for mesothelioma (dotted arrow).

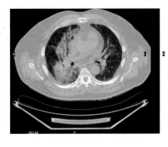 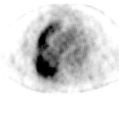 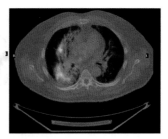

**Figure 4.19** Radiation pneumonitis: axial CT, FDG-PET, and fused FDG-PET/CT slices obtained 4 months after radiotherapy for right lung cancer. The images show the characteristic, intense FDG-uptake pattern with a sharply demarcated linear boundary, consistent with radiation pneumonitis.

therapeutically augmented with granulocyte-colony-stimulating factor (GCSF) or similar agents. This is reflected in a uniform pattern of moderately increased bone marrow uptake throughout the axial and proximal appendicular skeleton, which can persist for several months, or even as long as one year after therapy (Figure 4.14). It is important to distinguish this from the heterogeneous pattern of uptake that is seen with diffuse bone marrow involvement by lymphoma or metastatic carcinoma.

Mild post-chemotherapy uptake can sometimes be seen in the thymus or spleen. Again, this is self-limited. While brain activity is usually unaffected, a persistent pattern of decreased cerebral cortical activity has been described in some patients receiving chemotherapy; this was accompanied by cognitive abnormalities (25).

**Radiation therapy.** Local radiation to the spine causes a well-defined zone of decreased bone marrow uptake that can persist for years after therapy. Radiation pneumonitis is seen as moderate, or occasionally even intense, uptake with a sharply demarcated linear boundary, usually appearing several months after treatment (Figure 4.19). CT will show patchy consolidation in the same distribution. Multiple follow-up PET/CT studies may be required to definitively exclude superimposed areas of tumor recurrence.

## Endnote

1. In the remainder of this chapter, uptake will be described in terms that are defined in terms of comparative activity ratios. Thus, "mild" will refer to uptake that is 20% or less that of the cerebral cortex or basal ganglia, "moderate" to uptake greater than 20% but less than 60%, and "intense" to uptake that is 60% or more. Assuming a typical brain SUV of approximately 10, the equivalent raw SUV measurements would be: "mild," $\leq 2.0$; "moderate," 2.0–6.0; and "intense," $\geq 6.0$.

## References

1. Warburg O. On respiratory impairment in cancer cells. *Science* 1956;**124** (3215):269–70.

2. Warburg O, Wind F, Negelein E. The metabolism of tumors in the body. *J Gen Physiol* 1927;**8**(6):519–30.

3. Carruthers A. Facilitated diffusion of glucose. *Physiol Rev* 1990;**70**(4): 1135–76.

4. Uldry M, Thorens B. The SLC2 family of facilitated hexose and polyol transporters. *Pflugers Arch* 2004; **447**(5):480–9. Erratum in: *Pflugers Arch* 2004;**448**(2):259–60.

5. Crane RK, Dorando FC. On the mechanism of Na+-dependent glucose transport. *Ann N Y Acad Sci* 1980; **339**:46–52.

6. Moran JK, Lee HB, Blaufox MD. Optimization of urinary FDG excretion during PET imaging. *J Nucl Med* 1999; **40**:1352–7.

7. Anderson JW, Herman RH, Tyrrell JB, Cohn RM. Hexokinase: a compartmented enzyme. *Am J Clin Nutr* 1971;**24**(6):642–50.

8. Purich DL, Fromm HJ, Rudolph FB. The hexokinases: kinetic, physical, and regulatory properties. *Adv Enzymol Relat Areas Mol Biol* 1973;**39**:249–326.

9. Torizuka T, Tamaki N, Inokuma T *et al.* In vivo assessment of glucose metabolism in hepatocellular carcinoma with FDG-PET. *J Nucl Med* 1995;**36**(10):1811–17.

10. Britz-Cunningham SH, Millstine JW, Gerbaudo VH. Improved discrimination of benign and malignant lesions on FDG PET/CT, using comparative activity ratios to brain, basal ganglia, or cerebellum. *Clin Nucl Med* 2008;**33**(10):681–7.

11. Boerner AR, Voth E, Theissen P *et al.* Glucose metabolism of the thyroid in autonomous goiter measured by F-18-FDG-PE. *Exp Clin Endocrinol Diabetes* 2000;**108**(3):191–6.

12. Park CH, Lee EJ, Kim JK, Joo HJ, Jang JS. Focal F-18 FDG uptake in a nontoxic autonomous thyroid nodule. *Clin Nucl Med* 2002;**27**(2):136–7.

13. Ramos CD, Chisin R, Yeung HW, Larson SM, Macapinlac HA. Incidental focal thyroid uptake on FDG positron emission tomographic scans may represent a second primary tumor. *Clin Nucl Med* 2001;**26**(3):193–7.

14. Kang KW, Kim SK, Kang HS *et al.* Prevalence and risk of cancer of focal thyroid incidentaloma identified by 18F-fluorodeoxyglucose positron emission tomography for metastasis evaluation and cancer screening in healthy subjects. *J Clin Endocrinol Metab* 2003;**88**(9):4100–4.

15. Gerbaudo VH, Julius B. Anatomo-metabolic characteristics of atelectasis in F-18 FDG-PET/CT imaging. *Eur J Radiol* 2007;**64**(3):401–5.

16. Kamel EM, McKee TA, Calcagni ML *et al.* Occult lung infarction may induce false interpretation of 18F-FDG PET in primary staging of pulmonary malignancies. *Eur J Nucl Med Mol Imaging* 2005;**32**(6):641–6.

17. Nguyên VT, Mossberg KA, Tewson TJ *et al.* Temporal analysis of myocardial glucose metabolism by 2-[18F]fluoro-2-deoxy-D-glucose. *Am J Physiol* 1990;**259**(4 Pt 2):H1022–31.

18. Choi Y, Brunken RC, Hawkins RA *et al.* Factors affecting myocardial 2-[F-18]

fluoro-2-deoxy-D-glucose uptake in positron emission tomography studies of normal humans. *Eur J Nucl Med* 1993;**20**(4):308–18.

19. Gontier E, Fourme E, Wartski M *et al.* High and typical 18F-FDG bowel uptake in patients treated with metformin. *Eur J Nucl Med Mol Imaging* 2008;**35**(1):95–9.

20. Ozülker T, Ozülker F, Mert M, Ozpaçaci T. Clearance of the high intestinal (18)F-FDG uptake associated with metformin after stopping the drug. *Eur J Nucl Med Mol Imaging* 2010;**37**(5):1011–17.

21. Oh JR, Song HC, Chong A *et al.* Impact of medication discontinuation on increased intestinal FDG accumulation in diabetic patients treated with metformin. *Am J Roentgenol* 2010;**195**(6):1404–10.

22. Lerman H, Metser U, Grisaru D *et al.* Normal and abnormal 18F-FDG endometrial and ovarian uptake in pre- and postmenopausal patients: assessment by PET/CT. *J Nucl Med* 2004;**45**(2):266–71.

23. Parysow O, Mollerach AM, Jager V *et al.* Low-dose oral propranolol could reduce brown adipose tissue F-18 FDG uptake in patients undergoing PET scans. *Clin Nucl Med* 2007;**32**(5):351–7.

24. Williams G, Kolodny GM. Method for decreasing uptake of 18F-FDG by hypermetabolic brown adipose tissue on PET. *Am J Roentgenol* 2008;**190**(5):1406–9.

25. Aluise CD, Sultana R, Tangpong J *et al.* Chemo brain (chemo fog) as a potential side effect of doxorubicin administration: role of cytokine-induced, oxidative/nitrosative stress in cognitive dysfunction. *Adv Exp Med Biol* 2010;**678**:147–56.

# Brain

## 5

### Laura L. Horky and Wei Chen

In the USA, over 44,500 people are diagnosed with primary brain tumors each year, approximately 20,500 of which are malignant (1). Primary brain tumors were the cause of death of approximately 12,920 people in 2009, according to an estimate by the American Cancer Society (2). Over 140,000 people in the USA are diagnosed each year with brain metastases, most commonly from lung, breast, and colon cancer primaries (3, 4). Nuclear imaging plays an important role in the diagnosis and management of both primary and metastatic brain tumors. This chapter will review the brain tumor pathology and clinical management and will discuss the role of nuclear imaging with a particular emphasis on the most common clinical indication for nuclear brain tumor imaging: evaluate for tumor recurrence versus post-radiation necrosis.

## Staging

### Gliomas

Gliomas are derived from glia which comprise 90% of the cells within the brain and play an important role in cellular homeostasis. Gliomas are subdivided into astrocytic, oligodendroglial, and mixed oligoastrocytic types (Table 5.1).

The WHO classification separates gliomas into Grades I–IV on the basis of histological features. Since they are often heterogeneous, gliomas are classified based on the most malignant sample of tissue analyzed. Low grade gliomas (Grades I–II) are characterized by high cellularity, pleomorphism, and a low cellular proliferation rate or mitotic index. High grade gliomas (Grade III–IV) have high cellularity and pleomorphism and a high mitotic index. Grade IV astrocytomas (also called

glioblastoma multiforme or GBM) are characterized by endothelial proliferation and/or necrotic features. Low-grade gliomas are further classified into three subtypes: pilocytic astrocytoma (grade I), astrocytoma (grade II), and oligodendroglioma (grade II). High-grade gliomas include grade III anaplastic astrocytoma and anaplastic oligodendroglioma, and grade IV glioblastoma (5).

Grade I astrocytomas, also known as pilocytic astrocytomas, are most common in children and young adults and are associated with a favorable prognosis, with an 85% survival rate at 20 years (6). Because they are well-circumscribed tumors, they are often treated with surgery alone. Malignant transformation is rare.

Grade II gliomas account for 5–10% of all adult brain tumors. These tumors are infiltrative and typically are associated with an intact blood–brain barrier. Therefore, they do not enhance on MRI and are often ill-defined on anatomic studies. Their proliferation index is low at only 2–4%. Though once considered benign, they are now classified as malignant, due to their high potential of malignant transformation (7). These tumors may be treated surgically, however, due to their infiltrative nature, complete resection is not possible. Radiotherapy also plays a role in management, although optimal timing of radiation therapy is not well established for these tumors. Astrocytomas and oligodendrogliomas, both types of grade II gliomas, are often indistinguishable on MRI. They are associated with different outcomes; therefore, an accurate diagnosis is important. Oligodendrogliomas respond more effectively than astrocytomas to chemotherapy and have a better overall prognosis. The 5-year survival of patients with astrocytomas is

**Table 5.1** WHO classification of glial tumors.

| Grade I | Grade II | Grade III | Grade IV |
|---|---|---|---|
| Pilocytic astrocytoma | Diffuse astrocytoma | Anaplastic astrocytoma | Glioblastoma multiforme |
| Fibrillary astrocytoma | Oligodendroglioma | Anaplastic oligodendroglioma | |
| | Oligoastrocytoma | Anaplastic oligoastrocytoma | |

approximately 37%, compared with 70% in patients with oligodendrogliomas (8). One of the keys in nuclear imaging, as will be discussed in a later section, is to distinguish low- from high-grade portions of a tumor in order to detect malignant transformation and to provide biopsy guidance.

Grade III and Grade IV gliomas are together classified as malignant or "high grade" gliomas. The median survival for grade III astrocytomas is 2–3 years, as compared with approximately 12 months for Grade IV gliomas (9). Grade IV gliomas (GBM) are the most common glioma type, accounting for 40–50% of all gliomas. High-grade gliomas often evolve from low-grade gliomas but some, particularly GBM, present *de novo* in their high-grade form. The current standard of care for high-grade gliomas includes biopsy or subtotal resection followed by concurrent radiotherapy and low-dose chemotherapy (temozolomide) for a period of 6 weeks, followed by a protracted course of high-dose temozolomide (10). High-grade gliomas almost inevitably recur after treatment. Routine MRI surveillance is performed (usually bimonthly), and progression is suspected when growth of a contrast-enhancing lesion is observed. An enlarging contrast-enhanced lesion may represent tumor progression or radiation-induced necrosis (also called pseudoprogression). Nuclear imaging plays a key diagnostic role in distinguishing between these possibilities.

## Brain metastases

Metastatic brain tumors are even more common than primary brain tumors and are associated with the death of over 100,000 people per year (11). The median survival for patients with brain metastases is less than 1 year, and many of these patients die from systemic disease. Brain metastases are detected in 20–40% of cancer patients, and the frequency of brain metastases has increased in recent years as a function of prolonged survival in patients with primary extracranial tumors. The most frequent tumor types that metastasize to the brain are lung, breast, colon, and malignant melanoma, in descending order (4). Surgery and/or radiation are the primary treatments for brain metastases. Solitary metastatic lesions are typically well-circumscribed and often resectable. It has been shown that patients who have surgery plus whole-brain irradiation survive longer than those who receive surgery alone (12, 13, 14). If lesions are multiple or not treatable by surgery, radiation therapy is the preferred treatment.

## Radiation injury

Radiation is a standard component of therapy for high-grade gliomas and is also used selectively in patients with brain metastases, as well as in other brain tumors such as surgically inaccessible meningiomas. Radiation therapy options include whole brain radiation (WBRT), stereotactic radiosurgery (SRS), and intensity modulated radiotherapy (IMRT). SRS is often used in lesions that are not surgically accessible. It is also used for the treatment of recurrent tumors after the patient has previously been treated with whole brain radiation.

Stereotactic radiosurgery is a targeted approach that concentrates radiation on the lesion, minimizing the damage to the normal brain parenchyma. This approach results in a higher radiation dose to the region of interest and induces radiation necrosis in 20% of patients as opposed to 5% of patients treated with WBRT; the risk is even higher in patients who have had both WBRT and SRS at various stages in their therapy (15). The risk of radiation necrosis also increases when the patient also receives chemotherapy, but actual figures are not clearly established at present (16).

Necrosis may occur after radiation or chemotherapy, and on MRI is often indistinguishable from residual or recurrent tumor. Seventy percent of cases of radiation necrosis occur within the first 2 years after radiation. The incidence of late-delayed radiation necrosis is 5–37% and increases as a function of radiation dose (11, 17). Radiation injury may occur from hours to years after treatment and is classified as early (hours to weeks), early delayed (weeks to months), and late delayed (four months to several years) (16). Early radiation necrosis is caused by edema, demyelination, necrosis, and vascular proliferation. From approximately 4 months to several years, the pathologic basis of radiation necrosis includes vascular necrosis and vascular proliferation, edema, hemorrhagic necrosis of the gray and white matter, demyelination and axonal swelling, and reactive gliosis. Chronic radiation necrosis is a result of reactive gliosis, vascular inflammation, and cyst formation. Acute and early delayed radiation necrosis are reversible, whereas late and chronic radiation necrosis are usually not (16, 17).

## Imaging options
### Magnetic resonance imaging (MRI)

MRI with and without contrast is considered the gold standard for initial evaluation and follow-up of brain tumors, both primary and metastatic. There is no associated radiation exposure to the patient, and the test is generally well tolerated by patients. Standard MRI sequences demonstrate the number, size, and location of lesions, as well as the state of the surrounding brain. The presence of edema, mass effect, and hemorrhage can be clearly determined. Contrast enhancement is dependent on the integrity of the blood–brain barrier. Low-grade gliomas are typically minimally or non-contrast enhancing, due to an intact blood–brain barrier. High-grade gliomas are typically contrast-enhancing on MRI, due to disruption of the blood–brain barrier. They often cross the midline to involve both cerebral hemispheres. Ring-enhancing lesions, necrosis, and increased relative cerebral blood volume (rCBV) are associated with GBM. On MR spectroscopy, elevation in the choline (Cho) peak and depression of the N-acetylaspartate (NAA) peak indicate the presence of tumor, and the Cho/NAA ratio has been used to determine glioma grade. Also, the presence of a lactic acid peak is associated with a higher grade (18).

Different MRI sequences are useful, depending on the glioma grade. In the case of a non-contrast-enhancing low-grade glioma, T2WI and FLAIR images are the preferred sequences to estimate the extent of tumor infiltration. For metastases and high-grade gliomas as well as other tumors such as meningiomas, post-contrast images often best demonstrate the lesions (T1 post-contrast or 3-D SPGR sequences). It should be noted, however, that Grade III gliomas and even glioblastomas may present as non-contrast enhancing tumors. Histologic sampling is needed to make a diagnosis. Standard T1 post-contrast MRI cannot distinguish recurrent tumor from post-radiation necrosis because both are contrast-enhancing. More advanced sequences such as MR spectroscopy and perfusion and diffusion sequences may increase the accuracy of MRI for distinguishing tumor from radiation necrosis, but as we will see, metabolic imaging often provides superior specificity. MRI is, however, an indispensable guide for the interpretation of nuclear brain images. There is high background cortical uptake in FDG brain PET, in order to evaluate the FDG avidity of a contrast-enhancing lesion, particularly one in a region of high background metabolism, fusion to a contrast MRI is very helpful [19]. For brain metastases in particular, PET-MRI co-registration was shown to improve the sensitivity of PET in distinguishing recurrence from post-radiation necrosis from 65% to 86% in one series (specificity unchanged at 80%)[20, 21].

## Nuclear medicine imaging of brain tumors

Nuclear imaging of brain tumors provides functional information about tumor blood flow, glucose metabolism, and other metabolic characteristics such as protein transport, mitosis, and hypoxia. A variety of radiotracers are available for tumor characterization. Each tracer provides certain clues about tumor behavior, and selection of the proper tool for each case is vital.

## Single photon emission computed tomography (SPECT)

Prior to the advent of PET imaging, SPECT imaging was a vital modality in nuclear brain imaging. With SPECT imaging, multiple 2-D images are acquired by a gamma camera that circles around the patient, and the images are then tomographically reconstructed to create a 3-D image dataset. In state-of-the-art SPECT–CT imaging, these images are combined with CT images that are acquired in the same session. Tracers used for brain tumor SPECT imaging include [201]thallium and Technetium-99m sestamibi ([99m]Tc-sestamibi). These tracers still have an important role in the modern management of brain tumor patients.

[201]**Thallium** is a potassium analog and an indicator of perfusion and sodium-potassium pump activity. It was initially used in the mid 1970s for cardiac imaging studies to evaluate myocardial perfusion and viability, and it soon found applications in brain imaging as well. It is only taken up by viable cells

and is thus a good discriminator between tumor recurrence and radiation necrosis. It is primarily a 69–83 keV X-ray emitter, which is a relatively low energy. The disadvantage of a low energy emitter from an imaging perspective is that the lesion must be large for its signal to be detected, particularly if the lesion is deep within the brain. Its half life is 73 hours, and the dose administered is approximately 4 mCi; the long half life limits the dose. This provides a satisfactory signal in lesions of at least 1.5 cm. [201]Thallium does not cross the blood–brain barrier, and therefore the target/background signal ratio is favorable. As this tracer does not cross the blood–brain barrier, it is used only to assess lesions that are contrast enhancing on MRI, and not for low-grade gliomas when the blood–brain barrier is usually intact [22].

[201]Thallium SPECT was shown to have a specificity of 100% in one study to distinguish recurrent tumor from radiation necrosis at 6 or more weeks after radiation therapy [23, 24]. False-positive thallium uptake can be seen in acute or subacute hemorrhage [25] and within the first 6 weeks after radiation, where thallium accumulates in mobilized inflammatory cells such as macrophages [23]. There are different methods for interpretation of thallium images, but comparison of uptake in the lesion to that of the normal contralateral cortex appears to provide the highest predictive power in distinguishing tumor from radiation necrosis [26].

[99m]**Tc-sestamibi** is another gamma imaging tracer, which is useful in brain-tumor imaging. Sestamibi is bound to Technetium-99m, which has imaging characteristics superior to those of thallium. Its energy is 140 keV and its half life is 6 hours. The short half life permits a higher dose administration (20–25 mCi), another favorable imaging characteristic. Sestamibi was originally used in cardiac, parathyroid, and breast imaging. It is an isonitrile that is taken up by mitochondria as a function of their negative electrical potential [22]. It is useful in brain-tumor imaging because the background uptake is negligible. Like thallium, it does not accumulate in normal brain parenchyma where the blood–brain barrier is intact. While thallium can be used for tumor grading, there is no clear association between tumor grade and sestamibi uptake [27]. Unlike thallium, sestamibi accumulates in the choroid plexus, which is responsible for cerebrospinal fluid (CSF) production and is found in the lateral, third, and fourth ventricles. Because of this uptake pattern, care must be taken when assessing paraventricular lesions. This is not troublesome if the images are interpreted with or fused to a recent MRI for precise anatomic localization. Sestamibi may be preferred over thallium for SPECT imaging if the lesion is smaller than 1.5 to 2.0 cm due to its favorable imaging characteristics. However, it should be noted that the sensitivity of SPECT is limited for lesions smaller that approximately 2.0 cm, and false-negative interpretations may be frequent at smaller sizes [28]. For certain lesions that are not characteristically FDG-avid, Thallium SPECT imaging is preferred over FDG-PET. These include lobular breast

carcinoma and some renal cell carcinomas. FDG avidity is usually determined by assessing avidity of the primary tumor on an initial staging PET scan.

# Positron emission tomography (PET)

## FDG-PET

$^{18}$F-fluorodeoxyglucose (FDG), is the workhorse of oncologic imaging. FDG-PET was first used in humans for the purpose of functional brain mapping (29, 30). Shortly after, FDG-PET was used for the assessment of gliomas, the first oncologic application of FDG-PET in humans (31). It is the preferred imaging tracer for brain tumors, because the resolution of PET is superior to that of SPECT imaging, allowing accurate assessment of lesions as small as approximately 0.5 cm$^3$ (approximate diameter of 7–10 mm). It is preferred because of its associated higher resolution (PET versus SPECT camera) rather than the properties of the tracer. FDG-PET provides a measure of glucose uptake and metabolism (31). FDG-PET has been shown to be useful in predicting primary brain-tumor grade and survival (32), determining the most highly metabolic tissue for biopsy planning (33, 34), and monitoring low-grade gliomas for malignant degeneration (35).

In general, high FDG uptake correlates with increased glucose metabolism. High-grade gliomas have high glucose metabolism whereas low-grade tumors have low levels of glucose metabolism. Cut-off levels of FDG in tumor relative to normal brain have been determined to allow differentiation between high- and low–grade brain tumors. A tumor to white matter ratio of greater than 1.5 and a tumor to cortex ratio of greater than 0.6 correlate with high-grade malignancy (primary tumors and brain metastases), with a sensitivity of 100% and a specificity of 67% for gliomas and a sensitivity of 94% and a specificity of 77% for all brain tumors (32). With a few exceptions, it has been shown in gliomas that high FDG avidity is associated with a shorter survival, and is therefore a useful prognostic indicator. In one group of 166 patients with low-grade tumors classified by FDG uptake, 94% of patients with tumor uptake less than or equal to that of normal white matter survived for at least 1 year, and 19% survived for at least 5 years. In contrast, among 165 patients with high-grade tumors, the median survival was only 11 months, with only 29% surviving for more than 1 year, and none surviving 5 years (36).

High FDG uptake in certain low-grade tumors such as pilocytic astrocytomas, neuromas and benign pituitary adenomas (not included in the aforementioned study) are exceptions to the rule (37, 38). Pilocytic astrocytoma, the most benign type of glioma, can have a variable appearance on FDG-PET, ranging from uptake below that of normal white matter to higher than normal gray matter. These are found usually in pediatric patients, and are associated with high survival rates, but they may have high-grade imaging features on both MRI and PET (37). On MRI, they may be contrast enhancing, attributable to

**Table 5.2** $^{18}$F-fluorodeoxyglucose (FDG) avidity in brain lesions.

| High | Variable | Low |
|---|---|---|
| Grade III and IV gliomas | Metastases (lung, breast, squamous cell carcinoma, melanoma) | Grade II glioma |
| Pilocytic astrocytoma | Oligoastrocytoma | PNET (Primitive neurectodermal tumor) |
| Medulloblastoma | Meningioma | Neurinoma |
| Primary CNS lymphoma | Craniopharyngioma | Delayed radiation necrosis |
| Pineoblastoma | | |
| Pituitary adenoma | | |
| Central neurocytoma | | |

fenestrated endothelial cells and a leaky blood–brain barrier (39). High metabolism on FDG-PET has been attributed to high proliferative activity of capillary endothelial cells (40, 41, 42). This endothelial proliferation does not correlate with glial proliferation, and overall FDG uptake is not an accurate predictor of grade or outcome for this tumor.

Meningiomas may also have variable FDG uptake; higher uptake tends to correlate with the aggressiveness of the tumor, and uptake tends to be higher in atypical than in typical meningiomas (43). This will be discussed in further detail in case #4.

The FDG uptake characteristics of different brain-tumor types are summarized in Table 5.2.

FDG uptake in metastases is even more variable than in primary brain tumors. Di Chiro et al. demonstrated in an early study that in 2 of 6 patients with brain metastases, FDG uptake was less than that of the white matter. Such lesions may go undetected on FDG-PET, particularly if attempting to distinguish radiation necrosis from tumor recurrence (43). As will be demonstrated in the case studies in this chapter, certain tumors such as lobular breast cancer, renal cell carcinoma, and mucinous cancers are not characteristically highly FDG avid and can easily be missed in the brain, which is one of the most highly metabolic organs in the body. Because of the variable uptake of metastases and the high background physiologic uptake of the brain, FDG-PET should not be used as a screening tool for identifying brain metastases when a whole body oncologic scan is performed. MRI is a more sensitive tool than FDG–PET for detecting brain lesions.

As discussed earlier, a false-negative interpretation on FDG-PET may result if the lesion is below the resolution of PET (7–8 mm, depending on the inherent metabolic activity of the lesion and the metabolic activity of the background tissue). Some histological types such as CNS lymphoma and glioblastoma multiforme are intensely FDG avid, and PET is occasionally sensitive for even smaller lesions of these histological types. Alternately, false-positive interpretations may also occur. Inflammatory and infectious lesions may be intensely FDG-avid, including recent post-radiation changes, abscesses, and granulomatous disease, i.e., neurosarcoidosis (44). In the case of inflammatory lesions, glycolytic activity in granulocytes and macrophages account for the uptake. Brain tumor-related epilepsy is not uncommon, and a seizure during the FDG uptake would appear FDG-avid and may give the false appearance of an FDG-avid tumor.

Dual-phase FDG-PET imaging appears promising as a method of increasing the sensitivity and specificity of FDG-PET in distinguishing tumor recurrence from post-radiation necrosis. It was shown that images acquired at 180–480 minutes after FDG injection were more helpful than images acquired at the routine time point of 1 hour after injection (45). This technique capitalizes on the differing FDG tracer kinetics between normal brain and tumor. On standard 1-hour imaging, the kinetics of gray matter and tumor are similar. At delayed time points, however, FDG tracer kinetics significantly differ between normal cortex and tumor. Tumor has higher levels of hexokinase, and FDG uptake continues for a longer time period. Also, some FDG-6-phosphate is dephosphorylated over time, preferentially in normal cortex, and therefore tumor appears more FDG avid as the background fades. This results in improved tumor-to-background distinction (45). A case example will be illustrated in a later section.

## Other PET tracers

## Amino acid tracers

Amino acid tracers are a class of radiotracers that play an important role in brain-tumor characterization, particularly for biopsy guidance, distinguishing recurrent tumor from post-radiation necrosis, and in distinguishing benign from malignant lesions (46). Among the major advantages of amino acid tracers over FDG and thallium are that increased uptake is seen in low-grade gliomas, uptake is not dependent on a damaged blood–brain barrier, the background uptake is negligible, and uptake is not cell cycle-specific (47).

Brain-tumor transport of amino acids is typically high relative to normal brain tissue, resulting in a favorable tumor-to-background uptake ratio for brain tumors. Amino acids are transported through the blood–brain barrier and into the cell via the large neutral amino acid transporter, which is densely present on endothelial cell membranes (48). While $^{11}$C-methionine is incorporated into proteins and metabolized, many other amino acid tracers such as O-2–18F-fluoroethyl-L-tyrosine (FET) and 3,4-dihydroxy-6–18F-fluoro-L-phenylalanine (F-DOPA) are transport-only amino acid analogs which are not incorporated into proteins or metabolized (37). In fact, it has been shown that amino acid transport is bidirectional, and higher-grade gliomas demonstrate more rapid influx and efflux of F-DOPA, as opposed to low-grade gliomas (49). F-DOPA has proven to be a valuable tracer in for brain-tumor imaging. The application of F-DOPA in brain-tumor imaging was discovered serendipitously in a patient who was undergoing a scan for Parkinson's disease, with the incidental discovery of a brain tumor (50).

$^{11}$C-methionine was developed as an amino acid tracer for brain-tumor imaging over a decade ago (51). $^{11}$C-methionine has a short half life of only 20 minutes and therefore can only be used in centers with an in-house cyclotron. Methionine uptake tends to correlate with tumor grade and prognosis; higher-grade tumors tend to have higher methionine uptake than lower-grade tumors. Methionine is not taken up by all low-grade gliomas, however, and uptake levels cannot be used reliably for tumor grading (52).

### Mitotic indicator

3′-deoxy-3′-$^{18}$F-fluorothymidine (FLT) is a surrogate marker for cellular proliferation, and its uptake correlates with the histological proliferation marker Ki67. It is phosphorylated by the enzyme thymidine kinase-1 (TK-1) and subsequently trapped intracellularly. FLT demonstrates low or undetectable uptake in low-grade tumors and high uptake in high-grade tumors. Low-grade gliomas are not well demonstrated with FLT, and like FDG it is therefore useful for tumor grading. FLT will be discussed in further detail in the clinical cases (53, 54).

## Other applications of PET

## Biopsy planning

As previously stated, brain tumors are often heterogeneous in their histological composition and are classified according to the highest grade portion of the surgical specimen. The patient's therapy is based on the tumor's grade, and in certain centers, a patient may be eligible for certain therapeutic trials based on tumor grade. FDG-PET has been shown to provide superior biopsy guidance versus CT, in that lesions with higher metabolic activity provided better diagnostic accuracy than contrast-enhancing foci (34, 55). More recently it was demonstrated that $^{11}$C-methionine outperforms FDG in PET-guided biopsy planning. Thirty-two patients with unresectable gliomas underwent both FDG- and methionine-PET scans prior to biopsy. When tumor uptake was greater than normal cortical uptake, FDG was used for biopsy guidance. When tumor uptake was less than or equal to normal cortical uptake and tumor could not be distinguished from background, methionine was used. When methionine served as a guide, 100% of the 61 biopsies of methionine-positive tissue yielded diagnostic results. Likewise, 100% of the nine methionine-negative biopsies were non-diagnostic. It was concluded from this study that if only one tracer is used for preoperative planning for biopsy guidance, it should be methionine (56). Subsequently, FET-PET with MRI co-registration was demonstrated to be 93% sensitive and 94% specific for tumor, as opposed to 96% sensitivity and 53% specificity using MRI alone (57).

# References

1. North American Brain Tumor Coalition. *CBTRUS (2005) Statistical Report: Primary Brain Tumors in the United States, 1998–2002.* [Web page www.nabraintumor.org/facts.html] 2005 [cited 2010 March 1].

2. American Cancer Society. *Cancer Facts & Figures Report 2009.* [Web page http://www.scribd.com/doc/21686287/ Cancer-Facts-and-Figures-Report-2009] 2009 [cited 2010 March 1].

3. Medline Plus. *Medical Encyclopedia: Metastatic brain tumor.* [Web page http://www.nlm.gov/medlineplus/print/ ency/article/000769.htm] 2006 [cited 2010 March 1].

4. Arnold SM, Patchell RA. Diagnosis and management of brain metastases. *Hematol – Oncol Clin N Am* 2001;**15**(6):1085–107.

5. Kleihues P, Burger PC, Scheithauer BW. The new WHO classification of brain tumours. *Brain Pathol* 1993;**3**(3):255–68.

6. Kayama T, Tominaga T, Yoshimoto T. Management of pilocytic astrocytoma. *Neurosurg Rev* 1996;**19**(4):217–20.

7. Lang FF, Gilbert MR. Diffusely infiltrative low-grade gliomas in adults. *J Clin Oncol* 2006;**24**(8):1236–45.

8. Central Brain Tumor Registry of the United States. *CBTRUS. Statistical Report: Primary Brain Tumors in the United States 1995–1999.* [Web page http://www. cbtrus.org/reports/2002/2002report.pdf] 2002 [cited 2010 March 1].

9. Smith JS, Jenkins RB. Genetic alterations in adult diffuse glioma: occurrence, significance, and prognostic implications. *Front Biosci* 2000;**5**:D213–31.

10. Stupp R Mason WP, van den Bent MJ et al. Radiotherapy plus concomitant and adjuvant temozolomide for glioblastoma. *N Engl J Med* 2005;**352**(10):987–96.

11. Sawaya, R. Brain metastasis: steel knife or gamma knife? *Ann Surg Oncol* 2000;**7**(5):323–4.

12. Patchell RA, Tibbs PA, Walsh JW et al. A randomized trial of surgery in the treatment of single metastases to the brain. *N Engl J Med* 1990;**322**(8):494–500.

13. Vecht CJ, Haaxma-Reiche H, Noordijk EM et al. Treatment of single brain metastasis: radiotherapy alone or combined with neurosurgery? *Ann Neurol* 1993;**33**(6):583–90.

14. Rock JP, Haines S, Recht L et al. Practice parameters for the management of single brain metastasis. *Neurosurg Focus* 2000;**9**(6):ecp2.

15. Nguyen TD, DeAngelis LM. Brain metastases. *Neurol Clin* 2007;**25**(4):1173–92, x–xi.

16. Hustinx R, Pourdehnad M, Kaschten B, Alavi A. PET imaging for differentiating recurrent brain tumor from radiation necrosis. *Radiol Clin North Am* 2005;**43**(1):35–47.

17. Langleben DD, Segall GM. PET in differentiation of recurrent brain tumor from radiation injury. *J Nucl Med* 2000;**41**(11):1861–7.

18. Law M, Yang S, Wang H et al. Glioma grading: sensitivity, specificity, and predictive values of perfusion MR imaging and proton MR spectroscopic imaging compared with conventional MR imaging. *Am J Neuroradiol* 2003;**24**(10):1989–98.

19. Wong TZ, Turkington TG, Hawk TC, Coleman RE. PET and brain tumor image fusion. *Cancer J* 2004;**10**(4):234–42.

20. Chao ST, Suh JH, Raja S, Lee SY, Barnett G. The sensitivity and specificity of FDG PET in distinguishing recurrent brain tumor from radionecrosis in patients treated with stereotactic radiosurgery. *Int J Cancer* 2001;**96**(3):191–7.

21. Grossman RI, Yousem DM *Neuroradiology: the Requisites.* Requisites series. St. Louis: Mosby, 1994. xiv, 544 pp.

22. Thrall JH, Ziessman HA. *Nuclear Medicine.* 2nd edn. St. Louis: Mosby, 2001, x, 419 pp.

23. Lorberboym M, Mandell LR, Mosesson RE et al. The role of thallium-201 uptake and retention in intracranial tumors after radiotherapy. *J Nucl Med* 1997;**38**(2):223–6.

24. Tie J, Gunawardana DH, Rosenthal MA. Differentiation of tumor recurrence from radiation necrosis in high-grade gliomas using 201Tl-SPECT. *J Clin Neurosci* 2008; **15**(12):1327–34.

25. Tomura N, Hirano H, Kato K et al. Unexpected accumulation of thallium-201 in cerebral infarction. *J Comput Assist Tomogr* 1998;**22**(1):126–9.

26. Ortega-Lozano SJ, del Valle-Torres DM, Gómez-Río M, Llamas-Elvira JM. Thallium-201 SPECT in brain gliomas: Quantitative assessment in differential diagnosis between tumor recurrence and radionecrosis. *Clin Nucl Med* 2009;**34**(8):503–5.

27. Benard F, Romsa J, Hustinx R. Imaging gliomas with positron emission tomography and single-photon emission computed tomography. *Semin Nucl Med* 2003; **33**(2):148–62.

28. Martin WH, Delbeke D, Patton JA et al. FDG-SPECT: correlation with FDG-PET. *J Nucl Med* 1995; **36**(6):988–95.

29. Reivich M, Kuhl D, Wolf A et al. The [18F]fluorodeoxyglucose method for the measurement of local cerebral glucose utilization in man. *Circ Res* 1979;**44**(1):127–37.

30. Phelps ME, Huang SC, Hoffman EJ et al. Tomographic measurement of local cerebral glucose metabolic rate in humans with (F-18)2-fluoro-2-deoxy-D-glucose: validation of method. *Ann Neurol* 1979;**6**(5):371–88.

31. Di Chiro G, DeLaPaz RL, Brooks RA et al. Glucose utilization of cerebral gliomas measured by [18F] fluorodeoxyglucose and positron emission tomography. *Neurology* 1982;**32**(12):1323–9.

32. Delbeke D, Meyerowitz C, Lapidus RL et al. Optimal cutoff levels of F-18 fluorodeoxyglucose uptake in the differentiation of low-grade from high-grade brain tumors with PET. *Radiology* 1995;**195**(1):47–52.

33. Hanson MW, Glantz MJ, Hoffman JM et al. FDG-PET in the selection of brain lesions for biopsy. *J Comput Assist Tomogr* 1991;**15**(5):796–801.

34. Levivier M, Goldman S, Pirotte B *et al.* Diagnostic yield of stereotactic brain biopsy guided by positron emission tomography with [18F] fluorodeoxyglucose. *J Neurosurg* 1995;**82**(3):445–52.

35. Francavilla TL, Miletich RS, Di Chiro G *et al.* Positron emission tomography in the detection of malignant degeneration of low-grade gliomas. *Neurosurgery* 1989;**24**(1):1–5.

36. Padma MV, Said S, Jacobs M *et al.* Prediction of pathology and survival by FDG PET in gliomas. *J Neurooncol* 2003;**64**(3):227–37.

37. Herholz K, Herscovitch P, Heiss WD. *NeuroPET: Positron Emission Tomography in Neuroscience and Clinical Neurology.* Berlin: Springer-Verlag, 2004, xv, p. 297.

38. De Souza B, Brunetti A, Fulham MJ *et al.* Pituitary microadenomas: a PET study. *Radiology* 1990;**177**(1):39–44.

39. Sato K, Rorke LB. Vascular bundles and wickerworks in childhood brain tumors. *Pediatr Neurosci* 1989;**15**(3):105–10.

40. Murovic JA, Nagashima T, Hoshino T, Edwards MS, Davis RL. Pediatric central nervous system tumors: a cell kinetic study with bromodeoxyuridine. *Neurosurgery* 1986;**19**(6):900–4.

41. Fulham MJ, Melisi JW, Nishimiya J, Dwyer AJ, Di Chiro G. Neuroimaging of juvenile pilocytic astrocytomas: an enigma. *Radiology* 1993;**189**(1):221–5.

42. Roelcke U, Radü EW, Hausmann O *et al.* Tracer transport and metabolism in a patient with juvenile pilocytic astrocytoma. A PET study. *J Neurooncol* 1998;**36**(3):279–83.

43. Di Chiro G, Hatazawa J, Katz DA, Rizzoli HV, De Michele DJ. Glucose utilization by intracranial meningiomas as an index of tumor aggressivity and probability of recurrence: a PET study. *Radiology* 1987;**164**(2):521–6.

44. Aide N, Benayoun M, Kerrou K *et al.* Impact of [18F]-fluorodeoxyglucose ([18F]-FDG) imaging in sarcoidosis: unsuspected neurosarcoidosis discovered by [18F]-FDG PET and early metabolic response to corticosteroid therapy. *Br J Radiol* 2007;**80**(951):e67–71.

45. Spence AM, Muzi M, Mankoff DA *et al.* 18F-FDG PET of gliomas at delayed intervals: improved distinction between tumor and normal gray matter. *J Nucl Med* 2004;**45**(10):1653–9.

46. Jager PL, Vaalburg W, Pruim J *et al.* Radiolabeled amino acids: basic aspects and clinical applications in oncology. *J Nucl Med* 2001;**42**(3):432–45.

47. Sasajima T, Miyagawa T, Oku T *et al.* Proliferation-dependent changes in amino acid transport and glucose metabolism in glioma cell lines. *Eur J Nucl Med Mol Imaging* 2004;**31** (9):1244–56.

48. Kracht LW, Friese M, Herholz K *et al.* Methyl-[11C]-l-methionine uptake as measured by positron emission tomography correlates to microvessel density in patients with glioma. *Eur J Nucl Med Mol Imaging* 2003;**30** (6):868–73.

49. Schiepers C, Chen W, Cloughesy T, Dahlbom M, Huang SC. 18F-FDOPA kinetics in brain tumors. *J Nucl Med* 2007;**48**(10):1651–61.

50. Heiss WD, Wienhard K, Wagner R *et al.* F-Dopa as an amino acid tracer to detect brain tumors. *J Nucl Med* 1996;**37**(7):1180–2.

51. Herholz K, Hölzer T, Bauer B *et al.* 11C-methionine PET for differential diagnosis of low-grade gliomas. *Neurology* 1998;**50**(5): 1316–22.

52. Ogawa T, Shishido F, Kanno I *et al.* Cerebral glioma: evaluation with methionine PET. *Radiology* 1993; **186**(1):45–53.

53. Chen W, Cloughesy T, Kamdar N *et al.* Imaging proliferation in brain tumors with 18F-FLT PET: comparison with 18F-FDG. *J Nucl Med* 2005; **46**(6):945–52.

54. Salskov A, Tammisetti VS, Grierson J, Vesselle H. FLT: measuring tumor cell proliferation in vivo with positron emission tomography and 3'-deoxy-3'-[18F]fluorothymidine. *Semin Nucl Med* 2007;**37**(6):429–39.

55. Pirotte B, Goldman S, Bidaut LM *et al.* Use of positron emission tomography (PET) in stereotactic conditions for brain biopsy. *Acta Neurochir (Wien)*, 1995;**134**(1–2):79–82.

56. Pirotte B, Goldman S, Massager N *et al.* Comparison of 18F-FDG and 11C-methionine for PET-guided stereotactic brain biopsy of gliomas. *J Nucl Med* 2004;**45**(8):1293–8.

57. Pauleit D, Floeth F, Hamacher K *et al.* O-(2-[18F]fluoroethyl)-L-tyrosine PET combined with MRI improves the diagnostic assessment of cerebral gliomas. *Brain* 2005; **128**(Pt 3):678–87.

A 75-year-old female who presented to her local hospital with a 5-day history of intermittent right hand and foot tingling, likely secondary to seizures. The patient was unable to have an MRI, due to metal hardware in her ear. A contrast CT of the head revealed enhancing lesions in the left internal capsule and left insula (Figure 5.1B, D). Contrast CT of the chest, abdomen, and pelvis reportedly did not reveal a primary malignancy.

PET/CT of the brain and body was performed to characterize the metabolic activity of the brain lesions and to detect a possible extracranial primary lesion.

## PET/CT acquisition and processing parameters

1. Dedicated brain FDG-PET (arms down).
2. Whole body FDG-PET.

After fasting for a period of 6 hours, the patient was injected intravenously with 21.5 mCi of FDG. Then after an uptake period of 1 hour, PET imaging was performed from the vertex of the skull through the thighs. When possible, it is preferable to image the body with arms up over the head. Dedicated PET of the brain was also obtained, with arms down. Non-contrast helical CT imaging was performed over the same range without breath-hold, for attenuation correction of PET images and anatomic correlation, but not for primary interpretation as it is not of standard diagnostic quality.

## Findings and differential diagnosis

Two intensely FDG-avid masses with surrounding edema within the left insula (SUVmax 16.1) and left basal ganglia (SUVmax 14.6) are highly suspicious for malignancy.

Metabolic activity within the right cerebral and bilateral cerebellar hemispheres is normal.

No FDG-avid disease is identified within the neck, chest, abdomen, or pelvis.

Primary CNS lymphoma, multifocal glioblastoma multiforme, or an infectious process such as an abscess may have this appearance on PET. Metastatic melanoma or small cell lung cancer could also have this appearance, with an occult primary lesion. On CT, the homogeneous enhancing pattern and the involvement of the deep structures is most compatible with primary CNS lymphoma.

## Diagnosis and follow-up

Biopsy of left insular lesion revealed primary diffuse large B-cell lymphoma of the CNS. The patient then received methotrexate chemotherapy at her local hospital.

## Discussion and teaching points

Primary CNS lymphoma (PCNSL) is an aggressive form of non-Hodgkin's lymphoma that may arise within the brain, spinal cord, meninges, or eyes. CHOP, the common treatment for systemic lymphoma, is generally not effective due to poor penetration of the blood–brain barrier. Methotrexate, which crosses the blood–brain barrier, is one effective treatment option. Cranial or craniospinal radiation therapy is also used additionally to prolong survival. Median overall survival is now approximately 30–40 months (1–4).

Primary CNS lymphoma is intensely FDG-avid. Other intensely FDG-avid pathologic types include glioblastoma

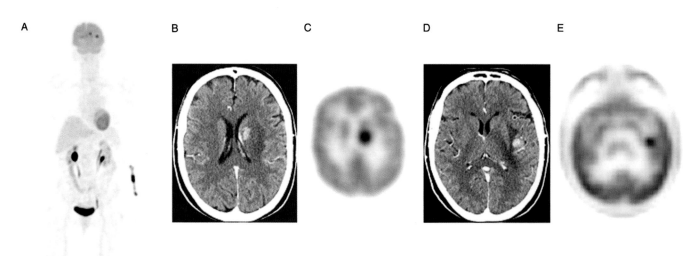

**Figure 5.1** 1 (A) Maximum intensity projection (MIP) image; (B and D) axial brain MRI slices; (C and E) axial FDG-PET brain images.

multiforme (GBM) and melanoma (sometimes), and poorly differentiated lung cancer. Lymphoma tends to have a high tumor-to-cortex SUV ratio.

FDG-PET aids in the differential diagnosis of lymphoma from benign lesions, including inflammatory lesions (toxoplasmosis) in the setting of HIV, which are often indistinguishable on MRI. Lymphoma is intensely FDG-avid whereas toxoplasmosis is not FDG-avid, with SUV often below that of the contralateral cortex (5). In several studies of AIDS patients, SUV of PCNSL, metastases, and GBM are typically 1.5–2 times that of the normal contralateral cortex whereas the SUV of toxoplasmosis tends to be lower than that of the contralateral cortex (6–8).

## Take-home message

- Primary CNS lymphoma is typically intensely FDG-avid.
- The degree of FDG avidity may help distinguish lymphoma from toxoplasmosis, which is not characteristically FDG-avid but may have the same appearance on MRI.
- Whole body PET/CT may be used in the setting of a newly diagnosed brain lesion in order to assess the grade of the lesion and to look for possible primary lesions outside of the CNS.

## References

1. Abrey LE, Yahalom J, DeAngelis LM. Treatment for primary CNS lymphoma: the next step. *J Clin Oncol* 2000;**18**(17):3144–50.

2. Batchelor T, Carson K, O'Neill A *et al.* Treatment of primary CNS lymphoma with methotrexate and deferred radiotherapy: a report of NABTT 96–07. *J Clin Oncol*, 2003; **21**(6):1044–9.

3. Abrey LE, DeAngelis LM, Yahalom J. Long-term survival in primary CNS lymphoma. *J Clin Oncol* 1998;**16**(3):859–63.

4. Nelson DF, Martz KL, Bonner H *et al.* Non-Hodgkin's lymphoma of the brain: can high dose, large volume radiation therapy improve survival? Report on a prospective trial by the Radiation Therapy Oncology Group (RTOG): RTOG 8315. *Int J Radiation Oncol Biol Physics* 1992;**23**(1):9–17.

5. Roelcke U, Leenders KL. Positron emission tomography in patients with primary CNS lymphomas. *J Neuro-Oncol* 1999;**43**(3):231–6.

6. Davis WK, Boyko OB, Hoffman JM *et al.* [18F]2-fluoro-2-deoxyglucose-positron emission tomography correlation of gadolinium-enhanced MR imaging of central nervous system neoplasia. *Am J Neuroradiol* 1993;**14**(3):515–23.

7. Pierce MA, Johnson MD, Maciunas RJ *et al.* Evaluating contrast-enhancing brain lesions in patients with AIDS by using positron emission tomography. *Ann Intern Med* 1995;**123**(8):594–8.

8. Heald AE, Hoffman JM, Bartlett JA, Waskin HA. Differentiation of central nervous system lesions in AIDS patients using positron emission tomography (PET). *Int J STD AIDS* 1996;**7**(5):337–46.

A 60-year-old female with history of stage IIIA invasive lobular breast cancer and a 5 mm left parietal brain metastasis. She is status post-stereotactic radiosurgery (22 Gy) 18 months previously as well as chemotherapy. Baseline MRI revealed an 8 mm left parietal contrast-enhancing lesion that increased from 5 mm at the time of radiosurgery. The patient was

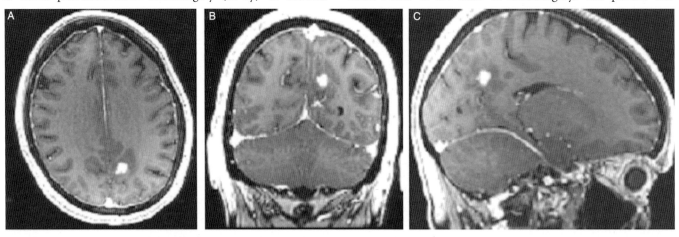

**Figure 5.2** Magnetic resonance images (A, axial; B, coronal; C, sagittal).

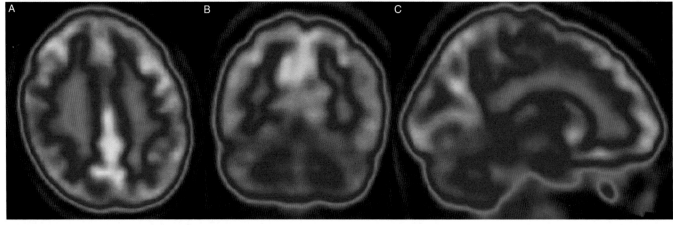

**Figure 5.3** Early FDG-PET-MRI fusion images (A, axial; B, coronal; C, sagittal).

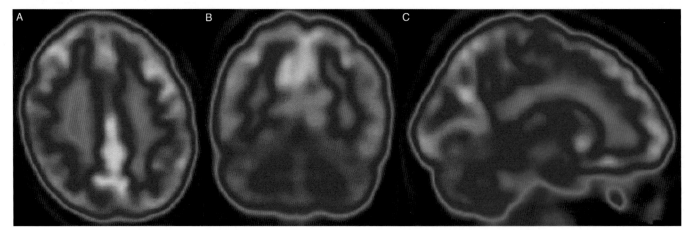

**Figure 5.4** Delayed FDG-PET-MRI fusion images (A, axial; B, coronal; C, sagittal).

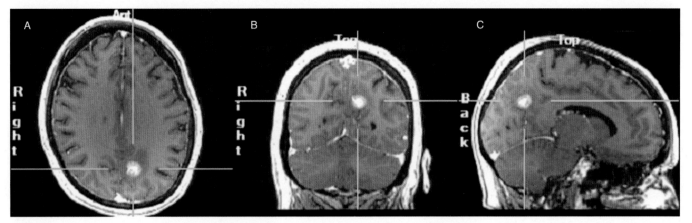

**Figure 5.5** Contrast-enhanced MRI (A, axial; B, coronal; C, sagittal), performed 6 months after MRI in Fig. 5.2.

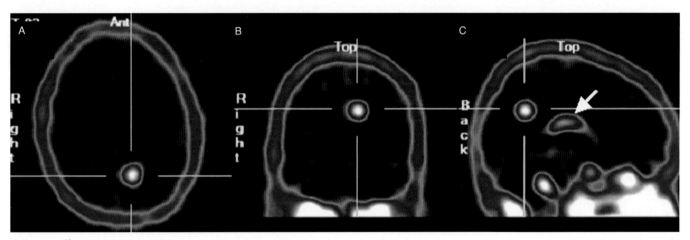

**Figure 5.6** $^{99m}$Tc-sestamibi brain SPECT (A, axial; B, coronal; C, sagittal).

referred to Nuclear Medicine for an FDG-PET scan to evaluate for post-radiation (XRT) necrosis versus tumor recurrence.

## FDG-PET acquisition and processing parameters

The patient had no dietary restrictions and was encouraged to eat prior to the study. Blood glucose was measured to be 104 mg/dL. Twenty mCi of FDG was injected intravenously, and the patient rested in a quiet room for 60 minutes. (10–12 mCi is the standard dose for brain-only PET, but 20 mCi is the standard dose for brain plus whole body imaging.) Approximately 1 hour following tracer administration, PET of the brain was performed using a 3-D mode brain acquisition protocol. Non-contrast low-dose helical CT imaging was performed over the same range for attenuation correction of the PET images. Whole body PET/CT imaging was also performed (not shown). In addition, delayed brain PET/CT was performed using the same acquisition protocol approximately 4 hours later, at 5 hours post-tracer injection. Images were correlated with and fused to a recent contrast-enhanced MRI (Figures 5.2–5.4).

## Findings and initial follow-up

Initial and delayed PET imaging phases demonstrate no FDG avidity corresponding to the area of contrast enhancement in the left parietal lobe. However, the sensitivity of this test has significant limitations due to its location near metabolically active cortex, the subcentimeter lesion size, and the histopathology of lobular breast cancer, which is characteristically not highly FDG avid.

Six months later, the lesion increased in size to 12 mm. The patient then underwent brain SPECT imaging with $^{99m}$Tc-sestamibi.

## $^{99m}$Tc-Sestamibi SPECT acquisition and processing parameters

The patient was injected with 25.5 mCi of $^{99m}$Tc-sestamibi, and 20 minutes later SPECT images were acquired using a SPECT camera equipped with a low-energy high-resolution parallel-hole (LEHRP) collimator, with the following parameters: matrix $128 \times 128$, Offset zoom: 2.69, Dual-head detectors; patient in supine position; 360° rotation, 64 views, 30 seconds per view, and non-circular and continuous acquisition. Images were reconstructed by filtered back projection, using a Butterworth filter with order of 5. Chang attenuation coefficient of 0.12 was used.

SPECT images were compared with a recent contrast-enhanced MRI.

## Findings

A well-defined focus of abnormal uptake in the posterior left parieto-occipital region of the brain (Figure 5.6) correlates precisely with the enhancing lesion seen in the MRI (Figure 5.5). Physiologic tracer accumulation is noted within the choroid plexus and the pituitary gland (Figure 5.6C: arrow).

## Diagnosis and follow-up

One month later, the lesion was surgically resected, and the pathology revealed metastatic breast adenocarcinoma.

## Discussion and teaching points

The FDG-PET study was technically limited by the lesion size. The typical size threshold is approximately 8–10 mm. The incidence of false-negative findings increases with smaller lesions.

On repeat imaging 6 months later, an FDG-PET might have been positive due to the increased size of the lesion. However, due to the background cortical activity that can obscure the FDG avidity of the lesion as well as the typically low FDG avidity in lobular breast cancer, the mechanism of which is unknown (1, 2, 3), $^{99m}$Tc-sestamibi SPECT was considered the technique of choice and was performed instead.

Thallium imaging is also useful in the assessment of brain metastases, because it is positive in all histologic types of breast cancer (4), but its size threshold is larger than for PET. This is because thallium has a lower energy than $^{99m}$Tc-sestamibi (69 keV and 81 keV peaks, versus 140 keV for $^{99m}$Tc-sestamibi). Furthermore, the half life of $^{99m}$Tc-sestamibi is 6 hours, whereas it is 73.1 hours for thallium. The long half life is dose-limiting (i.e., dose for $^{99m}$Tc-sestamibi is approximately 25 mCi, versus 4 mCi for thallium). A higher dose translates into a larger signal.

## Take-home message

- Lobular breast cancer may not be FDG-avid.
- FDG-PET may not demonstrate viable metastases due to tumor histology or to poor metabolic distinction on a background of high metabolic activity within normal gray matter.
- $^{99m}$Tc-sestamibi has the following advantages over FDG-PET:
  - No background uptake in cortex.
  - Better binding to lobular breast cancer cells.
- Limitations of $^{99m}$Tc-sestamibi:
  - Physiologic uptake in choroid plexus can be confounding, but this can often be overcome by fusion to MRI.
  - Lesion should be at least 10–15 mm, due to lower resolution of SPECT.

In this case, the lesion was only 12 mm but was intense enough to be clearly visualized.

## References

1. Avril N, Schelling M, Dose J, Weber WA, Schwaiger M. Utility of PET in breast cancer. *Clin Positron Imaging* 1999;**2**(5):261–71.

2. Crippa F, Seregni E, Agresti R, Chiesa C *et al.* Association between [18F] fluorodeoxyglucose uptake and postoperative histopathology, hormone receptor status, thymidine labelling index and p53 in primary breast cancer: a preliminary observation. *Eur J Nucl Med* 1998;**25**(10):1429–34.

3. Buck A, Schirrmeister H, Kühn T, Shen C *et al.* FDG uptake in breast cancer: correlation with biological and clinical prognostic parameters. *Eur J Nucl Med Mol Imaging* 2002;**29**(10):1317–23.

4. Cimitan M, Volpe R, Candiani E *et al.* The use of thallium-201 in the preoperative detection of breast cancer: an adjunct to mammography and ultrasonography. *Eur J Nucl Med* 1995; **22**(10):1110–17.

A 50-year-old female with right posterior frontal melanoma metastasis resected 2 years ago, followed by stereotactic radiosurgery (SRS) (22 Gy) one month later, and repeat SRS 10 months later, due to increasing lesion enhancement on MRI, thought to represent tumor. The patient now presents with increased enhancement on MRI, approximately 1 year after SRS to evaluate for tumor recurrence versus post-radiation necrosis.

## Acquisition and processing parameters

The patient had no dietary restrictions and was encouraged to eat prior to the study. Blood glucose was measured to be 99 mg/dL. Twelve mCi of $^{18}$F-FDG was injected intravenously, and the patient rested in a quiet room for 60 minutes. Approximately 1 hour following tracer administration, PET of the brain was performed using a 3-D brain acquisition protocol. Non-contrast low-dose helical CT imaging was performed over the same range for attenuation correction of the PET images.

$^{99m}$Tc-sestamibi SPECT was acquired 20 minutes post-injection of 25.5 mCi, using a SPECT camera equipped with a LEHRP collimator.

$^{201}$Thallium SPECT images were acquired 30 minutes after IV injection of 3.9 mCi. $^{201}$Thallium images were fused to a recent MRI, using Hermes fusion software.

PET: Indeterminate (Lesion size 8 × 11 mm on MRI).

## Findings

The initial FDG-PET scan was read as equivocal because the lesion was not clearly FDG avid (Figure 5.7D–F). This was difficult to interpret due to the proximity to physiologically active cortex. Subsequent $^{201}$thallium and $^{99m}$Tc-sestamibi scans 24 hours and 2 months later, respectively, were negative, though sensitivity was limited due to the small lesion size (Figure 5.8B; Figure 5.9B). Five months later on repeat thallium imaging, a focus of intensely increased thallium uptake in the right frontal lobe corresponded (Figure 5.10D–F) to the 2 cm enhancing lesion on the correlating MRI (Figure 5.10A–C). The uptake was greater than twice the uptake of the scalp and highly suspicious for melanoma metastasis.

## Diagnosis and follow-up

Right frontal craniotomy was performed three weeks after the repeat thallium scan. Pathology revealed metastatic melanoma with extension to the meninges. The patient subsequently underwent whole-brain radiation therapy to treat the leptomeninges plus temozolomide chemotherapy. MRI performed 18 months later demonstrated no evidence of metastatic melanoma.

## Discussion and teaching points

Like many tumors, melanoma is highly thallium-avid, whether in the brain or elsewhere in the body (1). Thallium is transported into cells via the sodium potassium adenosine triphosphate Na+/K+ ATPase (2, 3). This transporter is functional only in viable tissue, and not in scar. It is therefore a useful tool to distinguish tumor from scar. Distance to the lesion from the detector is an important factor in visualization, and lesions deep within the brain are typically difficult to detect. It is clear from this example that even a superficial cortical lesion can not be well seen if the lesion is too small. Also, the size of the lesion is an important factor, and it is not advisable to attempt to image lesions smaller than 1–1.5 cm with thallium, since the false-negative rate will be high. The lesion in this case was not detected when it measured 11 × 8 mm, but it was well seen when it doubled in size 7 months later.

Sestamibi binds to melanoma because like all tumors it is dense in mitochondria. The tumor was not detected with $^{99m}$Tc-sestamibi due to its somewhat small size (ideal minimal diameter is 15 mm).

Melanoma is typically intensely FDG-avid but is often difficult to detect on FDG-PET because of high background cortical activity. In this case, the lesion lies along the cortex and can be obscured by functional activity. Necrosis should appear as a cold defect, however, and the lack of this defect (on MRI–PET co-registered images) should raise the suspicion of tumor.

## Take-home message

- $^{201}$Thallium or $^{99m}$Tc-sestamibi may be a better choice than FDG-PET in the assessment of recurrent melanoma metastasis, because background cortical activity on FDG-PET may obscure uptake in a lesion. Metastases tend to occur at the gray–white junction, so this is a common problem.
- $^{201}$Thallium and $^{99m}$Tc-sestamibi are only effective, however, when the lesion is large enough to detect. The usual threshold for SPECT imaging is 1.5 to 2.0 cm.

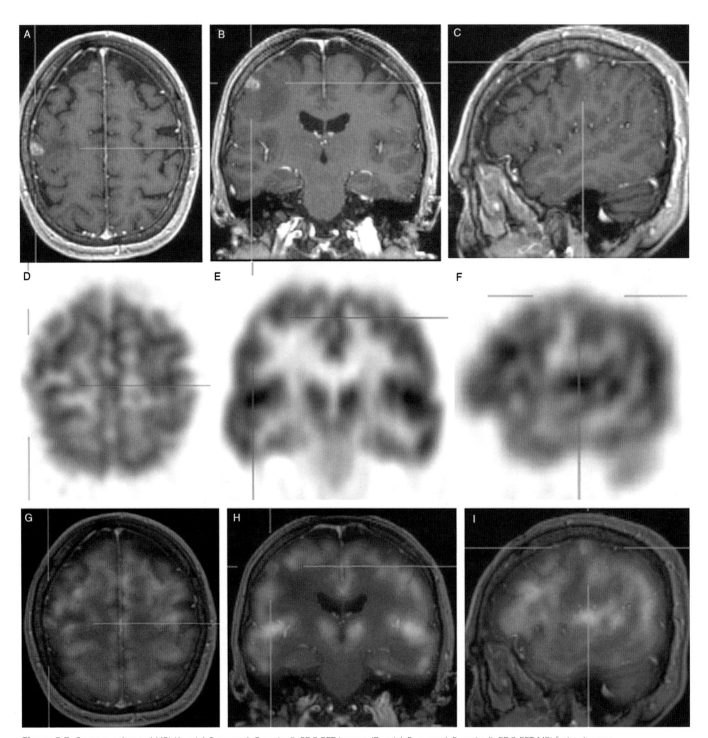

**Figure 5.7** Contrast-enhanced MRI (A, axial; B, coronal; C, sagittal), FDG-PET images (D, axial; E, coronal; F, sagittal), FDG-PET-MRI fusion images (F, axial; H, coronal; I, sagittal).

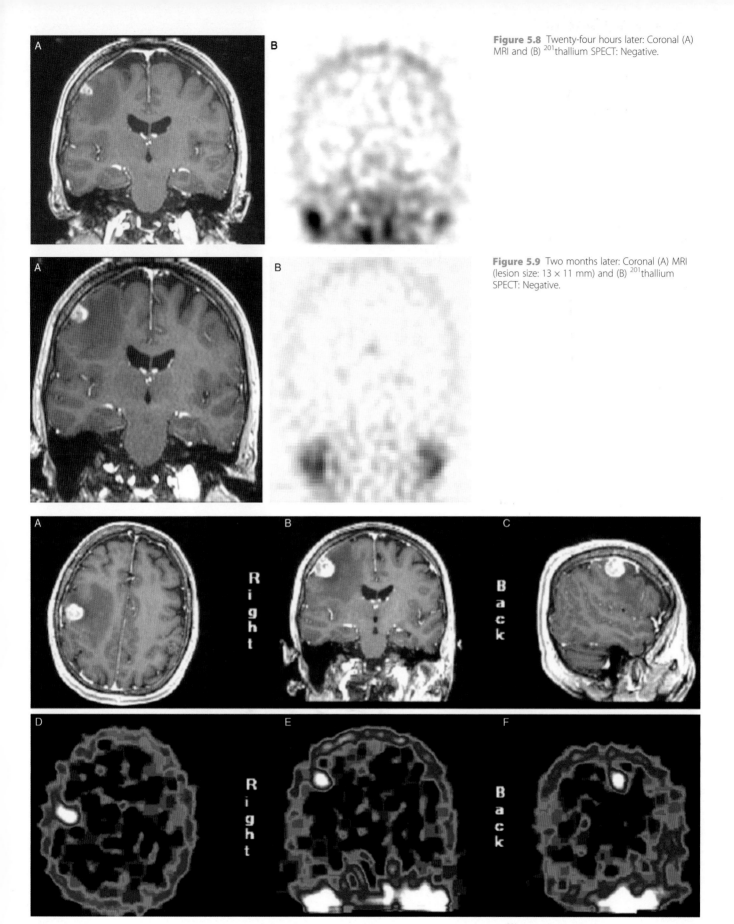

**Figure 5.8** Twenty-four hours later: Coronal (A) MRI and (B) $^{201}$thallium SPECT: Negative.

**Figure 5.9** Two months later: Coronal (A) MRI (lesion size: 13 × 11 mm) and (B) $^{201}$thallium SPECT: Negative.

**Figure 5.10** Five months later: Contrast-enhanced MRI (A, axial; B, coronal; C, sagittal) (lesion size: 22 × 22 mm), and $^{201}$thallium SPECT (D, axial; E, coronal; F, sagittal).

# References

1. Rettenbacher L, Koller J, Kässmann H, Galvan G. Detection of melanoma metastases with thallium-201 scintigraphy. *J Nucl Med* 1998;**39** (5):798–802.

2. Sessler MJ, Geck P, Maul FD, Hör G, Munz DL. New aspects of cellular thallium uptake: Tl+-Na+-2Cl(-)-cotransport is the central mechanism of ion uptake. *Nuklearmedizin* 1986; **25**(1):24–7.

3. Sehweil A, McKillop JH, Ziada G *et al.* The optimum time for tumour imaging with thallium-201. *Eur J Nucl Med* 1988;**13**(10):527–9.

A 49-year-old female with meningioma diagnosed 30 years ago, status resection and multiple courses of radiation plus repeat surgery for recurrence (histology consistent with malignant meningioma). She now presents to evaluate for recurrence versus post-radiation necrosis 2 years after Gamma knife radiation.

## Acquisition and processing parameters

Six mCi of In-111 OctreoScan (Octreotide) were injected IV, and SPECT images of the brain were performed 24 hours later. Images were compared with a recent MRI of the brain.

## Findings

Moderate uptake is noted in the right parietal high convexity which correlates with the $42 \times 31 \times 34$ mm contrast-enhancing lesion on MRI. The findings are concerning for recurrent malignant meningioma.

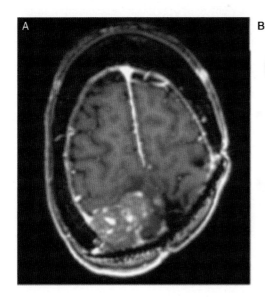 

**Figure 5.11** (A) Axial 3-D MPRAGE T1 Post-Contrast MRI and (B) [111]In octreotide SPECT.

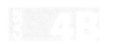

An 80-year-old female with a history of right temporal lobe meningioma status post-resection 10 years ago. Pathology at that time was compatible with a benign meningioma, despite multifocal necrosis. The tissue was devoid of features such as patternless growth and frequent mitoses, and therefore could not be classified as an atypical meningioma. The MIB-1 (proliferation index) was elevated at 7%, however. MIB-1 labeling indices greater than 3% have been associated with recurrence (1). The patient underwent stereotaxic radiosurgery (49 Gy) for recurrence 1.5 years ago. She is referred to assess for recurrence versus post-radiation necrosis.

## Acquisition and processing parameters

Approximately 60 minutes following IV administration of 10.5 mCi of FDG, PET of the brain in 3-D mode was performed as described previously. PET/CT images of the brain were obtained at 1 hour and again 4 hours after tracer injection. Images were compared with a recent brain MRI.

## Findings

Early 1-hour PET images show an area of photopenia in the right temporal lobe that correlates with the known resection cavity. In addition there is an area of increased tracer activity in the right anterior temporal lobe, at the anterior aspect of the resection cavity (SUV max of 12.6, as compared with SUV max of 11.7 in the contralateral cortex). There is normal metabolism elsewhere throughout the remainder of the cerebral cortex and the deep nuclei of the brain. Asymmetric, moderately decreased metabolism in the right posterior temporal and occipital cortex likely represents post-treatment changes. A small photopenic focus in the right cerebellum corresponds to known PICA infarct, also seen on MRI.

Delayed PET images show a hypermetabolic focus in the right anterior temporal pole that has become more intense, with a SUVmax of 16. The contralateral cortex SUVmax has slightly decreased to 11.1. The area of increased tracer uptake seen in the anterior right temporal lobe, corresponding to the region of contrast enhancement on recent MRI, continues to accumulate radiotracer on delayed images and is concerning for disease recurrence.

## Diagnosis and follow-up

Surgical resection revealed a Grade III anaplastic meningioma.

## Discussion and teaching points

Meningiomas are the most common primary brain tumor aside from glial tumors and account for approximately 15% of all intracranial malignancies. They are extra-axial and arise from the arachnoid meningothelial cells in the middle layer of meninges ensheathing the brain. They may occur in the intracranial vault or in the spinal dura. Most commonly they are found in the cerebral convexities, parasagittal regions, and adjacent to the sphenoid wing.

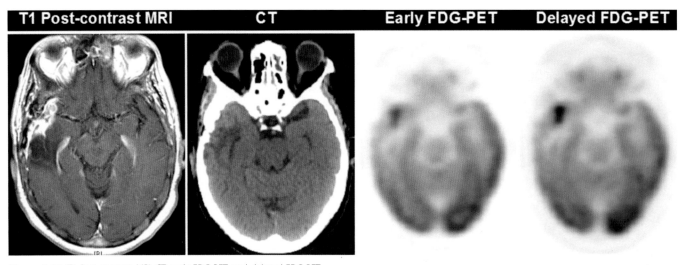

**Figure 5.12** T1 Post-contrast MRI, CT, early FDG-PET, and delayed FDG-PET.

**Table 5.3** World Health Organization classification of meningiomas, including disease prevalence, and survival.

| Grade | Type | Prevalence | Survival | Time to relapse | Survival after relapse |
|-------|------|-----------|----------|-----------------|------------------------|
| I | Benign | 90% | N/A | N/A | |
| II | Atypical | 7% | 11.9 years | 11.5 years | 0.4 years |
| III | Malignant/ anaplastic | 2% | 3.3 years | 2.7 years | 0.6 years |

According to the WHO classification system (3), meningiomas are classified as follows:

Grade I: Benign (90%).

Grade II: Atypical (7%).

Grade III: Malignant/Anaplastic (2%).

Overall survival, time to relapse, and survival after relapse based on histology are shown in the following Table 5.3 summarizing data from a recent review (4).

Meningiomas are often asymptomatic and are found incidentally. The majority of small, asymptomatic meningiomas, 63% in one series of 43 patients, do not grow on follow-up imaging. The remaining 37% in the study demonstrated moderate growth, with an average of 4 mm per year. Stable, asymptomatic meningiomas are managed by observation and serial imaging. Those that demonstrate growth, most often seen in younger patients, are managed more aggressively. Treatment is also advised for symptomatic meningiomas, which occur 2–3 times more often in females (2). Surgery is often curative, particularly in uncomplicated cases in which complete resection is possible. Radiation therapy is an alternate treatment strategy for meningiomas that are not amenable to surgery and a complementary treatment in the case of an incomplete resection (5, 6). Somatostatin analogs and angiogenesis inhibitors are examples of promising, targeted molecular therapies for meningiomas (7).

The MRI characteristics of meningiomas are often diagnostically accurate (extra-axial location, well-perfused, contrast enhancing) (8), and nuclear imaging is therefore not often required at initial diagnosis.

FDG-PET is useful, however, for grading menigiomas. FDG-PET correlates with glycolytic metabolism, cell density, and metabolic rate, and therefore, uptake values are higher in high-grade meningiomas and recurrent meningiomas. Di Chiro *et al.* demonstrated that glucose utilization rates for recurrent meningiomas were 4.5 mg/dL per min $\pm$ 1.9, as opposed to 1.9 mg/dL per min $\pm$ 1.0 for non-recurrent meningiomas (9).

Meningiomas strongly express somatostatin receptors (SSTR2), which are a molecular imaging target for [68Ga]-DOTA-D Phe$^1$-Tyr$^3$ Octreotide (DOTATOC) PET/CT (10–12) (see Chapter 2). The gamma emitter $^{111}$-Indium-Octreotide also binds to somatostatin receptors and is effective in tumors measuring at least 1.5 cm, and has wider clinical use (13). Amino acid PET tracers such as $^{11}$C-methionine and 2–$^{18}$F-Fluoro-L-tyrosine (TYR) show high uptake in meningiomas, and the latter has been shown to correlate with the mitotic index Ki-67 (14, 15).

Nuclear imaging is often requested at the time of possible recurrence, which may radiographically mimic radiation necrosis on MRI. At this time, Octreotide SPECT imaging and FDG-PET are most commonly used. Octreotide is useful if the tumor cells express somatostatin receptors 2A (sst2A) and to a lesser extent 5 (sst5).

## Take-home message

- Octreotide SPECT imaging is useful for somatostatin-expressing meningiomas, and is effective in tumors measuring at least 1.5 cm in size.
- FDG-PET imaging, including dual-phase imaging, may also be useful. Benign meningiomas may be less FDG avid and harder to detect with FDG-PET than more aggressive meningiomas. For this reason, FDG imaging can be useful for grading of meningiomas.

# References

1. Abramovich CM, Prayson RA. MIB-1 labeling indices in benign, aggressive, and malignant meningiomas: a study of 90 tumors. *Hum Pathol* 1998;**29**(12):1420–7.

2. Buetow MP, Buetow PC, Smirniotopoulos JG. Typical, atypical, and misleading features in meningioma. *Radiographics* 1991;**11**(6):1087–106.

3. Perry A, Louis DN, Scheithauer BW *et al.* Meningiomas. In DN Louis et al. (Eds.), *WHO Classification of Tumors of the Central Nervous System*, 4th edn. Lyon: IARC, 2007, pp. 146–172.

4. Yang SY, Park CK, Park SH *et al.* Atypical and anaplastic meningiomas: prognostic implications of clinicopathological features. *J Neurol Neurosurg Psychiatry* 2008;**79**(5):574–80.

5. Herscovici Z, Rappaport Z, Sulkes J, Danaila L, Rubin G. Natural history of conservatively treated meningiomas. *Neurology* 2004;**63**(6):1133–4.

6. Goldsmith, B, McDermott MW. Meningioma. *Neurosurg Clin N Am* 2006;**17**(2):111–20, vi.

7. Norden AD, Drappatz J, Wen PY. Advances in meningioma therapy. *Curr Neurol Neurosci Rep* 2009;**9**(3):231–40.

8. Modha A, Gutin PH. Diagnosis and treatment of atypical and anaplastic meningiomas: a review. *Neurosurgery* 2005;**57**(3):538–50; discussion 538–50.

9. Di Chiro G, Hatazawa J, Katz DA, Rizzoli HV, De Michele DJ. Glucose utilization by intracranial meningiomas as an index of tumor aggressivity and probability of recurrence: a PET study. *Radiology* 1987;**164**(2):521–6.

10. Dutour A, Kumar U, Panetta R *et al.* Expression of somatostatin receptor subtypes in human brain tumors. *Int J Cancer* 1998;**76**(5):620–7.

11. Henze M, Schuhmacher J, Hipp P *et al.* PET imaging of somatostatin receptors using [68GA]DOTA-D-Phe1-Tyr3-octreotide: first results in patients with meningiomas. *J Nucl Med* 2001;**42**(7):1053–6.

12. Gehler B, Paulsen F, Oksüz MO *et al.* [68Ga]-DOTATOC-PET/CT for meningioma IMRT treatment planning. *Radiat Oncol* 2009;**4**:56.

13. Nathoo N, Ugokwe K, Chang AS *et al.* The role of 111indium-octreotide brain scintigraphy in the diagnosis of cranial, dural-based meningiomas. *J Neurooncol* 2007;**81**(2):167–74.

14. Iuchi T, Iwadate Y, Namba H *et al.* Glucose and methionine uptake and proliferative activity in meningiomas. *Neurol Res* 1999;**21**(7):640–4.

15. Rutten I, Cabay JE, Withofs N *et al.* PET/CT of skull base meningiomas using 2–18F-fluoro-L-tyrosine: initial report. *J Nucl Med* 2007;**48**(5):720–5.

A 60-year-old male with a history of right frontotemporal GBM with oligodendroglial features, status post-chemoradiation 2 years ago, followed by recurrence, chemotherapy, and stereotactic radiosurgery 2.5 months previously. Now presents with increased contrast enhancement on MRI in the right temporal lobe, which could either indicate tumor progression or radiation necrosis (Figure 5.13).

## Acquisition and processing parameters

A dual-phase FDG-PET/CT 3-D brain imaging protocol was used, as described in a prior case. The blood glucose at the time of injection was 124 mg/dL, and 12.4 mCi of FDG were administered intravenously.

Early images were acquired 1 hour after injection, and delayed images were acquired 5 hours later, at 6 hours post-injection.

## Findings

On the early images, the SUVmax of the lesion is 8.0, and the SUVmax of the normal contralateral gray matter is 9.5. On the delayed images, the SUVmax of the lesion increases to 10.5; an increase of 31%. The SUVmax of the gray matter decreases to 9.0; a decrease of 5%. These findings are suspicious for tumor recurrence involving both the anterior and posterior margins of the resection cavity in the right temporal lobe.

## Diagnosis and follow-up

This patient was not a surgical candidate. MRI performed 4 months after the PET scan demonstrated markedly progressive disease. The patient died from progressive disease 2 weeks afterward.

## Discussion and teaching points

Recurrent GBM is typically intensely FDG-avid. In this case, FDG uptake on the early images was more intense than the ipsilateral treated cortex but not more intense than the normal contralateral gray matter. Stereotactic radiosurgery is associated with a high incidence of pseudoprogression, and FDG-PET is particularly difficult to interpret in the first several months after radiosurgery due to FDG-avid post-treatment inflammation, which can be moderately to intensely FDG-avid.

In this case, dual-phase imaging was helpful, because inflammation tends to be stable between the early and delayed scans (1). The delayed images demonstrated an increase in FDG avidity in the lesion, relative to a decrease in FDG avidity of the normal contralateral gray matter. This pattern of change is most suspicious for tumor recurrence.

Spence et al. were the first to demonstrate that delayed FDG-PET imaging increased the sensitivity of PET for detecting gliomas by providing greater image contrast between tumor and normal gray matter (2).

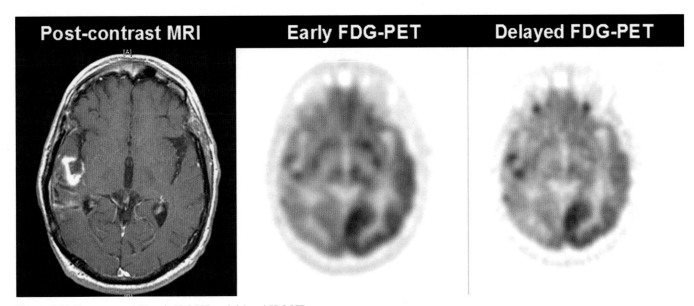

**Figure 5.13** Post-contrast MRI, early FDG-PET, and delayed FDG-PET.

## Take-home message

- Recurrent GBM is typically intensely FDG avid.
- Dual-phase FDG imaging can be useful in distinguishing recurrence from post-radiation necrosis.

- Tumor tends to increase in FDG avidity whereas normal brain parenchyma may become less FDG avid.
- The target-to-background ratio for tumor may improve on delayed images.

## References

1. Kubota K, Itoh M, Ozaki K *et al.* Advantage of delayed whole-body FDG-PET imaging for tumour detection. *Eur J Nucl Med* 2001;**28** (6):696–703.

2. Spence AM, Muzi M, Mankoff DA *et al.* 18F-FDG PET of gliomas at delayed intervals: improved distinction between tumor and normal gray matter. *J Nucl Med* 2004; **45**(10):1653–9.

A 40-year-old male presents for evaluation of possible recurrent brain tumor. His history began 5 years ago when he had a gross total resection for a left frontal lobe oligodendroglioma grade II. The patient did not receive any further chemotherapy nor did he receive radiation therapy. From that point he had been followed conservatively with serial MRI scans. His recent MRI revealed that his left frontal lobe lesion was "slightly larger." MR spectroscopy showed a slightly elevated choline peak, consistent with a residual abnormality. FDG-PET and a thallium brain SPECT were negative.

## Acquisition and processing parameters

The patient was asked to fast for at least 4 hours before image acquisition. F-DOPA synthesis was carried out using a previously reported procedure (1). The chemical and radiochemical purities of the product isolated from the semi-preparative HPLC system were further confirmed by an analytical HPLC method (specific activity: ~ 5 Ci/mmol) and were both > 99%. The product was made isotonic with sodium chloride and sterilized by passing through a 0.22 µm Millipore filter into a sterile multi-dose vial.

The patient was injected intravenously with 2 MBq/kg (0.054 mCi/kg) of F-DOPA intravenously and imaging was started immediately after injection. The unenhanced CT scan was performed first (120 kV, 80 mAs, 1 s tube rotation, 3-mm slice collimation). The CT images were used to generate the transmission maps for attenuation correction of the PET acquisitions. Immediately after the CT scan, and without changing the patient's position, PET emission scan was started for 30 minutes in the 3-D mode. Image data acquired between 10 and 30 minutes were summed to obtain a 20-minute static image. This time window was based on a previous report that the highest tracer uptake in the tumor generally occurs between 10 min and 30 min after F-DOPA injection (2). PET images were reconstructed using iterative techniques with ordered-subset expectation maximization consisting of six iterations with eight subsets (3). A Gaussian filter was used with a full width at half maximum of 4 mm.

## Findings

Contrast-enhanced MRI T1, MRI T2, and F-DOPA-PET are shown in Figure 5.14A, B, C, respectively. There is a small curvilinear area of enhancement within the resection site. Posterior to this area of enhancement, there is a parasagittal area of T2 hyperintensity/T1 hypointensity, which appears to be associated with swelling of the gyrus, suggestive of residual/recurrent non-enhancing tumor. F-DOPA-PET scan reveals an intensely positive lesion in the corresponding left frontal lobe. Based on the MRI scan alone, there is a possibility that this is residual/recurrent tumor. However, with the F-DOPA-PET scan result, a recurrent tumor becomes a much more likely diagnosis.

## Diagnosis and follow-up

Left frontal craniotomy with resection of left frontal lesion was performed. Pathology revealed features of a well-differentiated oligodendroglioma. However, several foci of more anaplastic character were seen and the Ki-67 proliferation index was high at 5–10%. This, together with the easily found mitoses, suggested that the tumor might be evolving into an anaplastic oligodendroglioma.

## Discussion and teaching points

After the initial surgical resection, patients with low-grade gliomas are often followed clinically with serial MRI scans. Recurrent low-grade gliomas are often difficult to diagnose based on MRI scans. As these recurrent low-grade tumors can have uptakes equal to or even lower than the normal brain tissue, they are also often difficult to diagnose with FDG-PET or thallium SPECT, as demonstrated in this case. In this patient, tumor was not diagnosed with conventional MRI, FDG-PET, or thallium SPECT scans (not shown) even when features of evolving into anaplastic oligodendroglioma were already present.

F-DOPA-PET as a PET biomarker of amino acid uptake has been investigated in brain tumor imaging (2). F-DOPA is transported into tumor cells via amino acid transporters (see Chapter 1). Previous reports showed that F-DOPA-PET provides excellent visualization of high-grade as well as low-grade brain tumors with higher sensitivity and specificity than FDG-PET scans (2, 4–6).

## Take-home message

- After surgical resection, follow-up of patients with low-grade gliomas can be challenging.
- Conventional imaging with MRI can often be difficult to diagnose recurrent low-grade or even low-grade glioma evolving into higher-grade tumors.
- F-DOPA-PET imaging studies amino acid transport in brain tumors.
- Compared with FDG-PET, F-DOPA-PET imaging has higher lesion-to-target ratio, and thus is a superior non-invasive predictor of malignancy in indeterminate brain gliomas (both of the low and high grades of tumors).

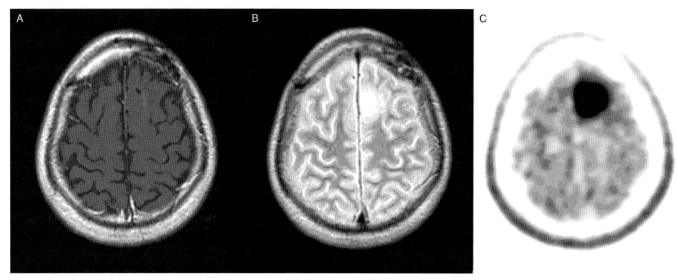

**Figure 5.14** (A) Contrast-enhanced axial MRI T1; (B) axial MRI T2; (C) axial F-DOPA-PET.

## References

1. Namavari M, Bishop A, Satyamurthy N, Bida G, Barrio JR. Regioselective radiofluorodestannylation with $[^{18}F]F_2$ and $[^{18}F]CH_3COOF$: a high yield synthesis of 6-$[^{18}F]$fluoro-L-dopa. *Appl Radiat Isot* 1992;**43**:989–96.

2. Chen W, Silverman DH, Delaloye S *et al.* 18F-FDOPA PET imaging of brain tumors: comparison study with 18F-FDG PET and evaluation of diagnostic accuracy. *J Nucl Med* 2006; **47**(6):904–11.

3. Nuyts J, Michel C, Dupont P. Maximum-likelihood expectation-maximization reconstruction of sinograms with arbitrary noise distribution using NEC-transformations. *IEEE Trans Med Imaging* 2001;**20**(5):365–75.

4. Heiss WD, Wienhard K, Wagner R *et al.* F-Dopa as an amino acid tracer to detect brain tumors. *J Nucl Med* 1996;**37**(7):1180–2.

5. Becherer A, Karanikas G, Szabo M *et al.* Brain tumour imaging with PET: a comparison between [18F]fluorodopa and [11C]methionine. *Eur J Nucl Med Mol Imaging* 2003;**30**:1561–7.

6. Ledezma CJ, Chen W, Sai V *et al.* (18)F-FDOPA PET/MRI fusion in patients with primary/recurrent gliomas: initial experience. *Eur J Radiol* 2009; **71**:242–8.

A 31-year-old male who was in his usual state of good health until 2 months before presentation when he suffered a grand mal seizure. An MRI scan identified a brain lesion. The patient subsequently had a biopsy. The biopsy specimen was evaluated at two different medical centers and the conclusion was no "abnormal tissue versus a possible ganglioglioma". In retrospect, the patient had had some episodes of headache and blurry vision and subtle neurological findings. The patient presented for further evaluation for the nature of his brain lesion.

## Acquisition and processing parameters

The patient was consented to participate in multiple PET tracer scans including FDG, FLT, and F-DOPA. FLT was synthesized by modifying a previously published procedure (1). Briefly, no-carrier-added $^{18}$F-fluoride ion was produced by an 11 MeV proton bombardment of 95% oxygen-18 enriched water via $^{18}$O (p,n) $^{18}$F nuclear reaction. This aqueous $^{18}$F-fluoride ion (~18,500 MBq) was treated with potassium carbonate and Kryptofix 2.2.2. Water was evaporated by azeotropic distillation with acetonitrile. The dried K$^{18}$F/Kryptofix residue thus obtained was reacted with the precursor of FLT [5'-O-(4, 4'-dimethoxytrityl)-2, 3'-anhydrothymidine] and then hydrolyzed with dilute HCl. The crude $^{18}$F-labeled product was purified by semi-preparative HPLC (Phenomenex Aqua column; 25 cm × 1 cm; 10% ethanol in water; flow rate: 5.0 mL/min) to give chemically and radiochemically pure FLT in 555–1110 MBq (6–12% radiochemical yield, decay corrected) amounts per batch. The chemical and radiochemical purities of the product isolated from the semi-HPLC system were confirmed by an analytical HPLC method (Phenomenex Luna C-18 column: 25 cm × 4.1 mm; 10% ethanol in water; flow rate: 2.0 mL/min; 287 nm UV and radioactivity detection; specific activity: ~ 74 Bq/mmol) and found to be > 99%. The product was made isotonic with sodium chloride and sterilized by passing through a 0.22 μm Millipore filter into a sterile multi-dose vial. The final product was sterile and pyrogen free.

For each scan, FDG-, FLT-, and F-DOPA-PET scans were performed on consecutive days. For each scan, 2.10 MBq/kg (0.056 mCi/kg) was injected intravenously. FLT-PET imaging was started immediately after injection while FDG-PET was started after a 45-minute uptake period. No specific dietary instruction was given to the patients except for instructing them to drink plenty of water before and after the PET study (to accelerate FLT or FDG excretion). The unenhanced CT scan was performed first (120 kV, 80 mAs, 1-s tube rotation, 3-mm slice collimation). The CT images were used to generate the transmission maps for attenuation correction of the PET acquisitions. Immediately after the CT scan, and without changing the patient's position, the PET emission scan was started. An emission acquisition sequence in 3-D mode over 60 minutes was obtained. PET images were reconstructed using iterative techniques with ordered-subset expectation maximization consisting of six iterations with eight subsets (2). A Gaussian filter was used with a full width at half maximum of 4 mm.

For region of interest analysis (ROI), FLT data were summed between 30 and 60 minutes to obtain static images. The PET slice with the maximum tumor uptake was chosen for ROI analysis and the two adjacent axial slices one plane above and one plane below the chosen slice, were included to improve count statistics. A circular ROI (diameter 1.0 cm, 16 pixels) was placed over the area of the tumor. The radiotracer concentration in the ROIs was normalized to the injected dose per patient's body weight to derive the standardized uptake values (SUVs, g/mL).

## Findings

MRI T2, FDG-PET, F-DOPA-PET, and FLT-PET, are presented in Figure 5.15A, B, C, and D, respectively. On the MRI scan, a large T2 hyperintense signal is seen in the right frontal lobe. There is a cystic area adjacent to this. There is no evidence of any contrast enhancement (not shown). There is midline shift. The MRI scan characteristics are suggestive of a low-grade tumor, presumptively astrocytoma, although the biopsy was inconclusive. FDG-PET revealed an area of non-discrete border, with glucose metabolism falling between that of normal gray matter and white matter. This could represent a low-grade tumor. F-DOPA-PET scan revealed an intensely PET-positive lesion in the corresponding right frontal lobe. However, FLT-PET showed no increased uptake in the area corresponding to the MRI T2 lesion.

## Diagnosis and follow-up

Because biopsy yielded non-diagnostic tissue, and the patient had mass effect on his MRI, it was felt suitable to have an open resection for two purposes: (1) to obtain sufficient tissue for an accurate diagnosis, and (2) to relieve some of the mass effect. Right frontal craniotomy with resection of the lesion was performed. Pathology revealed features of a grade II, well-differentiated oligodendroglioma. The patient was subsequently followed by his neuro-oncologist for treatment and management of his low-grade glioma.

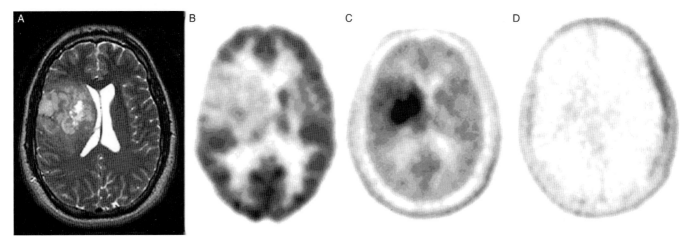

**Figure 5.15** (A) Axial MRI T2; (B) FDG-PET; (C) FDOPA-PET; (D) FLT-PET.

## Discussion and teaching points

The thymidine analog 3′-deoxy-3′-$^{18}$F-fluorothymidine (FLT) was developed as a PET tracer to image proliferation *in vivo* (3) (see Chapter 1). FLT uptake has been shown to reflect the activity of thymidine kinase-1 (TK1), an enzyme expressed during the DNA synthesis phase of the cell cycle (4). TK1 activity is high in proliferating cells and low in quiescent cells. Owing to the phosphorylation of FLT by TK1, negatively charged FLT monophosphate is formed, resulting in intracellular trapping and accumulation of radioactivity (5, 6). In a previously published study in 25 patients with gliomas, FLT tumor uptake was well correlated with the proliferation index Ki-67 (7). However, FLT does not penetrate the blood–brain barrier, thus no uptake is seen in low-grade gliomas with intact blood–brain barrier (7).

## Take-home message

- A low-grade glioma with an intact blood–brain barrier typically shows no FDG uptake or mild uptake less than or equal to white matter (8).
- F-DOPA-PET imaging shows high uptake in newly diagnosed low-grade gliomas with an intact blood–brain barrier.
- With poor ability to penetrate the blood–brain barrier, FLT-PET shows no increased uptake in newly diagnosed low-grade gliomas with an intact blood–brain barrier.

## References

1. Blocher A, Kuntzsch M, Wei R *et al.* Synthesis and labeling of 5′-O-(4,4′-dimethoxytrityl)-2,3′-anhydrothymidine for [$^{18}$F]FLT preparation. *J Radioanal Nucl Chem* 2002;**251**:55–8.

2. Nuyts J, Michel C, Dupont P. Maximum-likelihood expectation-maximization reconstruction of sinograms with arbitrary noise distribution using NEC-transformations. *IEEE Trans Med Imaging* 2001;**20**(5):365–75.

3. Shields A, Grierson J, Dohmen B *et al.* Imaging proliferation in vivo with F-18 FLT and positron emission tomography. *Nature Med* 1998;**4**:1334–6.

4. Rasey JS, Grierson JR, Wiens LW *et al.* Validation of FLT uptake as a measure of thymidine kinase-1 activity I A549 carcinoma cells. *J Nucl Med* 2002;**43**:1210–17.

5. Toyohara J, Waki A, Takamatsu S *et al.* Basis of FLT as a cell proliferation marker: comparative uptake studies with [$^{3}$H]thymidine and [$^{3}$H] arabinothymidine, and cell-analysis in 22 asynchronously growing tumor cell lines. *Nucl Med Biol* 2002;**29**:281–7.

6. Schwartz JL, Grierson JR, Rasey JS *et al.* Rates of accumulation and retention of 3′-deoxy3′-fluorothymidine (FLT) in different cell lines. *J Nucl Med* 2001;**42**:283–90.

7. Chen W, Cloughesy T, Kamdar N *et al.* Imaging proliferation in brain tumors with $^{18}$F-FLT PET: comparison with FDG. *J Nucl Med* 2005;**46**:945–52.

8. Padma MV, Said S, Jacobs M *et al.* Prediction of pathology and survival by FDG-PET in gliomas. *Journal of Neuro-oncology* 2003;**64**:227–37.

A 41-year-old female with recurrent glioblastoma. An MRI scan showed a contrast-enhancing around the original resection site in the right temporal lobe, suggesting tumor progression. As significant responses were seen in patients with recurrent high-grade gliomas treated with anti-angiogenic therapy, bevacizumab (1–4), this patient was started with bevacizumab (10 mg/kg) and irinotecan (125 mg/m$^2$) combination therapy.

## Acquisition and processing parameters

A baseline MRI scan and FLT-PET were performed within 3 days before the start of the treatment. Subsequently, repeat MRI scan and FLT-PET were performed at 6 weeks after starting the treatment.

The PET slice with the maximum tumor uptake was chosen for ROI analysis and the two adjacent axial slices one plane above and one plane below the chosen slice, were included to improve count statistics. A circular ROI (diameter 1.0 cm, 16 pixels) was placed over the area of the tumor. The radiotracer concentration in the ROI was normalized to the injected dose per patient's body weight to derive the standardized uptake values (SUVs, g/mL). PET images were aligned with first MRI scan. The same ROI from the first FLT-PET were placed on the second FLT-PET to measure the change of the PET uptake.

## Findings

Baseline (Figure 5.16A) and 6 weeks post-treatment (Figure 5.16B), MRI T1 with contrast and FLT-PET were performed. On the baseline MRI scan, a contrast-enhancing T1 signal is seen in the right temporal lobe. FLT-PET showed high uptake in the corresponding region. The follow-up MRI scan showed little changes whereas the follow-up FLT-PET scan showed significantly reduced PET uptake (approx 50% reduction in SUV), suggesting treatment response.

## Diagnosis and follow-up

Because MRI showed stable disease and FLT-PET suggested response, patient was continued on the bevacizumab and irinotecan treatment. Subsequent MRI showed reduction in tumor size at 3 months after starting treatment.

## Discussion and teaching points

Considering that FLT tumor uptake correlates well with the proliferation index Ki-67 (5), FLT-PET might play an

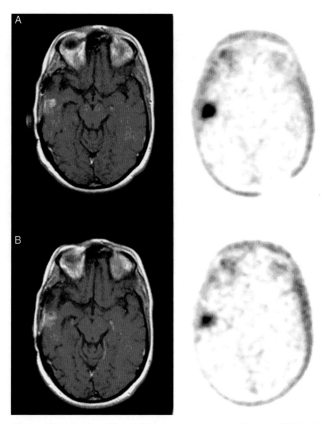

**Figure 5.16** Baseline (A) and 6 weeks post-treatment (B), axial MRI T1 with contrast (left) and FLT-PET images (right).

important role as a surrogate biomarker for evaluating treatment response. This can only be done in tumors with a broken blood–brain barrier, usually recurrent high-grade gliomas as FLT does not penetrate the blood–brain barrier (5). Indeed, it was reported in a pilot study that FLT-PET can serve as an imaging biomarker for predicting treatment response in patients with recurrent malignant gliomas (6). Changes in FLT tumor uptake stratified the patient population into two subgroups: FLT responders with a median survival of 10.8 months, while non-responders lived one third as long, with a median survival of only 3.4 months ($P = 0.003$). The majority (56%) of patients with metabolic response, but none (0%) of the non-responders, were alive at the end of the study. FLT-PET responses at 6 weeks after starting treatment were more significant predictors of overall survival ($P = 0.002$), than the MRI responses (6).

## Take-home message

- PET biomarkers may serve as early predictors of treatment response.

FLT-PET shows promise in predicting overall survival in recurrent high-grade gliomas treated with the anti-angiogenic agent bevacizumab in combination with irinotecan. Further larger-scale study is needed.

## References

1. Vredenburgh JJ, Desjardins A, Hernon JE *et al.* Phase II trial of bevacizumab and irinotecan in recurrent malignant glioma. *Clin Cancer Res* 2007;**13**:1253–9.

2. Vredenburgh JJ, Desjardins A, Herndon JE *et al.* Bevacizumab plus irinotecan in recurrent glioblastoma multiforme. *J Clin Oncol* 2007;**25**:4722–9.

3. Desjardins A, Reardon DA, Herndon JE *et al.* Bevacizumab plus irinotecan in recurrent WHO grade 3 malignant gliomas. *Clin Cancer Res* 2008;**14**:7068–73.

4. Friedman HS, Prados MD, Wen PY *et al.* Bevacizumab alone and in combination with irinotecan in recurrent glioblastoma. *J Clin Oncol* 2009;**27**:4733–40.

5. Chen W, Cloughesy T, Kamdar N *et al.* Imaging proliferation in brain tumors with $^{18}$F-FLT PET: comparison with FDG. *J Nucl Med* 2005;**46**:945–52.

6. Chen W, Delaloye S, Silverman DHS *et al.* Predicting treatment response of malignant gliomas to bevacizumab and irinotecan by imaging proliferation with [$^{18}$F] fluorothymidine positron emission tomography: a pilot study. *J Clin Oncol* 2007;**25**;4714–21.

**Chapter**

# 6

# Head, neck, and thyroid

Heiko Schöder and Ravinder Grewal

## Introduction

Head and neck squamous cell carcinoma (HNSCC) is the sixth most common cancer worldwide. In the USA it accounts for approximately 2% of all cancers and 2% of cancer-related deaths. Nevertheless, HNSCC is an important topic in oncologic imaging, because imaging findings can aid significantly in the detection, staging, and treatment evaluation of these tumors. Patients presenting with primary tumors that are confined at the time of initial diagnosis (T1/2N0M0) have an excellent cure rate. Unfortunately, at the time of initial diagnosis many patients already have regional nodal metastases (45%) or even distant metastases (10%). Also noteworthy is the approximately 5% annual rate of second primaries in HNSCC patients, mostly occurring in the upper aerodigestive tract. The most appropriate treatment approach for HNSCC varies with the disease stage and disease site in the head and neck. Concurrent chemoradiotherapy has become a widely used means for the definitive treatment of locoregionally advanced HNSCC.

Probably 98% of PET studies in patients with head and neck cancer are performed using FDG as the radiotracer. The widespread clinical introduction of FDG-PET/CT in the workup of patients with HNSCC has improved staging accuracy and patient management (1). Today, essentially all patients are examined on combined PET/CT scanners. Studies have shown that combined PET/CT improves the detection of focal FDG uptake in the head and neck and its clear characterization as either benign or malignant. For the overall assessment of disease status, combined PET/CT is more accurate then either modality alone (2–4). This translates into improved patient care (2, 5). The clinical indications of PET/CT in head and neck cancer include: the detection of an unknown primary tumor in patients presenting with neck node metastases; tumor staging (lymph nodes, distant disease); radiotherapy planning; treatment response assessment, usually after concurrent chemoradiotherapy, and sometimes also in patients with advanced disease treated with targeted therapies; and the detection of recurrent disease.

In patients with thyroid cancer, there are fewer indications of FDG-PET/CT (6). They include the assessment of disease extent in patients with differentiated thyroid cancer after total thyroidectomy who present with elevated thyroglobulin (Tg) marker levels but negative radioiodine scan (or where high Tg levels are not sufficiently explained by minor abnormalities on the iodine scan), and patients with Hürthle cell, poorly differentiated, or anaplastic thyroid carcinoma. The latter disease entities are exquisitely FDG-avid.

## References

1. Lonneux M, Hamoir M, Reychler H et al. Positron emission tomography with [18F]fluorodeoxyglucose improves staging and patient management in patients with head and neck squamous cell carcinoma: a multicenter prospective study. *J Clin Oncol* 2010;**28**:1190–5.

2. Schöder H, Yeung HW, Gonen M, Kraus D, Larson SM. Head and neck cancer: clinical usefulness and accuracy of PET/CT image fusion. *Radiology* 2004;**231**:65–72.

3. Branstetter BF 4th, Blodgett TM, Zimmer LA et al. Head and neck malignancy: is PET/CT more accurate than PET or CT alone? *Radiology* 2005;**235**:580–6.

4. Gordin A, Golz A, Daitzchman M et al. Fluorine-18 fluorodeoxyglucose positron emission tomography/ computed tomography imaging in patients with carcinoma of the nasopharynx: diagnostic accuracy and impact on clinical management. *Int J Radiat Oncol Biol Phys* 2007;**68**:370–6.

5. Connell CA, Corry J, Milner AD et al. Clinical impact of and prognostic stratification by, F-18 FDG PET/CT in head and neck mucosal squamous cell carcinoma. *Head Neck* 2007;**29**:986–95.

6. Robbins RJ, Larson SM. The value of positron emission tomography (PET) in the management of patients with thyroid cancer. *Best Pract Res Clin Endocrinol Metab* 2008;**22**:1047–59.

# Neck metastases from an unknown primary tumor

A 63-year-old male was found to have bilateral neck lymph-adenopathy on an annual physical exam. Physical exam of the head and neck failed to show any clear abnormality in oral cavity and oropharynx.

## Acquisition and processing parameters

Following a 6-hour fasting period, 12.3 mCi of FDG was injected intravenously. The plasma glucose at the time of FDG injection was 103 mg/dL. After a 75 min uptake period, low-dose CT (140 kVp, 80 mA, 0.8 s per CT rotation, pitch of 1.75 : 1 and reconstructed slice thickness of 3.8 mm) and PET emission images were obtained from the mid skull to the upper thighs on a Discovery LS PET/CT. PET data were acquired for 5 min per bed position. The CT data were reconstructed using an iterative algorithm and a 512 × 512 matrix for 70 cm trans-axial field of view. The PET images were reconstructed using an iterative algorithm and a 128 × 128 matrix. The CT data were used to generate the transmission maps for attenuation correction of the PET emission images and for anatomic localization. Standardized uptake values (SUV) were normalized to patient body weight; the highest activity concentration (SUVmax) in a given disease site is recorded.

## Findings and differential diagnosis

There are enlarged lymph nodes in the bilateral neck. These show intense FDG uptake (SUVmax 9.9 right neck, SUVmax 5.9 left neck) (Figure 6.1A–F). A small soft tissue nodule at the left base of the tongue at the left side of the epiglottis shows

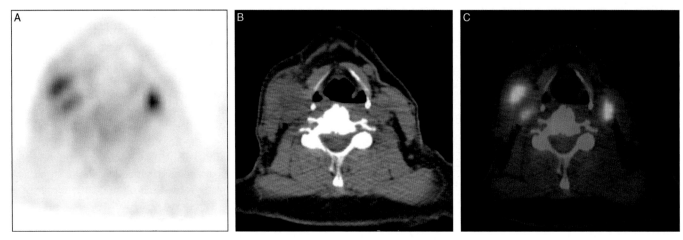

**Figure 6.1A–C** Transaxial FDG-PET, CT, and fusion images (A, B, C) showing abnormal FDG uptake in bilateral neck lymph nodes.

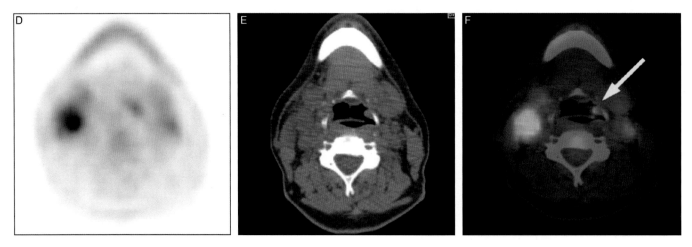

**Figure 6.1D–F** Transaxial FDG-PET, CT, and fusion images (D, E, F) showing focal increased FDG uptake in a small soft tissue nodule at the left base of tongue (arrow).

mild FDG uptake with SUVmax 3.2 (D, E, F with arrow). In this patient with metastatic lymph nodes from an unknown primary, this finding is suspicious for a primary tumor at the left base of tongue. There are no other abnormalities in the head and neck.

## Diagnosis and follow-up

Fine needle biopsy from the left base of tongue, performed after the PET/CT, showed malignant cells, squamous cell carcinoma, proving the diagnosis. The PET/CT finding was clearly abnormal, and there is virtually no other differential diagnosis in this case.

The patient underwent combined modality treatment with concurrent intensity modulated radiation therapy (IMRT) and cisplatin chemotherapy. A PET/CT approximately 12 weeks after the end of therapy showed residual 2.5 cm cystic node in the right neck, level 3, with mild FDG uptake in the rim, and no uptake centrally. This finding was not considered suspicious, but instead thought to be a necrotic node. A follow-up scan 4 months later showed the same findings (not shown here). However, due to lack of lymph node involution, the patient underwent right neck dissection of levels 2–4. The histopathologic specimen showed the 2.5 cm right neck node with necrosis, fibrosis, acute inflammation, and punctuate calcifications. No viable tumor was identified.

## Discussion and teaching points

Carcinoma of unknown primary accounts for 3–15% of all cancer diagnoses and for approximately 1–2% of head and neck cancers (see Chapter 17). For practical purposes this entity should be defined as the combination of no history of previous malignancy, no clinical or laboratory evidence for primary neoplasm, neck mass that is histologically or cytologically proven to be carcinoma. Occurrence of nodal metastases in neck levels 1–3 increases the likelihood for a primary HNSCC. However, in 5–40% of cases a primary malignancy is never identified during diagnostic evaluation and long-term follow-up.

FDG-PET, and in particular PET/CT, has emerged as the single imaging test to evaluate these patients (1). Other imaging studies rarely contribute valuable information, and it is extremely unlikely that these will identify a primary tumor that cannot be detected by PET/CT. If the PET/CT study is positive, biopsies can be obtained from the suggested location. If the PET/CT is negative, panendoscopy with biopsy sampling from suspected locations (based on the location of the lymph node and statistical considerations) can be performed. Potential reasons for false-negative PET studies include a small primary tumor (although lesions as small as 4 mm can be detected as long as they demonstrate intense FDG uptake); low metabolic activity (cystic, necrotic tumor, or lymph nodes) or the primary tumor was accidentally removed at time of neck dissection.

## Take-home message

- If thorough clinical exam, including office endoscopy, by a dedicated head and neck surgeon or oncologist fails to show a primary tumor in patients with neck nodal metastases, FDG-PET/CT should be considered as the next diagnostic step.
- PET/CT should be done before biopsies are obtained, in order to avoid false-positive scan findings. Biopsies should be directed to sites of suspicious FDG uptake. In the past, many patients with unknown primary were subjected to "blind" or "random" biopsies from the nasopharynx, oropharynx, base of tongue, bilateral tonsillectomy, etc. In the era of PET/CT this random search for the site of primary disease can no longer be justified.
- In patients who have undergone thorough clinical exam and imaging prior to PET/CT, the scan will identify the site of the primary tumor in approximately 30% of cases. Of note these are then cases, in which all other modalities, short of "random biopsies," failed to show the site of primary disease.

## Reference

1. Schöder H, Yeung HW. Positron emission imaging of head and neck cancer, including thyroid carcinoma. *Semin Nucl Med* 2004;34:180–97.

A 49-year-old male with history of non-seminomatous germ cell tumor approximately 20 years earlier, now presenting with left tonsillar carcinoma. FDG-PET/CT was done for staging of disease and radiotherapy planning.

## Acquisition and processing parameters

Following a 6-hour fasting period, 14.8 mCi of FDG was injected intravenously. The plasma glucose at the time of FDG injection was 92 mg/dL. After a 79 min uptake period, low-dose CT (140 kVp, 80 mA, 0.8 s per CT rotation, pitch of 1.75 : 1 and reconstructed slice thickness of 3.8 mm) and PET emission images were obtained from the mid skull to the upper thighs on a Discovery LS PET/CT. PET data were acquired for 5 min per bed position. The CT data were reconstructed using an iterative algorithm and a $512 \times 512$ matrix for 70 cm transaxial field of view. The PET images were reconstructed using an iterative algorithm and a $128 \times 128$ matrix. The CT data were used to generate the transmission maps for attenuation correction of the PET emission images and for anatomic localization. Standardized uptake values (SUV) were normalized to patient body weight; the highest activity concentration (SUVmax) in a given disease site is recorded.

## Findings and differential diagnosis

Increased abnormal FDG uptake (SUV 8.9) is identified in the left palatine tonsil, corresponding to the known primary tumor. A left lateral retropharyngeal lymph node also shows abnormal tracer uptake (SUV 3.1), suspicious for a metastatic

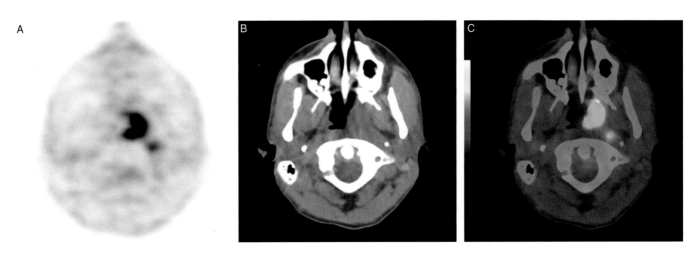

**Figure 6.2 A–C** Transaxial FDG-PET, CT, and fusion images (A, B, C) show clearly abnormal FDG uptake in the tumor in the left palatine tonsil as well as a left retropharyngeal lymph node. A 6 × 10 mm right retromandibular (level 2) lymph node and a 8 × 10 mm left level 2 node have mild FDG uptake.

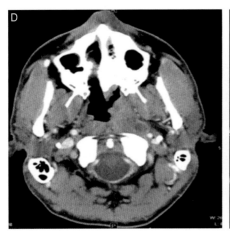

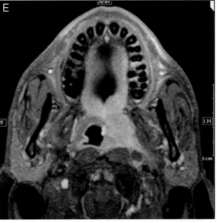

**Figure 6.2 D, E** Both findings are also well recognized on contrast enhanced transaxial CT (D) and T1-weighted MR image (E).

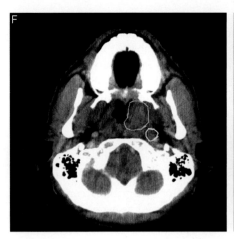
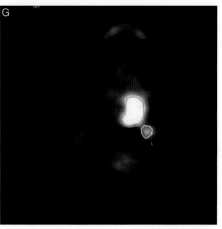

**Figure 6.2F, G** Selected images from the radiotherapy plan are shown in F and G.

node. A 6 × 10 mm right retromandibular (level 2) lymph node and a 8 × 10 mm left level 2 node have mild FDG uptake with SUVmax of 2.4 and 1.7 respectively. These are possibly metastatic, but may be reactive.

## Discussion and teaching points

This patient was clinically staged as T3N2B tonsillar carcinoma. The patient was successfully treated with concurrent chemoradiotherapy with 70 Gy IMRT to the left tonsil and neck and three cycles of cisplatin chemotherapy. A follow-up PET/CT, approximately 10–12 weeks after the end of chemoradiotherapy, showed no residual disease. Unfortunately, 3 years later, this patient developed a third primary carcinoma elsewhere in the head and neck.

FDG-PET/CT is increasingly being used for the staging of head and neck cancer. The primary emphasis is in the staging of lymph node metastases and distant disease outside the neck. The primary tumor can usually be better assessed by high-resolution CT or MRI studies, in particular when addressing questionable perineural spread, bone invasion, and skull base invasion, etc.

The presence of nodal metastases is an independent prognostic factor for survival in patients with head and neck cancer; it decreases the overall survival by approximately one-half (1). The prognosis worsens additionally with the number of lymph nodes involved, with extracapsular spread of nodal disease (2), and with metastases located in the lower neck. The presence and extent of nodal metastases may affect patient management. Early removal of neck nodal metastases also has prognostic implications (3). Accurate nodal staging of the neck is therefore important. The clinical neck exam and anatomic imaging studies suffer from a lack of sensitivity and specificity in assessing the extent of nodal disease (reviewed in reference 4). With CT and MRI, lymph nodes are primarily characterized based on size criteria, although newer MR techniques are emerging. In addition to nodal size, other parameters, such as grouped location, central necrosis, and contrast enhancement, can be used to guide CT and MRI interpretation, but nevertheless, their false-negative rates range from 10% to 30%.

Numerous studies have compared the accuracy of anatomic imaging modalities and FDG-PET for the detection of nodal metastases in the neck (5–7). A recent meta-analysis confirmed the superiority of FDG-PET or PET/CT over structural imaging alone (8). Nevertheless, PET cannot identify microscopic disease. Therefore, the need for neck dissection should be decided based on clinical concerns and statistical considerations of disease spread to neck lymph nodes at various levels; imaging studies, including PET, may confirm the need for neck dissection, but a negative study cannot exclude disease spread with certainty. This situation bears some similarity to breast cancer imaging with PET, and similarly, sentinel node mapping is now emerging as a new tool in the management of HNSCC (9). Reasons for false-positive findings include reactive lymph node enlargement and non-specific FDG uptake in nodes, for instance related to viral infections, granulomatous infections (10), etc. Reasons for false-negative PET studies may include a small tumor burden in metastatic nodes, cystic degeneration of metastatic nodes only surrounded by a small rim of viable tumor tissue, low tracer uptake in the metastatic node, and imaging artifacts. Nodal metastases in close proximity to the primary tumor may not be detectable as separate hypermetabolic focus when the primary shows very intense tracer uptake.

Another indication for staging PET/CT is the detection of distant metastatic disease outside the neck as well as the detection of second, synchronous primary tumors (11). Distant metastases are rare in patients with head and neck cancers, but the frequency increases with higher T-stage, size, and number of tumor-involved lymph nodes. Patients with nodal metastases in the lower neck or supraclavicular region have a higher chance for distant metastases, too. In general, patients with HNSCC have a higher propensity for synchronous second primaries as compared with many other malignancies. Based on our own experience, a second primary or distant metastases outside the neck will be detected in 3–8% of cases, depending on the stage and location of the primary tumor.

The role of PET/CT for radiotherapy planning in the head and neck is under investigation (12–16). To be meaningful, both the CT and PET must be acquired in an identical radiotherapy set-up position, including a flat tabletop, and immobilization mask. The data are then imported into the radiotherapy planning software. Studies have shown that the addition of PET data to standard treatment planning with CT alone improves (decreases) inter-observer variability in target design. Differences between CT-based target design and PET-based target design are not unidirectional; i.e., in some cases the PET-based volume is larger, in other cases smaller than the CT-based volume. This might occur because PET detects lymph node metastases not recognized by CT, and differentiates better between tumor spread and normal soft tissue or mucous retention (in paranasal sinuses). Prospective randomized studies investigating patient outcome in a PET/CT-based target design as compared with standard treatment planning are lacking. In patients undergoing chemoradiotherapy, the metabolic tumor volume at staging may be associated with worse treatment outcome (17).

## Take-home message

- FDG-PET/CT improves the staging of HNSCC with regard to lymph node involvement and distant disease outside the neck. Therefore, staging PET/CT is particularly

recommended in patients with large primary tumors and clinical lymph node metastases in the lower neck – factors that increase the statistical probability for distant disease. In patients who are candidates for primary tumor surgery, the PET/CT may add information in some cases, but may not be needed as a routine staging test. In contrast, all patients with locoregional advanced disease, who are usually treated with concurrent chemoradiotherapy, should undergo baseline PET/CT for staging and radiotherapy planning.

- Depending on the location and nature of the primary tumor, high-resolution CT or MRI with IV contrast remains essential, in particular for assessing bone (skull base) invasion and perineural spread of disease.

- The incorporation of PET findings into radiotherapy planning requires clinical expertise in PET imaging, recognition of potential artifacts, imaging physics, knowing about sources of false-positive and false-negative FDG uptake. Close cooperation between the radiation oncologist and PET/CT readers is recommended for successful implementation of PET/CT-based radiotherapy planning.

## References

1. O'Brien C, Smith J, Soong S et al. Neck dissection with and without radiotherapy – prognostic factors, patterns of recurrence and survival. Am J Surg 1986;**152**:456–63.

2. Snyderman NL, Johnson JT, Schramm VL, Jr et al. Extracapsular spread of carcinoma in cervical lymph nodes. Impact upon survival in patients with carcinoma of the supraglottic larynx. Cancer 1985;**56**:1597–9.

3. Haddadin KJ, Soutar DS, Oliver RJ et al. Improved survival for patients with clinically T1/T2, N0 tongue tumors undergoing a prophylactic neck dissection. Head Neck 1999;**21**:517–25.

4. Schöder H, Yeung HW. Positron emission imaging of head and neck cancer, including thyroid carcinoma. Semin Nucl Med 2004;**34**:180–97.

5. Hannah A, Scott AM, Tochon-Danguy H et al. Evaluation of 18 F-fluorodeoxyglucose positron emission tomography and computed tomography with histopathologic correlation in the initial staging of head and neck cancer. Ann Surg 2002;**236**:208–17.

6. Yamamoto Y, Wong TZ, Turkington TG, Hawk TC, Coleman RE. Head and neck cancer: dedicated FDG PET/CT protocol for detection – phantom and initial clinical studies. Radiology 2007;**244**:263–72.

7. Ng SH, Yen TC, Chang JT et al. Prospective study of [18F] fluorodeoxyglucose positron emission tomography and computed tomography and magnetic resonance imaging in oral cavity squamous cell carcinoma with palpably negative neck. J Clin Oncol 2006;**24**(27):4371–6.

8. Kyzas PA, Evangelou E, Denaxa-Kyza D, Ioannidis JP. 18F-fluorodeoxyglucose positron emission tomography to evaluate cervical node metastases in patients with head and neck squamous cell carcinoma: a meta-analysis. J Natl Cancer Inst 2008;**100**:712–20.

9. Civantos FJ, Zitsch RP, Schuller DE et al. Sentinel lymph node biopsy accurately stages the regional lymph nodes for T1-T2 oral squamous cell carcinomas: results of a prospective multi-institutional trial. J Clin Oncol 2010;**28**:1395–400.

10. Schöder H, Carlson DL, Kraus DH et al. 18F-FDG PET/CT for detecting nodal metastases in patients with oral cancer staged N0 by clinical examination and CT/MRI. J Nucl Med 2006;**47**:755–62.

11. Stokkel MP, Moons KG, ten Broek FW et al. 18F-fluorodeoxyglucose dual-head positron emission tomography as a procedure for detecting simultaneous primary tumors in cases of head and neck cancer. Cancer 1999;**86**:2370–7.

12. Ciernik IF, Dizendorf E, Baumert BG et al. Radiation treatment planning with an integrated positron emission and computer tomography (PET/CT): a feasibility study. Int J Radiat Oncol Biol Phys 2003;**57**:853–63.

13. Schwartz DL, Ford EC, Rajendran J et al. PET/CT-guided intensity modulated head and neck radiotherapy: a pilot investigation. Head Neck 2005;**27**:478–87.

14. Vernon MR, Maheshwari M, Schultz CJ et al. Clinical outcomes of patients receiving integrated PET/CT-guided radiotherapy for head and neck carcinoma. Int J Radiat Oncol Biol Phys 2008;**70**:678–84.

15. Schinagl DA, Vogel WV, Hoffmann AL et al. Comparison of five segmentation tools for 18F-fluoro-deoxy-glucose-positron emission tomography-based target volume definition in head and neck cancer. Int J Radiat Oncol Biol Phys 2007;**69**:1282–9.

16. Greco C, Nehmeh SA, Schöder H et al. Evaluation of different methods of 18F-FDG-PET target volume delineation in the radiotherapy of head and neck cancer. Am J Clin Oncol 2008;**31**:439–45.

17. La TH, Filion EJ, Turnbull BB et al. Metabolic tumor volume predicts for recurrence and death in head-and-neck cancer. Int J Radiat Oncol Biol Phys 2009;**74**:1335–41.

A 53-year-old male with a clinical diagnosis of base of tongue cancer. Two months prior to clinical presentation the patient noted bilateral neck lymph node swelling after what was thought to be a common cold. This did not resolve, eventually leading to lymph node biopsy, which showed malignant cells. The clinical exam demonstrated a firm base of tongue mass and bilateral neck lymphadenopathy; the clinical stage was assigned as T2N2C (right N2A, left N1), stage IV.

Biopsy from the right tongue base showed poorly differentiated invasive squamous cell carcinoma. Multimodality treatment with concurrent intensity modulated radiation therapy (IMRT) and chemotherapy (cisplatin and bevacizumab) was selected as appropriate treatment option. Following our institutional guidelines, 11 weeks after completion of therapy, the patient underwent FDG-PET/CT to assess treatment response.

## Acquisition and processing parameters

Following a 6-hour fasting period, 12.1 mCi of FDG was injected intravenously. After a 90 min uptake period, low-dose CT (140 kVp, 80 mA, 0.8 s per CT rotation, pitch of 1.75 : 1 and reconstructed slice thickness of 3.8 mm) and PET emission images were obtained from the mid skull to the upper thighs on a Discovery LS PET/CT. PET data were acquired for 5 min per bed position. The CT data were reconstructed using an iterative algorithm and a 512 × 512 matrix for 70 cm transaxial field of view. The PET images were reconstructed using an iterative algorithm and a 128 × 128 matrix. The CT data were used to generate the transmission maps for attenuation correction of the PET emission images and for anatomic localization.

The plasma glucose at the time of FDG injection was 88 mg/dL. Standardized uptake values (SUV) were normalized to patient body weight; the highest activity concentration (SUV-max) in a given disease site is recorded.

## Findings and differential diagnosis

The baseline study had shown abnormal FDG uptake at the base of tongue, and this is no longer seen following treatment. Instead, however, there is intense FDG uptake in the epiglottis, which appears thickened, as well as in the pre-epiglottic space. There is also new intense FDG uptake in the region of the right glossotonsillar sulcus, extending to the right side of the posterior tongue. This is in fact more intense than in the baseline scan (SUV 7.7, prior 5.4). The area of abnormal uptake here is also larger. CT findings suggest ulceration. The previously noted FDG uptake in bilateral neck lymph nodes including levels 2 bilaterally and level 3 on the right side of the neck has resolved. Although a few residual enlarged nodes are seen on the CT component of the scan, these have no abnormal tracer uptake. Laryngeal edema is considered to be a post-treatment effect.

## Diagnosis and follow-up

Based on negative FDG-PET/CT findings, the patient was observed. A subsequent PET/CT scan approximately 5 months later showed resolution of inflammation and ulceration at the right lateral tongue. Unfortunately, at that time the patient had developed (asymptomatic) metastatic disease in

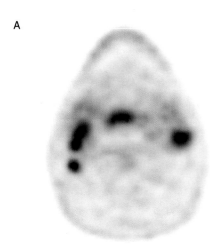
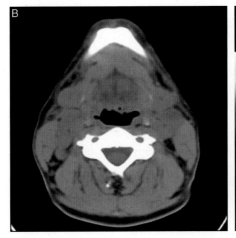
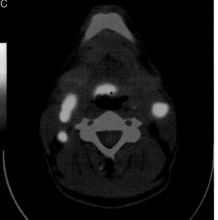

**Figure 6.3A–C** Baseline transaxial FDG-PET, CT, and fusion images (A, B, C) show the abnormal FDG uptake in the primary tumor at the base of tongue as well as bilateral neck lymph node metastases.

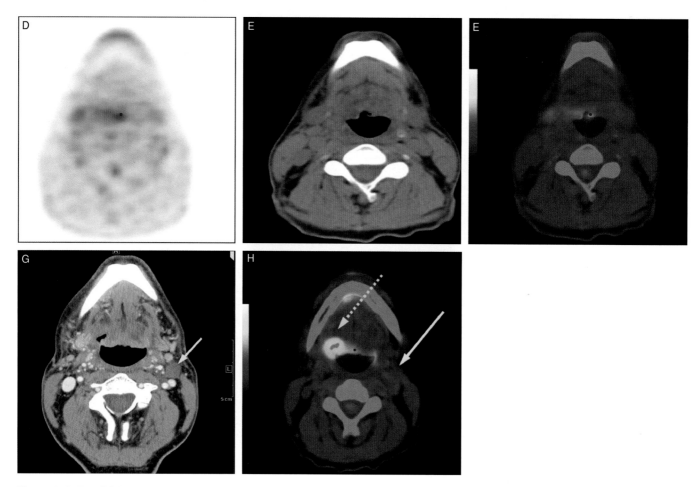

**Figure 6.3D–F and G–H** Post-treatment scan done 11 weeks after the end of therapy (D, E, F) showing that the abnormal FDG uptake in neck nodes and primary site has resolved. However, transaxial contrast enhanced CT (G, arrow) shows a residual 1.4 × 1.4 cm lymph node in the left neck, level 2, which has no abnormal FDG uptake (H). There is a new area of ulceration with intense FDG uptake along the right posterior lateral tongue and glossotonsillar sulcus, consistent with treatment-induced changes (G, H, dotted arrow).

mediastinal lymph nodes and in the bilateral lungs. This was proven by bronchoscopy.

## Discussion and teaching points

Patients with locoregionally advanced head and neck cancer that is surgically unresectable, and patients in whom definitive treatment is administered with an attempt at organ-preservation (e.g., oropharyngeal and laryngeal carcinomas), undergo treatment with concurrent chemoradiotherapy. Randomized studies have shown that this regimen leads to excellent outcome in the majority of patients (1–2).

Non-specific findings, including residual enlarged neck nodes, are commonly encountered after chemoradiotherapy. Complete response rates in irradiated cervical lymph nodes vary between 59% and 83% and to some degree are related to nodal size, dose of radiotherapy, as well as the time point when response is determined: complete response rates are almost 100% in N1 disease, higher in N2 than in N3 disease, and better when the largest metastatic node is < 3 cm (3). In N2–N3 disease, residual cancer in neck nodes has been reported in

16–39% of patients achieving a clinical complete response (no overt residual neck mass) (3–6). Early studies demonstrated better outcomes when radiotherapy was followed by neck dissection, leading to the practice of "planned neck dissection" for all patients with N2–N3 disease on presentation (regardless of the response to treatment) as well as for patients with N1 disease and persistent palpable lymph nodes after irradiation. However, in light of the improved locoregional control rates with concurrent chemoradiotherapy this may no longer be necessary (7). Several recent studies have consistently shown that a negative FDG-PET/CT after chemoradiotherapy excludes residual disease with a very high negative predictive value in the range of 95–98% (8–10). Therefore, many patients with residual enlarged lymph nodes after the end of therapy do not need to undergo neck dissection. The positive predictive value is lower, in the range of 30–50%; however, this is still considerably better than with CT or MRI alone. Readers must be familiar with the many reasons for false-positive FDG findings in the head and neck, in particular post-therapy inflammation and ulceration, as in this case. Scan interpretation should primarily rest on visual interpretation. While semiquantitative SUV analysis may be helpful to demonstrate the magnitude of treatment-induced changes, there is no clear cut off (either as absolute SUV or percent change compared with the baseline study) that can distinguish residual malignancy post-treatment from treatment-induced inflammation or infection. Persistent high uptake after CRT does not necessarily indicate residual/recurrent disease, but is generally a marker of poor clinical outcome because it is inversely related to quality of life and indicates persistent inflammation, infection, development of fibrosis, or other treatment sequelae (11).

## Take-home message

- Concurrent chemoradiotherapy in the modern era leads to excellent outcome in the majority of patients. Residual disease after completion of this regimen can occur but this is a rare event. In contrast, post-treatment inflammation is a common phenomenon.

- Residual disease is extremely unlikely in lymph nodes with short axis of 1.0 cm or less. The additional information from FDG imaging increases the accuracy of imaging after chemoradiotherapy by reducing the usually large number of false-positive cases that are encountered when decisions are solely made based on nodal size. PET interpretation should rely on comparison of tracer uptake in nodes as compared with adjacent neck tissues.

- Our interdisciplinary group of head and neck surgeons, medical oncologists and imaging experts recommends that FDG-PET/CT be performed at approximately 10–12 weeks after chemoradiotherapy, which strikes a balance between resolving post-treatment inflammation and the surgical need for early decision to avoid operating in heavily fibrotic tissues. Our current algorithm is outlined in reference (10).

## References

1. Forastiere AA, Goepfert H, Maor M *et al.* Concurrent chemotherapy and radiotherapy for organ preservation in advanced laryngeal cancer. *N Engl J Med* 2003;**349**:2091–8.

2. Denis F, Garaud P, Bardet E *et al.* Final results of the 94–01 French Head and Neck Oncology and Radiotherapy Group randomized trial comparing radiotherapy alone with concomitant radiochemotherapy in advanced-stage oropharynx carcinoma. *J Clin Oncol* 2004;**22**:69–76.

3. McHam SA, Adelstein DJ, Rybicki LA *et al.* Who merits a neck dissection after definitive chemoradiotherapy for N2-N3 squamous cell head and neck cancer? *Head Neck* 2003;**25**:791–8.

4. Brizel DM, Prosnitz RG, Hunter S *et al.* Necessity for adjuvant neck dissection in setting of concurrent chemoradiation for advanced head-and-neck cancer. *Int J Radiat Oncol Biol Phys* 2004;**58**:1418–23.

5. Frank DK, Hu KS, Culliney BE *et al.* Planned neck dissection after concomitant radiochemotherapy for advanced head and neck cancer. *Laryngoscope* 2005;**115**:1015–20.

6. Argiris A, Stenson KM, Brockstein BE *et al.* Neck dissection in the combined-modality therapy of patients with locoregionally advanced head and neck cancer. *Head Neck* 2004;**26**:447–55.

7. Schöder H, Fury M, Lee N, Kraus D. PET monitoring of therapy response in head and neck squamous cell carcinoma. J Nucl Med 2009;**50** Suppl 1: 74S–88S.

8. Porceddu SV, Jarmolowski E, Hicks RJ *et al.* Utility of positron emission tomography for the detection of disease in residual neck nodes after (chemo) radiotherapy in head and neck cancer. *Head Neck* 2005;**27**:175–81.

9. Yao M, Smith RB, Graham MM *et al.* The role of FDG PET in management of neck metastasis from head-and-neck cancer after definitive radiation treatment. *Int J Radiat Oncol Biol Phys* 2005;**63**:991–9.

10. Ong SC, Schoder H, Lee NY *et al.* Clinical utility of 18F-FDG PET/CT in assessing the neck after concurrent chemoradiotherapy for locoregional advanced head and neck cancer. *J Nucl Med* 2008;**49**:532–40.

11. Dornfeld K, Hopkins S, Simmons J *et al.* Posttreatment FDG-PET uptake in the supraglottic and glottic larynx correlates with decreased quality of life after chemoradiotherapy. *Int J Radiat Oncol Biol Phys* 2008;**71**:386–92.

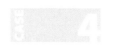

A 65-year-old female with increasing nasal congestion. A local ENT specialist prescribed a nasal spray and decongesting medication, but her symptoms progressed. Ultimately, the patient was seen by five different physicians. A neck CT was eventually ordered and showed a 4.5 cm soft tissue mass in the nasopharynx causing occlusion of the eustachian tube with fluid accumulation in the middle ear and mastoid process. There was tumor extension into the sphenoid sinus and skull base with invasion of clivus, petrous apices, and prepontine cistern.

## Acquisition and processing parameters

Following a 6-hour fasting period, 12.8 mCi of FDG was injected intravenously. The plasma glucose at the time of FDG injection was 104 mg/dL. After a 79 min uptake period, low-dose CT (140 kVp, 80 mA, 0.8 s per CT rotation, pitch of 1.75 : 1 and reconstructed slice thickness of 3.8 mm) and PET

emission images were obtained from the mid skull to the upper thighs on a Discovery STE PET/CT. PET data were acquired for 5 min per bed position. The CT data were reconstructed using an iterative algorithm and a $512 \times 512$ matrix with a 70 cm transaxial field of view. The PET images were reconstructed using an iterative algorithm and a $128 \times 128$ matrix. The CT data were used to generate the transmission maps for attenuation correction of the PET emission images and for anatomic localization. Standardized uptake values (SUV) were normalized to patient body weight; the highest activity concentration (SUVmax) in a given disease site is recorded.

## Findings and differential diagnosis
## Diagnosis and follow-up

The patient was staged as T4N1M0; right cranial nerve VI palsy was diagnosed. Due to locally advanced disease, the

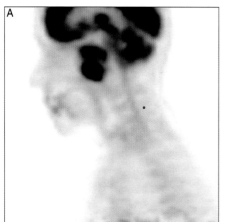
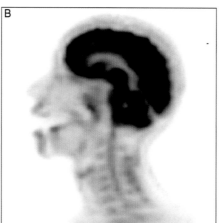

**Figure 6.4A, B** (A) Initial staging sagittal FDG-PET emission images show abnormal FDG uptake in a large nasopharyngeal primary extending inferiorly to the level of the soft palate. In (B) 4 weeks after induction chemotherapy there is evidence of significant reduction in size and metabolic activity in the mass.

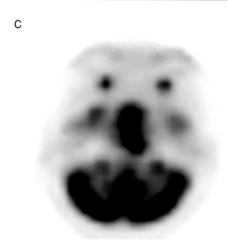
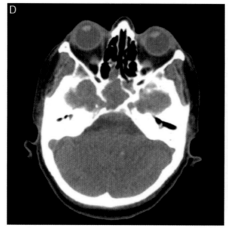
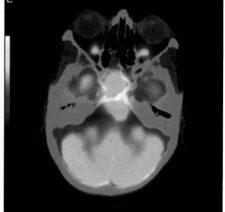

**Figure 6.4C–E** Initial staging transaxial FDG-PET, CT, and fusion images (C, D, E) demonstrate abnormal FDG uptake (SUVmax 15.4) in the nasopharyngeal mass with extension into the sphenoid sinus, skull base, and prepontine cistern.

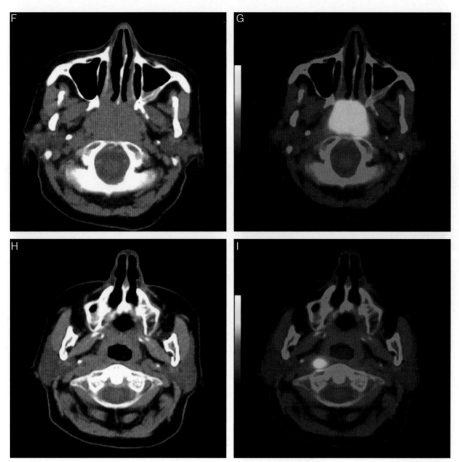

**Figure 6.4F–I** Additional CT and fusion images (F, G, H, I) demonstrate the full extent of the large nasopharyngeal soft tissue mass and abnormal FDG uptake in a right retropharyngeal lymph node consistent with metastasis. Other hypermetabolic metastatic lymph nodes (not shown) were seen in the right neck level 2 (retromandibular, SUV 3.8) and levels 5A (SUV 9.0) (not shown). A left retropharyngeal lymph node had an SUV of 4.1 (not shown). No hypermetabolic nodes in the left lateral neck (normal-sized non-FDG-avid nodes are seen on the CT component of this study).

patient underwent induction chemotherapy with TPF (docetaxel, cisplatin, 5-fluorouracil) to reduce the tumor volume. This was followed by 70 Gy IMRT to the nasopharynx and to the neck bilaterally, with concurrent cisplatin chemotherapy. There was rapid response to induction chemotherapy, and complete response to the subsequent concurrent chemoradiotherapy. Approximately 2.5 years later, the patient is still free of disease.

## Discussion and teaching points

Nasopharyngeal cancer (NPC) is a unique disease entity that shows a clinical behavior and histopathology that is different from that of other squamous cell carcinomas of the head and neck. It occurs endemically in Southeast Asia. MRI is considered the imaging modality of choice for staging NPC (1), because it has excellent soft tissue contrast, demonstrates perineural tumor spread, skull base invasion and intracranial spread, identifies disease spread into the parapharyngeal space (associated with worse prognosis), and differentiates disease from mucous retention secondary to obstruction in the paranasal sinuses. Bilateral neck lymph node involvement is common in NPC (up to 80% of cases), secondary to the primary tumor location close to the midline. The probability for distant metastasis outside the neck increases with tumor

size and N stage. Bone, lung, or mediastinum and liver are the most common sites of metastatic spread. Nodal involvement and distant spread are evaluated well by PET/CT (2–4). The intensity of FDG uptake in NPC provides prognostic information (5). PET/CT is also an excellent test for response assessment and for the detection of recurrent disease in the nasopharynx. On post-therapy scans, there is often mild residual FDG uptake due to inflammation. Its intensity will decline over several months. Recurrent disease can be detected and staged with PET/CT. Treatment-induced osteoradionecrosis is a reason for false-positive FDG uptake in the skull base. Overall, combined assessment with MRI and FDG-PET/CT is probably the best approach in staging and follow-up of NPC (6). This patient presented with advanced disease. Induction chemotherapy was used to reduce tumor volume for subsequent concurrent chemoradiotherapy with curative intent. The patient showed a complete clinical response. However, the high initial FDG uptake and extent of disease at presentation may indicate an overall poor prognosis.

## Take-home message

- Primary staging of nasopharynx cancer should include FDG-PET/CT and MRI.
- PET/CT is valuable in assessing response to induction chemotherapy and concurrent chemoradiotherapy.

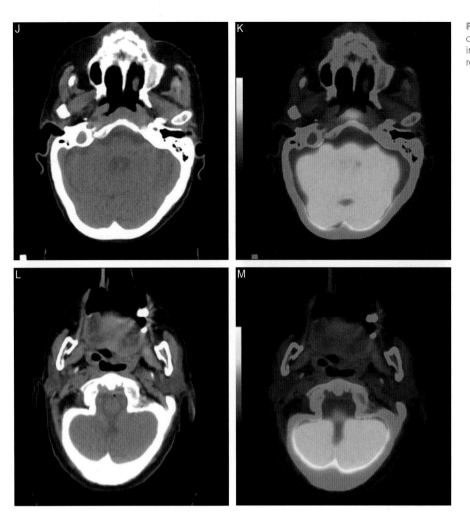

**Figure 6.4J–M** Following induction chemotherapy, the mass is significantly reduced in size and FDG uptake, and the hypermetabolic retropharyngeal lymph node is no longer identified.

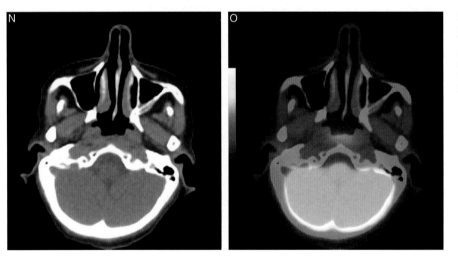

**Figure 6.4N–O** Subsequently, the patient underwent concurrent chemoradiotherapy. The follow-up scan approximately 7 months after the end of treatment shows very mild residual FDG uptake in the nasopharynx; this indicates non-specific post-treatment inflammation, which can last for many months.

- Non-specific post-treatment changes are common; mild residual uptake will resolve over the course of several weeks or even months after the end of therapy.

Changes in imaging appearance, rather than a single finding by itself, are therefore key to recognize recurrence early.

# References

1. Chong VF, Ong CK. Nasopharyngeal carcinoma. *Eur J Radiol* 2008;**66**:437–47.

2. Yen RF, Hung RL, Pan MH *et al.* 18-fluoro-2-deoxyglucose positron emission tomography in detecting residual/recurrent nasopharyngeal carcinomas and comparison with magnetic resonance imaging. *Cancer* 2003;**98**:283–7.

3. Liu FY, Chang JT, Wang HM *et al.* [18F]fluorodeoxyglucose positron emission tomography is more sensitive than skeletal scintigraphy for detecting bone metastasis in endemic nasopharyngeal carcinoma at initial staging. *J Clin Oncol* 2006;**24**:599–604.

4. Chang JT, Chan SC, Yen TC *et al.* Nasopharyngeal carcinoma staging by (18)F-fluorodeoxyglucose positron emission tomography. *Int J Radiat Oncol Biol Phys* 2005;**62**:501–7.

5. Xie P, Yue JB, Fu Z, Feng R, Yu JM. Prognostic value of 18F-FDG PET/CT before and after radiotherapy for locally advanced nasopharyngeal carcinoma. *Ann Oncol* 2010;**21**:1078–82.

6. Comoretto M, Balestreri L, Borsatti E *et al.* Detection and restaging of residual and/or recurrent nasopharyngeal carcinoma after chemotherapy and radiation therapy: comparison of MR imaging and FDG PET/CT. *Radiology* 2008;**249**:203–11.

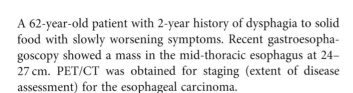

A 62-year-old patient with 2-year history of dysphagia to solid food with slowly worsening symptoms. Recent gastroesophagoscopy showed a mass in the mid-thoracic esophagus at 24–27 cm. PET/CT was obtained for staging (extent of disease assessment) for the esophageal carcinoma.

## Acquisition and processing parameters

Following a 6-hour fasting period, 14.5 mCi of FDG was injected intravenously. The plasma glucose at the time of FDG injection was 76 mg/dL. After a 65 min uptake period, low-dose CT (140 kVp, 80 mA, 0.8 s per CT rotation, pitch of 1.75 : 1 and reconstructed slice thickness of 3.8 mm) and PET emission images were obtained from the mid skull to the upper thighs on a Discovery STE PET/CT. PET data were acquired

for 5 min per bed position. The CT data were reconstructed using an iterative algorithm and a 512 × 512 matrix for 70 cm transaxial field of view. The PET images were reconstructed using an iterative algorithm and a 128 × 128 matrix. The CT data were used to generate the transmission maps for attenuation correction of the PET emission images and for anatomic localization. Standardized uptake values (SUV) were normalized to patient body weight; the highest activity concentration (SUVmax) in a given disease site is recorded.

## Findings and differential diagnosis

This case illustrates the incidental finding of obstruction of all left paranasal sinuses, an admixture of mucosal swelling, inflammation, and mucous retention. There is intense tracer

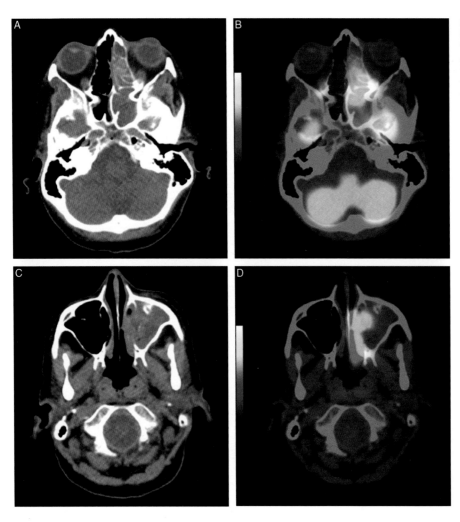

**Figure 6.5A–D** Baseline transaxial CT and FDG-PET/CT fusion images show extensive hypermetabolic mucosal swelling in the left sphenoid and ethmoid sinuses (A, B), as well as nasal cavity and left maxillary sinus (C, D). There is post-obstructive fluid (mucous) retention in all left paranasal sinuses (pansinusitis).

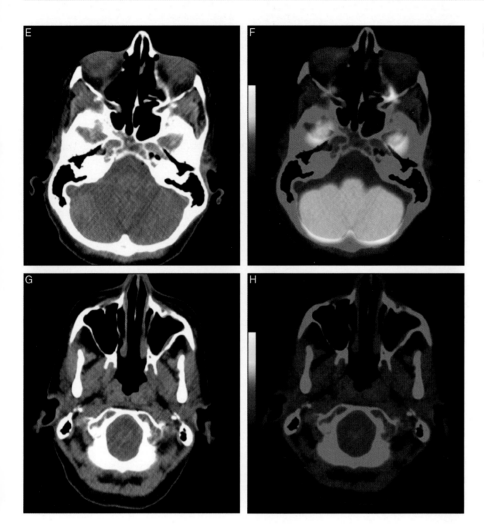

accumulation in mucosal thickening involving the left nasal cavity and maxillary sinus, with outlet obstruction of left maxillary, frontal, ethmoid, and sphenoid sinuses. The maximum SUV is 14.5 (Figure 6.5A–D). Several hypermetabolic and enlarged lymph nodes are seen in the left neck, level 2. A representative node measures approximately $1.5 \times 1.5$ cm and has an SUV of 6.9 (not shown). Normal size right cervical lymph nodes have no tracer uptake. Right paranasal sinuses are clear. These findings are non-specific but suggestive of left pansinusitis. The patient was treated with antibiotics. The follow-up images (E, F, G, H) show complete resolution of disease in the paranasal sinuses.

## Diagnosis and follow-up

The primary esophageal carcinoma was clearly identified on PET (not shown), which was done for staging and as baseline for subsequent chemoradiotherapy. Left pansinusitis was suspected on PET/CT. Further questioning and review of electronic medical records revealed that the patient was undergoing treatment with antibiotics for severe sinusitis at the time of the PET/CT. A subsequent PET/CT scan 2 months later (for response assessment of the esophageal cancer) showed complete resolution of left sinusitis (as well as response in the esophageal primary tumor).

## Discussion and teaching points

FDG uptake is a non-specific phenomenon. Numerous reasons for false-positive uptake, related to inflammation or infection, have been described (1–3). In the head and neck this may include sinusitis (although rarely as severe and advanced as in the present case), variable uptake in the lymphoid tissues of Waldeyer's ring, and reactive lymph nodes as part of bacterial or viral infections.

## Take-home message

- False-positive FDG uptake in the head and neck can occur for many reasons, including uptake in physiologic lymphoid tissue, brown adipose tissue, in Waldeyer's ring, and at sites of inflammation or infection (1–3). Readers must be familiar with a large number of normal variants in FDG uptake in the head and neck.

- Many other radiotracers have been proposed for head and neck cancer imaging, and variably have been advocated as showing greater specificity than FDG. As more data emerge, most of these newer agents also suffer from non-specific uptake at sites of inflammation and infection, or are of limited value for tumor staging due to their high physiologic uptake in neck soft tissues (4–6).
- Up-to-date clinical information (clinical findings, level of suspicion, treatment regimen, time of last treatment) and joint review of all current imaging data (structural and functional) is pertinent to minimize the number of false-positive scan interpretations. As for all imaging tests, interpretation should emphasize sensitivity or specificity, depending on the clinical situation and available data (e.g., residual viable tumor is rare in enlarged lymph nodes with no or only minimal FDG uptake after concurrent chemoradiotherapy; see Case 3).

## References

1. Schöder H, Yeung HW. Positron emission imaging of head and neck cancer, including thyroid carcinoma. *Semin Nucl Med* 2004;**34**:180–97.

2. Blodgett TM, Fukui MB, Snyderman CH *et al.* Combined PET-CT in the head and neck: part 1. Physiologic, altered physiologic, and artifactual FDG uptake. *Radiographics* 2005;**25**:897–912.

3. Fukui MB, Blodgett TM, Snyderman CH *et al.* Combined PET-CT in the head and neck: part 2. Diagnostic uses and pitfalls of oncologic imaging. *Radiographics* 2005;**25**:913–30.

4. Troost EG, Vogel WV, Merkx MA *et al.* 18F-FLT PET does not discriminate between reactive and metastatic lymph nodes in primary head and neck cancer patients. *J Nucl Med* 2007;**48**:726–35.

5. Krabbe CA, van der Werff-Regelink G, Pruim J, van der Wal JE, Roodenburg JL. Detection of cervical metastases with (11)C-tyrosine PET in patients with squamous cell carcinoma of the oral cavity or oropharynx: a comparison with (18)F-FDG PET. *Head Neck* 2010;**32**:368–74.

6. Ito K, Yokoyama J, Kubota K *et al.* (18)F-FDG versus (11)C-choline PET/CT for the imaging of advanced head and neck cancer after combined intra-arterial chemotherapy and radiotherapy: the time period during which PET/CT can reliably detect non-recurrence. *Eur J Nucl Med Mol Imaging* 2010;**37**(7):1318–27.

# Detection of recurrence

A 49-year-old male with cancer of the retromolar trigone. The patient underwent left composite mandibulectomy, left partial maxillectomy, wide resection of left retromolar trigone tumor with partial pharyngectomy and palatectomy and left modified radical neck dissection. The surgical defect was covered with a rectus abdominis myocutaneous flap. This was followed by post-operative radiation therapy. At 3 months follow-up, there were no signs of recurrence and the free flap appeared normal. Approximately 2 months later, the patient presented with left facial pain and swelling. PET was done to assess for recurrence.

## Acquisition and processing parameters

Following a 6-hour fasting period, 11.2 mCi of FDG was injected intravenously. The plasma glucose at the time of FDG injection was 84 mg/dL. After a 69 min uptake period, low-dose CT (140 kVp, 80 mA, 0.8 s per CT rotation, pitch of 1.75:1 and reconstructed slice thickness of 3.8 mm) and PET emission images were obtained from the mid skull to the upper thighs on a Biograph PET/CT. PET data were acquired for 5 min per bed position. The CT data were reconstructed using an iterative algorithm and a 512 × 512 matrix for 70 cm transaxial field of view. The PET images were reconstructed using an iterative algorithm and a 128 × 128 matrix. The CT data were used to generate the transmission maps for attenuation correction of the PET emission images and for anatomic localization. Standardized uptake values (SUV) were normalized to patient body weight; the highest activity concentration (SUVmax) in a given disease site is recorded.

## Findings and differential diagnosis

The patient is status post-left mandibulectomy, left partial maxillectomy; partial pharyngectomy and palatectomy as well as status post-left neck dissection. The surgical defect was covered with a myocutaneous flap. Restaging PET/CT shows intense FDG uptake in soft tissues along the anterior portion of the flap, beginning at the mandibulectomy margin and extending along the left hemimandible and into the left floor of the mouth. There also is a small fluid collection with some gas pockets in the anterior/inferior portion of the flap. Previously noted FDG uptake in right neck soft tissue has largely resolved. Small right neck nodes show mild FDG uptake (for instance SUV 3.1 in a 5 mm right level 2 node). This is likely reactive.

## Discussion and teaching points

FDG-PET/CT is an excellent tool for detection of recurrent HNSCC; the intensity of FDG uptake has prognostic value (1–2). This patient presented with recent left facial pain and swelling, within weeks after completing chemoradiotherapy. This finding is non-specific for either recurrence or infection. The scan showed intense FDG uptake along the myocutaneous flap, a small fluid collection and gas pockets – necrotic tumor (less likely) and infection (more likely) were considered as differentials. The fluid collection with gas pockets was biopsied

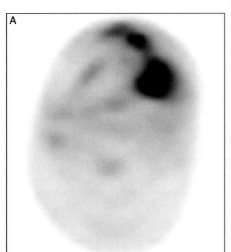
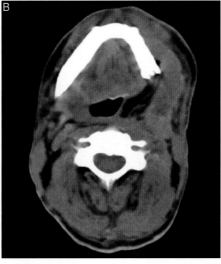
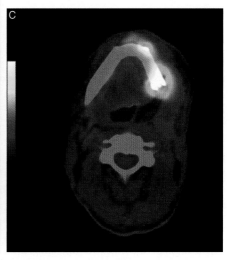

**Figure 6.6A–C** Restaging transaxial FDG-PET, CT, and fusion images show abnormal FDG uptake at the mandibulectomy margin.

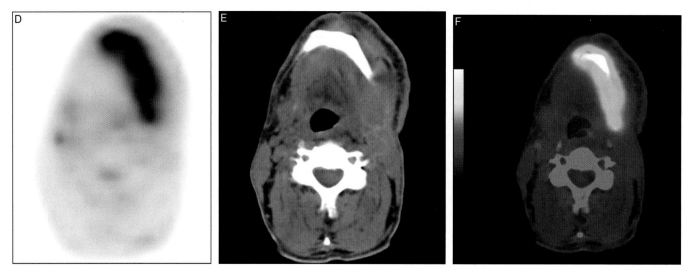

**Figure 6.6D–F** FDG uptake along the myocutaneous flap.

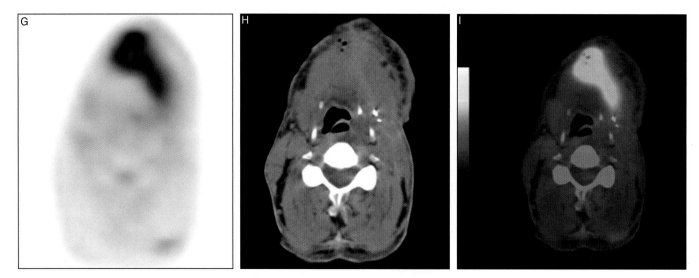

**Figure 6.6G–I** Small fluid collection with pockets of gas at the anterior margin of the flap in the midline.

and showed gram-positive and gram-negative bacteria. The patient was treated with IV antibiotics and recovered fully. The flap remained vital.

The follow-up regimen after head and neck cancer surgery varies among institutions. Some institutions perform PET/CT based on strict regimens or algorithms in the first 2 years after therapy (e.g., 3, 6, 12, 24 months), whereas in many other practices PET/CT is only ordered based on clinical suspicion. The frequency at which PET/CT is done may reflect the level of clinical expertise of the surgeon or oncologist, protocol requirements, and disease-specific criteria. In some instances, "surveillance PET" may be indicated for patients at high risk for locoregional recurrence (3–4).

## Take-home message

- FDG-PET/CT is an excellent tool for detection of recurrent HNSCC; the intensity of FDG uptake has prognostic value.
- Clinical information is essential for image interpretation and to guide patient management; PET/CT should be used to guide biopsies to sites of suspected recurrence (or, in this case, infection).
- Readers have to be aware of the many reasons for false-positive FDG scans in HNSCC, including infection (current case) and various treatment sequelae, such as osteoradionecrosis.

# References

1.  Wong RJ, Lin DT, Schöder H *et al.* Diagnostic and prognostic value of [(18) F]fluorodeoxyglucose positron emission tomography for recurrent head and neck squamous cell carcinoma. *J Clin Oncol* 2002;**20**:4199–208.

2.  Kunkel M, Förster GJ, Reichert TE *et al.* Detection of recurrent oral squamous cell carcinoma by [18F]-2-fluorodeoxyglucose-positron emission tomography: implications for prognosis and patient management. *Cancer* 2003;**98**:2257–65.

3.  Salaun PY, Abgral R, Querellou S *et al.* Does 18fluoro-fluorodeoxyglucose positron emission tomography improve recurrence detection in patients treated for head and neck squamous cell carcinoma with negative clinical follow-up? *Head Neck* 2007;**29**:1115–20.

4.  Lowe VJ, Boyd JH, Dunphy FR *et al.* Surveillance for recurrent head and neck cancer using positron emission tomography. *J Clin Oncol* 2000;**18**:651–8.

# Recurrent differentiated thyroid cancer

A 56-year-old male with papillary thyroid cancer, status post-thyroidectomy, with persistent elevated thyroglobulin levels. Disease was refractory to multiple treatments with $^{131}$Iodine ($^{131}$I).

## Acquisition and processing parameters

Recombinant human TSH (rh-TSH; Thyrogen) was administered intramuscularly on 2 consecutive days (0.9 mg each) on the 2 days preceding the PET scan. On the day of PET,

following a 6-hour fasting period, 12.5 mCi of FDG was injected intravenously. After a 75 min uptake period, low-dose CT (140 kVp, 80 mA, 0.8 s per CT rotation, pitch of 1.75 : 1 and reconstructed slice thickness of 3.8 mm) and PET emission images were obtained from the mid skull to the upper thighs on a Discovery LS PET/CT. PET data of the head and neck were acquired for 5 min per bed position, in the torso for 3 min per bed position. The CT data were reconstructed using an iterative algorithm and a 512 × 512 matrix for 70 cm transaxial

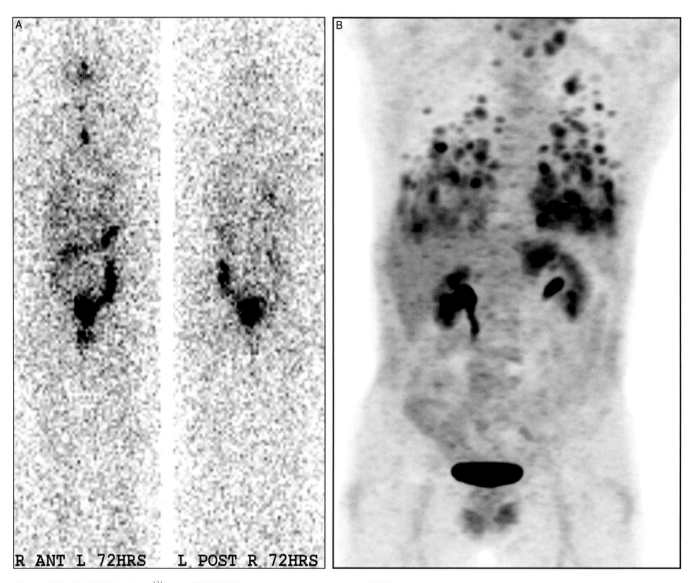

**Figure 6.7A, B** (A) Whole-body $^{131}$I scan; (B) FDG-PET maximum intensity projection (MIP).

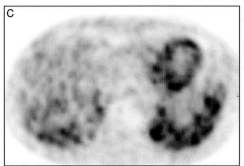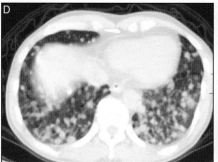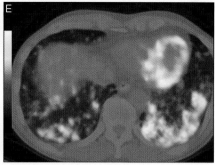

**Figure 6.7C–E** Transaxial FDG-PET, CT, and fusion images of the chest.

field of view. The PET images were reconstructed using an iterative algorithm and a $128 \times 128$ matrix. The CT data were used to generate the transmission maps for attenuation correction of the PET emission images and for anatomic localization. The plasma glucose at the time of FDG injection was 112 mg/dL. Standardized uptake values (SUV) were normalized to patient body weight; the highest activity concentration (SUVmax) in a given disease site is recorded.

## Findings and differential diagnosis

Planar images of an [131]I scan (Figure 6.7A) show no clear evidence of disease. Linear uptake in the mediastinum was attributed to swallowed salivary activity in the esophagus. The MIP image of the FDG-PET/CT (Figure 6.7B) shows a hypermetabolic neck (left greater than right) and supraclavicular adenopathy, for example: left level 2 node with SUV 2.6, **left supraclavicular node** with SUV 4.7, right thoracic inlet node with SUV 3.8. Abnormal FDG uptake is also present in the left thyroid bed, and in numerous hypermetabolic lung nodules. FDG-PET, CT, and fusion images of the chest (Figure 6.7C, D, E) show numerous hypermetabolic lung nodules consistent with metastases with SUV ranging from 6.2 to 9.1.

## Diagnosis and follow-up

This patient has papillary thyroid cancer with recurrent disease in the neck, and with metastatic disease to neck lymph nodes and the bilateral lungs. The disease was refractory to treatment with [131]I; the patient has therefore entered an experimental protocol.

## Discussion and teaching points

In cases with differentiated thyroid carcinoma FDG-PET/CT is indicated for patients with elevated thyroglobulin levels but negative [131]I scan after thyroidectomy or during subsequent follow-up. It is now clearly established that FDG-PET and PET/CT define the extent of disease in these patients. In one large study (1) of 64 patients with elevated serum thyroglobulin (n = 48) or clinical suspicion of metastases (n = 16) and negative [131]I scans, the positive predictive value of FDG-PET was 83%, with a negative predictive value of 25%. Recent studies have shown high sensitivity of combined FDG-PET/

CT (2, 3). FDG-PET findings may affect patient management in 30–40% of cases (1, 4). In a study of 125 patients with elevated thyroglobulin levels, negative [131]I scans, and positive FDG-PET, the single strongest predictor of survival during 41 months of follow-up in multivariate analysis was the volume of FDG-avid disease (5). A subsequent study in 400 patients from the same group (6) confirmed the prognostic value of FDG-PET in patients with demonstrated or suspected recurrent thyroid cancer; suspicion for recurrence was based on clinical and imaging findings or elevated thyroglobulin levels (suppressed Tg > 10). Patients with positive FDG-PET scans had a 7.3-fold higher risk of dying from thyroid cancer as compared with patients with negative PET. SUVmax also had a strong prognostic value for survival.

In general, the fraction of true-positive FDG scans increases with rising thyroglobulin levels (1, 2), but no clear cut-off level for thyroglobulin has been established to define when FDG-PET should be done. In patients with FDG-positive disease, premedication (stimulation) with rh-TSH increases the number of detected disease sites (7).

Among other histologic entities of thyroid carcinoma, FDG-PET/CT is of value in Hürthle cell carcinoma (see next Case), as well as for poorly differentiated and anaplastic carcinoma (to assess disease spread, prognostic information, and response assessment). In patients with medullary thyroid cancer after thyroidectomy, the detection of recurrent or metastatic disease on FDG-PET is related to the level of calcitonin (tumor marker) and possibly calcitonin doubling time at the time of imaging. This is likely a reflection of the tumor burden. However, the radiolabeled amino acid F-DOPA has emerged as the preferred radiotracer for imaging of medullary thyroid cancer; it has significantly higher sensitivity than FDG.

## Take-home message

- FDG-PET/CT is indicated in patients with differentiated thyroid carcinoma, elevated thyroglobulin levels, and negative [131]I scans.
- PET can be used to define the true extent of metastatic disease and to monitor response to therapy.
- The intensity of FDG uptake in metastatic lesions provides prognostic information.

# References

1. Schluter B, Bohuslavizki KH, Beyer W *et al.* Impact of FDG PET on patients with differentiated thyroid cancer who present with elevated thyroglobulin and negative 131I scan. *J Nucl Med* 2001;**42**:71–6.

2. Palmedo H, Bucerius J, Joe A *et al.* Integrated PET/CT in differentiated thyroid cancer: diagnostic accuracy and impact on patient management. *J Nucl Med* 2006;**47**:616–24.

3. Finkelstein SE, Grigsby PW, Siegel BA *et al.* Combined [18F] Fluorodeoxyglucose positron emission tomography and computed tomography (FDG-PET/CT) for detection of recurrent, 131I-negative thyroid cancer. *Ann Surg Oncol* 2008;**15**:286–92.

4. Shammas A, Degirmenci B, Mountz JM *et al.* 18F-FDG PET/CT in patients with suspected recurrent or metastatic well-differentiated thyroid cancer. *J Nucl Med* 2007;**48**:221–6.

5. Wang W, Larson SM, Fazzari M *et al.* Prognostic value of [18F] fluorodeoxyglucose positron emission tomographic scanning in patients with thyroid cancer. *J Clin Endocrinol Metab* 2000;**85**:1107–1113.

6. Robbins RJ, Wan Q, Grewal RK *et al.* Real-time prognosis for metastatic thyroid carcinoma based on 2-[18F] fluoro-2-deoxy-D-glucose-positron emission tomography scanning. *J Clin Endocrinol Metab* 2006;**91**:498–505.

7. Leboulleux S, Schroeder PR, Busaidy NL *et al.* Assessment of the incremental value of recombinant thyrotropin stimulation before 2-[18F]-Fluoro-2-deoxy-D-glucose positron emission tomography/computed tomography imaging to localize residual differentiated thyroid cancer. *J Clin Endocrinol Metab* 2009;**94**:1310–16.

# Hürthle cell carcinoma

A 30-year-old female with Hürthle cell carcinoma, status post total thyroidectomy. Histopathology showed a 10.8 cm widely invasive carcinoma with extensive blood vessel invasion, and with involvement of extrathyroidal fibroadipose tissue. Metastatic lymph nodes were identified in the bilateral neck in levels 2, 3, 4, and 5. FDG-PET/CT was ordered for post-operative staging and evaluation of the extent of disease

## Acquisition and processing parameters

Following a 6-hour fasting period, 14.5 mCi of FDG was injected intravenously. The plasma glucose at the time of FDG injection was 79 mg/dL. After a 75 min uptake period, low-dose CT (140 kVp, 80 mA, 0.8 s per CT rotation, pitch of 1.75 : 1 and reconstructed slice thickness of 3.8 mm) and PET emission images were obtained from the mid skull to the upper thighs on a Discovery STE PET/CT. PET data of the head and neck were acquired for 5 min per bed position, in the torso for 3 min per bed position. The CT data were reconstructed using an iterative algorithm and a $512 \times 512$ matrix for 70 cm transaxial field of view. The PET images were reconstructed using an iterative algorithm and a $128 \times 128$ matrix. The CT data were used to generate the transmission maps for attenuation correction of the PET emission images and for anatomic localization. Standardized uptake values (SUV) were normalized to patient body weight; the highest activity concentration (SUVmax) in a given disease site is recorded.

## Findings and differential diagnosis

The patient is status post-thyroidectomy. FDG-PET maximum intensity projection (MIP) images (Figure 6.8A) provide a general assessment of the extent of disease, with metastatic lesions in the neck, chest, liver, and pelvic bones. In detail, there are multiple foci of markedly elevated FDG uptake in the thyroid bed, consistent with local disease recurrence (SUVmax 52.3). Markedly hypermetabolic lymph nodes are seen in the bilateral neck (Figure 6.8B, C, D) at multiple levels and in the supraclavicular regions, including a left level 5a node measuring $1.3 \times 1.1$ cm with SUVmax of 107, a left retropharyngeal node (SUVmax 71), a left supraclavicular node measuring $2.1 \times 1.6$ cm (SUVmax 96) and a right level 2 node (SUVmax 47). There is extensive hypermetabolic lymphadenopathy in the mediastinum with FDG uptake of similar intensity (Figure 6.8E, F, G). The largest mass in the subcarinal region measures $5.6 \times 2.8$ cm (SUVmax 97). Multiple bilateral lung nodules show intense FDG uptake. The largest nodule is located in the medial left lower lobe ($2.4 \times 2.3$ cm, SUVmax 78). The other nodules

are of punctuate size. There is no abnormal FDG uptake in the soft tissue organs and lymph nodes of the abdomen and pelvis. A lytic lesion in the right iliac bone shows abnormal FDG uptake (SUVmax 15), consistent with metastases.

## Diagnosis and follow-up

The patient has widespread metastatic Hürthle cell carcinoma to lymph nodes, lungs, and bones. The presentation is characteristic for widely metastatic disease; there is no other leading differential diagnosis. The patient entered a clinical research protocol employing experimental therapy with a VEGF inhibitor. However, no major response was seen on follow-up scans, and disease eventually progressed. The patient died from widely metastatic Hürthle cell carcinoma approximately 8 months later.

## Discussion and teaching points

Hürthle cell carcinoma is an uncommon aggressive differentiated thyroid cancer; it usually has low avidity for iodine. This means that scans with [123]I, [124]I, or [131]I, are often negative or do not show the full extent of disease. In addition, if treated with [131]I, these patients show low response rates. FDG-PET/CT has been proposed as an optimal imaging test in patients with Hürthle cell carcinoma (1, 2), in order to define the full extent of the disease after total thyroidectomy, to obtain prognostic information, and also to monitor the response to modern experimental therapies. In a study of 44 patients with Hürthle cell carcinoma (1) FDG-PET had a sensitivity of 95.8% and a specificity of 95%. Intense FDG uptake was a marker of poor prognosis. In another study (2), FDG-PET provided additional information on the extent of disease, leading to a change in patient management in 50% of cases. We recommend FDG-PET/CT in Hürthle cell carcinoma after total thyroidectomy in patients with unexpected (persistent) elevated thyroglobulin levels after total thyroidectomy, and/or when thyroglobulin levels are out of proportion to the extent of disease seen on the [131]I scan. In addition, we recommend it in all patients with histopathologic features of aggressiveness, including significant (i.e., more than one microscopic focus) vascular invasion, and in patients with primary tumor size greater than 4 cm. Although Hürthle cell carcinoma shows features of de-differentiation in that it has low iodine avidity, thyroglobulin appears to maintain its utility as an indicator of disease burden. Thus, regardless of findings on [131]I images, FDG-PET/CT will show more disease in the subset of patients with significantly elevated thyroglobulin levels, although this relationship is not linear and no clear cut-off level has been established.

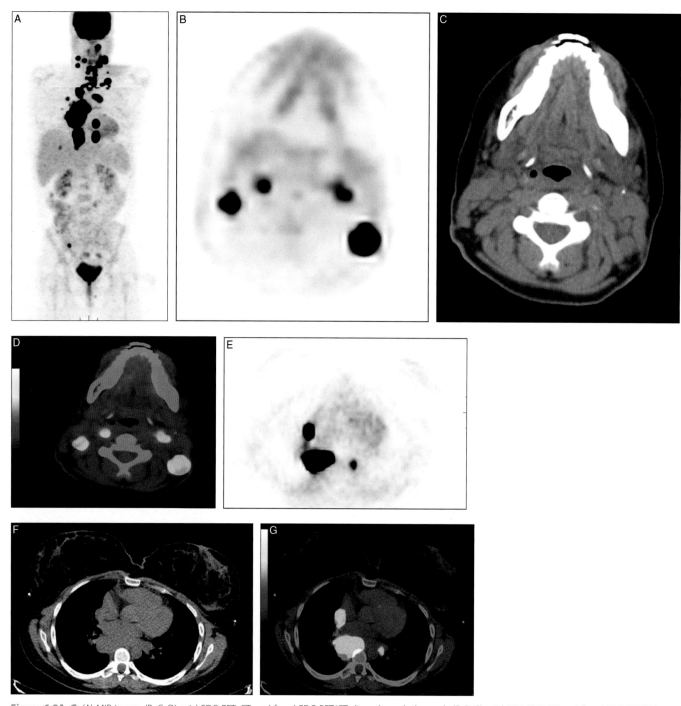

**Figure 6.8A–G** (A) MIP image; (B, C, D) axial FDG-PET, CT, and fused FDG-PET/CT slices through the neck; (E, F, G) axial FDG-PET, CT, and fused FDG-PET/CT images of the chest and mediastinum.

## Take-home message

- Hürthle cell carcinoma is an aggressive subtype of differentiated thyroid cancer. It generally has low avidity for iodine in the diagnostic and therapeutic setting. FDG-PET/CT has emerged as an optimal imaging test to define the true extent of disease in these patients.

- PET/CT should be performed when post-thyroidectomy levels of thyroglobulin continue to be high or are out of proportion to the extent of disease seen on the $^{131}$I scan. It should also be done routinely in patients with aggressive histopathologic features.

- PET/CT should be employed for response assessment as part of protocols testing experimental therapies in these patients.

## References

1. Pryma DA, Schoder H, Gonen M *et al.* Diagnostic accuracy and prognostic value of 18F-FDG PET in Hurthle cell thyroid cancer patients. *J Nucl Med* 2006;**47**:1260–6.

2. Lowe VJ, Mullan BP, Hay ID, McIver B, Kasperbauer JL. 18F-FDG PET of patients with Hurthle cell carcinoma. *J Nucl Med* 2003;**44**:1402–6.

**Chapter**

# 7

# Lung and pleura

Victor H. Gerbaudo

## Lung cancer

In 2011 the total number of expected cancer cases in the USA is 1,596,670 with 571,950 estimated deaths from cancer. The expected number of new lung cancer cases is 221,130 (115,060 men and 106,070 women), of which a total of 156,940 are expected to die from the disease (85,600 men and 71,340 women) (1). These data place lung cancer as the second most commonly diagnosed malignancy, and as the leading cause of cancer-related deaths in both men and women in the USA (1).

Amongst the known risk factors for developing lung cancer, cigarette smoking occupies the first place in importance (more than 90% of cases), followed by occupational and environmental exposure to radon, asbestos, second-hand smoke, chromium, arsenic, cadmium, organic chemicals, air pollution, radiation, and a previous history of tuberculosis. In those that develop lung cancer at a younger age, genetic susceptibility is also considered an important contributing risk factor (1).

## Histology

The tumor cell type and the stage at presentation affect the prognosis and survival after treating lung cancer patients. Accurate diagnosis with confirmed cell type is of utmost importance. Lung cancers are divided into two main histologic types: non-small cell lung cancer (NSCLC) and small-cell lung cancer (SCLC). The histologic classification of lung cancer has undergone several revisions since the original 1967 recommendation proposed by the World Health Organization (WHO). The most significant update took place in 1999, followed by a slight change in 2004 (2–5). The revised cellular classification for NSCLC and SCLC summarizing the 1999 and 2004 WHO recommendations is presented in Table 7.1.

## Non-small cell lung cancer (NSCLC)

Non-small cell lung cancers amount to 85% of lung neoplasia, and are further subdivided into eight subtypes (Table 7.1). The following paragraphs will expand on the most common

subtypes, namely: squamous cell carcinoma, adenocarcinoma, large cell carcinoma, and carcinoids (3–5).

### Squamous cell carcinoma (SCC)

This histologic type used to be the most frequent of all lung cancers, however, recently adenocarcinomas occupy the first place in incidence. SCC accounts for 20–30% of all cases of lung malignancy. It develops in the proximal airways, where the cells undergo squamous metaplasia to carcinoma in situ. Their invasive phase follows with the tumor growing beyond the basement membrane into the bronchial lumen. Their average volume doubling time is approximately 3 months, and they metastasize at a slower rate than adenocarcinomas. SCCs are central tumors associated with hilar adenopathy and mediastinal widening in chest radiographs. This in part explains their tendency to present with hemoptysis, and they are frequently diagnosed by sputum cytology.

### Adenocarcinoma

Adenocarcinomas are the most frequent histologic type of lung cancer, accounting for 40% of all cases of lung neoplasia. These tumors are characterized by a glandular type of architecture, arising from the bronchiolar or alveolar epithelia in areas of infection or scar tissue (scar carcinoma), with approximately three-quarters of them presenting as a solitary pulmonary nodule (SPN) in the lung periphery of the upper lobes. As shown in Table 7.1, the revised WHO histologic classification of lung cancer lists different subtypes of adenocarcinomas to include: mixed, acinar, papillary, bronchioloalveolar, and solid adenocarcinoma with mucin production. The doubling time of adenocarcinomas is approximately 6 months, but they tend to metastasize faster than SCC.

### Bronchioloalveolar carcinoma (BAC)

Bronchioloalveolar carcinoma is a well-differentiated, peripheric subtype of adenocarcinoma, not associated with pleural invasion, vascular structures, or lung stroma. BACs arise from type-2 pneumocytes and they account for 2–5% of all

*A Case-Based Approach to PET/CT in Oncology*, ed. Victor H. Gerbaudo. Published by Cambridge University Press.
© Cambridge University Press 2012.

**Table 7.1** Revised histologic classification of non-small cell lung cancer (NSCLC) and small cell lung cancer (SCLC) by the World Health Organization and the International Association for the Study of Lung Cancer. Adapted from references 2–7.

| Lung cancer type | Histologic type | Histologic subtype |
|---|---|---|
| **Pre-invasive lesions** | Squamous dysplasia/carcinoma in situ<br>Atypical adenomatous hyperplasia<br>Diffuse idiopathic pulmonary neuroendocrine hyperplasia | |
| **NSCLC** | Adenocarcinoma | Adenocarcinoma, mixed subtype<br>Acinar<br>Papillary<br>Bronchioloalveolar carcinoma*<br>• Non-mucinous<br>• Mucinous<br>• Mixed mucinous and non-mucinous or indeterminate<br>Solid adenocarcinoma with mucin production<br>• Fetal<br>• Mucinous<br>• Mucinous cystadenocarcinoma<br>• Signet-ring<br>• Clear-cell |
| | Squamous cell carcinoma | Papillary<br>Clear cell<br>Small cell<br>Basaloid |
| | Large cell carcinoma | Large cell neuroendocrine<br>• Combined large cell neuroendocrine<br><br>Basaloid<br>Lymphoepithelioma-like<br>Clear cell<br>Large cell with rhabdoid features |
| | Adenosquamous carcinoma | |
| | Carcinomas with pleomorphic, sarcomatoid, or sarcomatous elements | Carcinomas with spindle and/or giant cells<br>• Pleomorphic carcinoma<br>• Spindle cell carcinoma<br>• Giant cell carcinoma<br><br>Carcinosarcoma<br>Pulmonary blastoma<br>Others |
| | Carcinoid | Typical<br>Atypical |
| | Carcinomas of salivary gland type | Mucoepidermoid<br>Adenoid cystic<br>Epithelial–myoepithelial |
| | Unclassified carcinoma | |
| **SCLC** | Small cell carcinoma<br>Combined small cell carcinoma | • with neoplastic squamous components<br>• with glandular components |

*See 2011 proposed new classification of bronchioloalveolar carcinomas on page 130.

lung cancer cases. This tumor grows along the alveolar or bronchiolar walls in a pattern called **lepidic**. There are two distinct subtypes of BAC: (1) mucinous and (2) non-mucinous BAC. The mucinous subtype accounts for 40% of cases, and presents as multifocal or diffuse lung disease or with a progressive pneumonic consolidation pattern. The latter is due to its high rate of mucin production filling the alveoli. The non-mucinous subtype tends to present as a peripheral SPN in 60% of cases, with a ground-glass opacity pattern secondary to the lepidic growth characteristic of this tumor.

In February 2011, the International Association for the Study of Lung Cancer, together with the American Thoracic Society and the European Respiratory Society proposed a revised international multidisciplinary classification of lung adenocarcinomas (6). This new classification proposes that the terms BAC and mixed adenocarcinoma with BAC features should no longer be used. The authors recommend that the nomenclature of BACs be replaced with **adenocarcinoma in situ** (AIS: ≤ 3 cm in size with pure lepidic growth; mostly non-mucinous, and without stromal, vascular, or pleural invasion) and **minimally invasive adenocarcinoma** (MIA: ≤ 5 mm invasion, with predominant lepidic growth; mostly non-mucinous), in order to identify a subset of patients with a 100% or near 100% disease-free survival if the lesion is completely resected. In addition, invasive adenocarcinomas (> 3 cm in size and/or > 5 mm invasion and/or multiple nodules and/or military spread) are classified based on the most predominant subtype. **Invasive lepidic predominant** replaces the former term of mixed subtype with non-mucinous BAC features, and **invasive mucinous adenocarcinoma** includes the former mucinous BAC.

### Large cell carcinoma

This very aggressive subtype of adenocarcinoma accounts for 10–15% of lung tumors, and they present as a large (approximately 4 cm) peripheral mass, with an approximate doubling time of 3 months. Metastases appear early in the course of the disease, and their prognosis is dismal.

### Carcinoids

Carcinoids are neuroendocrine neoplasms accounting for approximately 2% of all lung cancers, and they arise from the bronchial walls. They are classified as typical and atypical carcinoids. **Typical carcinoids** are central in location, invasive, 50% may be calcified, and metastases are not common. Hemoptysis, cough, wheezing, and recurrent pneumonia are symptoms mostly related to their central location and rich vascular supply. In fact, their high degree of vascularity is often responsible for significant bleeding following biopsy. In addition, their tendency to block the bronchial lumen courses with atelectasis and consolidation. Two percent of typical carcinoids may present as a peripheral nodule, with round, well-defined or slightly irregular borders, and only 10% may be calcified. Carcinoid syndrome (flushing, diarrhea, wheezing, and hypotension) is uncommon, and takes place in those patients with liver metastasis. **Atypical carcinoids** are more aggressive, with half of the patients presenting with nodal metastasis. They may present as a lung nodule or a mass usually larger than the ones produced by their typical counterparts.

## Small-cell lung cancer

Small-cell lung cancers (7) are tumors of bronchial origin, associated with cigarette smoking. They constitute the third most common histologic type of lung cancer, accounting for 15–20% of all cases. They are a carcinoma of the neuroendocrine type, often responsible for causing paraneoplastic syndromes. A SCLC is usually a central tumor associated with hilar or perihilar lesions, arising from the main or lobar bronchi, which can infiltrate peribronchially and may cause obstruction of the airways. The tumor volume doubling time is approximately 30 days, and it is characterized for systemic metastasis early in the disease process. In 1950, the Veterans Administration Lung Study group classified SCLC into **limited stage disease** (40%) to one hemithorax, and its corresponding lymph nodes, and into **extensive stage disease**, consistent with disease spreading beyond the previously mentioned boundaries. In 1989, the International Association for the Study of Lung Cancer (IASLC) updated the **limited disease** classification to include tumors in one hemithorax with regional lymph nodes metastasis in ipsilateral hilar, contralateral mediastinal, and ipsilateral and contralateral supraclavicular nodes. Positive and negative ipsilateral pleural effusions without other concurrent extrathoracic systemic disease, were also considered limited disease. Recent data analysis of 8088 SCLC patients from an international database of the IASLC has concluded that the revised 2010 TNM (tumor, node, metastasis) staging system should now be applied to SCLC (Tables 7.2 and 7.3) as well.

## Tumor, node, metastasis (TNM) classification

Accurate disease staging in patients with lung cancer is essential to classify them into prognostic subgroups in order to allow delivery of stage-specific therapies. The most important prognostic indicators in lung cancer are the extent of disease and lymph node involvement. The American Joint Committee for Cancer's TNM staging system takes into account the extent of primary tumor spread (T), the presence and location of thoracic lymph node involvement (N), and the presence or absence of distant metastases (M).

The lung cancer tumor, node, metastasis staging system was revised in 2009, and published in the 7th edition of the AJCC manual in 2010 (8). The lung cancer staging system was modified based on the results of a large IASLC analysis of 100,869 lung cancer patients worldwide (9). Of these, 18,018 cases met the T descriptor inclusion criteria, 38,265 had information on clinical N staging, and 8371 had pathologic N staging records. The updated staging system is believed to better correlate with survival, as well as to be more in line with present management paradigms (Tables 7.3 and 7.4). The revised TNM classification, the updated anatomic groupings, and corresponding 5-year survival rates are shown in Tables 7.2, 7.3, and 7.4 respectively. With the exception of N status, changes were made to T and M modifiers. Briefly, the most salient modifications of the revised TNM system, which apply to all lung cancers (NSCLC, including carcinoids, and SCLC), with the exception of sarcomas and other rare tumors, include: (a) the T1 and T2 tumors based on size cut-offs of 2, 3, 5, and

**Table 7.2** Revised tumor, node, metastasis (TNM) classification for lung cancer (now applicable to non-small cell lung cancer (NSCLC), small cell lung cancer (SCLC) and Carcinoids. Adapted from reference 8.

| T (Primary tumor) | N (Lymph nodes) | M (Distant metastasis) |
| --- | --- | --- |
| **TX**: cannot be assessed, or proven by malignant cells in sputum or bronchial washings, with negative imaging studies | **NX**: regional nodes cannot be assessed | **M0**: No distant metastasis |
| **T0**: no evidence of primary | **N0**: No nodal metastasis | **M1**: Distant metastasis |
| **Tis**: In situ | **N1**: nodal metastasis or direct involvement of ipsilateral peribronchial and/or hilar and intrapulmonary nodes | – **M1a**: additional tumor nodules in the contralateral lung, or pleural nodules or malignant pleural or pericardial effusions |
| **T1**: ≤ 3 cm (**T1a** ≤ 2 cm; **T1b**: >2 cm but ≤ 3 cm); surrounded by lung or visceral pleura, without invading proximal to a lobar bronchus | **N2**: metastasis in ipsilateral mediastinal and/or subcarinal nodes | – **M1b**: all other distant metastasis |
| **T2**: > 3 cm but < 7 cm (**T2a**: > 3 cm, ≤ 5 cm; **T2b**: > 5 cm, ≤ 7 cm) or<br>– involving main bronchus ≥ 2 cm from the carina;<br>– with visceral pleura invasion,<br>– producing atelectasis or obstructive pneumonitis affecting less than the entire lung | **N3**: metastasis in contralateral mediastinal, hilar, ipsilateral or contralateral supraclavicular or scalene nodes | |
| **T3**: > 7 cm, **or**<br>– invasive tumor, including Pancoast tumors, affecting chest wall, diaphragm, phrenic nerve, parietal pericardium, mediastinal pleura, **or**<br>– lesion in main bronchus < 2 cm from the carina (without affecting it), **or**<br>– tumor producing atelectasis or whole lung obstructive pneumonitis, **or**<br>– separate tumor in the *same* lobe | | |
| **T4**:<br>– any tumor size, that invades mediastinal structures, recurrent laryngeal nerve, heart, trachea, vertebral body, carina;<br>– separate tumor (s) in another ipsilateral lobe.<br>– Pancoast tumor invading brachial plexus, vertebral body, spinal canal, or subclavian vessels | | |

7 cm are divided into a and b, respectively; (b) separate tumor nodules in same lobe are downstaged from T4 to T3; (c) separate tumor nodules in different lobes of the same lung are downstaged from M1 to T4, (d) additional tumor in the contralateral lung, and cases affected with malignant pleural or pericardial effusions and nodules, are classified as M1a; (f) distant metastatic disease is reclassified as M1b; (g) visceral pleural invasion is precisely defined; and (h) the concept of nodal zones has been adopted to better classify those cases in which bulky nodal disease extends beyond individual nodal stations.

## Staging work-up

As stated previously, accurate disease staging in patients with lung cancer is essential to classify them into prognostic subgroups in order to allow delivery of stage-specific therapies.

The most important prognostic indicators in lung cancer are the extent of disease and lymph node involvement. Therefore, the standard staging work-up of patients with NSCLC in the USA calls for a complete history and physical examination, including smoking history (pack/year), complete blood cell count, liver and renal function tests, electrolytes, sputum cytology (especially in patients with central tumors), past exposure to environmental carcinogens, and family history of lung cancer. Common symptoms include cough, hemoptysis, recurrent respiratory infections, weight loss, chest pain, symptoms and signs of superior vena cava obstruction, focal neurologic symptoms, osseous pain, and the presence of paraneoplastic syndrome symptomatology (especially in those patients with SCLC). All the information gathered from these tests is then used to guide the imaging studies that will be discussed in the following section.

**Table 7.3** Revised anatomic staging of lung cancer (applicable to non-small cell lung cancer (NSCLC), small cell lung cancer (SCLC) and carcinoids) and corresponding treatment options. Adapted from references 8, 9, and 24–26.

| Stage | TNM description | Management options |
|---|---|---|
| 0 | Tis N0 M0 | In situ disease |
| I | IA: T1a N0 M0<br>T1b N0 M0<br>IB: T2a N0 M0 | – Surgery (lobectomy or limited resection)<br>– Radiation therapy or stereotactic radiosurgery alone when ineligible for surgical resection [e.g., poor performance status (ECOG score $\leq$ 2)] and/or comorbidities<br>– Radiofrequency ablation of peripheral lesions in inoperable patients<br>– Some IBs: adjuvant chemotherapy |
| II | IIA: T2b N0 M0<br>T1a N1 M0<br>T1b N1 M0<br>T2a N1 M0<br>IIB: T2b N1 M0<br>T3 N0 M0 | – Surgery and post-operative adjuvant chemotherapy |
| III<br>Locally<br>Advanced<br>Disease | IIIA: T1a N2 M0<br>T1b N2 M0<br>T2a N2 M0<br>T2b N2 M0<br>T3 N1 M0<br>T3 N2 M0<br>T4 N0 M0<br>T4 N1 M0 | – Surgery in selected patients<br>– neoadjuvant concurrent chemoradiotherapy (better) or chemotherapy followed by radiation, in order to reduce tumor bulk and to eradicate micrometastatic disease<br>– Post-operative adjuvant chemotherapy |
| | IIIB: T1a N3 M0<br>T1b N3 M0<br>T2a N3 M0<br>T2b N3 M0<br>T3 N3 M0<br>T4 N2 M0<br>T4 N3 M0 | – Surgery in selected patients<br>– Concurrent neoadjuvant radiochemotherapy in selected patients with good performance status<br>– Adjuvant chemotherapy in patients with good performance status |
| IV<br>Advanced<br>Disease | T1–4 N0–3 M1a<br>or M1b | – Chemotherapy or symptom-targeted palliative therapy, or both, to improve quality of life and symptom control<br>– Combination of cytotoxic and cytostatic therapy (bevacizumab, erlotinib, etc.) |

**Table 7.4** Anatomic staging of lung cancer and corresponding 5-year survival rates after treatment. Survival data adapted from references 7 and 8.

| Stage | TNM description | Clinical stage (pre-operative) | Surgical stage (post-operative) |
|---|---|---|---|
| | | 5-year survival rate | |
| I | IA<br>IB | 50%<br>43% | 73%<br>58% |
| II | IIA<br>IIB | 36%<br>25% | 46%<br>36% |
| III<br>Locally advanced disease | IIIA<br>IIIB | 19%<br>7% | 24%<br>9% |
| IV<br>Advanced disease | IV | 2% | 13% |

## Imaging

The main role of imaging is to define the location and extent of the disease, of the primary tumor, nodal involvement, and systemic metastasis, in an attempt to minimize the use of invasive futile procedures. Various imaging modalities are used to stage lung cancer, all of which have advantages and limitations. Conventional imaging modalities include those discussed below.

## Chest radiography

Anteroposterior and lateral chest radiographs are the baseline and first imaging studies performed in patients with suspected lung cancer. This is a good test when it is normal, ruling out lung cancer in these cases. However, its overall sensitivity is limited, not only for the diagnosis, but also for staging the disease. An SPN might be missed before it reaches 8–10 mm in diameter. Quekel and colleagues (10) showed that approximately 19% (49 out of 259 patients) of NSCLC presenting as an SPN in chest radiographs were missed, having a definitive impact on prognosis. Although the missed rate was unrelated to nodule location, most of the lesions that were not visualized were close to superimposed anatomical structures. The average diameter of missed lesions was 16 mm, compared with 40 mm for those that were detected. Missed lesions on chest radiographs tend to be apical in location, peripheral, isodense to the surrounding lung parenchyma, perihilar, retrocardiac, or behind the diaphragm.

## Computed tomography (CT) imaging

A CT scan of the chest and upper abdomen should include the liver and adrenals as the minimum standard for a staging work-up of patients with lung cancer. CT provides more specific information about the location, density, and edge characteristics of lung lesions detected on plain films and may detect unsuspected lymphadenopathy, synchronous parenchymal lesions, or invasion of the chest wall, mediastinum, and other critical structures.

## Positron emission tomography/computed tomography (PET/CT)

In order to overcome the known limitations of anatomic imaging modalities, anatomo-metabolic imaging with FDG-PET/CT has now been incorporated to the imaging armamentarium for the diagnosis, staging, and monitoring response to lung cancer therapy. The role of PET/CT is discussed extensively at the end of this introduction and exemplified in the cases that follow.

## Magnetic resonance imaging (MRI)

The role of MRI in lung cancer is limited to the characterization of tumors that might be invading vital mediastinal structures, paravertebral and spinal structures, to the assessment of vertebral bone marrow disease, and to characterize the degree of involvement of different tissue planes and vascular structures in the thoracic inlet region, all of which might affect tumor resectability. In those patients that have focal neurologic findings, MRI is preferred over CT for the detection and characterization of CNS metastasis (11).

## Bone scintigraphy

In the past, radionuclide bone scintigraphy was used in asymptomatic patients with unsuspected bone metastasis in the early stage of the disease; however, its cost effectiveness was never proven. Considering that the skeletal system is a common site of metastases, some clinicians still use bone scanning in stage III patients with focal skeletal pain or with suspicious laboratory results of hypercalcemia or hyperphosphatemia and elevated alkaline phosphatase. The fact that FDG-PET/CT imaging has been shown to be as sensitive as bone scintigraphy to detect bony metastases, and that it has the advantage of staging non-osseous disease in one imaging session, it is displacing the use of bone scanning in lung cancer patients. An important exception is the need to characterize some non-FDG avid osteoblastic lesions observed on PET/CT.

## Invasive staging techniques

Regardless of the imaging technique being used to diagnose and stage lung cancer, all modalities should serve as a guide to direct tissue sampling, and not as a substitute for often necessary, invasive staging techniques, as described below.

## Trans-thoracic needle aspiration (TTNA)

Trans-thoracic needle aspiration (TTNA) is often used to assess peripheral lung lesions with a high diagnostic sensitivity of 88–92%, however, when the biopsy is negative, malignancy cannot be ruled out. Therefore, negative results should always be considered indeterminate until arriving to a benign histological diagnosis. TTNA is utilized to biopsy liver, bone, adrenals, or any other possible metastatic focus detected during clinical staging of the disease. Fine needle aspiration biopsies may be performed with ultrasound or CT guidance (12, 13).

## Bronchoscopy

Bronchoscopy is used to sample central parenchymal lesions using different kinds of techniques, such as transbronchial needle aspiration (TBNA), transbronchial brushing, and broncho-alveolar lavage. Bronchoscopy permits direct lesion visualization, the assessment of the extent of airway obstruction, and transbronchial lesion sampling. The technique may be performed alone or in combination with CT fluoroscopy, or with endobronchial ultrasound (EBUS) probes to confirm the exact location to be biopsied. Mediastinal, hilar nodes and the primary or metastatic tumors can also be sampled by the way of bronchoscopy. The diagnostic yield of TBNA is proportional to the size of the lesion being sampled, and the expertise of the operator. The diagnostic accuracy of fiber-optic bronchoscopy is approximately 90%. When lesions are not visible cytologic material may be obtained by irrigating and lavaging the suspicious area.

## Mediastinoscopy

Mediastinoscopy is considered the gold standard technique for mediastinal lymph nodes staging with a specificity of 100%, and with sensitivity rates approaching 90% (14, 15). It is usually performed to characterize the status of enlarged mediastinal lymph nodes detected in CT images in patients who are candidates for potentially curative surgical resection of lung cancer. During mediastinoscopy, a mediastinoscope is inserted through a pretracheal suprasternal incision into the mediastinal space, allowing access to the paratracheal (level 2R and 2L), tracheobronchial (4R and 4L), azygous, and subcarinal nodes (level 7). However, when CT images reveal enlarged level 5 [subaortic, aortopulmonary (A-P) window] and/or level 6 (para-aortic) nodes, which are common sites of metastases from left upper lobe lung tumors, and cannot be reached using routine cervical mediastinoscopy, the **Chamberlain procedure** or **anterior-second interspace mediastinotomy** may be used. This procedure involves the entry to the mediastinum through an incision in the parasternal second left intercostal space, opening access to level 5 and 6 nodes. An alternative procedure, and less popular, is the so-called **extended mediastinoscopy**. Exploration of the mediastinum is somewhat more difficult with the extended technique, and therefore it is contraindicated in patients with a previous sternotomy, or in those with a dilated or much calcified aortic arch. **Esophageal endoscopic ultrasound** with fine needle aspiration can be used to evaluate mediastinal nodes in the lower mediastinum, i.e., level 7 (subcarinal), level 8 (paraesophageal), and level 9 (pulmonary ligament), as well as the left adrenal gland and the left lobe of the liver. Presently, PET imaging has substantially decreased the need for mediastinoscopy at initial staging. On the other hand, mediastinal restaging after induction therapy for NSCLC still remains a challenge. De Leyn and colleagues (16) compared the performance of FDG-PET/CT to remediastinoscopy, and reported that post-induction re mediastinoscopy had significantly lower sensitivity, because of the limitations imposed by the adhesions and fibrosis resulting from the previous mediastinoscopy.

## Thoracoscopy

Thoracoscopy is a minimally invasive procedure used to sample lesions that remain undiagnosed after bronchoscopy or CT-guided biopsy (17, 18). The technique allows visualization of intrathoracic structures and of the pleural space. It may be used for diagnostic or therapeutic purposes. As a diagnostic tool, it is used to biopsy parenchymal, mediastinal, and/or pleural-based lesions. Thoracoscopic evaluation of the parietal pleura is used in patients with pleural effusions of unknown etiology and negative cytology in an attempt to differentiate

malignant from infectious lesions. Therapeutic thoracoscopy is performed to achieve pleurodesis, or with the aid of video assisted thoracic surgery (VATS) techniques, to perform segmentectomies, lobectomies, lung volume reduction surgery, and bullectomies. Complications of thoracoscopy include bleeding, infection, and iatrogenic laceration of lung parenchyma.

## Thoracentesis

Thoracentesis is used diagnostically and therapeutically to determine the cause of a pleural effusion, and/or to drain large effusions, respectively.

## Thoracotomy

Although the great majority of lung tumors are diagnosed and staged prior to surgery, a small number are still diagnosed during thoracotomy. Not infrequently, tumors are upstaged during surgery by visualizing more extensive disease than predicted during clinical staging.

## Treatment overview

Treatment options are based on the type and stage of lung cancer and are presented in Table 7.3. These include surgery, chemotherapy, radiation therapy; in advanced-stage disease and non-squamous histology, these are combined with new targeted, cytostatic therapies such as bevacizumab (Avastin, a monoclonal antibody anti-vascular endothelial growth factor (VEGF)) and erlotinib (Tarceva, a tyrosine kinase inhibitor) (19).

Early-stage cancers are usually treated surgically. Recent studies have shown improved survival in early-stage disease when platinum-based chemotherapy is offered following surgical resection. With more advanced disease (stages IIIa and IIIb) treatment decisions are made on a patient-by-patient basis. Options include surgery and a combination of chemotherapy and radiotherapy in the neoadjuvant and/or adjuvant settings, in order to reduce tumor bulk and to eradicate micrometastatic disease. Systemic disease (stage IV) can be treated with chemotherapy and radiation and with surgical resection of solitary metastasis when appropriate (19).

Chemotherapy alone or combined with radiation therapy is the treatment of choice for SCLC. This cell type is highly radiosensitive, and therefore chemotherapy can be complemented with consolidative radiation treatment of the thorax and prophylactic cranial irradiation (PCI) in patients with limited disease at presentation. Concurrent chemoradiotherapy has been shown to prolong survival in limited stage disease (20, 21). Some patients with stage I disease may be treated surgically followed by chemotherapy in the adjuvant setting (21). In extensive-stage disease, which is usually characterized by the presence of systemic disease at presentation, treatment is based on chemotherapy. Radiation therapy is used to treat bone and brain metastases. Prophylactic cranial irradiation is sometimes offered to those that respond well to chemotherapy, as described for limited-stage tumors, in an attempt to prevent disease relapse in the brain. Prophylactic cranial irradiation has been shown to improve overall relapse in the CNS and therefore is recommended for patients that have achieved a complete or near-complete remission following initial treatment.

Treatment options for recurrent disease include chemotherapy for local relapse, radiation therapy for metastases, and brachytherapy for endobronchial disease if additional external radiation cannot be tolerated. Rarely, surgical resection is considered to treat a recurrent solitary metastasis. The treatment of a locally recurrent NSCLC follows the same guidelines as for primary tumor stages I through III. If surgery was the primary line of treatment, radiation therapy is used. If the recurrence manifests as distant metastases, patients are treated as stage IV with a focus on palliation.

## The role of PET and PET/CT in the evaluation of lung cancer

PET imaging with FDG has become an integral part of today's clinical and surgical oncology armamentarium, because it provides visual access to the pathobiology of malignant processes in vivo. The proper clinical assessment of tumor invasion and metastasis calls for coupled anatomical and functional imaging information. Relying solely on parameters such as lesion size and shape only scratches the surface while attempting to understand the malignant behaviors of lung malignancies. The clinical success of PET imaging centers on its ability to investigate tumoral biologic behavior as opposed to relying solely on lesion morphology.

The recent introduction of hybrid imaging modalities such as PET/CT has allowed for the near-optimal co-registration of structure and function. The superior anatomical detail provided by CT is complemented by the biological significance of the findings detected in the PET images. Its end product, the combined image, grants greater accuracy and confidence in the interpretation of both the anatomic and metabolic information, when compared with PET or CT alone, and to PET and CT images displayed side-by-side. The fused anatomo-metabolic image overcomes the limitations of either modality alone.

Lung malignancies have distinctive anatomo-metabolic behaviors. FDG-PET/CT imaging of lung cancer has proven superior to assess the metabolic burden of the disease in its anatomic context. It is also a powerful tool to clarify the significance of high FDG uptake in otherwise normal structures. This imaging technique has improved the non-invasive: (a) characterization of the benign or malignant nature of indeterminate solitary pulmonary lesions and the guidance of biopsy procedures to metabolically active tumor of heterogeneous composition, thereby minimizing sampling errors; (b) assessment of T status, chest wall and mediastinal organ invasion; (c) characterization of nodal disease; (d) detection of distant metastatic disease and recurrence; and (e) assessment of the morphologic and metabolic tumoral response to cytotoxic and cytostatic cancer therapies.

The following sections will expand on the contribution of PET/CT to the diagnosis, staging, and monitoring response to therapy of lung cancer. Emphasis will be placed on the synergistic role played by fusion imaging as anatomy meets function in the setting of tumor aggressiveness.

## Diagnosis
## Morphologic characterization of a solitary pulmonary nodule

In the USA more than 100,000 patients are diagnosed with a solitary pulmonary nodule (SPN) every year. Although the majority of these nodules are benign, an SPN might constitute the first sign of lung cancer (22). The incidence of malignancy in SPN ranges from 10–70%, depending on the patient population being addressed (23, 24).

By definition, an SPN is an oval or round parenchymal opacity observed in the chest radiograph, which used to be called a "coin lesion," of less than 3 cm in diameter, and surrounded by normal lung in the absence of adenopathy, atelectasis, or a lung infection. However, characterizing the lesion as benign or malignant is not as simple as its definition, posing a difficult diagnostic challenge in daily clinical practice. The majority of SPNs constitute benign pathologic processes, such as granulomatous infections like tuberculosis, coccidioidomycosis, histoplasmosis, cryptococcosis, aspergillosis, or benign tumors such as hamartomas. However, up to 50% of SPNs might represent a lung cancer primary or lung metastasis from other histologic types (25). The clinical practice guidelines of the American College of Chest Physicians list adenocarcinomas as being the most common cause of malignant SPNs (almost 50%), followed by SCC (22%), metastasis from other primaries (8%), undifferentiated NSCLC (7%), and SCLC and BAC accounting for approximately 4% each. The remainder 12% is due to large cell carcinoma, carcinoid, adenoid cystic carcinoma, teratomas, adenosquamous carcinoma, and lymphomas (26). Therefore, it is very important to be able to non-invasively and accurately differentiate benign from malignant disease in order to select those patients who will benefit from potentially curable resection of their malignant tumors. The 5-year survival after nodule resection may be as high as 80% if the nodule is detected when it is 1 cm in diameter or smaller (22), with early resection minimizing the chance that the lesion will metastasize. On the other hand, when lesions are characterized as benign, or when metastatic disease has been detected during the SPN work-up, the morbidity and expense of unnecessary surgical procedures is minimized.

A combination of clinical and radiographic information should always be used to assess the probability of malignancy in patients with an SPN. Estimating pre-test probability facilitates the selection and interpretation of subsequent diagnostic tests. Swensen *et al.* (27) developed quantitative models to estimate the probability of malignancy in an SPN. The model used logistic regression to identify independent predictors of malignancy, showing that the clinical history and the radiographic patterns of SPNs provide useful information about the probability of malignancy of radiographically indeterminate lesions. In their model, age, cigarette-smoking status, history of cancer, diameter, spiculation, and upper lobe location of the SPNs were independent predictors of malignancy.

The clinical risk of malignancy increases with age (> 35 years old), with cigarette smoking and number of cigarettes smoked daily, and with a previous history of cancer. In addition, the benign or malignant nature of an SPN can be characterized radiographically based on lesion **size, location, margin, density, calcification pattern, growth rate, cavitation,** and **degree of contrast enhancement**.

The likelihood of malignancy approaches 90% when the **diameter** of the lesion exceeds 2 cm, and decreases to approximately 25–35% for lesions smaller than 1 cm in diameter. The majority of primary lung malignancies seem to have a predilection for the **upper lobes**, whereas metastases to the lung are usually basal and subpleural in location. Nodules with **irregular, spiculated** or **lobulated margins** are most likely malignant when compared with only a small fraction (approximately 20%) of nodules with smooth margins (28–30). A pleural tail, which is an opacity extending from the nodule to the pleural surface, represents fibrosis, and is most often observed with bronchioloalveolar carcinomas (BAC) and/or with adenocarcinomas. Those tumors characterized by a lepidic growth pattern or intratumoral bleeding might be surrounded by a halo of ground-glass opacity. Most malignant lesions have **soft tissue density**. As part of the Early Lung Cancer Action Project (ELCAP), Henschke and colleagues reported on the frequency and significance of part solid and non-solid nodules compared with solid nodules. The malignancy rate was 63% for part solid and 18% for non-solid nodules. After correcting for nodule size, the malignancy rate was significantly higher for part-solid nodules. Part-solid or non-solid nodules were predominantly BACs or adenocarcinomas with bronchioloalveolar features, whereas solid nodules were predominantly adenocarcinomas (31). The presence of fat in an SPN is a benign finding, and is usually consistent with a hamartoma or a lipoma, and occasionally with lipoid pneumonia. Prior infection may manifest as homogeneous, central, concentric, or laminar **calcification** in an SPN, whereas a popcorn pattern is typical of a hamartoma. Lastly, the eccentric and stippled patterns of calcification are considered indeterminate, because they may be associated with primary malignancy or metastasis, or found in SPNs of benign etiology, and therefore further evaluation is of utmost importance. A nodular-walled lung cavity with a thickness of ≥ 16 mm strongly suggests malignancy, whereas a thin, smooth wall may indicate a lung abscess or a benign lesion (32).

One of the hallmarks of cancer is the unnecessary and uncontrolled **growth** of tumor cells, and therefore, the degree

of malignancy of an SPN may be estimated by its rate of growth, expressed as the time it takes for the lesion's volume to double in size. One doubling time corresponds to the time it takes for the nodule's diameter to increase by 26%. With some exceptions [i.e., bronchioloalveolar tumors (> 3 years)], and certain metastases (faster growth), most carcinomas double in volume between 30 days and 1.5 years (24). If the SPN doubles in volume in less than 1 month this is suggestive of an acute infectious process, whereas if the doubling time exceeds 18 months this is more consistent with a granuloma, a carcinoid, or a hamartoma. It should be kept in mind that the doubling time of some benign and malignant lesions may overlap, and therefore, the above criteria should only be considered as a complementary parameter or tool to be analyzed in the context of the patient's clinical history, and not as the definite rule to characterize a lesion as malignant or benign. Lesion size stability for 2 years is generally accepted to be consistent with a benign process, underscoring the importance of comparing present imaging results with those from previous studies. Serial chest radiographs facilitate estimation of the growth rate of a nodule. Comparison should be done with radiographs or CT scans obtained preferably beyond 2 years to be able to detect subtle increases in size that otherwise would remain unappreciated, especially in very small lesions (33).

The described morphologic patterns of SPNs are not 100% specific for malignancy as some degree of undesired overlap with benign lesion patterns exists, with approximately one-third of SPNs remaining radiographically indeterminate in daily clinical practice. When relying on conventional imaging criteria to characterize SPNs, 25–39% of malignant lesions are incorrectly diagnosed as benign (34). On the other side of the spectrum, many benign lesions are categorized as malignant leading to unnecessary invasive procedures in order to arrive to a definitive diagnosis. In fact, approximately 60% of indeterminate lung nodules treated surgically are benign (35).

Based on the above, it is clear that there is not a perfect management approach to non-invasively differentiate benign from malignant nodules by relying on morphological imaging criteria alone, but fortunately in recent years the use of PET and PET/CT imaging has helped improve the diagnostic accuracy to characterize pulmonary lesions.

## Metabolic characterization of SPN

By taking advantage of its inherent capacity to investigate the metabolic behavior of a lesion, FDG-PET has proven to be a superior non-invasive predictor of malignancy in indeterminate SPNs. The degree of FDG uptake in a lesion depends on the number of viable tumor cells, on the malignant cell type, the degree of anaplasia and proliferative capacity, on the presence and number of inflammatory cells, and on lesion size. All these factors contribute to the ability of the technique to differentiate a malignant from a benign process.

Lowe and colleagues (36) studied 89 patients with indeterminate SPNs using FDG-PET. PET data were analyzed semiquantitatively by calculating the lesions' average SUV (SUVavg), and visually by comparing the lesions' uptake to the activity in the mediastinal blood pool. Sixty SPNs were malignant and 29 were benign. Using semiquantitative analysis (SUVavg cut-off 2.5), PET had an overall sensitivity and specificity for detection of malignant nodules of 92% and 90%, respectively. Visual analysis provided a slightly higher, although not statistically significant, sensitivity of 98% and a lower specificity of 69%. When analyzing 34 SPNs smaller than 1.5 cm, the sensitivity and specificity using SUV values were 80% and 95%, respectively, compared with 100% and 74%, respectively, for visual analysis.

Gould *et al.*'s meta-analysis of 40 studies ($n$ = 1474 pulmonary lesions) showed that for the total number of lesions the mean sensitivity was 96%, with highly variable specificities that ranged from 0–100% (mean 73%). For pulmonary nodules only ($n$ = 450), the mean sensitivity and specificity were 94% and 86%, respectively. The authors indicated that when the pre-test probability of malignancy is low in patients with a pulmonary nodule, a negative FDG-PET carries a 1% post-test probability of malignancy. Thus, in this population, watchful waiting to ensure nodule stability or resolution is probably safe. In contrast, in a high-risk patient a negative PET carries a 14% post-test probability of malignancy, and therefore, histologic confirmation is warranted (37). Only eight studies in this meta-analysis included and evaluated lesions smaller than 1 cm. However, based on the reported findings, the authors recommended that any degree of FDG activity in a lesion smaller than 1 cm should be considered worrisome for malignancy until proven otherwise (37).

Although lesions with very low FDG uptake (less than mediastinal blood pool activity) may be benign, it should be kept in mind that false-negative results may be encountered due to various reasons including lesion size, lesion biology, and respiratory motion, amongst others.

Radiologic characterization of SPNs smaller than 1 cm in diameter is certainly a challenge, and with newer state-of-the-art CT and PET/CT systems these findings are quite common. For the most part nodules smaller than 1 cm tend to be benign, yet some may carry a 4% chance of being malignant if they are located in a non-primary lobe (38), while the results of other studies have shown that approximately 18–25% may be malignant (39, 40). When the lesion size falls under the resolution of the PET scanner (~8 mm), the recovery of counts arising from it is significantly affected by the partial volume effect (see Chapter 1). The recommendation is that caution should be exercised when attempting to characterize lesions smaller than 8 mm in diameter with PET. FDG-PET or PET/CT are suboptimal for the characterization of subcentimeter nodules because uptake in them decreases when their diameter is less than twice the spatial resolution of the PET scanner. A limited number of studies have been published addressing the accuracy of FDG-PET to characterize nodules smaller than 1 cm in diameter. Herder and colleagues (41) conducted a retrospective analysis in 35 patients with 36 SPNs to evaluate the diagnostic accuracy of FDG-PET in radiologically indeterminate SPNs that were 1 cm or smaller on spiral CT. The prevalence of malignancy was 39%. PET was false-negative in one lesion (1 cm in diameter), and false-positive in five, yielding a sensitivity of 93%, a specificity of 77%, a positive predictive value of 72%, and a negative predictive value 94%. This retrospective study suggested that FDG-PET imaging could be a useful tool in differentiating benign from malignant SPNs 1 cm or smaller in diameter at clinical presentation. Recently, Divisi and co-investigators showed that FDG-PET/CT improves the characterization of potentially malignant pulmonary nodules smaller than 1 cm when compared with CT alone. They compared the value of FDG-PET/CT versus CT to characterize 57 lesions of 5 mm to 9.9 mm in diameter. The sensitivity and specificity of FDG-PET/CT was 95% and 72%, respectively, compared with 73% and 64%, respectively for CT alone (42).

Some primary lung malignancies such as bronchioloalveolar carcinomas, carcinoids or well-differentiated adenocarcinomas, may not be very metabolically active, and thus false-negative in FDG-PET (43, 44). Bryant and Cerfolio (45) studied 585 patients for SPN characterization with FDG-PET/CT. The investigators reported that lesions with SUVmax ranging from 0 to 2.5 still carried a 24% chance of being malignant. These included 11 cases of bronchioloalveolar carcinomas, 4 carcinoids and 2 metastases from renal cell carcinoma. O et al. shared similar results about the clinical significance of small pulmonary nodules with little or no FDG uptake on PET/CT images of patients with non-thoracic malignancies. They found that more than 19% of these lesions turned out to be malignant (46).

In order to increase the sensitivity of the technique, Matthies *et al.* proposed the use of dual time point FDG imaging to characterize the benign or malignant nature of lesions with an SUV close to the cut-off value of 2.5. Using a cut-off of 10% increase in lesion SUV between the two imaging sessions, the sensitivity increased from 80% to 100% at the expense of a decline in specificity from 94% to 89% (47). Unfortunately, the results from other investigators have not been as encouraging, and the use of dual time imaging still remains controversial in everyday clinical practice. Cloran and colleagues assessed the accuracy of dual time point FDG-PET imaging in those lesions with baseline SUVmax lower than 2.5. They evaluated 130 studies in 113 patients with 152 lesions. Using a SUVmax increase of 10% as the cut-off, the sensitivity was only 61%, and the specificity 58%, which yielded an accuracy of 60% (48).

Thoracic PET images are acquired across many respiratory cycles, and therefore respiratory motion, if not corrected for, has a limiting effect on the quality of the images. As lesions (especially small ones) move during the acquisition, their metabolic size is overestimated, and the intensity of uptake is underestimated (49, 50). The use of respiratory gating has been helpful, yet not simple enough to be applied clinically on a daily basis. The technique increases PET image quality during free- or shallow breathing by dividing the respiratory cycle into multiple phases and sorting the acquired events into temporal bins (usually between 6 and 10). Although the number of recorded counts per bin is smaller, and the images are noisier, it improves spatial resolution and quantification of uptake in small lesions (49, 50). In other words, the lesion SUV recovered is closer to what it is supposed to be, and this can have important implications when the degree of lesion uptake is borderline malignant in uncorrected images. Recently, Werner and co-investigators shared their clinical experience using respiratory gating during FDG-PET/CT and its effect on lesion size and tracer uptake in patients with pulmonary nodules (51). The investigators found that respiratory gating improved SUV and volume estimates in solitary pulmonary nodules. Respiratory gating reduced the measured volume of lung lesions by 44.5% ($P = 0.025$), with the lesion volumes in gated images being closer to those estimated from CT images. On the other hand the lesion SUVmax increased by 22.4% and the SUVavg by 13.3%, but the increase was not size-dependent. They attributed this size-independent effect to the number of lesions examined and the limited distribution of lesion sizes in their sample (51).

Highly FDG-avid lesions are usually considered malignant, but false-positive results are not uncommon in patients with infectious and/or inflammatory processes such as active tuberculosis, sarcoidosis, and fungal infections (e.g., histoplasmosis, coccidiodiomycosis, etc.) (52–54). Therefore, FDG-positive nodules always require further histologic assessment.

Most studies referred to in the previous paragraphs were conducted using dedicated PET scanners. The role of integrated PET/CT has not been systematically evaluated in this setting, when in fact this technology may further improve the characterization of SPNs in high-risk patients. The use of hybrid imaging systems brings about the best of both worlds. CT provides the anatomic landscape and the means for attenuation correction of the PET emission data, thus reducing acquisition times by about 40%. On the other hand, PET images provide information regarding the metabolic and biologic behavior of the lesion in question. Conclusions can be drawn by combining the information provided by both sets of images. In the author's opinion, the fused PET/CT image is certainly more than the CT and the PET images alone, as it overcomes the limitations of each when used independently (55, 56). For example, a practical approach is that a finding should be considered positive when lesions appear malignant on either the PET and/or the CT images. It is relatively simple to interpret the nature of an SPN that is positive by both CT and PET criteria. What do you do when the imaging finding is incongruent between CT and PET? For example, a ground-glass opacity with irregular margins opening into an obvious pleuropulmonary tail on CT, but non-FDG avid on PET. It is in cases like this when the reader needs to rely on the morphologic imaging phenotype (lesion size and shape) and on the patient's clinical history, to reliably judge the significance of the lack of lesion FDG uptake in this probable

bronchioloalveolar carcinoma. Lardinois and colleagues published the first comprehensive study comparing the value of PET/CT versus PET or CT alone in NSCLC (57). Their results showed that PET/CT provided more and better anatomic detail improving the staging accuracy versus PET or CT alone. Later on in 2007, the UCLA group reported their results on the accuracy of PET/CT for the characterization of SPN (58). They studied 52 patients referred for SPN characterization with lesion sizes ranging from 7 mm to 3 cm. PET/CT correctly characterized 39 of the 42 lesions as malignant or benign, compared with 3 out of 42 by PET and CT alone. The sensitivity and specificity for CT were 93% and 31%, for PET, 69% and 85%, and for PET/CT, 97% and 85%, respectively. The authors stressed the fact that using a SUVmax cut-off of 2.0 or lean body mass correction did not improve the accuracy of the technique (58). This was yet another example illustrating the synergistic value of the combination of anatomic and metabolic information to take advantage of the sensitivity of CT and the specificity of PET, to improve accuracy.

Blood flow in malignant pulmonary nodules has been shown to be higher than in benign nodules (59). A greater degree of contrast enhancement of a solitary pulmonary nodule is highly suspicious of malignancy, and it is directly related to its vascularity. In 2000, Swensen and co-investigators (60) reported the results of a prospective 7-center study of solid lung nodule enhancement with iodinated contrast in 356 patients with a 48% prevalence of malignancy. Using dynamic CT and an early phase enhancement level cut-off greater than 15 Hounsfield units (HU), the investigators reported a sensitivity, specificity, and accuracy of 98%, 58%, and 77% respectively. Malignant nodules enhanced significantly more than granulomas and benign neoplasms, whereas nodule enhancement less than 15 HU was highly predictive of a benign lesion.

Recently, by combining contrast wash-in and wash-out characteristics on dynamic helical CT acquisitions, investigators have achieved better specificities during the evaluation of SPN hemodynamics. Jeong and colleagues (61) characterized malignant nodules using a wash-in of ≥ 25 HU and a washout between 5 and 31 HU. When both wash-in of 25 HU and washout of 5–31 HU were applied for malignancy, the sensitivity, specificity, and accuracy were 81–94%, 90–93%, and 85–92%, respectively. Benign nodules were characterized using a wash-in of < 25 HU, a wash-in of ≥ 25 HU in combination with a wash-out of > 31 HU, or a wash-in of ≥ 25 HU and persistent enhancement without wash-out (71–95% negative predictive value). PET/CT increases diagnostic accuracy in these patients. In fact, the combination of lesion FDG uptake and the degree of contrast enhancement improves SPN characterization, as shown by the work of Yi and colleagues (62). In a recent retrospective study the investigators compared dynamic helical CT and PET/CT in 119 patients with indeterminate SPNs (malignant nodules size ranged from 9 to 30 mm, with only 8 nodules being smaller than 1 cm). The results showed a sensitivity, specificity, and accuracy of 81%, 93%, and 85%, respectively, for predicting malignancy with dynamic helical CT, versus 96%, 88%, and 93%, respectively with PET/CT. The authors concluded from their findings that PET/CT should be the test of choice for characterizing lung nodules, and that all malignant nodules may be interpreted correctly by at least one of the two techniques (62).

It is safe to say that despite the considerable technical advances of imaging techniques in recent years, the diagnostic work-up and management of patients with SPNs still relies on clinical perspectives, and that no single clinically based diagnostic algorithm can be applied to all cases. Clinicians need to rely on the complementary information arising from both imaging modalities (PET and CT) in the context of the patient's clinical pre-test probability of malignancy.

FDG-PET has been shown to be cost-effective to establish the differential diagnosis of lung nodules $\geq$ 8 mm when clinical and morphological findings are incongruent (low-risk patient with a "probably malignant" CT pattern), or in high-risk patients with an indeterminate nodule. At a low probability of cancer and a negative PET, observation would be optimal, as survival is not necessarily affected by the surveillance period. On the other hand, Gould et al. recommend surgery for high-risk patients, if the CT findings are possibly malignant, unless the risk for surgical complications is very high. If the CT shows a benign pattern, FDG-PET should be performed, followed by surgery if the SPN is FDG positive, without evidence of metastatic disease. If the PET is negative, needle biopsy is more effective than surveillance (63).

The 2007 American College of Chest Physicians (ACCP) guidelines (64) for the diagnosis and treatment of lung cancer recommend the use of FDG-PET for the characterization of SPN:

- in patients with a low to moderate pre-test probability of malignancy (5–60%) and an indeterminate SPN (8–10 mm in diameter), and
- in those patients with a moderate to high pre-test probability of malignancy (> 60%), and an FDG-avid SPN, in whom surgical diagnosis is preferred when clinically appropriate.

The Society of Nuclear Medicine 2008 recommendation (65) is that FDG-PET/CT should be obtained in the diagnostic work-up of SPNs:

- to detect potential malignant lesions early in the course of the disease,
- to exclude the possibility of malignancy in indeterminate lesions in low-risk patients,
- to improve healthcare outcomes by avoiding futile surgeries in low-risk patients and enabling curative surgeries in high-risk patients.

## Tumor status

Accurate disease staging in patients with lung cancer is essential to choose the appropriate therapy, and it has prognostic information. FDG images have low spatial resolution and therefore they do not provide or add much to the assessment of disease extent or resectability status. CT continues to be considered the modality of choice to assess tumor (T) status (lesion size, relationship to neighbouring structures, mediastinal invasion, and/or chest wall compromise). Recently, studies conducted to evaluate the role of hybrid imaging with FDG-PET/CT have crystallized its promising value to assess T status (57, 66). Lardinois and colleagues (57) showed that FDG-PET/CT imaging improves the diagnostic accuracy of NSCLC staging. In a prospective study of 50 patients with proven or suspected NSCLC the investigators compared the role of PET/CT versus PET and CT alone to assess TNM status. PET/CT provided additional information in 41% of the patients diminishing the number of equivocal findings. PET/CT assigned the correct T stage in 88% of the patients compared with 40% by PET alone and 58% by CT alone. The incorrect T stage was assigned by PET/CT in only 2% of the cases, compared with approximately 20% by CT and PET alone. PET/CT improved the detection of chest wall and mediastinal invasion, and provided a more accurate assessment of N and M stage. Similar results were published the same year by Antoch and colleagues (66). The combination of anatomic and physiologic information in one image overcomes the limitations of either modality alone. In this regard, PET/CT becomes the technique of choice to more accurately define the extent of invasion, to detect the presence of additional pulmonary nodules in the same or a different lobe, and to differentiate tumor from atelectasis (55). The latter is particularly important in radiation therapy planning when a tumor is associated with lung collapse, in which the metabolic information from PET leads to a change in the radiation field in approximately 30% of cases (67). However, fine detail is still a limitation, because the technique is still unable to distinguish contiguity of tumor with the mediastinum (resectable disease) from direct invasion of mediastinal structures (unresectable disease).

## Prognostic value of the primary tumor's metabolic activity

The fact that FDG uptake in primary lung lesions is a function of the number of cancer cells, cellular proliferation and tumor growth, and expression of GLUT receptors, all of which have been correlated with poor outcome, has led several investigators to study the prognostic value of FDG uptake in primary lung tumors.

Ahuja et al. (68) studied the prognostic value and the potential of FDG-PET to guide therapeutic options. Their univariate analysis results indicated that the overall survival of patients with a primary tumor SUV > 10 was significantly shorter than for those with an SUV < 10. Multivariate analysis confirmed that the lesion SUV provided independent and additional prognostic information to the clinical stage and the lesion size.

Cerfolio and colleagues (69) published their results from a study of 315 patients in whom an SUV > 10 in their primary tumor was an independent predictor of progression-free survival, as well as an independent predictor of stage and tumor differentiation. The authors concluded that those patients with the same disease stage but with a higher primary tumor SUV were more likely to have progression of their disease and a shorter overall survival.

## Node status

Dillemans and colleagues (70) compared the accuracy of CT versus mediastinoscopy to stage the mediastinum in 561 patients. The investigators reported a sensitivity, a specificity, and an accuracy of 69%, 71%, and 71%, respectively for CT to detect mediastinal metastasis. On the other hand, mediatinoscopy had a sensitivity of 72%, a specificity of 100%, and an accuracy of 89%. The CT sensitivity was lower in left-sided and central tumors.

FDG-PET detects tumor in normal size lymph nodes (< 1 cm in the short axis) and excludes tumor involvement in large lymph nodes, because it interrogates the biologic behavior of lesions and does not rely on nodal size. Unlike mediatinoscopy, PET provides full sampling of the mediastinum, changing the node (N) stage in approximately 20% of the patients.

Toloza *et al.* (71) published a review of the literature on the performance of CT, endoscopic ultrasound (EUS) and PET for staging the mediastinum. PET scanning was more accurate than CT scanning or EUS for detecting mediastinal metastases. The CT sensitivity was 57% and the specificity 82%, compared with 84% and 89%, respectively for PET, and 78% and 71%, respectively for EUS. Gould and colleagues (72) arrived at similar conclusions when comparing the usefulness of PET and CT to stage the mediastinum. For CT, the median sensitivity and specificity were 61% and 79%, respectively, compared with FDG-PET, which had a median sensitivity and specificity of 85% and 90%, respectively. In addition, the authors stressed the fact that PET was more sensitive (up to 100%) but less specific (78%) when CT showed lymph node enlargement.

Gupta and co-investigators (73) studied the accuracy of PET according to nodal size. PET had a sensitivity of 97%, a specificity of 82%, and an accuracy of 95% for detecting metastasis in lymph nodes < 1 cm in size. For nodes between 1 and 3 cm in size the values were 100%, 91%, and 95%, respectively. The PPV and NPV for PET were 86% and 98% respectively, compared with 47% and 82% for CT.

de Langen and colleagues (74) conducted a meta-analysis to evaluate the relationship between nodal size and the probability of malignancy. Their results showed that for non-FDG avid nodes measuring 10–15 mm on CT, the post-test probability of N2 disease was 5%, and therefore, safe for these patients to undergo thoracotomy without mediastinoscopy. When non-FDG avid nodes measured ≥ 16 mm on CT, the post-test probability of malignancy was 21%, stressing the fact that in this patient cohort mediastinoscopy should precede thoracotomy.

The use of combined PET/CT imaging for N staging allows for more precise localization of mediastinal lymph nodes metastasis by being able to reveal the exact location of single or small nodes, and involved supraclavicular nodes, with an accuracy of 93%, compared with 89% for PET, and 63% for CT alone (66).

It must be remembered that not all hot nodes are metastatic; inflammatory/reactive nodes can be FDG avid as well. Therefore, nodal sampling is indicated so that patients free of metastatic disease are able to undergo surgery, that otherwise would be denied due to false-positive findings.

Finally, yet importantly, is the interesting relationship that exists between the primary tumor size and intensity of uptake and the presence of nodal metastases. In patients with NSCLC, FDG uptake by the primary tumor has been shown to be a strong predictor of intratumoral lymphatic vessel invasion and lymph node metastasis. Vesselle and colleagues (75) reported that FDG avidity by the primary tumor and tumor size are to be taken into consideration when reporting PET studies in patients with lung cancer, because they affect the likelihood of malignant involvement in hypermetabolic nodes. The size of the lung tumor significantly influenced the incidence of malignant mediastinal adenopathy, with larger primaries being more likely to have nodal involvement than smaller tumors. Later on Higashi and co-investigators (76) confirmed these findings by reporting a significant correlation between FDG uptake in the primary lesion, the incidence of intratumoral lymphatic vessel invasion, and nodal involvement in patients with NSCLC. Patients with a low to moderate FDG uptake in the primary lesion had significantly less intratumoral lymphatic vessel invasion and lymph node metastasis than those with a high FDG uptake.

## Metastasis status

Approximately 21% of patients with NSCLC will have distant metastatic disease at presentation (77). The frequency of occult metastasis from adenocarcinomas is approximately 67%, from large cell carcinomas in the order of 12%, and 21% from squamous cell types (78). In the great majority of cases metastatic disease starts with lymphatic spread from the primary tumor to N1 (parenchymal, hilar, and peribronchial nodes), from there to N2 (mediastinal nodes), to finally arrive to the ipsilateral supraclavicular and/or contralateral N3 nodes. Primary tumors may also metastasize to the pleura by the way of retrograde lymphatic spread. Satellite nodes, now called "additional" parenchymal tumors, in the same or another ipsilateral lung lobe, also constitute metastasis secondary to lymphatic or airway spread from the primary tumor. The invasion of vascular structures by the primary tumor gives rise to hematopoietic metastases to distant sites. The most common sites of lung cancer metastases include the adrenal glands, bones, liver, and brain; however, every other organ may be affected.

FDG-PET is probably the most sensitive imaging technique for the detection of extracerebral metastasis from lung cancer. PET detects distant metastases missed by CT or excludes false-positive sites detected by CT in up to approximately 24% of patients. A 2004 review of the literature concluded that FDG-PET detected up to 20% more distant metastases than other imaging methods, and that a change in patient management takes place in 9–64% of patients, mainly by reducing the number of futile surgeries (79). A meta-analysis conducted by Hellwig *et al.* (80) of a total of four studies with 336 patients, found the sensitivity, specificity, and accuracy of FDG-PET for the detection of systemic metastasis to be 94%, 97%, and 96%, respectively. The investigators stated that the technique changed therapeutic management in 18% of cases, with unexpected extrathoracic systemic disease found in 12% of patients. The sensitivity, specificity, and accuracy for the detection of adrenal metastasis were 96%, 99%, and 98%, respectively. FDG-PET has similar sensitivity (90–92%) and higher specficity (98–99%) than bone scintigraphy for the detection of osteoclastic bone metastasis, and its sensitivity is lower in the presence of osteoblastic lesions (due to their lower cellularity and glycolytic metabolism) (81). As far as the detection of liver metastasis is concerned, FDG-PET has a sensitivity of 97%, a specificity of 88%, and an accuracy of 92%, compared with 93%, 75%, and 85% for CT, with FDG-PET adding new information in 23.5% of the cases (82). In contrast, the diagnostic accuracy of PET is inferior to MRI and CT for the detection of brain metastasis due to the high cortical FDG uptake (sensitivity ~60%, specificity ~99%).

The incidence of occult metastasis increases with stage, and was reported by MacManus and colleagues as ranging from 7.5% when the pre-PET stage is I to approximately 24% in pre-PET stage III (83).

One of the most important contributions of PET/CT to metastasis staging is to detect extrathoracic lesions more accurately, and to be able to determine the clinical significance of a single focal abnormality by localizing it to a specific anatomical structure, and therefore characterizing its physiologic or pathologic nature. In this manner, once the lesion is localized it may serve as a guidance tool to biopsy it (see Chapter 20). However, of utmost importance is that not all extrathoracic FDG-avid lesions found in lung cancer patients are in fact metastasis. A prospective study of 350 patients conducted by Lardinois and colleagues found that 71 (21%) patients had extrapulmonary FDG-avid lesions (84). Sixty-nine of these lesions were biopsied, and 37 (54%) were found to be metastatic, whereas 32 (46%) were not. Of the latter, 26 (37% of total) lesions were benign or inflammatory, and the remainder 6 (9% of total) were unsuspected second primaries or recurrence from a previous malignancy. Therefore, extrathoracic lesions should be biopsied if their malignant nature would in fact alter patient management.

## Monitoring response to therapy

The greatest contribution provided by FDG-PET when used to monitor metabolic response to treatment, is its predictive value of treatment outcome and patient survival. In addition, it does not rely on lesion size or shape to characterize response, and PET information is not confounded by tissue changes (necrosis/fibrosis) following therapy. Evaluating response to treatment using morphological criteria has several limitations. The most important one is that conventional response evaluation criteria in solid tumors (RECIST) do not always correlate with histopathological response and with final treatment outcome, and that morphologic changes are often preceded by biologic response to therapy (85). Monitoring response to therapy using FDG-PET may be done during or after therapy, both in the neoadjuvant or the adjuvant settings or a combination thereof. The published sensitivities and specificities of FDG-PET to assess histopathological response to lung cancer treatment range from 81% to 97%, and 64% to 100%, respectively (86). The results of all these studies have confirmed that FDG-PET predicts response earlier than conventional imaging modalities, with outcomes being predicted as early as after one course of neoadjuvant chemotherapy (87, 88).

## Detection and staging of recurrent lung cancer

To this date several studies have demonstrated that FDG-PET and PET/CT are able to very accurately detect and stage recurrent disease after surgery, chemotherapy, and/or radiotherapy, before conventional imaging modalities do. Sensitivities and specificities range from 90 to 100% and 62 to 92%, respectively (89–96).

Hellwig and colleagues showed that FDG-PET imaging improves the detection of recurrent lung cancer and also provides prognostic information by selecting those patients that will benefit from additional treatment (96).

## FDG-PET of small cell lung cancer

There is no reliable and available evidence to support the use of FDG imaging for the diagnosis and staging of SCLC. Its role remains uncertain and further research is certainly underway. The number of studies that has been published is limited, with a small number of patients, and these lack histologic confirmation of disease or have used inconsistent reference standards.

Investigations have dealt mainly with the role of FDG-PET in staging, on its impact on patient management, on monitoring treatment response, and on elucidating its prognostic value.

These studies have shown that adding PET to conventional staging methodologies results in a change in management in 9–30% of cases (97–102). PET has been found to influence clinical stage migration by detecting lymph node and distant metastases, or by characterizing the benign nature of a finding in conventional imaging. Upstaging from limited to extensive disease has been reported to occur in approximately in 0–33% of cases, and downstaging in 0–17% (97–102).

In a recent study of 20 patients that evaluated the role of FDG-PET/CT to monitor response to SCLC therapy, Fischer *et al.* (103) indicated that a significant difference in relative change in tumor FDG-uptake and tumor volume was observed between responding and non-responding patients. The investigators did not find a significant difference between qualitative and semi-quantitative analysis of the PET images when attempting to assess response. The authors concluded that although response evaluation by PET/CT is feasible, it is uncertain whether it adds further information to the one provided by conventional imaging criteria.

Metabolic activity of SCLC has been shown to be an independent prognostic factor. Lee and colleagues (104) studied the prognostic value of tumoral FDG uptake in 76 consecutive patients with pathologically proven SCLC. A high tumoral SUVmax was associated with poor survival. Furthermore, the SUVmax was able to identify prognostic subgroups amongst patients with extensive disease and limited disease. These results are important and call for confirmation with well-designed prospective studies.

## Malignant pleural mesothelioma

Malignant pleural mesothelioma (MPM) is a very aggressive neoplasm of mesothelial cells with an annual incidence of approximately 3,000 patients in the USA, and a male to female ratio of approximately 4 : 1 (105, 106). The clinical manifestation of the disease occurs approximately 30–40 years (range 15–60 years) after exposure to asbestos fibers, with the majority of patients developing the disease at an average age of 60 years (107–109). Mesothelioma may also arise after exposure to non-asbestos mineral fibers such as erionite and tremolite, therapeutic radiation, and diethylstilbestrol. It has been proposed that exposure to the Simian Virus 40 in contaminated polio vaccines may also be a source of the disease, but this has recently been contested (110, 111).

The three main histologic subtypes of MPM are epithelioid (50–60%), sarcomatoid (10%), and a combination of both, called biphasic or mixed subtype (30–40%) (112).

The pattern of tumor invasion is first locoregional as small plaques affecting the parietal pleura. This leads to pleural thickening and subsequent fusion, and finally to encasement, compression and/or invasion of the lung parenchyma. The tumor continues growing to invade the chest wall, the mediastinal organs, the contralateral lung, the diaphragm, and the peritoneum.

Early diagnosis and an accurate staging of the disease are essential to classify patients into prognostic subgroups and to plan therapy (113, 114). Proper staging reduces the risk of finding unresectable tumor during surgery, and prevents the morbidity associated with unnecessary operations on those with extrapleural disease. MPM is considered unresectable when there is mediastinal, contralateral pleura, transdiaphragmatic,

spinal and/or diffuse chest wall invasion with or without rib destruction, and with or without associated systemic metastases. Unfortunately, the non-invasive selection of patients that could benefit from therapy is still a challenge. The first diagnostic step is to be able to differentiate between benign and malignant pleural disease, as well as between resectable and non-resectable disease. Because of its complex biology and growth pattern, imaging MPM is a challenging clinical task for all modalities, all of which have specific advantages and limitations.

## CT and MRI

Computed tomography (CT) plays a central role and together with chest radiography, is the first-line imaging technique used for the diagnosis and staging of MPM. The typical CT findings that suggest MPM are rind-like pleural thickening, mediastinal pleural involvement, pleural nodularity, and pleural thickness greater than 1 cm (115). Not uncommon are unilateral pleural effusions, pleural plaque soft tissue growth, and nodules in the pleural fissures, as well as evidence of local invasion and mediastinal or hilar adenopathy.

MRI plays a complementary role for the staging of MPM. It is used primarily to clarify equivocal findings on CT, and to characterize transdiaphragmatic invasion, as well as extension of the disease into the chest wall and the pericardium.

CT and MRI are successful at predicting tumor resectability; but they have limitations when attempting to characterize pleural lesions as benign or malignant (116, 117).

## FDG-PET and PET/CT

Fortunately the majority of mesotheliomas are FDG avid. In general the intensity of uptake ranges from moderate to high depending on the cell type (118, 119). Epithelioid MPM is generally less metabolically active than the other two cell types, and unfortunately in some epithelial tumors uptake can be very mild or even null (118, 120).

FDG-PET imaging has been shown to be very accurate to non-invasively characterize pleural lesions as benign or malignant. The reported sensitivity, specificity, and accuracy range from 88–100%, 75–95%, and 89–98%, respectively (118–122). One of its main drawbacks is that neither the pattern nor the intensity of radiotracer uptake can differentiate MPM from other pleural malignancies. This is an important limitation as it has treatment implications. The technique's specificity is less than perfect and therefore false-positive findings may be encountered. False-positive uptake in FDG-PET images has been described in asbestos-related plaques, tuberculous pleuritis, benign inflammatory pleuritis, parapneumonic effusions, and bronchopleural fistulas (118, 121, 122). FDG-PET and PET/CT reduce the number of unnecessary surgical procedures in patients with a negative test; however, a negative FDG-PET does not absolutely rule out MPM. As stated before, some epithelioid tumors may not be FDG avid.

FDG-PET and PET/CT imaging complement CT and MRI in the assessment of intrathoracic disease extent and tumor resectability. Both FDG-PET and PET/CT face known limitations when attempting to assess the nature of subtle, yet unresectable, invasive disease (113). The low spatial resolution of PET, coupled with the irregular, non-spherical growth and invasion patterns of MPM, make T staging quite challenging. PET/CT is superior to PET alone for staging MPM, with limitations when dealing with T4 and N2 disease. However, it is more accurate than CT and MRI for the detection of extrathoracic metastasis (113).

Intrathoracic lymph node involvement occurs in 22–50% of cases (123, 124). FDG-PET and PET/CT are superior to conventional imaging modalities to stage N disease, but not without limitations. This advantage is marginal, with an unacceptable number of false-negative and false-positive results. FDG-PET's disappointing sensitivity to stage N2 disease has been reported to be as low as 19% (125), with the highest being 38% and a specificity of 78% (126). Intrapleural nodal uptake needs to be high enough in order to be distinguished from the surrounding pleural uptake. On the other hand, extrapleural (N2) nodes (which have independent prognostic value) with micrometastases can be a source of false-negative findings (127). Therefore, histological confirmation of nodal disease is a must with a negative or positive FDG-PET.

Systemic metastases from malignant pleural mesothelioma can affect the adrenal glands, liver, bone, kidneys, the contralateral lung, abdominal wall and lymph nodes, the peritoneum, the brain, and the leptomeninges (127–129). FDG-PET and PET/CT imaging accurately detect or confirm the presence or absence of systemic metastases. FDG-PET/CT detects more extensive disease involvement, and identifies occult distant metastases not seen in CT and MRI.

Malignant pleural mesothelioma recurrence can present as locoregional (12–88%) and/or distant disease (9–100%) (130–132). Conventional imaging modalities have great difficulty in differentiating recurrent tumor from benign post-therapeutic changes. Granulation tissue can present with a nodular pattern simulating recurrence in CT or MRI images. FDG-PET/CT has been shown to have greater accuracy in this setting. Gerbaudo et al. recently showed that FDG-PET/CT is highly accurate to diagnose and to assess the extent of locoregional and distant MPM relapse, with impact on patient management after treatment failure of MPM (130). In their 50-patient study, FDG-PET/CT was 97.6% sensitive, 75% specific and 94% accurate to characterize the presence or absence of recurrent MPM.

Last but not least, high levels of tumoral FDG uptake and tumor morphologic and metabolic bulk are associated with an unfavorable prognosis in patients with MPM.

The cases that follow are real-life clinical scenarios that will highlight and apply the concepts that have been discussed about the role of FDG-PET and PET/CT in the management of patients with lung and pleural malignancies.

# References

1. Siegel R, Ward E, Brawley D, Jemal A. Cancer Statistics, 2011: the impact of eliminating socioeconomic and racial disparities on premature cancer deaths. *CA Cancer J Clin* 2011;**61**:212–36.

2. Travis WD, Colby TV, Corrin B, Shimosato Y, Brambilla E. In Collaboration with Sobin LH and Pathologists from 14 Countries. World Health Organization International Histological Classification of Tumours. *Histological Typing of Lung and Pleural Tumours*. 3rd Edn. Berlin: Springer-Verlag, 1999.

3. Travis WD, Brambilla E, Muller-Hermelink HK, Harris CC (Eds). *World Health Organization Classification of Tumours. Pathology and Genetics of Tumours of the Lung, Pleura, Thymus and Heart*. Lyon: IARC Press, 2004.

4. Travis WD, Garg K, Franklin WA *et al*. Evolving concepts in the pathology and computed tomography imaging of lung adenocarcinoma and bronchioloalveolar carcinoma. *J Clin Oncol* 2005;**23**:3279–87.

5. Travis WD, Garg K, Franklin WA *et al*. Bronchioloalveolar carcinoma and lung adenocarcinoma: the clinical importance and research relevance of the 2004 World Health Organization pathologic criteria. *J Thorac Oncol* 2006;**1**(9 Suppl):S13–19.

6. Travis WD, Brambilla E *et al*. International Association for the Study of Lung Cancer/American Thoracic Society/European Respiratory Society International Multidisciplinary Classification of Lung Adenocarcinoma. *J Thorac Oncol* 2011;**6**(2):244–85.

7. Hirsch FR, Matthews MJ, Aisner S *et al*. Histopathologic classification of small cell lung cancer. Changing concepts and terminology. *Cancer* 1988;**62**(5):973–7.

8. Edge SB, Byrd DR, Compton CC *et al*. (Eds.). Lung. In *AJCC Cancer Staging Manual*. 7th Edn. New York, NY: Springer, 2010, pp. 253–70.

9. Godlstraw P, Crowley J, Chanskey K *et al*. The IASLC Lung Cancer Staging Project: proposals for the revision of the TNM stage groupings in the forthcoming (seventh) edition of the TNM classification of malignant tumours. *J Thorac Oncol* 2007;**2**(8):706–14.

10. Quekel LG, Kessels AG, Goei R, van Engelshoven JM. Miss rate of lung cancer on the chest radiograph in clinical practice. *Chest* 1999;**115**(3):720–4.

11. Silvestri GA, Gould MK, Margolis ML *et al*.; American College of Chest Physicians. Noninvasive staging of non-small cell lung cancer: ACCP evidenced-based clinical practice guidelines (2nd edition). *Chest* 2007;**132** (3 Suppl):178S–201S.

12. Yung RC. Tissue diagnosis of suspected lung cancer: selecting between bronchoscopy, transthoracic needle aspiration, and resectional biopsy. *Respir Care Clin N Am* 2003;**9**(1):51–76.

13. Lacasse Y, Wong E, Guyatt GH, Cook DJ. Transthoracic needle aspiration biopsy for the diagnosis of localised pulmonary lesions: a meta-analysis. *Thorax* 1999;**54**(10):884–93.

14. De Leyn P, Lerut T. Cervical mediastinoscopy. *Multimedia Manual of Cardiothoracic Surgery* 2005. [Web page http://mmcts.ctsnetjournals.org/cgi/reprint/2005/0324/

mmcts.2004.000158.pdf] [Accessed December 2010].

15. De Leyn P, Vansteenkiste J, Cuypers P *et al.* Role of cervical mediastinoscopy in staging of non-small cell lung cancer without enlarged mediastinal lymph nodes on CT scan. *Eur J Cardiothorac Surg* 1997;**12**:706–12.

16. De Leyn P, Stroobants S, De Wever W *et al.* Prospective comparative study of integrated positron emission tomography-computed tomography scan compared with remediastinoscopy in the assessment of residual mediastinal lymph node disease after induction chemotherapy for mediastinoscopy-proven stage IIIA-N2 Non-small-cell lung cancer: a Leuven Lung Cancer Group Study. *J Clin Oncol* 2006;**24**(21):3333–9.

17. Harris RJ, Kavuru MS, Rice TW, Kirby KJ. The diagnostic and therapeutic utility of thoracoscopy. *Chest* 1995;**108**:828–41.

18. Landreneau RJ, Mack MJ, Hazelrigg SR *et al.* Video assisted thoracic surgery: basic technical concepts and intercostal approach strategies. *Ann Thorac Surg* 1992;**54**:800–7.

19. National Comprehensive Cancer Network. *NCCN (National Comprehensive Cancer Network) Guidelines.* [Web page http://www. nccn.org/professionals/physician_gls/ f_guidelines.asp] [Accessed 2010 January 17].

20. Jackman DM, Johnson BE. Small-cell lung cancer. *Lancet* 2005;**366**(9494):1385–96.

21. Simon GR, Turrisi A; American College of Chest Physicians. Management of small cell lung cancer: ACCP evidence-based clinical practice guidelines (2nd edition). *Chest* 2007;**132**(3 Suppl):324S–39S.

22. Lillington GA. Management of solitary pulmonary nodules. *Dis Mon.* 1991;**37**(5):271–318.

23. Khouri NF, Meziane MA, Zerhouni EA, Fishman EK. The solitary pulmonary nodule: assessment, diagnosis, and management. *Chest* 1987;**91**:128–33.

24. Ost D, Fein AM, Feinsilver SH. Clinical practice: the solitary pulmonary nodule. *N Engl J Med* 2003;**348**:2535–42.

25. Swensen SJ, Jett JR, Payne WS *et al.* An integrated approach to evaluation of the solitary pulmonary nodule. *Mayo Clin Proc* 1990;**65**:173–86.

26. Gould MK, Fletcher J, Iannettoni MD *et al.*; American College of Chest Physicians. Evaluation of patients with pulmonary nodules: when is it lung cancer?: ACCP evidence-based clinical practice guidelines (2nd edition). *Chest* 2007;**132** (3 Suppl):108S–30S.

27. Swensen SJ, Silverstein MD, Ilstrup DM, Schleck CD, Edell ES. The probability of malignancy in solitary pulmonary nodules. Application to small radiologically indeterminate nodules. *Arch Intern Med* 1997;**157**:849–55.

28. Swensen SJ, Viggiano RW, Midthun DE *et al.* Lung nodule enhancement at CT: multicenter study. *Radiology* 2000;**214**(1):73–80.

29. Gurney JW. Determining the likelihood of malignancy in solitary pulmonary nodules with Bayesian analysis. Part I. Theory. *Radiology* 1993;**186**(2):405–13.

30. Zerhouni EA, Stitik FP, Siegelman SS *et al.* CT of the pulmonary nodule: a cooperative study. *Radiology* 1986;**160**(2):319–27.

31. Henschke CI, Yankelevitz DF, Mirtcheva R *et al.*; ELCAP Group. CT screening for lung cancer: frequency and significance of part-solid and nonsolid nodules. *Am J Roentgenol* 2002;**178**(5):1053–7.

32. Woodring JH, Fried AM. Significance of wall thickness in solitary cavities of the lung: a follow-up study. *Am J Roentgenol* 1983;**140**(3):473–4.

33. Yankelevitz DF, Henschke CI. Does 2-year stability imply that pulmonary nodules are benign? *Am J Roentgenol* 1997;**168**(2):325–8.

34. Erasmus JJ, McAdams HP, Connolly JE. Solitary pulmonary nodules: Part II. Evaluation of the indeterminate nodule. *Radiographics* 2000;**20**(1):59–66.

35. Gupta NC, Maloof J, Gunel E. Probability of malignancy in solitary pulmonary nodules using fluorine-18-FDG and PET. *J Nucl Med* 1996;**37**:943–8.

36. Lowe VJ, Fletcher JW, Gobar L *et al.* Prospective investigation of PET in lung nodules (PIOPILN). *J Clin Oncol* 1998;**16**:1075–84.

37. Gould MK, Maclean CC, Kuschner WG, Rydzak CE, Owens DK. Accuracy of positron emission tomography for diagnosis of pulmonary nodules and mass lesions: a meta-analysis. *J Am Med Assoc* 2001;**285**:914–24.

38. Kim YH, Lee KS, Primack SL *et al.* Small pulmonary nodules on CT accompanying surgically resectable lung cancer: likelihood of malignancy. *J Thorac Imaging* 2002;**17**:40–6.

39. Chalmers N, Best JJ. The significance of pulmonary nodules detected by CT but not by chest radiography in tumor staging. *Clin Radiol* 1991;**44**:410–12.

40. Yuan Y, Matsumoto T, Hiyama A *et al.* The probability of malignancy in small pulmonary nodules coexisting with potentially operable lung cancer detected by CT. *Eur Radiol* 2003;**13**:2447–53.

41. Herder GJ, Golding RP, Hoekstra OS *et al.* The performance of (18)F-fluorodeoxyglucose positron emission tomography in small solitary pulmonary nodules. *Eur J Nucl Med Mol Imaging* 2004;**31**(9):1231–6.

42. Divisi D, Di Tommaso S, Di Leonardo G *et al.* 18-fluorine fluorodeoxyglucose positron emission tomography with computerized tomography versus computerized tomography alone for the management of solitary lung nodules with diameters inferior to 1.5 cm. *Thorac Cardiovasc Surg* 2010;**58**(7):422–6.

43. Higashi K, Ueda Y, Seki H *et al.* Fluorine-18-FDG PET imaging is negative in bronchioloalveolar lung carcinoma. *J Nucl Med* 1998;**39**:1016–20.

44. Erasmus JJ, McAdams HP, Patz EF, Jr *et al.* Evaluation of primary pulmonary carcinoid tumors using FDG PET. *Am J Roentgenol* 1998;**170**:1369–73.

45. Bryant AS, Cerfolio RJ. The maximum standardized uptake values on integrated FDG-PET/CT is useful in differentiating benign from malignant pulmonary nodules. *Ann Thorac Surg* 2006;**82**(3):1016–20.

46. O JH, Yoo IeR, Kim SH, Sohn HS, Chung SK. Clinical significance of small pulmonary nodules with little or no 18F-FDG uptake on PET/CT images of patients with nonthoracic malignancies. *J Nucl Med* 2007;**48**(1):15–21.

47. Matthies A, Hickeson M, Cuchiara A, Alavi A. Dual time point 18F-FDG PET

for the evaluation of pulmonary nodules. *J Nucl Med* 2002; **43**(7): 871–5.

48. Cloran FJ, Banks KP, Song WS, Kim Y, Bradley YC. Limitations of dual time point PET in the assessment of lung nodules with low FDG avidity. *Lung Cancer* 2010;**68**(1):66–71.

49. Erdi YE, Nehmeh SA, Pan T *et al*. The CT motion quantitation of lung lesions and its impact on PET measured SUVs. *J Nucl Med* 2004;**45**:1287–92.

50. Park SJ, Ionascu D, Killoran J *et al*. Evaluation of the combined effects of target size, respiratory motion and background activity on 3D and 4D PET/CT images. *Phys Med Biol* 2008;**53**(13):3661–79.

51. Werner MK, Parker JA, Kolodny GM, English JR, Palmer MR. Respiratory gating enhances imaging of pulmonary nodules and measurement of tracer uptake in FDG PET/CT. *Am J Roentgenol* 2009;**193**(6):1640–5.

52. Jones HA, Clark RJ, Rhodes CG *et al*. Positron emission tomography of 18FDG uptake in localized pulmonary inflammation. *Acta Radiol Suppl* 1991;**376**:148.

53. Chang JM, Lee HJ, Goo JM *et al*. False positive and false negative FDG-PET scans in various thoracic diseases. *Korean J Radiol* 2006;**7**(1):57–69.

54. Alavi A, Gupta N, Alberini JL *et al*. Positron emission tomography imaging in nonmalignant thoracic disorders. *Semin Nucl Med* 2002;**32**(4):293–321.

55. Gerbaudo VH, Julius B. Anatomo-metabolic characteristics of atelectasis in F-18 FDG-PET/CT imaging. *Eur J Radiol* 2007;**64**(3):401–5.

56. Britz-Cunningham SH, Millstine JW, Gerbaudo VH. Improved discrimination of benign and malignant lesions on FDG PET/CT, using comparative activity ratios to brain, basal ganglia, or cerebellum. *Clin Nucl Med* 2008;**33**(10):681–7.

57. Lardinois D, Weder W, Hany TF *et al*. Staging of non–small-cell lung cancer with integrated positron emission tomography and computed tomography. *N Engl J Med* 2003;**348**:2500–7.

58. Kim SK, Allen-Auerbach M, Goldin J *et al*. Accuracy of PET/CT in characterization of solitary pulmonary lesions. *J Nucl Med* 2007;**48**(2):214–20.

59. Yamashita K, Matsunobe S, Tsuda T *et al*. Solitary pulmonary nodule: preliminary study of evaluation with incremental dynamic CT. *Radiology* 1995;**194**:399–405.

60. Swensen SJ, Viggiano RW, Midthun DE *et al*. Lung nodule enhancement at CT: multicenter study. *Radiology* 2000;**214**(1):73–80.

61. Jeong YJ, Lee KS, Jeong SY *et al*. Solitary pulmonary nodule: characterization with combined washin and washout features at dynamic multi-detector row CT. *Radiology* 2005;**237**:675–83.

62. Yi CA, Lee KS, Kim B-T *et al*. Tissue characterization of solitary pulmonary nodule: comparative study between helical dynamic CT and integrated PET/CT. *J Nucl Med* 2006;**47**:443–50.

63. Gould MK, Sanders GD, Barnett PG *et al*. Cost-effectiveness of alternative management strategies for patients with solitary pulmonary nodules. *Ann Intern Med* 2003;**138**(9):724–35.

64. Alberts WM; American College of Chest Physicians. Diagnosis and management of lung cancer executive summary: ACCP evidence-based clinical practice guidelines (2nd Edition). *Chest*. 2007;**132**(3 Suppl):1S–19S.

65. Fletcher JW, Djulbegovic B, Soares HP *et al*. Recommendations on the use of 18F-FDG PET in oncology. *J Nucl Med* 2008;**49**(3):480–508.

66. Antoch G, Stattaus J, Nemat AT *et al*. Non-small cell lung cancer: dual-modality PET/CT in preoperative staging. *Radiology* 2003;**229**(2):526–33.

67. Dizendorf EV, Baumert BG, von Schulthess GK *et al*. Impact of whole-body 18E-EDG PET on staging and managing patients for radiation therapy. *J Nucl Med* 2003;**44**:24–9.

68. Ahuja V, Coleman RE, Herndon J, Patz EF Jr. The prognostic significance of fluorodeoxyglucose positron emission tomography imaging for patients with nonsmall cell lung carcinoma. *Cancer* 1998;**83**(5):918–24.

69. Cerfolio RJ, Bryant AS, Ohja B, Bartolucci AA. The maximum standardized uptake values on positron emission tomography of a non-small cell lung cancer predict stage, recurrence, and survival. *J Thorac Cardiovasc Surg* 2005;**130**(1):151–9.

70. Dillemans B, Deneffe G, Verschakelen J, Decramer M. Value of computed tomography and mediastinoscopy in preoperative evaluation of mediastinal nodes in non-small cell lung cancer. A study of 569 patients. *Eur J Cardiothorac Surg* 1994; **8**(1):37–42.

71. Toloza EM, Harpole L, McCrory DC. Noninvasive staging of non-small cell lung cancer: a review of the current evidence. *Chest* 2003;**123**(1 Suppl):137S–46S.

72. Gould MK, Kuschner WG, Rydzak CE *et al*. Test performance of positron emission tomography and computed tomography for mediastinal staging in patients with non-small-cell lung cancer: a meta-analysis. *Ann Intern Med* 2003;**139**:879–92.

73. Gupta NC, Graeber GM, Bishop HA. Comparative efficacy of positron emission tomography with fluorodeoxyglucose in evaluation of small (< 1 cm), intermediate (1 to 3 cm), and large (> 3 cm) lymph node lesions. *Chest* 2000;**117**(3):773–8.

74. de Langen AJ, Raijmakers P, Riphagen I, Paul MA, Hoekstra OS. The size of mediastinal lymph nodes and its relation with metastatic involvement: a meta-analysis. *Eur J Cardiothorac Surg* 2006;**29**(1): 26–9.

75. Vesselle H, Turcotte E, Linda W, Haynor D. Application of a neural network to improve nodal staging accuracy with F-18 FDG PET in non-small cell lung cancer. *J Nucl Med* 2003;**44**:1918–26.

76. Higashi K, Ito K, Hiramatsu Y *et al*. 18F-FDG uptake by primary tumor as a predictor of intratumoral lymphatic vessel invasion and lymph node involvement in non-small cell lung cancer: analysis of a multicenter study. *J Nucl Med* 2005;**46**(2):267–73.

77. Quint LE, Tummala S, Brisson LJ *et al*. Distribution of distant metastases from newly diagnosed non-small cell lung cancer. *Ann Thorac Surg* 1996;**62**(1):246–50.

78. Sider L, Horejs D. Frequency of extrathoracic metastases from bronchogenic carcinoma in patients with normal-sized hilar and mediastinal lymph nodes on CT. *Am J Roentgenol* 1988;**151**(5):893–5.

79. Facey K, Bradbury I, Laking G, Payne E. *Positron emission tomography (PET) imaging in cancer management. Ultra Rapid Review. Health Technology*

*Assessment.* Southampton: NHS R&D Programme, 2004.

80. Hellwig D, Ukena D, Paulsen F, Bamberg M, Kirsch CM; Onko-PET der Deutschen Gesellschaft fur Nuklearmedizin. [Meta-analysis of the efficacy of positron emission tomography with F-18-fluorodeoxyglucose in lung tumors. Basis for discussion of the German Consensus Conference on PET in Oncology 2000]. *Pneumologie* 2001;**55**(8):367–77.

81. Cook GJ, Houston S, Rubens R, Maisey MN, Fogelman I. Detection of bone metastases in breast cancer by 18FDG PET: differing metabolic activity in osteoblastic and osteolytic lesions. *J Clin Oncol* 1998;**16**(10):3375–9.

82. Hustinx R, Paulus P, Jacquet N *et al.* Clinical evaluation of whole-body 18F-fluorodeoxyglucose positron emission tomography in the detection of liver metastases. *Ann Oncol* 1998;**9**(4):397–401.

83. MacManus MP, Hicks RJ, Matthews JP *et al.* High rate of detection of unsuspected distant metastases by PET in apparent stage III non-small-cell lung cancer: implications for radical radiation therapy. *Int J Radiat Oncol Biol Phys* 2001;**50**(2):287–93.

84. Lardinois D, Weder W, Roudas M *et al.* Etiology of solitary extrapulmonary positron emission tomography and computed tomography findings in patients with lung cancer. *J Clin Oncol* 2005;**23**:6846–53.

85. Vansteenkiste J, Fischer BM, Dooms C, Mortensen J. Positron-emission tomography in prognostic and therapeutic assessment of lung cancer: systematic review. *Lancet Oncol* 2004;**5**:531–40.

86. de Geus-Oei LF, van der Heijden HF, Corstens FH, Oven WJ. Predictive and prognostic value of FDG-PET in nonsmall-cell lung cancer: a systematic review. *Cancer* 2007;**110**:1654–64.

87. Weber WA, Petersen V, Schmidt B *et al.* Positron emission tomography in non-small-cell lung cancer: prediction of response to chemotherapy by quantitative assessment of glucose use. *J Clin Oncol* 2003;**21**:2651–7.

88. Cerfolio RJ, Bryant AS, Winokur TS, Ohja B, Bartolucci AA. Repeat 18F-FDG-PET after neoadjuvant therapy is a predictor of pathologic response in patients with non-small cell lung cancer. *Ann Thorac Surg* 2004;**78**:1903–9.

89. Inoue T, Kim EE, Komaki R *et al.* Detecting recurrent or residual lung cancer with FDG-PET. *J Nucl Med* 1995;**36**(5):788–93.

90. Patz EF Jr, Lowe VJ, Hoffman JM *et al.* Persistent or recurrent bronchogenic carcinoma: detection with PET and 2-[F-18]-2-deoxy-D-glucose. *Radiology* 1994;**191**(2):379–82.

91. Bury T, Corhay JL, Duysinx B *et al.* Value of FDG-PET in detecting residual or recurrent nonsmall cell lung cancer. *Eur Respir J* 1999;**14**(6):1376–80.

92. Hicks RJ, Kalff V, MacManus MP *et al.* The utility of (18)F-FDG PET for suspected recurrent non-small cell lung cancer after potentially curative therapy: impact on management and prognostic stratification. *J Nucl Med* 2001;**42**(11):1605–13.

93. Higashi K, Ueda Y, Arisaka Y *et al.* 18F-FDG uptake as a biologic prognostic factor for recurrence in patients with surgically resected non-small cell lung cancer. *J Nucl Med* 2002;**43**(1):39–45.

94. Singnurkar A, Solomon SB, Gönen M, Larson SM, Schöder H. 18F-FDG PET/CT for the prediction and detection of local recurrence after radiofrequency ablation of malignant lung lesions. *J Nucl Med* 2010;**51**(12):1833–40. Erratum in: *J Nucl Med* 2011;**52**(1):106.

95. Shiono S, Abiko M, Sato T. Positron emission tomography/computed tomography and lymphovascular invasion predict recurrence in stage I lung cancers. *J Thorac Oncol* 2011;**6**(1):43–7.

96. Hellwig D, Gröschel A, Graeter TP *et al.* Diagnostic performance and prognostic impact of FDG-PET in suspected recurrence of surgically treated non-small cell lung cancer. *Eur J Nucl Med Mol Imaging* 2006; **33**(1):13–21.

97. Schumacher T, Brink I, Mix M *et al.* FDG-PET imaging for the staging and follow-up of small cell lung cancer. *Eur J Nucl Med* 2001;**28**:483–8.

98. Kamel EM, Zwahlen D, Wyss MT *et al.* Whole-body (18)F-FDG PET improves the management of patients with small cell lung cancer. *J Nucl Med* 2003;**44**:1911–17.

99. Bradley JD, Dehdashti F, Mintun MA *et al.* Positron emission tomography in limited-stage small-cell lung cancer: a prospective study. *J Clin Oncol* 2004;**22**:3248–54.

100. Shen YY, Shiau YC, Wang JJ, Ho ST, Kao CH. Whole-body 18F-2-deoxyglucose positron emission tomography in primary staging small cell lung cancer. *Anticancer Res* 2002;**22**:1257–64.

101. Fischer BM, Mortensen J, Langer SW *et al.* A prospective study of PET/CT in initial staging of small-cell lung cancer: comparison with CT, bone scintigraphy and bone marrow analysis. *Ann Oncol* 2007;**18**:338–45.

102. Azad A, Chionh F, Scott AM *et al.* High impact of 18F-FDG-PET on management and prognostic stratification of newly diagnosed small cell lung cancer. *Mol Imaging Biol* 2010;**12**:443–51.

103. Fischer BM, Mortensen J, Langer SW *et al.* PET/CT imaging in response evaluation of patients with small cell lung cancer. *Lung Cancer* 2006;**54**(1):41–9.

104. Lee YJ, Cho A, Cho BC *et al.* High tumor metabolic activity as measured by fluorodeoxyglucose positron emission tomography is associated with poor prognosis in limited and extensive stage small-cell lung cancer. *Clin Cancer Res* 2009;**15**(7):2426–32.

105. Connelly RR, Spirtas R, Myers MH, Percy CL, Fraumeni JF Jr. Demographic patterns for mesothelioma in the United States. *J Natl Cancer Inst* 1987;**78**(6):1053–60.

106. Price B, Ware A. Time trend of mesothelioma incidence in the United States and projection of future cases: an update based on SEER data for 1973 through 2005. *Crit Rev Toxicol* 2009;**39**(7):576–88.

107. Wagner JC, Sleggs CA, Marchand P. Diffuse pleural mesothelioma and asbestos exposure in the North Western Cape Province. *Br J Ind Med* 1960;**17**:260–7.

108. Bianchi C, Giarelli L, Grandi G *et al.* Latency periods in asbestos-related mesothelioma of the pleura. *Eur J Cancer Prev* 1997;**6**(2):162–6.

109. Travis WD. Sarcomatoid neoplasms of the lung and pleura. *Arch Pathol Lab Med* 2010;**134**(11):1645–58.

110. Lopez-Rios F, Illei PB, Rusch V, Ladanyi M. Evidence against a role for

SV40 infection in human mesotheliomas and high risk of false-positive PCR results owing to presence of SV40 sequences in common laboratory plasmids. *Lancet* 2004;**364**:1157–66.

111. Manfredi JJ, Dong J, Liu WJ *et al.* Evidence against a role for SV40 in human mesothelioma. *Cancer Res* 2005;**65**:2602–9.

112. Klebe S, Brownlee NA, Mahar A *et al.* Sarcomatoid mesothelioma: a clinical-pathologic correlation of 326 cases. *Mod Pathol* 2010;**23**(3):470–9.

113. Gerbaudo VH, Katz S, Nowak A, Francis R. Multimodality imaging review of malignant pleural mesothelioma diagnosis and staging. *PET Clinics* 2011;**6**(3): 275–98.

114. Nowak A, Francis R, Katz S, Gerbaudo VH. Multimodality imaging review of malignant pleural mesothelioma response to therapy assessment. *PET Clinics* 2011;**6**(3):299–311.

115. Metintas M, Ucgun I, Elbek O *et al.* Computed tomography features in malignant pleural mesothelioma and other commonly seen pleural diseases. *Eur J Radiol* 2002;**41**(1):1–9.

116. Yamamuro M, Gerbaudo VH, Gill RR *et al.* Morphologic and functional imaging of malignant pleural mesothelioma. *Eur J Radiol* 2007;**64** (3):356–66.

117. Gill RR, Gerbaudo VH, Jacobson FL *et al.* MR imaging of benign and malignant pleural disease. *Magn Reson Imaging Clin N Am* 2008;**16**(2):319–39.

118. Bénard F, Sterman D, Smith RJ *et al.* Metabolic imaging of malignant pleural mesothelioma with fluorodeoxyglucose positron emission tomography. *Chest* 1998;**114**:713–22.

119. Gerbaudo VH, Sugarbaker DJ, Britz-Cunningham S *et al.* Assessment of malignant pleural mesothelioma with 18 F-FDG dual-head gamma-camera coincidence imaging: comparison with histopathology. *J Nucl Med* 2002;**43**:1144–9.

120. Carretta A, Landoni C, Melloni G *et al.* 18-FDG positron emission tomography in the evaluation of malignant pleural diseases – a pilot study. *Eur J Cardiothorac Surg* 2000;**17**:377–83.

121. Bury T, Paulus P, Dowlati A *et al.* Evaluation of pleural diseases with FDG-PET imaging: preliminary report. *Thorax* 1997;**52**:187–89.

122. Schneider DB, Clary-Macy C, Challa S *et al.* Positron emission tomography with F18-fluorodeoxyglucose in the staging and preoperative evaluation of malignant pleural mesothelioma. *J Thorac Cardiovasc Surg* 2000;**120**:128–33.

123. Sugarbaker DJ, Flores RM, Jaklitsch MT *et al.* Resection margins, extrapleural nodal status, and cell type determine postoperative long-term survival in trimodality therapy of malignant pleural mesothelioma: results in 183 patients. *J Thorac Cardiovasc Surg* 1999;**117**:54–65.

124. Rusch VW. A proposed new international TNM staging system for malignant pleural mesothelioma from the International Mesothelioma Interest Group. *Lung Cancer* 1996;**14**:1–12.

125. Flores RM, Akhurst T, Gonen M, Larson SM, Rusch VW. Positron emission tomography defines metastatic disease but not locoregional disease in patients with malignant pleural mesothelioma. *J Thorac Cardiovasc Surg* 2003;**126**(1):11–16.

126. Erasmus JJ, Truong MT, Smythe WR *et al.* Integrated computed tomography-positron emission tomography in patients with potentially resectable malignant pleural mesothelioma: Staging implications. *J Thorac Cardiovasc Surg* 2005;**129**(6):1364–70.

127. Gerbaudo VH. 18F-FDG imaging of malignant pleural mesothelioma: scientiam impendere vero. . . [Editorial]. *Nucl Med Com* 2003;**24**:609–14.

128. Baldini EH, Recht A, Strauss GM et al. Patterns of failure after trimodality therapy for malignant pleural mesothelioma. *Ann Thorac Surg* 1997;**63**(2):334–8.

129. Oksuzoglu B, Yalcin S, Erman M, Dagdelen S. Leptomeningeal infiltration of malignant mesothelioma. *Med Oncol* 2002;**19**:167–9.

130. Gerbaudo VH, Mamede M, Trotman-Dickenson B, Hatabu H, Sugarbaker DJ. FDG PET/CT patterns of treatment failure of malignant pleural mesothelioma: relationship to histologic type, treatment algorithm, and survival. *Eur J Nucl Med Mol Imaging* 2011;**38**:810–21.

131. Baldini EH, Recht A, Strauss GM *et al.* Patterns of failure after trimodality therapy for malignant pleural mesothelioma. *Ann Thorac Surg* 1997;**63**(2):334–8.

132. Jänne PA, Baldini EH. Patterns of failure following surgical resection for malignant pleural mesothelioma. *Thorac Surg Clin* 2004;**14**(4):567–73.

A 62-year-old female non-smoker, without a previous history of cancer, in whom a chest X-ray revealed a 15-mm indeterminate left upper lobe lesion confirmed by CT. FDG-PET/CT was ordered to characterize the lesion and to plan the initial treatment strategy.

## Acquisition and processing parameters

Whole-body positron emission tomography was performed 70 min after the intravenous administration of 12 mCi of FDG in fasting conditions. Plasma glucose levels at the time of FDG injection were 105 mg/dL. The patient was encouraged to void before scanning, and images were obtained from the head to the proximal thighs with a combined PET/CT scanner. The patient was imaged in the supine position, without any specific breath-holding instructions. The unenhanced CT scan was performed first, from the patient's head to the proximal thighs, using the following acquisition parameters: 140 kVp, 75 mA, 0.8 s per CT rotation, pitch of 1.675 : 1, and a reconstructed slice thickness of 3.75 mm, for a total scanning time of 42.4 s. The CT data were reconstructed using a filtered back-projection algorithm and a $512 \times 512$ matrix, with a transaxial field of view of 50 cm. The CT images were used to generate the transmission maps for attenuation correction of the PET acquisitions and for anatomic localization.

Immediately after the CT scan, and without changing the patient's position, the tabletop moved automatically to the PET position. The emission scan was acquired in 3-D mode (septa in) starting at the mid-thighs toward the head, for six bed positions of 3 min each (47 image planes/bed position, 15.7 cm longitudinal field of view). PET data were reconstructed using an ordered-subset expectation maximization iterative algorithm (30 subsets, 2 iterations).

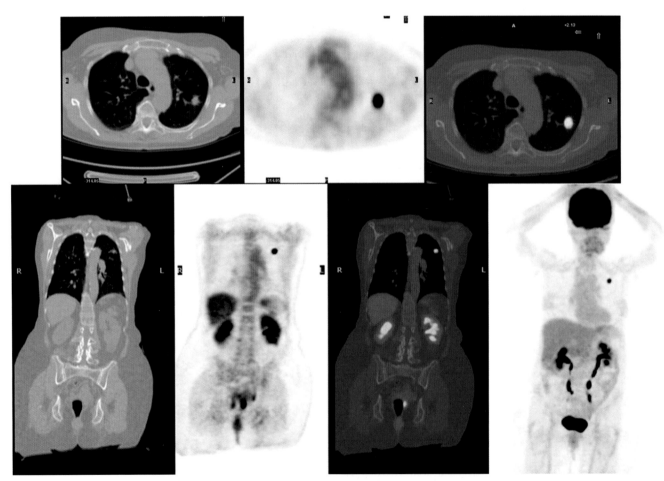

**Figure 7.1** Top row: Axial CT, FDG-PET, and fused FDG-PET/CT slices; bottom row: Coronal CT, FDG-PET, FDG-PET/CT slices and multiple intensity projection (MIP) image.

## Findings and differential diagnosis

Axial (top row) and coronal (lower row) CT, PET, and fused PET/CT slices and corresponding MIP image, demonstrate a spiculated, non-calcified FDG-avid nodule (uptake higher than in the mediastinal blood pool) in the left upper lobe measuring $14 \times 9$ mm with an SUVmax of 12.4. There is no evidence of FDG-avid hilar or mediastinal lymphadenopathy. There is mild emphysema. Below the diaphragm, the radiotracer is distributed physiologically in the gastrointestinal and genitourinary tracts. The differential diagnoses include primary lung cancer; metastatic tumor to the lung; coccidioidomycosis; histoplasmosis; tuberculosis; focal pneumonia; and hamartoma.

## Diagnosis and follow-up

The patient underwent left upper lobectomy, which revealed a moderately differentiated squamous cell carcinoma of 1.1 cm in its greatest dimension. The tumor did not invade the visceral pleura. The bronchial margin of excision was negative for tumor, with the lesion found to be 3.2 cm from the nearest bronchial resection margin. Lymphovascular invasion was not identified. The adjacent lung parenchyma had mild-to-moderate emphysematous change, chronic inflammation, and numerous pigment-laden macrophages. Six excised lymph nodes were negative for tumor. AJCC classification (7th edition): pT1a N0.

## Discussion and teaching points

Primary lung cancer and metastases from other histologic types make up to 50% of solitary pulmonary nodules (SPNs) (1, 2). Squamous cell carcinomas are the second most common cause of malignant SPNs. Therefore, it is very important to be able to non-invasively and accurately differentiate benign from malignant disease in order to select those patients who will benefit from potentially curable resection of their malignant tumors. On the other hand, when lesions are characterized as benign, or when metastatic disease has been detected during the SPN work-up, the morbidity and expense of futile surgery is minimized. Estimating pre-test probability of malignancy facilitates the interpretation of PET findings. The risk of malignancy increases with age ($> 35$ years old), with cigarette smoking, and with a previous history of cancer.

Morphologic evaluation of SPNs helps differentiate benign from malignant lesions when they have typical benign or malignant features, however, approximately one-third of malignant lesions are incorrectly diagnosed as benign (3–4). In addition, many benign lesions are categorized as malignant leading to unnecessary invasive procedures [e.g., approximately 60% of indeterminate lung nodules treated surgically are benign (5)].

PET has an overall sensitivity and specificity for detection of malignant nodules of 92% and 90%, respectively. The high net FDG uptake in neoplastic conditions enhances the ability of PET and PET/CT imaging to discriminate between benign and malignant lesions. When the pretest probability of

malignancy is low in patients with a pulmonary nodule, a negative FDG-PET carries a 1% post-test probability of malignancy. Thus, in this population a watch-and-wait approach is probably safe. In a high-risk patient a negative PET carries a 14% post-test probability of malignancy, and therefore, histologic confirmation is warranted (6). FDG-PET is cost-effective to establish the differential diagnosis of lung nodules $\geq 8$ mm when clinical and morphological findings are incongruent such as in this clinical case (low-risk patient with a "probably malignant" CT finding).

Although high FDG uptake (higher than mediastinal blood pool activity) is common in malignant lesions, false-positive results are not uncommon in patients with infectious and/or inflammatory processes. Inflammatory cells have upregulated and active glucose transporters, especially in the acute phase of inflammation. FDG uptake is not uncommon in granulation tissue and in both activated macrophages and neutrophils (7, 8). Sources of false-positives include active tuberculosis, sarcoidosis, and fungal infections (9–14). Therefore, FDG-positive nodules always require further histologic assessment.

## Take-home message

- Approximately one-third of malignant nodules are incorrectly classified as benign based on their morphologic characteristics alone.
- FDG-PET and PET/CT are superior to CT and MRI to predict malignancy in indeterminate SPNs.
- FDG-PET has been shown to be cost-effective to establish the differential diagnosis of lung nodules $\geq 8$ mm when clinical and morphological findings are incongruent (low-risk patient with a "probably malignant" CT pattern).
- The use of FDG-PET for the characterization of SPN is indicated:
  (a) to exclude the possibility of malignancy in patients with a low-to-moderate pre-test probability of cancer and an indeterminate SPN (8–10 mm in diameter), and in patients with a moderate-to-high pre-test probability and an FDG-avid SPN, in whom surgical diagnosis is preferred when clinically appropriate
  (b) to detect potential malignant lesions early in the course of the disease
  (c) to exclude the possibility of malignancy in indeterminate lesions in low-risk patients
  (d) to avoid futile surgeries in low-risk patients with negative findings and in those with evidence of systemic metastases
  (e) to enable curative surgeries in high-risk patients with a negative scan.
- A positive PET finding requires biopsy (less than perfect specificity).
- False-negative findings in PET: small lesion ($< 8$ mm), bronchioloalveolar carcinomas, and carcinoids. Negative findings in PET should be followed up clinically and with conventional imaging at 6- to 12-month intervals.

# References

1. Swensen SJ, Jett JR, Payne WS *et al.* An integrated approach to evaluation of the solitary pulmonary nodule. *Mayo Clin Proc* 1990;**65**:173–86.

2. Lillington GA. Systematic diagnostic approach to pulmonary nodules. In AP Fishman (Ed.), *Pulmonary Diseases and Disorders*. 2nd Edn. New York, NY: McGraw Hill, 1988, pp. 1945–54.

3. Erasmus JJ, McAdams HP, Connolly JE. Solitary pulmonary nodules: Part II. Evaluation of the indeterminate nodule. *Radiographics* 2000;**20**(1):59–66.

4. Siegelman SS, Khouri NF, Leo FP *et al.* Solitary pulmonary nodules: CT assessment. *Radiology* 1986;**160**(2):307–12.

5. Gupta NC, Maloof J, Gunel E. Probability of malignancy in solitary pulmonary nodules using fluorine-18-FDG and PET. *J Nucl Med* 1996;**37**:943–8.

6. Gould MK, Maclean CC, Kuschner WG, Rydzak CE, Owens DK. Accuracy of positron emission tomography for diagnosis of pulmonary nodules and mass lesions: a meta-analysis. *J Am Med Assoc* 2001;**285**(7):914–24.

7. Goerres GW, von Schulthess GK, Steinert HC. Why most PET of lung and head-and-neck cancer will be PET/CT. *J Nucl Med* 2004;**45**(*Suppl* **1**):66S–71S.

8. Lardinois D, Weder W, Hany TF *et al.* Staging of non-small-cell lung cancer with integrated positron-emission tomography and computed tomography. *N Engl J Med* 2003;**348**(25):2500–7.

9. Jones HA, Clark RJ, Rhodes CG *et al.* Positron emission tomography of 18FDG uptake in localized pulmonary inflammation. *Acta Radiol Suppl* 1991;**376**:148.

10. Zhuang H, Alavi, A. 18-fluorodeoxyglucose positron emission tomographic imaging in the detection and monitoring of infection and inflammation. *Semin Nucl Med* 2002;**32**(1):47–59.

11. Chang JM, Lee HJ, Goo JM *et al.* False positive and false negative FDG-PET scans in various thoracic diseases. *Korean J Radiol* 2006;**7**(1):57–69.

12. Goo JM, Im JG, Do KH *et al.* Pulmonary tuberculoma evaluated by means of FDG PET: findings in 10 cases. *Radiology* 2000;**216**:117–21.

13. Alavi A, Gupta N, Alberini JL *et al.* Positron emission tomography imaging in nonmalignant thoracic disorders. *Semin Nucl Med* 2002;**32**(4):293–321.

14. Yamada S, Kubota K, Kubota R, Ido T, Tamahashi N. High accumulation of fluorine-18-fluorodeoxyglucose in turpentine-induced inflammatory tissue. *J Nucl Med* 1995;**36**(7):1301–6.

A 65-year-old male with a history of chronic lymphocytic leukemia, 6 years status post bone marrow transplantation. Now presents with a right upper lobe nodule. FDG-PET/CT was obtained to characterize the benign or malignant nature of the lesion and to plan the initial treatment strategy.

## Acquisition and processing parameters

After fasting for a period of 6 hours, the patient was injected intravenously with 19 mCi of FDG, and an uptake phase of 60 min was allowed prior to imaging. Plasma glucose levels at the time of FDG injection were 85 mg/dL. The patient was encouraged to void before scanning, and images were obtained from the head to the proximal thighs with a combined PET/CT scanner. The patient was imaged in the supine position, with his arms down, because he was unable to place them above his head due to shoulder pain. Images were obtained without any specific breath-holding instructions. The unenhanced CT scan was performed first, from the patient's head to the proximal thighs, using the following acquisition parameters: 140 kVp, 75 mA, 0.8 s per CT rotation, pitch of 1.675 : 1, and a reconstructed slice thickness of 3.75 mm, for a total scanning time of 42.4 s. The CT data were reconstructed using a filtered back-projection algorithm and a $512 \times 512$ matrix, with a transaxial field of view of 50 cm. The CT images were used to generate the transmission maps for attenuation correction of the PET acquisitions and anatomic localization.

Immediately after the CT scan, and without changing the patient's position, the tabletop moved automatically to the PET position. The emission scan was acquired in 2-D mode (septa out) starting at the mid-thighs toward the head, for six bed positions of 4 min each (47 image planes/bed position, 15.7 cm longitudinal field of view). PET data were reconstructed using an ordered-subset expectation maximization iterative algorithm (30 subsets, 2 iterations).

## Findings and differential diagnosis

Multiple intensity projection PET image (arrow) and PET/CT fused axial slice (Figure 7.2) reveal a right upper lobe stellate mass with mild FDG uptake. On the basis of PET criteria alone, this would be more characteristic of a benign or inflammatory type lesion. However, given its CT characteristics, a well-differentiated adenocarcinoma with bronchioloalveolar carcinoma (BAC) features (i.e., pleuropulmonary tail), or tuberculoma cannot be excluded. There is physiologic radiotracer distribution in the genitourinary tract.

Based on the anatomo-metabolic characteristics of the lesion, the different diagnostic possibilities are primary lung cancer; tuberculosis; subacute abscess; and focal pneumonia.

## Diagnosis and follow-up

Pulmonary wedge resection and completion lobectomy revealed multifocal, moderately differentiated adenocarcinoma, of the bronchioloalveolar type, with focal mucin production. The tumor was surrounded by normal lung, and the bronchial margin of excision was negative for tumor. Lung lymphovascular invasion was not identified.

**Figure 7.2** FDG-MIP (left) and axial fused FDG-PET/CT slice (right).

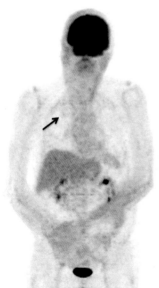
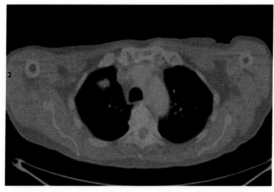

## Discussion and teaching points

Bronchioloalveolar carcinoma (now adenocarcinoma in situ) is considered a relatively uncommon subtype of well-differentiated adenocarcinoma, yet its incidence is rising (1). Localized forms of this tumor have the best prognosis. The tumor consists of a layer of columnar cells that grow along the alveolar or bronchiolar walls without invading the surrounding stroma, in a pattern called lepidic. These cells have low proliferative potential and longer doubling time when compared with other histologic types of lung cancer (2, 3). There are non-mucinous and mucinous subtypes of BAC, with the former commonly presenting as an SPN, and the latter usually presenting with diffuse or multifocal patterns. However, exceptions to the rule, as shown in this case, do exist.

There is a high percentage of false-negative FDG-PET scans in focal BAC. However, the sensitivity of FDG-PET increases in the setting of multifocal disease (4). In our experience and that of others, BACs in general, and the mucinous subtypes in particular, show mild to absent FDG uptake (3–5). A pre-operative tumor FDG SUV of 2.5 or greater has been reported recently as a powerful predictor of long-term mortality in patients with lymph node-negative, pure and mixed bronchioloalveolar carcinoma, who undergo complete surgical resection (6). Three-year survival was 49% in the FDG-avid group and 95% in the non-avid group ($P = 0.005$). Therefore, those patients with lesions that have high FDG uptake may benefit from adjuvant chemotherapy and more frequent clinical follow-up (6).

In the case shown, the information provided by the superior anatomical detail of CT, helped clarify the significance of low FDG uptake in the context of morphologic malignancy. Thus, the synergistic information derived from the PET/CT images provided a more detailed and complete characterization of a lung lesion than PET or CT alone, increasing the level of confidence in image interpretation.

## Take-home message

- Morphologic characteristics of the mucinous-BAC subtype include distinct nodule with ill-defined margins containing ground-glass opacity, multiple nodules or diffuse lung consolidation resembling pneumonia. May cause tethering of the pleura (pleuropulmonary tail) whether or not it is peripheral in location.
- False-negative findings in PET may be due to the small size of the nodule(s) ($< 8$ mm) and/or to the low metabolic activity of mucinous bronchioloalveolar carcinomas. Negative findings in PET should be followed up clinically and with conventional imaging at 6- to 12-month intervals. Patients with CT findings suggestive of lepidic growth should be followed with diagnostic CT with thin section images (high resolution CT) through the lesion. The conventional follow-up interval of 2 years to determine the benign nature of the nodule might be inadequate, as BACs can be stable for 7 years. An increase in lesion opacity may precede an increase in nodule size. Mucin may also contribute to the increasing opacity of the lesion.
- BACs have lower FDG uptake and lower Ki-67 scores than any other histologic subtype of lung cancer.
- False-positive results are due to inflammation or infection, thus a positive finding always requires biopsy.

## References

1. Barsky SH, Cameron R, Osann KE, Tomita D, Holmes EC. Rising incidence of bronchioloalveolar lung carcinoma and its unique clinicopathologic features. *Cancer* 1994;**73**(4):1163–70.
2. Kim BT, Kim Y, Lee KS *et al.* Localized form of bronchioloalveolar carcinoma: FDG PET findings. *Am J Roentgenol* 1998;**170**(4):935–9.
3. Sung YM, Lee KS, Kim BT, Han J, Lee EJ. Lobar mucinous bronchioloalveolar carcinoma of the lung showing negative FDG uptake on integrated PET/CT. *Eur Radiol* 2005;**15**(10):2075–8.
4. Heyneman LE, Patz EF. PET imaging in patients with bronchioloalveolar cell carcinoma. *Lung Cancer* 2002;**38**(3):261–6.
5. Higashi K, Ueda Y, Seki H *et al.* Fluorine-18-FDG PET imaging is negative in bronchioloalveolar lung carcinoma. *J Nucl Med* 1998; **39**(6):1016–20.
6. Raz DJ, Odisho AY, Franc BL, Jablons DM. Tumor fluoro-2-deoxy-D-glucose avidity on positron emission tomographic scan predicts mortality in patients with early-stage pure and mixed bronchioloalveolar carcinoma. *J Thorac Cardiovasc Surg* 2006;**132**(5):1189–95.

A 79-year-old female status post median sternotomy with aortic valve replacement, now presenting with a right upper lung lesion. FDG-PET/CT was ordered for initial treatment planning.

## Acquisition and processing parameters

After fasting for a period of 6 hours, the patient was injected intravenously with 21 mCi of FDG, and an uptake phase of 65 min was allowed prior to imaging. Plasma glucose levels at the time of FDG injection were 135 mg/dL. The patient was encouraged to void before scanning, and images were obtained from the head to the proximal thighs with a combined PET/CT scanner. The patient was imaged in the supine position and images were obtained without any specific breath-holding instructions. The unenhanced CT scan was performed first, from the patient's head to the proximal thighs, using the following acquisition parameters: 140 kVp, 75 mA, 0.8 s per CT rotation, pitch of 1.675:1, and a reconstructed slice thickness of 3.75 mm, for a total scanning time of 42.4 s. The CT data were reconstructed using a filtered back-projection algorithm and a 512 × 512 matrix, with a transaxial field of view of 50 cm. The CT images were used to generate the transmission maps for attenuation correction of the PET acquisitions and anatomic localization.

Immediately after the CT scan, and without changing the patient's position, the tabletop moved automatically to the PET position. The emission scan was acquired in 2-D mode (septa out) starting at the mid-thighs toward the head, for six bed positions of 4 min each (47 image planes/bed position, 15.7 cm longitudinal field of view). PET data were reconstructed using an ordered-subset expectation maximization iterative algorithm (30 subsets, 2 iterations).

## Findings and differential diagnosis

Unenhanced axial CT image (lung window) (Figure 7.4A) reveals the presence of an ill-defined, lobulated nodular opacity in the right upper lobe, measuring approximately

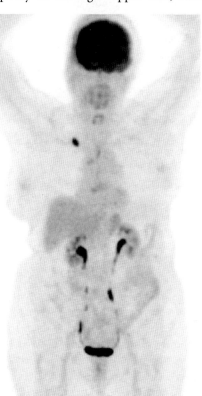

**Figure 7.3** FDG-MIP.

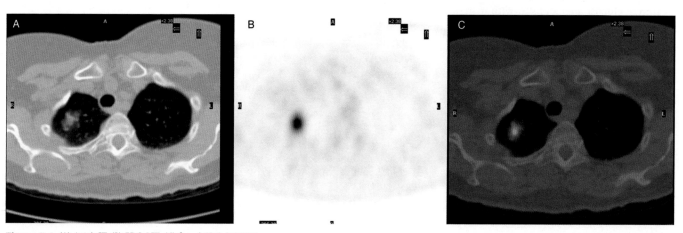

**Figure 7.4** (A) Axial CT; (B) FDG-PET; (C) fused FDG-PET/CT images.

2.5 cm, which is highly FDG avid in the location of the solid component of the nodule (Figures 7.3 and 7.4B, C). There is no mediastinal lymphadenopathy. There are no pleural effusions, and there is physiologic radiotracer distribution in the gastro-intestinal and genitourinary tracts (Figure 7.3). Differential diagnoses include: primary lung cancer; tuberculosis; subacute abscess, focal pneumonia, focal fibrosis, and atypical adeno-matous hyperplasia.

## Diagnosis and follow-up

Right upper lobectomy revealed a 2 cm, non-mucinous bronchioloalveolar carcinoma, with foci of invasive well-dif-ferentiated adenocarcinoma. The parenchymal resection margin and the pleura were free of tumor and there was no lymphovascular invasion.

## Discussion and teaching points

Bronchioloalveolar carcinoma is considered a relatively uncommon subtype of well-differentiated adenocarcinoma, yet its incidence is rising (1). Localized forms of this tumor have the best prognosis. The tumor consists of a layer of columnar cells that grow along the alveolar or bronchiolar walls without invading the surrounding stroma, in a pattern called lepidic. These cells have low proliferative potential and longer doubling time when compared with other histologic types of lung cancer (2, 3). There are non-mucinous and mucinous subtypes of BAC, with the former commonly presenting as a SPN, and the latter usually presenting with the diffuse or multi-focal patterns.

There is a high percentage of false-negative FDG-PET scans in the setting of focal BAC. However, the sensitivity of FDG-PET increases in the setting of multifocal disease (4, 5). In addition, we and others have observed that the intensity of FDG uptake tends to be lower in the mucinous subtypes, and that it increases in non-mucinous tumors with higher cellular densities (6) and higher Ki-67 proliferation indices (7). Vesselle and colleagues (7) reported that differences in lung tumor cell proliferation may give rise to matching differences in tumor glucose metabolism, with a significant positive cor-relation between FDG uptake and Ki-67 scores. In fact, the results of their prospective study revealed that bronchioloal-veolar carcinomas were found to have lower FDG uptake and lower Ki-67 scores than any other histologic subtype of lung cancer.

This case demonstrates high glycolytic activity in a non-mucinous mixed BAC with foci of invasive well-differenti-ated adenocarcinoma. Goudarzi and colleagues (8) showed that the intensity of lesion uptake is higher in mixed tumors. The investigators correlated tumor size, density, and glucose metabolism in 53 patients with 57 pathology-proven lesions (26 pure BACs and 31 adenocarcinomas with BAC components). The authors confirmed that pure BAC lesions tend to be smaller in size, and have lower FDG uptake and density than adenocarcinomas with BAC com-ponents. The authors argued that many BACs had low SUVs (< 2.0), but their low densities on CT helped establish the diagnosis.

As mentioned in the previous case, FDG uptake in BACs (pure and mixed) has prognostic value. A pre-operative tumor FDG SUV of 2.5 or greater was a powerful predictor of long-term mortality in patients with lymph node-negative, pure and mixed bronchioloalveolar carcinomas, who undergo complete surgical resection (9). Those patients with high FDG uptake may benefit from adjuvant chemotherapy or more frequent clinical follow-up (9).

## Take-home message

- Morphologic characteristics of the non-mucinous BAC subtype include distinct nodule with ill-defined margins containing ground-glass opacity. The nodule may contain air bronchograms or cystic air-filled pseudocavitations.
- False-negative findings in PET may be due to the small size of the nodule(s) (< 8 mm) and/or to the inherent low metabolic activity of BACs. Negative findings in PET should be followed up clinically and with conventional imaging at 6- to 12-month intervals. Patients with CT findings suggestive of lepidic growth should be followed with diagnostic CT with thin section images (HRCT) through the lesion. The conventional follow-up interval of 2 years to determine the benign nature of the nodule might be inadequate, as BACs can be stable for 7 years. The slow and difficult to detect increase in opacity may precede an increase in nodule size.
- BAC lesions tend to be smaller in size, have lower FDG uptake and density, than adenocarcinomas with BAC features.
- BACs have lower FDG uptake and lower Ki-67 scores than any other histologic subtype of lung cancer.
- False-positive results are due to inflammation or infection, thus a positive finding usually requires biopsy.

## References

1. Barsky SH, Cameron R, Osann KE, Tomita D, Holmes EC. Rising incidence of bronchioloalveolar lung carcinoma and its unique clinicopathologic features. *Cancer* 1994;**73**(4):1163–70.

2. Kim BT, Kim Y, Lee KS *et al.* Localized form of bronchioloalveolar carcinoma: FDG PET findings. *Am J Roentgenol* 1998;**170**(4):935–9.

3. Sung YM, Lee KS, Kim BT, Han J, Lee EJ. Lobar mucinous bronchioloalveolar carcinoma of the lung showing negative FDG uptake on integrated PET/CT. *Eur Radiol* 2005;**15**(10):2075–8.

4. Heyneman LE, Patz EF. PET imaging in patients with bronchioloalveolar cell carcinoma. *Lung Cancer* 2002;**38**(3):261–6.

5. Higashi K, Ueda Y, Seki H *et al.* Fluorine-18-FDG PET imaging is negative in bronchioloalveolar lung carcinoma. *J Nucl Med* 1998;**39**(6):1016–20.

6. Britz-Cunningham S, Anagnostopoulos C, Millstine J, Gerbaudo V. FDG uptake in bronchioloalveolar carcinoma correlates with lesion CT density and cytologic differentiation. *J Nucl Med* 2008;**49**:361P-b (Abstract).

7. Vesselle H, Salskov A, Turcotte E *et al.* Relationship between non-small cell lung cancer FDG uptake at PET, tumor histology, and Ki-67 proliferation index. *J Thorac Oncol* 2008;**3**(9):971–8.

8. Goudarzi B, Jacene HA, Wahl RL. Diagnosis and differentiation of bronchioloalveolar carcinoma from adenocarcinoma with bronchioloalveolar components with metabolic and anatomic characteristics using PET/CT. *J Nucl Med* 2008;**49**(10):1585–92.

9. Raz DJ, Odisho AY, Franc BL, Jablons DM. Tumor fluoro-2-deoxy-D-glucose avidity on positron emission tomographic scan predicts mortality in patients with early-stage pure and mixed bronchioloalveolar carcinoma. *J Thorac Cardiovasc Surg* 2006;**132**(5):1189–95.

A 45-year-old male who has suffered recurrent bouts of upper respiratory infections with cough. Patient was exposed to asbestos at work and was advised to obtain a chest X-ray for evaluation.

## Acquisition and processing parameters

After fasting for a period of 7.5 hours, the patient was injected intravenously with 20.5 mCi of FDG, and an uptake phase of 65 minutes was allowed prior to imaging. Plasma glucose levels at the time of FDG injection were 145 mg/dL. The patient was encouraged to void before scanning, and images were obtained from the head to the proximal thighs with a combined PET/CT scanner. The patient was imaged in the supine position and images were obtained without any specific breath-holding instructions. The unenhanced CT scan was performed first, from the patient's head to the proximal thighs, using the following acquisition parameters: 140 kVp, 75 mA, 0.8 s per CT rotation, pitch of 1.675 : 1, and a reconstructed slice thickness of 3.75 mm, for a total scanning time of 42.4 s. The CT data were reconstructed using a filtered back-projection algorithm and a 512 × 512 matrix, with a transaxial field of view of 50 cm. The CT images were used to generate the transmission maps for attenuation correction of the PET acquisitions and anatomic localization.

Immediately after the CT scan, and without changing the patient's position, the tabletop moved automatically to the PET position. The emission scan was acquired in 2-D mode (septa out) starting at the mid-thighs toward the head, for six bed positions of 4 minutes each (47 image planes/bed position, 15.7 cm longitudinal field of view). PET data were reconstructed using an ordered-subset expectation maximization iterative algorithm (30 subsets, 2 iterations).

## Findings and differential diagnosis

Postero-anterior chest film (Figure 7.5) demonstrates bilateral, hilar lymph node enlargement, and small nodular and micro-nodular opacities primarily in the right middle and upper lobes. The right hilum is larger than the left, with lung nodules being more numerous on the right side than on the left side. Unenhanced axial chest CT slices (Figure 7.6) show bilateral subpleural nodules. Nodules are present along the right minor fissure, and bronchovascular bundles, and most prominent toward the hilum.

Axial PET (Figure 7.7A) and fused PET/CT (Figure 7.7B) demonstrate intense and diffuse FDG uptake in the areas of peribronchovascular nodularity, being most prominent in the

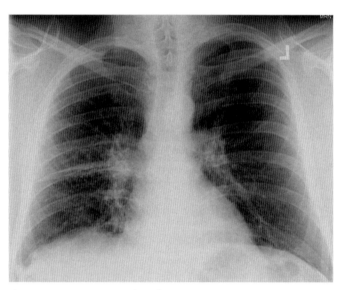

**Figure 7.5** Postero-anterior chest film.

**Figure 7.6** Axial CT slices in lung windows.

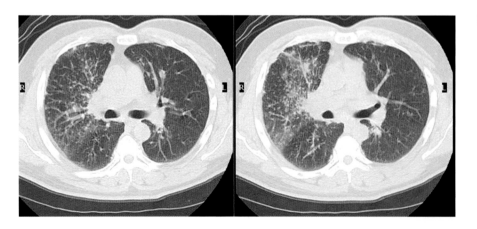

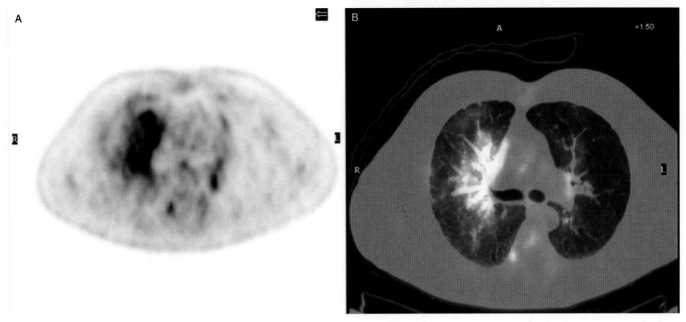

**Figure 7.7** (A) Axial FDG-PET; (B) axial fused FDG-PET/CT.

right hilum. Moderate FDG avidity is present in the areas of subpleural nodularity.

Right hilar lymphadenopathy is not separately defined, as it is covered by FDG avidity. Focal uptake along the left side of the mediastinum may represent a small amount of subpleural abnormality. These findings are suspicious for sarcoidosis. However, in the presence of micronodules with extensive distribution, hematogenous dissemination of tuberculosis (TB) cannot be excluded. This occurs during primary infection although the nodules infrequently become visible on imaging. Increasing summation of such nodules makes recognition of military TB more likely in primary progressive and recurrent disease presentations. In primary TB, asymmetric lymphadenopathy and pleural effusion may distinguish it from sarcoidosis. In cases of bilateral or unusually distributed lymphadenopathy, lymphoma and associated lymphomatous diseases may require exclusion. This is particularly applicable to patients with HIV disease and potential B symptoms, although TB can also cause fever and night sweats. FDG-avid septal thickening may be present along with subpleural nodularity, therefore, lymphangitic spread of carcinoma may also be considered. Differential diagnoses include sarcoidosis; military tuberculosis; lymphoma; and lymphangitic carcinomatosis.

## Diagnosis and follow-up

Right lower lobe wedge resection revealed atypical mycobacterial infection, characterized by granulomatous inflammation, and occasional acid-fast bacilli and caseating granulomas.

## Discussion and teaching points

Sarcoidosis most frequently presents with bilateral symmetric hilar lymphadenopathy. The characteristic locations of accompanying mediastinal lymphadenopathy are in the subcarinal space and right paratracheal region. Lymphadenopathy, in the absence of lung involvement, represents stage I disease. Peribronchial extension into the lung parenchyma results in thickening of central bronchovascular bundles. Sarcoidosis in lymph nodes and lung parenchyma comprises stage II disease. Lung disease may be seen in the absence of lymphadenopathy, as in stage III sarcoidosis. Extensive involvement of the interstitium can decrease aeration of alveolar airspaces enough to produce air-bronchograms. Bronchiectasis is seen primarily in the setting of end-stage changes in the lung, due to traction bronchiectasis accompanying fibrosis. Honeycombing and bronchiectasis may be difficult to differentiate by CT.

Differentiating non-infectious granulomatous disease due to sarcoidosis from infectious granulomatous disease due to TB and from lymphoma, is important to guide proper clinical management. Elevated serum angiotensin-converting enzyme levels may be used to follow sarcoidosis, but they are not specific for the diagnosis. In addition, lymphoma may initially respond to steroid therapy initiated for sarcoidosis. It is therefore mandatory to establish the pathologic diagnosis in cases like this.

Atypical mycobacterial infection usually presents with bronchiectasis and tree-in-bud opacities representing peribronchiolar inflammation and mucoid impaction. Mucoid impaction may be seen as both tubular and nodular opacities. It may be most confidently identified when these findings are combined in a branching pattern. Nodular and tubular opacities may spare the subpleural region even when the abnormality is extensive. In comparing the likelihood of military versus atypical TB, the former is usually bilateral while atypical TB may be unilateral.

It generally follows areas of bronchial dilatation and may be scattered in one or both lungs.

While FDG could be considered a probe of a specific altered process in cancer cells, by no means is it a marker of a tumor-specific process. Inflammatory cells also have upregulated glucose transporters, and therefore FDG uptake is not uncommon in granulation tissue, and in both activated macrophages and neutrophils (1, 2). In inflammatory processes, the low hexokinase/phosphatase ratio favors dephosphorylation, with the final outcome "generally" being a relatively low but noticeable FDG uptake compared with that in tumor. However, high levels of FDG avidity in the acute phase of infection/inflammation may be present, which can be mistaken for malignancy (3, 4). Infectious diseases (mycobacterial, fungal, and other bacterial infections), sarcoidosis, radiation pneumonitis, and post-surgical conditions are FDG avid (5, 6).

Image fusion combining PET and CT usually provides better localization of PET abnormalities, improving the characterization of lesions of unclear clinical significance on PET and CT viewed side-by-side. However, there are exceptions to the rule, such as in this case. The non-diagnostic CT scan obtained as part of the PET/CT may not provide adequate differentiation of aerogenous and hematogenous distribution of disease. In addition, FDG avidity may not improve this distinction either, as the intense and diffuse pattern of uptake could result in a larger or more confluent abnormality than that seen on CT. The anatomo-metabolic information from the PET/CT images served to guide biopsy to arrive to the final diagnosis.

## Take-home message

- Primarily interstitial lung disease can be seen with confluent FDG uptake when it is very avid. Thus, characterization of hilar lymphadenopathy may be compromised in this situation. Complementary imaging with contrast-enhanced diagnostic chest CT should be used to attain this distinction.
- Standard CT examinations for interstitial lung disease are performed with 1–2-mm thick slices without the use of intravenous contrast material. These images are referred to as high resolution CT (HRCT) images. Bulky lymphadenopathy could still be identified in hilar regions, and more modest lymphadenopathy could be adequately seen in paratracheal and subcarinal locations. When evaluation of hilar lymphadenopathy requires contrast material, one must be careful to not confuse tiny vessels, particularly veins, with micronodules.
- FDG-PET will likely assume increasing importance in assessing infection and inflammatory processes [fever of unknown origin (FUO), spinal osteomyelitis, vasculitis, TB, and sarcoidosis] (6–8).
- Proper interpretation of FDG images requires knowledge of the normal physiologic distribution of the tracer, frequently encountered physiologic variants, and benign pathologic causes of FDG uptake that can be confused with cancer (7, 8) (see Chapter 4).
- A positive finding in FDG-PET always requires biopsy confirmation.

## References

1. Yamada S, Kubota K, Kubota R, Ido T, Tamahashi N. High accumulation of fluorine-18-fluorodeoxyglucose in turpentine-induced inflammatory tissue. *J Nucl Med* 1995;**36**(7):1301–6.

2. Jones HA, Clark RJ, Rhodes CG et al. Positron emission tomography of 18FDG uptake in localized pulmonary inflammation. *Acta Radiol Suppl* 1991;**376**:148.

3. Zhuang H, Alavi, A. 18-fluorodeoxyglucose positron emission tomographic imaging in the detection and monitoring of infection and inflammation. *Semin Nucl Med* 2002;**32**(1):47–59.

4. Love C, Tomas MB, Tronco GG, Palestro CJ. FDG PET of infection and inflammation. *Radiographics* 2005;**25**:1357–68.

5. Chang JM, Lee HJ, Goo JM et al. False positive and false negative FDG-PET scans in various thoracic diseases. *Korean J Radiol* 2006;**7**(1):57–69.

6. Goo JM, Im JG, Do KH et al. Pulmonary tuberculoma evaluated by means of FDG PET: findings in 10 cases. *Radiology* 2000;**216**:117–21.

7. Zhuang H, Yu JQ, Alavi A. Applications of fluorodeoxyglucose-PET imaging in the detection of infection and inflammation and other benign disorders. *Radiol Clin North Am* 2005;**43**(1):121–34.

8. Alavi A, Gupta N, Alberini JL et al. Positron emission tomography imaging in nonmalignant thoracic disorders. *Semin Nucl Med* 2002;**32**(4):293–321.

A 68-year-old female with a previous history of carcinoma of the larynx treated with radiation therapy 3 years ago. She has apparently remained locally controlled and states that she last had an endoscopy about 2 or 3 months ago, which did not show any evidence of recurrence. Now she presents with an indeterminate left upper lobe nodule, persistent cough for the past few days and recent onset of lower abdominal pain. In addition, she noted dysuria and hematuria over the past few days and left hip pain. A FDG-PET/CT was ordered to characterize the SPN and to establish initial treatment strategy.

## Acquisition and processing parameters

After fasting for a period of 6 hours, the patient was injected intravenously with 18.6 mCi of FDG, and an uptake phase of 70 min was allowed prior to imaging. Plasma glucose levels at the time of FDG injection were 110 mg/dL. The patient was encouraged to void before scanning, and images were obtained from the head to the proximal thighs with a combined PET/CT scanner. The patient was imaged in the supine position and images were obtained without any specific breath-holding instructions. The unenhanced CT scan was performed first, from the patient's head to the proximal thighs, using the following acquisition parameters: 140 kVp, 75 mA, 0.8 s per CT rotation, pitch of 1.675 : 1, and a reconstructed slice thickness of 3.75 mm, for a total scanning time of 42.4 s. The CT data were reconstructed using a filtered back-projection algorithm and a 512 × 512 matrix, with a transaxial field of view of 50 cm. The CT images were used to generate the transmission maps for attenuation correction of the PET acquisitions and anatomic localization.

Immediately after the CT scan, and without changing the patient's position, the tabletop moved automatically to the PET position. The emission scan was acquired in 2-D mode (septa out) starting at the mid-thighs toward the head, for six bed positions of 4 minutes each (47 image planes/bed position, 15.7 cm longitudinal field of view). PET data were reconstructed using an ordered-subset expectation maximization iterative algorithm (30 subsets, 2 iterations).

## Findings and differential diagnosis

There is a small left upper lobe spiculated nodule that measures 9 mm with moderate FDG uptake (SUVmax = 5.6) (Figure 7.8 arrowhead and Figure 7.9). There is also intense focal uptake at the posterior wall of the left acetabulum without obvious CT correlate, concerning for metastasis (Figures 7.8 and 7.10, arrows). No other lung nodules are seen. There is no mediastinal, hilar, or axillary lymphadenopathy. There are no pleural or

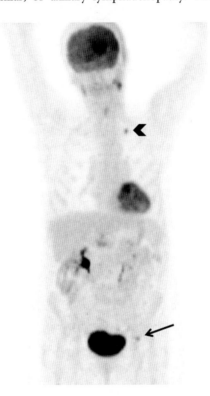

**Figure 7.8** Maximum intensity projection (MIP) image.

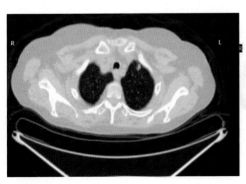
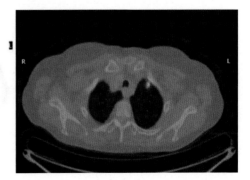

Figure 7.9 Axial CT, FDG-PET, and fused FDG-PET/CT slices at the level of the SPN.

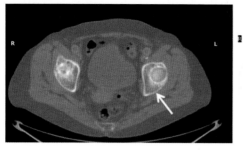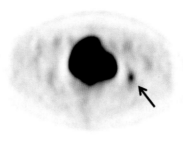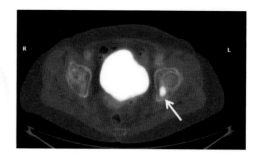

**Figure 7.10** Axial CT, FDG-PET, and fused FDG-PET/CT slices at the level of the acetabulum.

pericardial effusions. Below the diaphragm areas of FDG avidity represent physiologic uptake in the kidneys, collecting systems, and bowel loops. Differential diagnosis: given the small size of the SPN and the intensity of FDG uptake, the lesion should be considered a malignant lung neoplasm until proven otherwise with left acetabular metastasis, thus stage IV (M1b) lung cancer. Follow-up with a bone scan was recommended to evaluate for any additional sites of involvement. Bone scan results (not shown) confirmed a left acetabular focus of intense $^{99m}$Tc-methylene diphosphonate ($^{99m}$Tc-MDP) uptake consistent with metastasis. No other metastatic foci were noted.

## Diagnosis and follow up

A left acetabular biopsy showed metastatic NSCLC infiltrating marrow spaces with associated fibrosis, and bone marrow with maturing trilineage hematopoiesis. Immunohistochemistry results revealed the following staining profile in tumor cells: positive CK7, negative CK20 and TTF. These immunohistochemical features are consistent with origin from a lung primary, although other sites (e.g., breast, upper GI tract, pancreas, and ovary) cannot be excluded. The patient received palliative radiation therapy to the left hip followed by systemic chemotherapy consisting of a carboplatin and paclitaxel doublet.

## Discussion and teaching points

The skeleton is also a common site for lung cancer metastases. Osseous metastases are found in approximately 30% of lung cancer patients. They are mainly osteolytic and found in the vertebral column, the ribs, and the long bones (1). FDG-PET is a very accurate technique to evaluate for the presence of bone metastases in these patients. FDG-PET has similar sensitivity (90–92%) and higher specificity (98–99%) than bone scintigraphy for the detection of osteoclastic bone metastasis, and its sensitivity is lower in the presence of osteoblastic lesions (due to their lower cellularity and glycolytic metabolism) (2, 3).

Metastatic disease to bone usually starts at the marrow and later on affects the cortex. Therefore, and as shown in this case, discordant findings in bone between PET and CT do occur (focal uptake in the left acetabulum negative on CT). Metabolic evidence of metastasis may precede the amount of cortical bone derangement necessary for the lesion to be visualized on the CT images. On the other hand, there is also evidence that when there are discordant findings between the two modalities, the positive predictive value (PPV) of FDG-PET/CT diminishes (4). Taira and colleagues (4) recently retrospectively studied 59 patients with 113 lesions, to evaluate the PPV of FDG-PET/CT to characterize malignant bone lesions in which the metabolic and morphologic findings were discordant or concordant. A total of 47 lesions had concordant results in the PET and the CT examinations and of these, 46 were positive for malignancy (PPV = 98%). When analyzing discordant findings, only 19 of 31 lesions considered positive by PET but negative on CT, were actually malignant, thus lowering the PPV to 61%. Of 35 lesions considered positive by CT but negative by PET, only six were confirmed as being malignant (PPV = 17%). The authors stressed the fact that the PPV of all lesions with PET being positive was significantly higher than with positive findings on CT.

## Take-home message

- FDG-PET has similar sensitivity and higher specificity than bone scintigraphy to detect osteoclastic metastases to bone. Its sensitivity is lower in osteoblastic lesions.
- Metabolic evidence of osseous metastases may precede cortical bone derangement, giving place to a positive PET finding without obvious CT correlate.
- A positive FDG-PET finding always requires biopsy confirmation.
- FDG-PET is probably the most sensitive technique for the detection of extracerebral metastases from lung cancer.

## References

1. Patel AM, Peters SG. Clinical manifestations of lung cancer. *Mayo Clin Proc* 1993;**68**(3):273–7.

2. Cook GJ, Houston S, Rubens R, Maisey MN, Fogelman I. Detection of bone metastases in breast cancer by 18FDG PET: differing metabolic activity in osteoblastic and osteolytic lesions. *J Clin Oncol* 1998;**16**(10):3375–9.

3. Fogelman I, Cook G, Israel O, Van der Wall H. Positron emission tomography and bone metastases. *Semin Nucl Med* 2005;**35**(2):135–42.

4. Taira AV, Herfkens RJ, Gambhir SS, Quon A. Detection of bone metastases: assessment of integrated FDG PET/CT imaging. *Radiology* 2007;**243**(1):204–11.

A 71-year-old male undergoing PET/CT for restaging after left upper lobectomy and radiation for a T3N0Mx adenocarcinoma of the lung. The patient now presents with a new right lung mass. Past history is a right nephrectomy for renal cell carcinoma 4 years ago.

## Acquisition and processing parameters

After fasting for a period of 6 hours, the patient was injected intravenously with 20.2 mCi of FDG, and an uptake phase of 60 min was allowed prior to imaging. Plasma glucose levels at the time of FDG injection were 97.5 mg/dL. The patient was

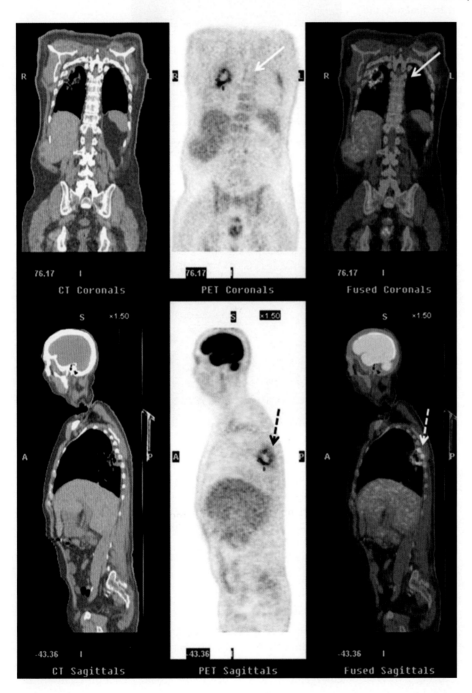

**Figure 7.11** Top row from left to right: Coronal CT, FDG-PET, and fused FDG-PET/CT images. Bottom row from left to right: Sagittal CT, FDG-PET, and fused FDG-PET/CT images.

encouraged to void before scanning, and images were obtained from the head to the proximal thighs with a combined PET/CT scanner. The patient was imaged in the supine position, with his arms placed above his head, in an attempt to reduce beam-hardening artifacts in the torso, and without any specific breath-holding instructions. The unenhanced CT scan was performed first, from the patient's head to the proximal thighs, using the following acquisition parameters: 140 kVp, 75 mA, 0.8 s per CT rotation, pitch of 1.675 : 1, and a reconstructed slice thickness of 3.75 mm, for a total scanning time of 42.4 s. The CT data were reconstructed using a filtered back-projection algorithm and a 512 × 512 matrix, with a transaxial field of view of 50 cm. The CT images were used to generate the transmission maps for attenuation correction of the PET acquisitions and anatomic localization.

Immediately after the CT scan, and without changing the patient's position, the tabletop moved automatically to the PET position. The emission scan was acquired in 2-D mode (septa out) starting at the mid-thighs toward the head, for six bed positions of 4 min each (47 image planes/bed position, 15.7 cm longitudinal field of view). PET data were reconstructed using an ordered-subset expectation maximization iterative algorithm (30 subsets, 2 iterations).

## Findings and differential diagnosis

In the right lower lung lobe there is a distinct halo of moderate FDG uptake surrounding a cavitary mass measuring 4.1 × 3.0 cm. FDG uptake extends posteriorly into the chest wall involving the adjacent rib (Figures 7.11 and 7.12: dotted arrows). No other lung parenchymal masses are seen. Minimal FDG uptake is noted within the right hilum. Paramediastinal radiation changes are noted, together with decreased marrow uptake in the thoracic vertebrae secondary to radiation treatment (Figure 7.11: white arrows). A focus of intense FDG uptake is noted within the left 6th rib laterally at the site of a healing fracture (Figure 7.12: arrowhead). The patient is status post-right nephrectomy, with herniation of the liver posteriorly into the right flank defect. Intense FDG uptake (SUVmax = 13) is seen in a 1.7 × 1.5 cm left adrenal gland nodule compatible with metastatic disease (Figures 7.13 and 7.14: black arrows). The remaining solid abdominal viscera are unremarkable. Differential diagnosis: stage IV (M1b) lung cancer.

## Diagnosis and follow-up

Fine needle aspiration biopsy of the right adrenal gland was positive for poorly differentiated malignant cells, consistent with metastasis from patient's known lung adenocarcinoma. Immunoperoxidase studies performed on paraffin cell block sections showed very rare neoplastic cells positive for CK7, TTF-1, and EMA, and negative for CK20. A surgical approach was not considered appropriate, and the patient was treated with Taxotere at 75 mg/sq m IV given every 3 weeks, and gefinitib as an oral agent at 250 mg p.o. QD.

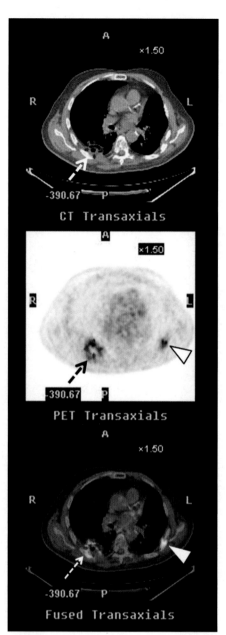

**Figure 7.12** Axial slices. Top: CT; middle: FDG-PET; and bottom: fused FDG-PET/CT images.

After chemotherapy the left adrenal mass was irradiated in order to prevent any tumor encroachment onto the left kidney; his only viable kidney. Later on the patient developed osseous metastasis in the L1 vertebral body, and received two full cycles of gemcitabine (at 640 mg/sq m at 10 mg/sq m per minute) and flavopiridol (60 mg/sq m) followed by restaging PET/CT (not shown) studies. The disease progressed and the patient died.

## Discussion and teaching points

The frequency of occult metastasis from adenocarcinomas is approximately 67% (1). Furthermore, adrenal metastases are fairly common, with approximately 35% of unilateral adrenal enlargement at CT being malignant. The differentials for

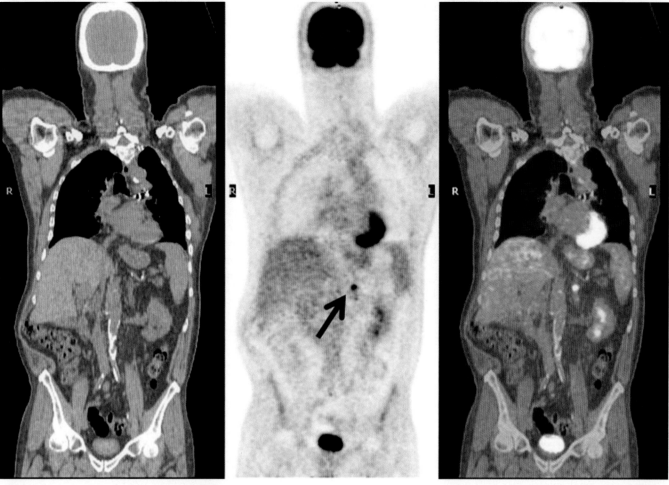

**Figure 7.13** Coronal CT, FDG-PET, and fused FDG-PET/CT images.

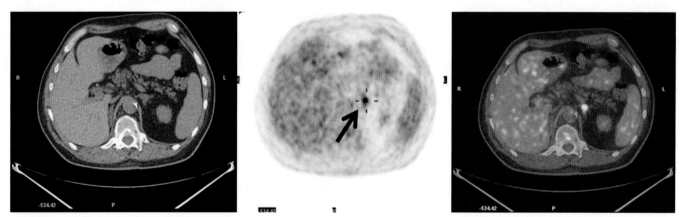

**Figure 7.14** Axial CT, FDG-PET, and fused FDG-PET/CT images.

benign enlarged adrenal glands include adenomas, hemorrhagic cysts, and adrenal hyperplasia.

The power of FDG-PET in this setting relies on its superiority to detect unsuspected distant metastases very accurately. FDG-PET is probably the most sensitive imaging technique for the detection of extracerebral metastasis from lung cancer. It detects distant secundarism missed by CT or excludes false-positive sites

detected by CT in up to approximately 24% of the patients, leading to a change in patient management in 9–64% of cases, mainly by reducing the number of unnecessary surgeries (2).

In a meta-analysis conducted by Hellwig *et al.* (3) the sensitivity, specificity and accuracy for the detection of adrenal metastasis were 96%, 99%, and 98%, respectively. Single-center studies have reported specificities as low as 84%, because some benign adrenal adenomas and/or certain inflammatory foci may take up the radiotracer as well (4–6). Of note, not all FDG-avid extrathoracic lesions are in fact metastases; 37% can be benign or inflammatory (7). Extrathoracic lesions should be biopsied if their malignant nature could in fact alter patient management. One of the most important contributions of FDG-PET/CT to metastasis staging is to detect more accurately extrathoracic lesions, and to be able to determine the clinical significance of a single focal abnormality by localizing it to a specific structure and in this manner characterize the finding as physiological or pathological in nature. Once the lesion is localized the PET/CT image may serve as a guidance tool for biopsy (see Chapter 20).

Some of the visual and semiquantitative methods that have been proposed to characterize adrenal gland uptake as malignant include: (a) visual analysis of adrenal activity higher than liver uptake (5, 8); (b) ratio of adrenal SUVmax to liver SUVmax $> 1$ (5, 8); (c) adrenal SUVmax $> 3.1$ (9); (d) ratio of adrenal SUVmax to liver SUVavg $> 2.5$ (increases specificity) (10); (e) adrenal size $> 3$ cm (10); and (f) adrenal Hounsfield units (HU) $> 10$ in unenhanced CT (8, 11). At our institution we consider malignant an adrenal-to-liver ratio higher than 2, and indeterminate, a ratio between 1 and 2, which calls for clinical follow-up.

## Take-home message

- FDG-PET and PET/CT are superior predictors of metastasis compared with conventional imaging modalities in this regard.
- Patients diagnosed with unresectable disease will be excluded from futile surgery.
- Adrenal adenomas can be FDG avid. Therefore, a positive PET finding should be biopsied if its malignant nature could alter patient management.

## References

1. Sider L, Horejs D. Frequency of extrathoracic metastases from bronchogenic carcinoma in patients with normal-sized hilar and mediastinal lymph nodes on CT. *Am J Roentgenol* 1988;**151**(5):893–5.

2. Facey K, Bradbury I, Laking G, Payne E. *Positron emission tomography (PET) imaging in cancer management. Ultra Rapid Review. Health Technology Assessment.* Southampton: NHS R&D Programme, 2004.

3. Hellwig D, Ukena D, Paulsen F, Bamberg M, Kirsch CM; Onko-PET der Deutschen Gesellschaft fur Nuklearmedizin. [Meta-analysis of the efficacy of positron emission tomography with F-18-fluorodeoxyglucose in lung tumors. Basis for discussion of the German Consensus Conference on PET in Oncology 2000]. *Pneumologie* 2001;**55**(8):367–77.

4. Yun M, Kim W, Alnafisi N *et al.* 18F-FDG PET in characterizing adrenal lesions detected on CT or MRI. *J Nucl Med* 2001;**42**(12):1795–9.

5. Blake MA, Slattery JM, Kalra MK *et al.* Adrenal lesions: characterization with fused PET/CT image in patients with proved or suspected malignancy – initial experience. *Radiology* 2006;**238**(3):970–7.

6. Erasmus JJ, Patz EF Jr, McAdams HP *et al.* Evaluation of adrenal masses in patients with bronchogenic carcinoma using 18F-fluorodeoxyglucose positron emission tomography. *Am J Roentgenol* 1997;**168**(5):1357–60.

7. Lardinois D, Weder W, Roudas M *et al.* Etiology of solitary extrapulmonary positron emission tomography and computed tomography findings in patients with lung cancer. *J Clin Oncol* 2005;**23**:6846–53.

8. Caoili EM, Korobkin M, Brown RK, Mackie G, Shulkin BL. Differentiating adrenal adenomas from nonadenomas using (18)F-FDG PET/CT: quantitative and qualitative evaluation. *Acad Radiol* 2007;**14**(4):468–75.

9. Metser U, Miller E, Lerman H *et al.* 18F-FDG PET/CT in the evaluation of adrenal masses. *J Nucl Med* 2006;**47**(1):32–7.

10. Brady MJ, Thomas J, Wong TZ *et al.* Adrenal nodules at FDG PET/CT in patients known to have or suspected of having lung cancer: a proposal for an efficient diagnostic algorithm. *Radiology* 2009;**250**(2):523–30.

11. Boland GW, Lee MJ, Gazelle GS *et al.* Characterization of adrenal masses using unenhanced CT: an analysis of the CT literature. *Am J Roentgenol* 1998;**171**(1):201–4.

A 74-year-old male with a history of chronic obstructive pulmonary disease and NSCLC, treated with talc pleurodesis for recurrent and symptomatic pleural effusions. FDG-PET/CT was obtained for restaging.

## Acquisition and processing parameters

After fasting for a period of 5 hours, the patient was injected intravenously with 20 mCi of FDG, and an uptake phase of 60 min was allowed prior to imaging. Plasma glucose levels at the time of FDG injection were 104 mg/dL. The patient was encouraged to void before scanning, and images were obtained from the head to the proximal thighs with a combined PET/CT scanner. The patient was imaged in the supine position, with his arms placed above his head, in an attempt to reduce beam-hardening artifacts in the torso, and without any specific breath-holding instructions. The unenhanced CT scan was performed first, from the patient's head to the proximal thighs, using the following acquisition parameters: 140 kVp, 75 mA, 0.8 s per CT rotation, pitch of 1.675 : 1, and a reconstructed slice thickness of 3.75 mm, for a total scanning time of 42.4 s. The CT data were reconstructed using a filtered back-projection algorithm and a 512 × 512 matrix, with a transaxial field of view of 50 cm. The CT images were used to generate the transmission maps for attenuation correction of the PET acquisitions and anatomic localization.

Immediately after the CT scan, and without changing the patient's position, the tabletop moved automatically to the PET position. The emission scan was acquired in 2-D mode (septa out) starting at the mid-thighs toward the head, for six bed positions of 4 min each (47 image planes/bed position, 15.7 cm longitudinal field of view). PET data were reconstructed using an ordered-subset expectation maximization iterative algorithm (30 subsets, 2 iterations).

## Findings and differential diagnosis

Unenhanced axial CT (Figure 7.15A), PET (Figure 7.15B) and fused PET/CT (Figure 7.15C) images show encasement of right lung by diffusely thickened and focally nodular right pleura with mild-to-moderate FDG avidity, suspicious for tumor recurrence. However, given the patient's history of prior pleurodesis, these findings are not specific for malignancy, since considerable FDG uptake can be associated with the resulting chronic inflammatory reaction associated with this procedure. Differential diagnoses include: metastasis to the pleura (M1a); malignant pleural mesothelioma; fibrous mesothelioma; talc pleurodesis; benign inflammatory pleuritis; benign asbestos-related plaques; parapneumonic effusion; and tuberculous pleuritis.

## Diagnosis

Pleural biopsy revealed metastatic lung adenocarcinoma to the pleura (stage IV–M1a).

## Discussion and teaching points

Adenocarcinoma is the most common histologic type of lung cancer that metastasizes to the pleura (1, 2). Metastatic deposits in the pleura occur via hematogenous seeding of the visceral pleura first, followed by cell migration and attachment to the parietal pleura (1).

In patients with suspicion of pleural malignancy there is a need for accurate distinction between benign and malignant lesions, as well as for the reliable differentiation between focal or multifocal invasive disease. Computed tomography (CT) and magnetic resonance imaging (MRI) have limitations when attempting to characterize pleural lesions as benign or

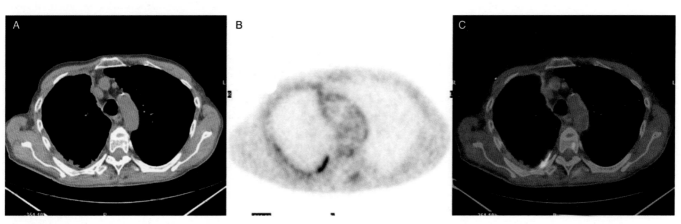

**Figure 7.15** (A) axial CT; (B) axial FDG-PET; (C) fused axial FDG-PET/CT.

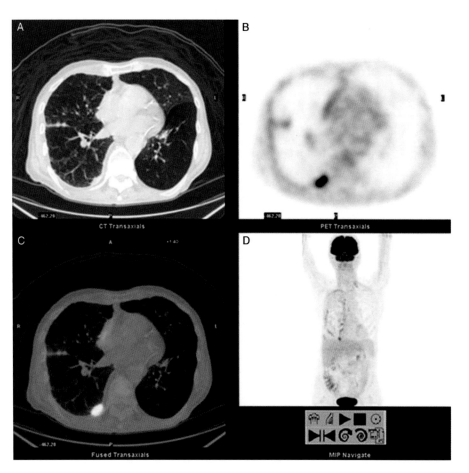

**Figure 7.16** Talc pleurodesis. A 55-year-old male with a history of lung adenocarcinoma and prior pleurodesis. There is diffuse thickening and nodularity of the pleura with increased FDG uptake (A, B, C). There is also nodularity of the major fissure (A, C). There is some septal thickening toward the right posterior basal parenchyma related to prior radiation therapy (A). There are small to medium-sized foci of moderately increased uptake throughout the pleura of the right lung (better visualized on the MIP image (D)). More focally at the right medial basilar pleura there is a more intense focus of FDG uptake (B and C) corresponding to a high-attenuation area of pleural thickening on CT (A). Given the patient's history of prior pleurodesis, these findings are not specific for recurrence of malignancy, since considerable FDG uptake can be associated with the resulting chronic inflammatory reaction caused by the instillation of talc in the pleural space.

malignant. The CT criteria for malignant pleural disease (diffuse or nodular pleural thickening and pleural effusion) have a sensitivity and specificity of 72% and 83%, respectively (3).

FDG-PET has been shown to accurately differentiate benign from malignant pleural-based lesions, and to be useful in the staging and pre-operative evaluation of disease extent (4). The typical FDG-PET appearance of malignant pleural disease is that of moderate-to-high FDG uptake involving the areas of thickened pleura observed on anatomic imaging. The commonly observed patterns of FDG uptake are focal, linear, and mixed (focal-linear). These patterns closely reflect the extent of pleural and parenchymal involvement observed in conventional imaging and surgery (5–7).

Unfortunately, the pattern or intensity of FDG lesion uptake can neither differentiate between different malignancies that metastasize to the pleura (i.e., lung, ovary, breast, prostate, and kidney adenocarcinomas, as well as sarcoma), nor distinguish metastatic disease to the pleura from a pleural primary (i.e., mesothelioma) (4).

Talc pleurodesis is performed for the management of persistent pneumothorax or pleural effusion. In patients treated with pleurodesis, the pleural space is obliterated by inducing a chronic inflammatory response through the instillation of talc, antibiotics, antiparasitic, or chemotherapeutic agents (8). Talc provides high-attenuation material on CT images that serves as

a reminder to think of this diagnosis. Other agents can cause the same pleural appearance without specific attenuation to suggest it. Increased FDG uptake is not uncommon in activated macrophages in a variety of inflammatory processes; therefore, areas of the pleura that have been subjected to talc pleurodesis might be difficult to distinguish from tumor on the basis of the intensity or the pattern of FDG uptake alone (5, 6). The inflammatory effects of pleurodesis are evident on FDG-PET imaging and may persist for years (9). Findings characteristic of pleurodesis include focal (single or multiple) patterns of uptake in both plaque-like and nodular areas of high attenuation pleural thickening, and although not as common, a diffuse pattern of uptake may also be present in some patients (9) (Figure 7.16). Other sources of false-positive results include benign inflammatory pleuritis; benign asbestos-related plaques; parapneumonic effusion, and tuberculous pleuritis (4, 5).

The less-than-perfect specificity of FDG in this subset of patients, stresses the importance of pleural biopsy to characterize anatomo-metabolic findings as malignant. In our practice the use of FDG-PET images has proven to be of great value for the selection of the most metabolically active site for needle or thoracoscopic biopsy (see Chapter 20). This approach, especially when performed in integrated PET/CT systems, increases the yield of positive biopsies by minimizing sampling errors.

## Take-home message

- FDG imaging is an accurate tool for the non-invasive metabolic characterization of pleural lesions as benign or malignant.
- The pattern or intensity of FDG lesion uptake can neither differentiate between different malignancies that metastasize to the pleura (i.e., lung, ovary, breast, prostate, kidney adenocarcinomas, and sarcoma), nor distinguish metastatic disease to the pleura from a pleural primary.

- Talc pleurodesis is FDG avid on PET and produces high-attenuation areas of pleural thickening on CT, which may remain unchanged on serial imaging for years.
- Other sources of false-positive results include benign inflammatory pleuritis; benign asbestos-related plaques; parapneumonic effusion; and tuberculous pleuritis.
- FDG-PET/CT imaging successfully guides biopsy to metabolically active sites, thus minimizing sampling errors.

## References

1. Sahn SA. State of the art. The pleura. *Am Rev Respir Dis* 1988;**138**(1):184–234.

2. Patel AM, Peters SG. Clinical manifestations of lung cancer. *Mayo Clin Proc* 1993;**68**(3):273–7.

3. Leung AN, Muller NL, Miller RR. CT in differential diagnosis of diffuse pleural disease. *Am J Roentgenol* 1990;**154**(3):487–92.

4. Bury T, Paulus P, Dowlati A *et al.* Evaluation of pleural diseases with FDG-PET imaging: preliminary report. *Thorax* 1997;**52**(2):187–9.

5. Gerbaudo VH, Sugarbaker DJ, Britz-Cunningham S *et al.* Assessment of malignant pleural mesothelioma with (18)F-FDG dual-head gamma-camera coincidence imaging: comparison with histopathology. *J Nucl Med* 2002;**43**(9):1144–9.

6. Gerbaudo VH, Britz-Cunningham S, Sugarbaker DJ, Treves ST. Metabolic significance of the pattern, intensity and kinetics of 18F-FDG uptake in malignant pleural mesothelioma. *Thorax* 2003;**58**(12):1077–82.

7. Gerbaudo VH. 18F-FDG imaging of malignant pleural mesothelioma: scientiam impendere vero . . . [Editorial]. *Nucl Med Com* 2003;**24**:609–14.

8. Adler RH, Sayek I: Treatment of malignant pleural effusion: a method using tube thoracostomy and talc. *Ann Thorac Surg* 1976;**22**(1):8–15.

9. Kwek BH, Aquino SL, Fischman AJ. Fluorodeoxyglucose positron emission tomography and CT after talc pleurodesis. *Chest* 2004;**125**(6):2356–60.

A 71-year-old female without prior history of malignancy presents with two indeterminate pulmonary nodules observed in a chest film and in a subsequent CT scan. FDG-PET/CT was obtained to characterize the nodules and for initial treatment strategy.

## Acquisition and processing parameters

After fasting for a period of 6.5 hours, the patient was injected intravenously with 19 mCi of FDG, and an uptake phase of 80 min was allowed prior to imaging. Plasma glucose levels at the time of FDG injection were 99 mg/dL. The patient was encouraged to void before scanning, and images were obtained from the head to the proximal thighs with a combined PET/CT scanner. The patient was imaged in the supine position, with her arms placed above her head, in an attempt to reduce beam-hardening artifacts in the torso, and without any specific breath-holding instructions. The unenhanced CT scan was performed first, from the patient's head to the proximal thighs, using the following acquisition parameters: 140 kVp, 75 mA, 0.8 s per CT rotation, pitch of 1.675 : 1, and a reconstructed slice thickness of 3.75 mm, for a total scanning time of 42.4 s. The CT data were reconstructed using a filtered back-projection algorithm and a $512 \times 512$ matrix, with a transaxial field of view of 50 cm. The CT images were used to generate the transmission maps for attenuation correction of the PET acquisitions and anatomic localization.

Immediately after the CT scan, and without changing the patient's position, the tabletop moved automatically to the PET position. The emission scan was acquired in 2-D mode (septa

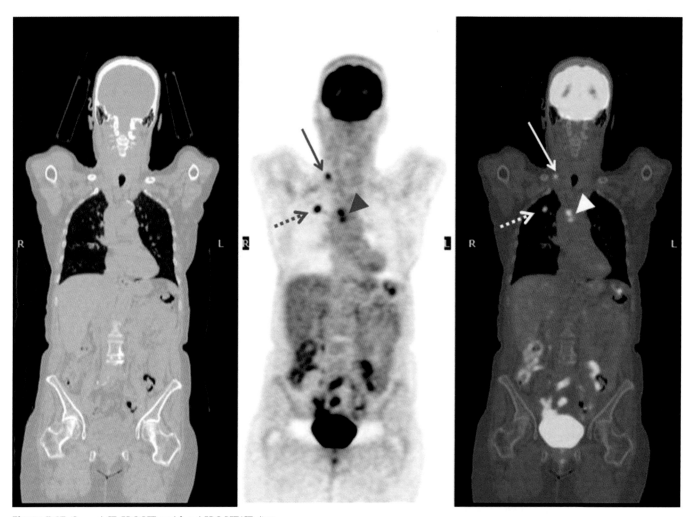

**Figure 7.17** Coronal CT, FDG-PET, and fused FDG-PET/CT slices.

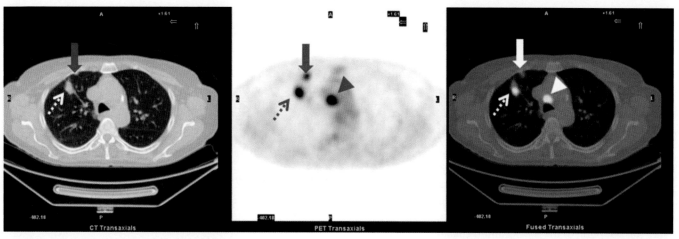

**Figure 7.18** Axial CT, FDG-PET, and fused FDG-PET/CT slices.

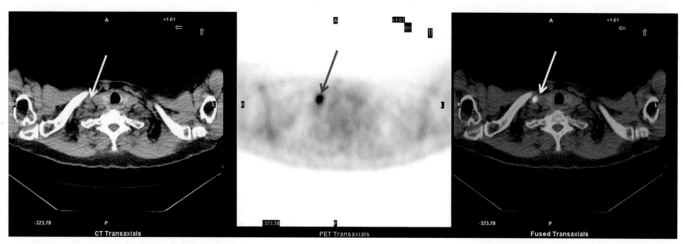

**Figure 7.19** Axial CT, FDG-PET, and fused FDG-PET/CT slices.

out) starting at the mid-thighs toward the head, for six bed positions of 4 min each (47 image planes/bed position, 15.7 cm longitudinal field of view). PET data were reconstructed using an ordered-subset expectation maximization iterative algorithm (30 subsets, 2 iterations).

## Findings and differential diagnosis

A highly FDG avid (SUVmax = 14.8) spiculated nodule measuring 2.2 × 1.3 cm is seen in the anterior segment of the right upper lung lobe (Figures 7.17 and 7.18: dotted arrows). A right subpleural 6 mm nodule demonstrates moderate FDG uptake (SUVmax = 3) despite its small size (Figure 7.18: thick arrows). No left lung nodule is seen. There is no evidence of pleural or pericardial effusions. In addition, there is a 1.4 × 0.8 cm right supraclavicular lymph node (N3) that is moderately FDG avid (SUVmax = 5.6) (Figures 7.18 and 7.19: arrows). There is intensely FDG-avid midline paratracheal adenopathy (N2) (SUVmax = 10) (Figures 7.17 and 7.18: arrowheads). There is a small hiatal hernia, and a small focus of atherosclerotic

calcification in the aortic arch. Below the diaphragm, the radiotracer is distributed physiologically in the gastrointestinal and genitourinary tracts, without significant lymphadenopathy. There are no FDG-avid or destructive bone lesions. Differential diagnosis: Stage IIIB lung cancer; metastatic disease from a non-lung primary; inflammatory disease.

## Diagnosis and follow-up

Supraclavicular node biopsy revealed metastasis from poorly differentiated squamous cell carcinoma of lung origin. The patient was treated surgically (right upper lobe wedge resection) followed by adjuvant chemotherapy consisting of carboplatin and Gemzar.

## Discussion and teaching points

As discussed in the introduction of this chapter, squamous cell carcinomas are highly FDG avid, especially those that are poorly differentiated; in most instances their uptake is higher than in adenocarcinomas. Despite the small size of the detected lesions in this patient, the intensity of uptake was significantly higher than mediastinal and background activity, and therefore, highly suspicious of being malignant.

FDG-PET and PET/CT are known for their superior accuracy to stage lung malignancies. PET/CT improves the detection of mediastinal disease, providing a more accurate assessment of N stage (1). Additional information is obtained in aproximately 41% of patients by better characterizing malignancy and by diminishing the number of equivocal findings. FDG-PET interrogates the biologic behavior of lesions and does not rely on nodal size, and as in this case, it detects tumor in normal-size lymph nodes and excludes metastatic involvement of large nodes. Unlike mediatinoscopy, FDG-PET provides full sampling of the mediastinum changing the N stage in approximately 20% of patients. In fact, the disease in this particular patient was upstaged from a probable stage IIIA: T3 (although small in size, there were two satellite lesions in the same lobe), N2 (paratracheal lymphadenopathy), M0, to a stage IIIB: T3, N3 (supraclavicular lymphadenopathy), M0. The use of combined PET/CT imaging for nodal staging allows for more precise localization of mediastinal lymph nodes as well as supraclavicular node metastases, with an accuracy of 93%, compared with 89% for PET alone and with 63% for CT alone (2).

As has already been stressed by all the experts sharing their knowledge in this book, highly FDG-avid lesions are most likely malignant, but false-positive results are not uncommon in patients with infectious and/or inflammatory processes that take up FDG (e.g., active tuberculosis, sarcoidosis, histoplasmosis, coccidioidomycosis, etc.), or in reactive, yet benign, lymphadenopathy. Therefore, FDG-positive lesions should always be examined histologically.

The treatment algorithms for stage IIIB are decided on a patient-by-patient basis. In this case the patient's treatment team elected to treat surgically followed by adjuvant chemotherapy. There is some evidence that patients with satellite lesion-based stage IIIB disease enjoy longer survival following surgical resection of the primary and of lymph node lesions whenever possible (3).

## Take-home message

- Squamous cell carcinomas are highly FDG-avid tumors.
- PET/CT improves the detection of mediastinal disease, providing a more accurate assessment of nodal stage.
- Unlike mediatinoscopy, FDG-PET provides full sampling of the mediastinum changing the nodal stage in approximately 20% of patients.
- FDG-PET/CT imaging precisely localizes supraclavicular node metastasis.
- False-positive results are not uncommon in patients affected by infectious and/or inflammatory processes that take up FDG, or that have reactive, yet benign, lymphadenopathy.
- FDG-positive lesions that could alter management should always be biopsied.

## References

1. Lardinois D, Weder W, Hany TF *et al.* Staging of non-small-cell lung cancer with integrated positron emission tomography and computed tomography. *N Engl J Med* 2003;**348**:2500–7.

2. Antoch G, Stattaus J, Nemat AT *et al.* Non-small cell lung cancer: dual-modality PET/CT in preoperative staging. *Radiology* 2003;**229**(2):526–33.

3. Detterbeck FC, Jones DR, Kernstine KH, Naunheim KS; American College of Physicians. Lung cancer. Special treatment issues. *Chest* 2003;**123**(1 Suppl): 244S–58S.

A 65-year-old male with a history of biopsy-proven epithelial subtype mesothelioma (MPM) of the right pleura. FDG-PET/CT scans were obtained for initial treatment strategy, and again after 6 cycles of cisplatin plus pemetrexed chemotherapy.

## Acquisition and processing parameters

The patient underwent FDG-PET/CT imaging at baseline and after treatment. Both scans were acquired using the same parameters. After fasting for a period of 6 hours, the patient was injected intravenously with 20.2 mCi for the baseline scan and 19.8 mCi of FDG for the post-treatment scan, with an uptake phase of 60 min in both occasions. Plasma glucose levels at the time of FDG injection were 109 mg/dL and 102 mg/dL, before and after therapy, respectively. The patient was encouraged to void before scanning, and images were obtained from the head to the proximal thighs with a combined PET/CT scanner. The patient was imaged in the supine position, without any specific breath-holding instructions. The unenhanced CT scans were performed first, from the patient's head to the proximal thighs, using the following acquisition parameters: 140 kVp, 75 mA, 0.8 s per CT rotation, pitch of 1.675 : 1, and a reconstructed slice thickness of 3.75 mm, for a total scanning time of 42.4 s. The CT data were reconstructed using a filtered back-projection algorithm and a 512 × 512 matrix, with a transaxial field of view of 50 cm. The CT images were used to generate the transmission maps for attenuation correction of the PET acquisitions and anatomic localization.

Immediately after the CT scans, and without changing the patient's position, the tabletop moved automatically to the PET position. The emission scans were acquired in 2-D mode (septa out) starting at the mid-thighs toward the head, for six

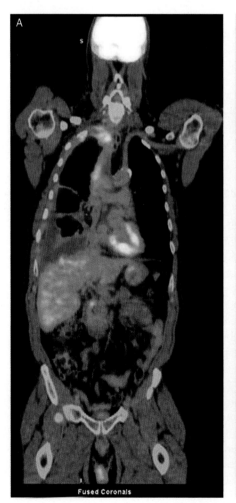
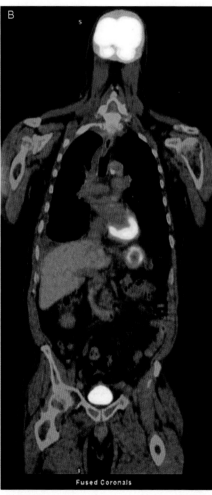

Fused Coronals

**Figure 7.20** (A) Baseline coronal FDG-PET/CT; (B) post-therapy coronal FDG-PET/CT.

bed positions of 4 min each (47 image planes/bed position, 15.7 cm longitudinal field of view). PET data were reconstructed using an ordered-subset expectation maximization iterative algorithm (30 subsets, 2 iterations).

## Findings and differential diagnosis

*Baseline scan findings* (Figure 7.20A): there is diffuse concentric pleural thickening in the right lung. The thickened pleura demonstrates intense tracer uptake consistent with the known diagnosis of mesothelioma. Medially, the thickened pleura is adjacent to the vascular structures of the mediastinum including the superior vena cava and the right pulmonary artery. Encasement of the vessels, in particular the superior vena cava by the tumor cannot be excluded. There is also infiltration of the mediastinal fat. The thickened pleura extends into the subcarinal space. Laterally, the tumor extends to the chest wall and interdigitates the intercostal spaces. There is a 1 cm FDG-avid right anterior diaphragmatic lymph node, likely a metastasis. There are no suspicious lung nodules. There is a right pleural effusion. Below the diaphragm the radiotracer is distributed physiologically in the gastrointestinal and genitourinary tracts. There is no significant lymphadenopathy. The extent of tumor invasion renders this case unresectable. The treatment team suggested six cycles of cisplatin plus pemetrexed and that a follow-up FDG-PET/CT be obtained to assess response to chemotherapy.

*Post-treatment scan findings* (Figure 7.20B): The pleural nodularity associated with intense FDG avidity along the right hemithorax in the baseline scan, now demonstrates only mild FDG avidity. The pleural disease abutting the mediastinum at the level of the aortic arch, now shows a significant decrease in FDG uptake. The mediastinal fat demonstrates markedly decreased stranding and infiltration. The right-sided diaphragmatic lymph node has decreased in size from 1 cm to 8 mm in transverse diameter and currently demonstrates no increased FDG avidity. There is a residual right pleural effusion that has decreased in size. Below the diaphragm, tracer is distributed physiologically in the gastrointestinal and genitourinary tracts. There is no significant lymphadenopathy and no FDG-avid disease.

## Diagnosis and follow-up

Marked interval improvement in right hemithorax pleural, mediastinal, and pericardial disease with marked decreased FDG avidity in these sites as described above. This is consistent with significant treatment response which was confirmed following subsequent successful extrapleural pneumonectomy. Thorough gross and extensive microscopic examination of the post-surgical specimen did not reveal any tumor. There were pathologic changes in the parietal and visceral pleura consisting of an inflammatory cell infiltration (by lymphocytes, plasma cells, and histiocytes), prominent vascularity, hemosiderin deposition, reactive mesothelial cell proliferation and extensive fibrosis. These changes are consistent with chemotherapy-induced regression of a biopsy-proven epithelial mesothelioma of the pleura. Three years after treatment the patient is doing very well and a recent follow-up PET/CT scan (not shown) excluded the presence of disease recurrence.

## Discussion and teaching points

The pattern of malignant pleural mesothelioma (MPM) invasion is first locoregional, presenting as small plaques on the parietal pleura. Diffuse thickening and subsequent fusion of the pleurae follow, which will eventually lead to encasement and possible invasion of the ipsilateral lung, as is the case of the patient being discussed. As the tumor grows, the chest wall, the mediastinal organs, the diaphragm and sometimes the contralateral lung and the peritoneum may be involved.

Defining the extent of disease at the time of diagnosis has important treatment and prognostic implications. Accurate tumor staging is key to being able to assess response to therapy. The Brigham and Women's Hospital surgical staging system (1) has been shown to stratify survival; it considers tumor histology, resectability, and nodal status with definition of four stages: stage I: disease confined within the capsule of the ipsilateral parietal pleura without adenopathy, lung, pericardium, diaphragm, or chest wall disease limited to previous biopsy sites. Stage II: same as stage I with positive resection margins, and/or positive intrapleural lymph nodes. Stage III: local extension of disease into chest wall or mediastinum; heart, or through the diaphragm, peritoneum; with or without extrapleural lymph node involvement; and stage IV: distant metastatic disease. As mentioned previously in this chapter, the disease is considered unresectable when there is evidence of mediastinal, contralateral pleura, transdiaphragmatic, spine and/or diffuse chest wall invasion with or without rib destruction, and with or without associated systemic metastases (Brigham stages III and IV) (2). FDG-PET/CT demonstrated unresectable disease in this patient who was then treated with chemotherapy.

FDG-PET has already earned its place in clinical oncology as an accurate imaging biomarker of cancer therapy in many tumor types (3), and it is also now being used to monitor mesothelioma response (4). FDG-PET is more accurate than conventional imaging modalities (e.g., CT and MRI) to differentiate viable tumor tissue from fibrosis or necrosis in residual tissues after treatment.

Ceresoli and colleagues were the first to share their experience with FDG-PET imaging to assess MPM response to chemotherapy. The investigators monitored response in 20 patients following 2 cycles of single agent pemetrexed, or pemetrexed in combination with carboplatin (5). The authors defined complete metabolic response as total resolution of FDG uptake within the tumor volume between scans. Partial response was defined as a reduction in tumor FDG uptake of 25% or more, whereas progressive disease corresponded to an increase in tumor SUV of $\geq 25\%$, or the appearance of any new FDG-avid lesions. Stable metabolic disease was considered when there was an increase or decrease in tumor SUV of < 25%. Their results showed that early metabolic response was significantly correlated with median time-to-tumor progression (TTP), which was 14 months for metabolic responders, and 7 months for non-responders ($P < 0.05$). In addition, patients with a metabolic response had a trend toward longer overall survival ($P = 0.07$). No correlation was found between TTP and CT response following two cycles of therapy.

Therapy-induced metabolic tumor volume changes derived from FDG images have been used as markers of response in MPM. Francis et al. used FDG-PET-derived volumetric analysis in 23 patients with MPM, at baseline and after one cycle of chemotherapy with cisplatin and gemcitabine (6). The investigators estimated the total tumor glycolytic volume (TGV) to assess response to therapy. Their results demonstrated a strong and significant correlation between the change in TGV after one cycle of chemotherapy and survival ($P = 0.015$). On the other hand, CT response using Modified RECIST criteria was not predictive of survival ($P = 0.131$).

Veit-Haibach and co-investigators have recently published their results from FDG-PET/CT acquired at baseline and after three cycles of first- or second-line pemetrexed and platinum chemotherapy in 41 patients (7). They compared the value of different PET/CT-derived response parameters to include SUVmax, SUVavg, PETvol, and tumor lesion glycolysis (TLG). Their results showed that volume-based measures [PETvol ($P = 0.0002$) and TLG ($P = 0.01$)], and CT response using modified RECIST criteria ($P = 0.001$), were predictive of overall survival. The lesion SUVmax ($P = 0.61$) or SUVavg ($P = 0.68$) were not.

In conclusion, the emerging evidence tells us that the assessment of tumor metabolic response is a viable technique to assess the effect of treatment in patients with MPM, and that it appears to have prognostic value.

## Take-home message

- FDG-PET and PET/CT imaging are complementary to CT and MRI to assess intrathoracic disease extent and tumor resectability. FDG-PET/CT's limitations become evident when attempting to assess subtle, yet unresectable invasive disease.
- FDG-PET/CT increases the accuracy of overall MPM staging, by detecting more extensive disease involvement, and identifying occult distant metastases not seen in CT and MRI.
- FDG-PET has already earned its place in clinical oncology as an accurate imaging biomarker of cancer therapy in many tumor types, including MPM.
- FDG-PET is more accurate than conventional imaging modalities to differentiate viable tumor tissue from fibrosis or necrosis in residual tissues after treatment.
- Therapy-induced metabolic tumor volume changes derived from FDG images can be used as markers of response in MPM.
- The assessment of tumor metabolic response is a viable technique to assess the effect of treatment in patients with MPM, and it appears to have prognostic value.

## References

1. Sugarbaker DJ, Flores RM, Jaklitsch MT et al. Resection margins, extrapleural nodal status, and cell type determine postoperative long-term survival in trimodality therapy of malignant pleural mesothelioma: results in 183 patients. J Thorac Cardiovasc Surg 1999;117(1):54–63.

2. Gerbaudo VH, Katz S, Nowak A, Francis R. Multimodality imaging review of malignant pleural mesothelioma diagnosis and staging. PET Clinics 2011;6(3):275–98.

3. Weber WA. Assessing tumor response to therapy. J Nucl Med 2009;50(Suppl 1):10S.

4. Nowak A, Francis R, Katz S, Gerbaudo VH. Multimodality imaging review of malignant pleural mesothelioma response to therapy assessment. PET Clinics 2011;6(3):299–311.

5. Ceresoli GL, Chiti A, Zucali PA et al. Early response evaluation in malignant pleural mesothelioma by positron emission tomography with [18F] fluorodeoxyglucose. J Clin Oncol 2006;24:4587–93.

6. Francis RJ, Byrne MJ, van der Schaaf AA et al. Early prediction of response to chemotherapy and survival in malignant pleural mesothelioma using a novel semiautomated 3-dimensional volume-based analysis of serial 18F-FDG PET scans. J Nucl Med 2007;48:1449–58.

7. Veit-Haibach P, Schaefer NG, Steinert H et al. Combined FDG-PET/CT in response evaluation of malignant pleural mesothelioma. Lung Cancer 2010;67(3):311–17.

Victor H. Gerbaudo and Ritu R. Gill

## Introduction

Esophageal cancer incidence has risen in the last decade, accounting for 16,698 new cases of which 14,710 succumbed to the disease in 2011 (1–3). It is an uncommon tumor that accounts for approximately 7% of all gastrointestinal malignancies. The great majority of patients present with advanced disease. **Squamous cell carcinoma** was the most common histological type and has an association with tobacco and alcohol abuse. Recently **adenocarcinoma** associated with Barrett's metaplasia and seen almost exclusively in middle-aged white men with gastroesophageal reflux disease (GERD), has become the most predominant form, accounting for 60% of all esophageal cancers in 1994. Thus, the majority of adenocarcinomas affect the distal esophagus. Curative surgical resection is the treatment of choice; overall survival however is determined by the stage at initial diagnosis. Early esophageal cancer has 5-year survival ranging from 57%–78%, with locally advanced disease having a dismal prognosis despite aggressive therapy (3, 4). Therefore accurate pre-operative staging is crucial, as it helps guide management and avoids unnecessary surgery.

Computed tomography has been the first-line imaging modality for staging; however, endoscopic ultrasound and FDG-PET, each with their individual strengths, have improved pre-operative staging. The staging criteria in esophageal cancer comprise tumor size, depth of local invasion, nodal involvement, and distant metastases. The current work-up of newly diagnosed esophageal cancer is based on all three imaging modalities; hence familiarity with the strengths and weaknesses of each of these should prove helpful. Optimization of the utilization of the imaging results for the management of esophageal cancer patients requires an understanding of the epidemiology, patho-physiology, and patterns of metastases and recurrence.

## Staging and treatment of esophageal cancer

Staging a malignancy helps guide management (either therapeutic or palliative) and has prognostic value. Esophageal cancer prognosis depends on the depth of tumor penetration, tumor location, histologic grade, distance to the proximal and distal edge of tumor from the incisors, the number of regional nodes involved, and the presence of distant metastasis (5, 6). The increasing incidence of adenocarcinoma of the esophagus has prompted changes to the current staging system. The American Joint Committee on Cancer (AJCC) staging is based on TNM classification, and has recently been revised and published in the 7th edition of the AJCC manual in 2010 (6) (Table 8.1). Briefly, the most salient modifications of the revised TNM system, which apply to all esophageal cancers, include: carcinoma in situ is redefined as high-grade dysplasia; regional lymph nodes are classified based on the number of metastatic nodes; M1a and M1b classifications are no longer used, as they have not been found useful; and anatomic stage/prognostic groupings are set according to the histologic type (squamous cell and adenocarcinoma; we direct the reader to reference (6) for more details regarding the latter).

The overall 5-year survival rate is less than 20%. The 5-year survival rate for patients with tumors confined to the esophageal wall is approximately 40% and significantly worsens to as low as 4% with tumors involving the adventitia of the esophagus (7). The likelihood of nodal spread increases with increasing tumor (T) stage, due to contiguous involvement of mediastinal structures and is associated with worsening prognosis. Nodal involvement is less than 1% in tumors limited to the mucosa, and steeply increases up to 50% in patients with submucosal involvement. The previous classification of involved abdominal lymph nodes as M1 disease was controversial, as positive abdominal lymph nodes do not appear to carry as grave a prognosis as distant metastases (8). Therefore, celiac axis nodes are now considered regional nodes, and are amenable to curative resection. Complete resection of the primary tumor and appropriate lymphadenectomy should be attempted if possible.

The therapeutic approach to be followed depends on the stage of the disease, the patients' performance status, and the

*A Case-Based Approach to PET/CT in Oncology*, ed. Victor H. Gerbaudo. Published by Cambridge University Press.
© Cambridge University Press 2012.

**Table 8.1** Revised tumor, node, metastasis (TNM) classification for esophageal cancer (adapted from reference 6).

| T (Primary tumor) | N (regional lymph nodes: include peri-esophageal cervical nodes down to celiac nodes) | M (Distant metastasis) |
|---|---|---|
| **TX**: tumor cannot be assessed | **NX**: regional nodes cannot be assessed | **M0**: no distant metastasis |
| **T0**: no evidence of tumor | **N0**: no nodal metastasis | **M1**: distant metastasis (includes non-regional lymph nodes) |
| **Tis**: high grade dysplasia | **N1**: regional nodal metastasis in 1–2 nodes | |
| **T1**: invasion of lamina propia, muscularis mucosae or submucosa | **N2**: regional nodal metastasis in 3–6 nodes<br>**N3**: regional nodal metastasis in ≥ 7 nodes | |
| **T1a**: invasion of lamina propia or muscularis mucosae | | |
| **T1b**: invasion of submucosa | | |
| **T2**: invasion of muscularis propia | | |
| **T3**: invasion of adventitia | | |
| **T4**: invasion of adjacent organs | | |
| **T4a**: invasion of pleura, pericardium, or diaphragm by resectable tumor | | |
| **T4b**: invasion of other organs by unresectable tumor | | |

preference and expertise of the treating team. Although at the time of writing there is no consensus about what the best treatment approach is, it is safe to categorize treatment of patients with esophageal cancer as "management of curable or potentially curable disease" and "therapy for incurable tumors." The former calls for esophagectomy of superficial esophageal malignancies (Tis, T1a, and T1b). More controversial is the management of more invasive yet curable cancers (e.g., stages II and III), which may include surgery without systemic therapy (generally when there is no regional lymph node involvement), or with neoadjuvant chemoradiotherapy (in patients with regional lymph node metastasis), or chemotherapy combined with radiation without resection (in patients with localized disease who are poor surgical candidates secondary to poor performance status). The group with incurable disease includes those with T4b lesions with or without M1 disease. Here the primary goal is to provide relief of symptoms secondary to obstruction (dysphagia and pain), as well as optimization of quality of life, while minimizing the toxic effects of systemic therapy. Treatment algorithms may include radiotherapy or chemotherapy or combined radiochemotherapy in those with invasive tumors but without systemic disease. In patients with metastatic disease but with good functional status, combination chemotherapy may be considered, whereas those with poor functional status can be treated with single-agent palliative therapy (9). Other palliative therapies include laser resection and esophageal stenting and dilatation.

## Barium swallow, computed tomography, magnetic resonance imaging and endoscopic ultrasound for the evaluation and staging of esophageal cancer

### Barium imaging (esophagogram)

Barium swallow studies tend to be the first-line modality in evaluation of dysphagia, although recently it is being replaced by endoscopy.

Esophageal cancer may present as polypoid, infiltrative, varicoid, or ulcerative lesions. Superficial spreading lesions tend to show a nodular mucosal pattern without a well-defined mass. Early esophageal cancers may have subtle findings on barium studies, and can be easily missed (10). Barium swallow examinations are very useful in evaluating complications such as tracheoesophageal fistula secondary to locally advanced disease, and are also valuable in patients with stenotic lesions which limit passage of the endoscope.

### Computed tomography

Computed tomography (CT) is the initial modality used for staging. CT may be used to define the local extent of tumor by delineating the extent of involvement of the esophageal wall by tumor and invasion of the peri-esophageal fat. CT, however, cannot reliably delineate the individual layers of the esophageal wall and therefore cannot distinguish between T1 and T2 lesions and has no role in Tis lesions. Infiltration of the tumor into the peri-esophageal fat representing T3 disease has poor prognosis, however, en bloc resection with curative intent can be attempted. The accuracy of CT in diagnosing direct mediastinal invasion ranges from 59% to 82% (5). Direct invasion of adjacent mediastinal structures such as the aorta or tracheobronchial tree signifies a T4b lesion that is considered nonresectable. Contiguous invasion of adjacent structures may be difficult to predict by CT due to its limited spatial resolution.

The normal esophageal wall is usually less than 3 mm thick at CT (11), and is considered abnormal if it is greater than 5 mm (12). Asymmetric and eccentric thickening of the esophageal wall is considered abnormal and concerning for malignancy and warrants further evaluation with endoscopy. CT is also limited in determining the exact depth of tumor infiltration of the esophageal wall, thus cannot differentiate between T1, T2, and T3 disease (13). However, CT can reliably exclude T4 disease, which is indicated by the loss of fat planes between the esophagus and adjacent mediastinal structures and displacement or indentation of adjacent structures (13). Aortic invasion is suggested if the angle of contact of the tumor and aorta is greater than 90° or if there is obliteration of the triangular fat space between the esophagus, aorta, and spine adjacent to the primary tumor (14). Multiplanar reformats (MPR) help to accurately quantify the craniocaudal extent of disease and are superior to axial images in assessing gastroesophageal junction (GEJ) tumors (15, 16). Multiplanar reformats can also help evaluate tracheo-bronchial fistulas. Pericardial invasion is suspected if pericardial thickening, pericardial effusion, or indentation of the heart with loss of the pericardial fat plane is seen (17). The reported sensitivity and specificity of CT for detecting mediastinal invasion in patients with esophageal cancer are 88–100% and 85–100%, respectively (14–17).

Although loss of fat planes can be useful in predicting invasion of adjacent structures, obliteration of subcutaneous fat in cachectic patients and evidence of prior inflammation and radiation therapy can confound this advantage.

Nodes that are larger than 1 cm in short-axis dimension are considered suspicious for metastatic disease, however size is known to be an insensitive parameter for determining nodal spread as micrometastases can be present in subcentimeter nodes and vice versa.

CT is also the modality of choice for evaluation for pulmonary nodules, and osseous metastases. Contrast-enhanced CT remains the mainstay in imaging patients with esophageal cancer to rule out hepatic metastases.

## Magnetic resonance imaging

Magnetic resonance imaging has a limited role in staging esophageal tumors due to poor signal-to-noise ratio and cannot reliably distinguish the different layers of the esophageal wall, which is crucial for accurate local staging. Its developing role, in its investigational phase, is the evaluation of therapeutic effectiveness using dynamic contrast-enhanced MRI (DCE-MRI).

## Endoscopic ultrasound

Endoscopic ultrasound (EUS) is considered the imaging modality of choice in assessing the T stage in esophageal cancer. The esophageal wall is visualized as five alternating layers of differing echogenicity, allowing accurate pre-operative determination of the depth of tumor invasion. The first layer is hyperechoic and represents the interface between the balloon and superficial mucosa. The second layer is hypoechoic and represents the lamina propria and muscularis mucosae. The third layer is hyperechoic and represents the submucosa. The fourth layer is hypoechoic and represents the muscularis propria. The fifth layer is hyperechoic and represents the interface between the serosa and surrounding tissues.

Endoscopic ultrasound can help to accurately diagnose T staging as follows: 75–82% for T1, 64–82% for T2, 89–94% for T3, and 88–100% for T4 disease (18, 19). EUS has been found to be more accurate than CT; in studies comparing both techniques for pre-operative T staging, the reported accuracies range from 76–89% versus 49–59% (20–22). Recent advances in technology and with the advent of high-frequency probes, it is now possible to distinguish mucosal (T1m) from submucosal (T1sm) invasion (23, 24) which is critical in identifying tumors suitable for ablative photodynamic therapy or endoscopic mucosal resection.

EUS relies on size greater than 10 mm, echo characteristics such as a homogeneous and hypoechoic central echo patterns and a clear border to help identify lymph node metastases (22). The technique is superior to CT to detect lymph node metastases, with a pre-operative accuracy for N staging ranging from 72% to 80%, compared with CT, with accuracies ranging from 46% to 58% (21, 22). The sensitivity and specificity of EUS in detecting lymph node metastases is location dependent, and EUS is better for the assessment of celiac than mediastinal lymph nodes (25, 26). EUS-guided fine-needle aspiration is the optimal modality for the detection and evaluation of the primary tumor and regional lymph node metastasis as an adjunct to imaging findings. It potentiates the value of EUS, especially in the region of the celiac axis (27–29).

The main disadvantage of EUS is that it is operator dependent; hence the accuracy is prone to significant interobserver variability confounded by the experience of the operator. Moreover, EUS does not play a role in the evaluation of distant metastases, and cannot be performed in stenotic tumors; additionally it carries a risk of perforation if synchronous dilatation is performed.

## FDG-PET and PET/CT of esophageal carcinoma

The value of PET imaging centers on its ability to assess tumoral biologic behavior regardless of lesion size and shape. Hybrid imaging modalities such as PET/CT capitalize on the superior anatomical detail provided by CT complemented by the biological significance of the findings detected in the PET images. In this manner the hardware-fused image affords higher accuracy and confidence in image interpretation when compared with PET or CT alone, or to mentally fused functional and anatomic images displayed side-by-side. In fact, it is now well known that the fused anatomo-metabolic product overcomes the limitations of either modality alone.

FDG-PET and PET/CT imaging of esophageal cancer have proven to be superior to other imaging modalities to assess the extent of disease in one whole body pass. They are also powerful tools used to clarify the significance of high FDG uptake in otherwise normal structures. These imaging techniques have improved the non-invasive characterization of the benign or malignant nature of esophageal lesions; the guidance of biopsy procedures to metabolically active tumor in order to minimize sampling errors (see Chapter 20); the assessment of the prognostic value of the metabolic T status; the detection of distant metastatic disease and recurrence; and the assessment of the anatomo-metabolic tumoral response to cancer therapy.

## Diagnosis and T status

Most esophageal cancers are highly FDG avid. Squamous cell cancers tend to take up more FDG than adenocarcinomas. However, when one considers the fact that many inflammatory lesions (i.e., esophagitis) can be FDG avid as well, and that lesions smaller than 6–8 mm might go undetected by PET, it becomes evident that PET is not the imaging modality of choice to diagnose esophageal cancer.

Kato *et al.* (30) studied 149 consecutive patients with esophageal cancer to assess the value of FDG-PET compared with computed tomography (CT) for the detection of lymph node involvement and the presence of distant metastases. The investigators reported that FDG avidity by the primary tumor was detected in 80% of the patients. Of these, 81 underwent surgical resection and FDG uptake was present in 41% of T1 lesions, 83% of T2 tumors, and 97% of T3 lesions, compared with 100% of T4 tumors.

FDG images have low intrinsic spatial resolution and therefore they do not provide or add much to the assessment of esophageal wall invasion in order to assign the correct T status of the lesion. Little and colleagues (31) studied 58 patients with superficial esophageal malignancies to assess the value of FDG-PET/CT to characterize the T stage and to differentiate Tis (high-grade dysplasia) from T1 lesions. The authors reported that increased FDG uptake correlated with increasing tumor depth in 45% of Tis cases compared with 69% of T1 lesions. However, FDG imaging could not distinguish between the two T stages, and they concluded that the technique is not indicated to stage superficial esophageal cancer.

As previously discussed in this chapter, EUS remains the modality of choice in this setting.

## Prognostic value of the primary tumor's metabolic activity

Kato and colleagues (32) compared Glut-1 expression with clinic-pathologic variables in 95 patients with esophageal cancer and found significant correlations between Glut-1 expression and tumor status ($P < 0.001$), N status ($P < 0.05$), M status ($P < 0.01$), and pathological stage ($P < 0.001$). Patients with Glut-1-positive tumors had significantly lower survival rates than patients with Glut-1-negative tumors (log-rank $P < 0.05$).

FDG uptake in primary esophageal lesions is a function of the number of cancer cells, cellular proliferation and tumor growth, and the expression of GLUT receptors, all of which have been correlated with poor outcome. To this end, investigators have studied the prognostic value of FDG uptake in primary esophageal tumors in patients without metastatic disease. Overexpression of glucose transporter 1 (GLUT-1) correlates with higher FDG uptake in esophageal cancer, with higher rates of tumor recurrence after treatment, and with poor prognosis (32, 33). For example, the SUVmax of squamous cell carcinomas has been shown to be a significant predictor of progression-free survival. Similarly the pre-operative SUVmax of adenocarcinomas is predictive of outcome after esophageal adenocarcinoma resection. Therefore, the available evidence tends to support the concept that high FDG uptake in histologically proven esophageal cancer could be used as a complementary variable for risk stratification and to identify patients who could benefit from neoadjuvant therapy prior to tumor resection (34). Furthermore, the results from a retrospective study of 50 patients with adenocarcinoma of the esophagus confirmed that esophageal tumor SUVmax predicts overall survival as well (35).

## Nodal status

FDG-PET does not increase the accuracy of EUS for locoregional nodal staging, and the latter remains the primary modality to assess, and when combined with EUS-guided fine-needle aspiration, to biopsy regional lymph nodes.

van Westreenen and colleagues (36) reported their results of a systematic review of the literature to evaluate the diagnostic performance of FDG-PET during the pre-operative staging of patients with esophageal cancer. Twelve studies were included in their meta-analysis. The pooled sensitivity and specificity for the detection of locoregional nodal disease were 51% (95% CI, 34–69%) and 84% (95% CI, 76–91%), respectively.

The sensitivity of FDG-PET to assess regional lymph nodes is limited for the following reasons: (1) nodal size: metabolically active micrometastatic disease may not be resolved due to the limited intrinsic spatial resolution of the PET or PET/CT scanner; (2) FDG activity in the primary tumor may obscure nodal uptake, especially when the nodes are located in close proximity to it; and (3) the number of affected peri-esophageal nodes may not be possible to be assessed by PET, due to the reasons discussed above.

Most studies conducted to evaluate the value of FDG imaging to stage the locoregional lymph nodes in esophageal cancer patients were performed using dedicated PET scanners. Recently Kato *et al.* (37) published their results of a study to assess the contribution of FDG-PET/CT compared with PET alone to evaluate the N status during the initial staging of 167 consecutive patients with squamous cell carcinomas of the esophagus that were treated with radical esophagectomy. For individual nodal group evaluation, PET/CT's sensitivity, specificity, accuracy, positive predictive value (PPV), and negative predictive value (NPV) were 46.0%, 99.4%, 95.1%, 87.0%, and 95.5%, respectively. On the other hand, PET had 32.9% sensitivity, 98.9% specificity, 93.1% accuracy, 74.7% PPV and 93.9% NPV. The authors concluded that the sensitivity and accuracy of PET/CT were significantly higher than those of dedicated PET, and that PET/CT had a higher sensitivity in lower thoracic regions compared with PET alone and CT. Lymph node staging (N0 vs. N1) was not significantly different, but staging per lymph nodal group was significantly better with PET/CT. More studies are needed to elucidate the advantages offered by PET/CT over dedicated PET in this setting. Until then, EUS remains the modality of choice to assess N stage in esophageal cancer patients.

## Metastasis status

Once esophageal cancer metastases are confirmed further staging is unnecessary. In fact, the poor long-term survival of esophageal cancer patients treated surgically is in part related to failure to detect distant metastases before treatment.

Endoscopic ultrasound and CT imaging of the chest and abdomen are typically performed to detect metastases. However, as has already been reported in almost every other tumor type, FDG-PET imaging is more accurate than conventional imaging modalities for the detection of non-regional lymphatic and hematogenous metastases from esophageal cancer.

In a study of 74 esophageal cancer patients, Flamen and co-investigators (38) showed that FDG-PET was more accurate (84%) than CT and EUS combined (64%) to detect distant metastatic disease. Moreover, FDG-PET provided additional diagnostic value by correctly upstaging 11 (15%) and downstaging 5 (7%) patients.

van Westreenen's meta-analysis (36) showed that the pooled sensitivity and specificity of FDG-PET for the detection of distant metastatic disease were 67% (95% CI, 58–76%) and 97% (95% CI, 90–100%), respectively.

Accurate M staging is of utmost importance in esophageal cancer, because its detection prevents patients from undergoing futile surgical procedures. Block and colleagues (39) showed that FDG-PET imaging detected distant metastases in patients who were initially considered to have resectable disease based on conventional staging. FDG-PET identified metastatic disease in all 17 patients, whereas CT was positive for metastases in only five. Histopathology results were consistent with lymph node metastases in 21 patients. PET was positive in 11 patients of these cases and CT only in six.

In contrast to the results described above, van Westreenen et al. (40) recently argued that although FDG-PET improves the selection of patients with esophageal cancer in need of curative surgery, this benefit is limited (only in 3% of their cohort) if the study is performed after a comprehensive diagnostic work-up that includes multidetector CT, EUS, and sonography of the neck.

## Recurrent disease

Law and colleagues (41) in their seminal paper described the patterns of disease recurrence observed in a study of 108 patients who had undergone curative surgery for squamous cell cancer of the thoracic esophagus. Recurrence was confirmed in 52% of the patients within a period of 2 years. Extrathoracic recurrence occurred in 41% of patients in contrast to 25% who recurred within the thoracic cavity. Systemic organ metastases were present in 26% and 11% recurred in the cervical lymph nodes. Although pre-operative chemotherapy lowered the recurrence rate from 60% to 30%, survival remained the same.

The high degree of anatomic distortion following esophageal cancer treatment renders very difficult the differentiation between scar tissue and viable tumor recurrence using conventional imaging modalities. Anatomical imaging modalities often encounter indeterminate findings when attempting to characterize the presence of esophageal cancer recurrence in the post-treatment phase. FDG imaging has advantages in this setting, but not without limitations, as follows.

Flamen et al. (42) reported preliminary results comparing FDG-PET with CT and EUS for the characterization of recurrence in 41 patients treated with curative resection of cancer of the esophagus or gastroesophageal junction. A total of 33 patients had nine perianastomotic, 12 regional and 19 distant recurrent lesions. Conventional imaging (CI) was more accurate to diagnose perianastomotic lesions (96% vs. 74% for PET), because of the high rate of false-positive PET findings in progressive anastomotic stenosis requiring repetitive endoscopic dilatation. On the other hand, PET was more sensitive (94% vs. 81% for CI) and accurate (87% vs. 81% for CI) and as specific (82%) compared with conventional modalities, for the diagnosis of regional and distant recurrences. Furthermore, PET provided additional information in 27% of the cases allowing for prompt and more successful management.

Similar results were obtained with FDG-PET/CT. Guo et al. (43) evaluated the role of FDG-PET/CT in 56 patients with suspicion of recurrent squamous cell carcinoma of the esophagus. The overall PET/CT sensitivity was 93.1%, with a specificity of 75.7%, and an accuracy of 87.2%. There were nine false-positive and five false-negative results. The specificity was lower at local sites of recurrence due to a high incidence of false-positive findings at the level of the anastomosis.

A recent PET/CT study conducted in 20 patients with suspicion of esophageal cancer recurrence, confirmed previous results by showing that FDG-PET/CT was true positive in 11 patients, false-positive in three and true-negative in six. The overall accuracy was 85%, with a negative predictive value of 100%, and a positive predictive value of 78.6%. False-positive findings occurred in chronic inflammation of mediastinal lymph nodes and in the anastomoses. PET/CT demonstrated distant metastasis in 10 patients. Management was changed in 12 (60%) patients due to the PET/CT results (44).

Based on the available evidence and until more clinical data are accrued, it seems appropriate to consider that FDG-PET and PET/

CT play a complementary role to conventional imaging modalities for the characterization of esophageal cancer recurrence.

## Monitoring response to therapy

Pre-operative chemotherapy or concurrent chemoradiation are standard treatment options before resection (45–47). The aim of neoadjuvant treatment is to attempt to control both local and distant disease. Patients who respond to these therapies have a better prognosis after surgery than those who do not (48, 49). An insufficient objective response is achieved in a good number of patients who do not benefit from neoadjuvant therapy, and subsequently they are placed at risk of treatment-related toxicities. Currently, there is no universally accepted and reliable method to monitor response of esophageal cancer to neoadjuvant therapy, and the most accurate means of determining treatment effect has been esophagectomy followed by histopathologic assessment.

Response to therapy is currently assessed with CT and EUS (50, 51). Radiologic assessment of lesion response to therapy is based on a measurable reduction in tumor size or in the number of malignant lesions during and after treatment. In this setting the major assumption is that the agent used for treatment is cytotoxic, leading to cell death and reduction in tumor bulk, and therefore to a reduction in the size of lesions. Routinely used clinical staging methods are not able to accurately differentiate viable tumor from inflammation, or from scar tissue induced by treatment, even in the presence of a confirmed histopathological response (52, 53).

Newer anti-cancer drugs have been developed with cytostatic mechanisms of action, where a reduction in the size of tumors is not necessarily expected initially (54). Thus, conventional imaging techniques alone are unsuitable to assess the effect of these agents, and therefore, other methods capable of evaluating tumor metabolic and biologic response are needed. As described throughout this book and in the oncologic literature, functional imaging using FDG-PET has facilitated the non-invasive evaluation of tumor pathophysiology, metabolism, and proliferation in vivo. In fact, alterations in tissue metabolism that generally precede morphologic change are reflected and captured by FDG-PET imaging. Treated malignant tissue may have reduced FDG activity because of both cell death and lower metabolism. Therefore, in most instances, FDG-PET is able to detect metabolic changes independently of the type of drug (cytotoxic or cytostatic) being used. Several preliminary studies using FDG-PET in the post-chemoradiation setting for esophageal cancer patients have been published demonstrating strong associations between an FDG-PET-based response, histologic response, and improved overall survival (55–70).

In the setting of response to treatment, FDG-PET has been evaluated using various methodologies, ranging from visual assessment, semi-quantitative indices of uptake [e.g., SUVmax or SUVavg, before or after treatment, delta SUV (30–50% change from baseline), tumor/background SUV ratios], to full kinetic analysis of FDG uptake (66). Metabolic changes between baseline and post-therapeutic FDG-PET have been shown to be useful for the evaluation of response to therapy in esophageal cancer patients (55–60). However, the degree of correlation between a reduction in tumor FDG uptake before and after therapy, and histopathologic response, remains controversial (55–65, 68). Some studies have shown a good correlation (55–60, 68) while others have not (61–65). These incongruent findings could be due to differences in study design (timing to image after therapy, FDG uptake time after injection, type of therapy, and differences in defining the pathologic response criteria), in the grading of the post-therapeutic inflammatory process, and in the tumor metabolic characteristics.

Whatever the reasons are, the reader should keep in mind that a reduction of tumoral FDG uptake after treatment is indicative of response to therapy and that it has prognostic value. Yet more importantly is that the sooner the normalization or reduction in FDG uptake occurs, the higher the probability that cure will be achieved, and therefore, the best indication of a favorable outcome. Furthermore, the sensitivity of the technique is affected by its limitation to resolve microscopic residual disease after treatment despite it being metabolically active. Its specificity is also less than perfect, as the degree of uptake observed after treatment is influenced by active inflammatory cells, especially after radiotherapy (68, 71). We have observed an inverse correlation between the number of inflammatory cells and residual viable cells in the tumor bed. This inverse relationship was almost linear and contributed to a wide range of percent changes in SUVmax and SUVavg after therapy (68). Therefore, the change in tumor FDG uptake between scans should be taken with caution, especially in patients where the post-therapeutic scan was performed after radiation therapy (68).

The cases that follow will highlight and apply the concepts that have been discussed about the role of PET and PET/CT in the management of patients with esophageal cancer.

## References

1. Siegel R, Ward E, Brawley O, Jemal A. Cancer statistics 2011: the impact of eliminating socioeconomic and racial disparities on premature cancer deaths. *CA Cancer J Clin* 2011; **61**:212–36.

2. Kobori O, Kirihara Y, Kosaka N, Hara T. Positron emission tomography of esophageal carcinoma using 11 C-choline and 18 F-fluorodeoxyglucose. *Cancer* 1999;**86**:1638–48.

3. Block MI, Patterson GA, Sundaresan RS *et al.* Improvement in staging of esophageal cancer with the addition of positron emission tomography. *Ann Thorac Surg* 1997;**64**:770–7.

4. Greene F, Fritz A, Balch C *et al.* (Eds.) *AJCC Cancer Staging Handbook Part III: Digestive System 9 – Esophagus.* 6th Edn. New York, NY: Springer-Verlag, 2002.

5. Iyer RB, Silverman PM, Tamm EP, Dunnington JS, DuBrow RA.

Diagnosis, staging, and follow-up of esophageal cancer. *Am J Roentgenol* 2003;**181**:785–93.

6. Edge SB, Byrd DR, Compton CC et al. (Eds.) Esophagus and esophagogastric junction. In *AJCC Cancer Staging Manual*. 7th Edn. New York, NY: Springer, 2010, pp. 103–115.

7. Iizuka T, Isono K, Kakegawa T et al. Parameters linked to ten-year survival in Japan of resected esophageal carcinoma. Japanese Committee for Registration of Esophageal Carcinoma Cases. *Chest* 1989;**96**(5):1005–11.

8. Korst RJ, Rusch VW, Venkatraman E et al. Proposed revision of the staging classification for esophageal cancer. *J Thorac Cardiovasc Surg* 1998;**115**(3):660–9; discussion 669–70.

9. Enzinger PC, Mayer RJ. Esophageal cancer. *N Engl J Med* 2003; **349**:2241–52.

10. Levine MS. Esophageal cancer radiologic diagnosis. *Radiol Clin North Am* 1997;**35**:265–79.

11. Noh HM, Fishman EK, Forastiere AA, Bliss DF, Calhoun PS. CT of the esophagus: spectrum of disease with emphasis on esophageal carcinoma. *RadioGraphics* 1995;**15**:1113–34.

12. Desai RK, Tagliabue JR, Wegryn SA, Einstein DM. CT evaluation of wall thickening in the alimentary tract. *RadioGraphics* 1991;**11**:771–83.

13. Rice TW. Clinical staging of esophageal carcinoma. CT, EUS, and PET. *Chest Surg Clin North Am* 2000;**10**:471–85.

14. Picus D, Balfe DM, Koehler RE, Roper CL, Owen JW. Computed tomography in the staging of esophageal carcinoma. *Radiology* 1983;**146**:433–8.

15. Wakelin SJ, Deans C, Crofts TJ et al. A comparison of computerised tomography, laparoscopic ultrasound and endoscopic ultrasound in the preoperative staging of oesophago-gastric carcinoma. *Eur J Radiol* 2002;**41**:161–7.

16. Wallace MB, Nietert PJ, Earle C et al. An analysis of multiple staging management strategies for carcinoma of the esophagus: computed tomography, endoscopic ultrasound, positron emission tomography, and thoracoscopy. *Ann Thorac Surg* 2002;**74**(4):1026–32.

17. Daffner RH, Halber MD, Postlethwait RW, Korobkin M, Thompson WM. CT of the esophagus. II. Carcinoma. *Am J Roentgenol* 1979;**133**:1051–5.

18. Reed CE, Eloubeidi MA. New techniques for staging esophageal cancer. *Surg Clin North Am* 2002;**82**:697–710.

19. Saunders HS, Wolfman NT, Ott DJ. Esophageal cancer: radiologic staging. *Radiol Clin North Am* 1997;**35**:281–94.

20. Hordijk ML, Zander H, van Blankenstein M, Tilanus HW. Influence of tumor stenosis on the accuracy of endosonography in preoperative T staging of esophageal cancer. *Endoscopy* 1993;**25**:171–5.

21. Kalantzis N, Kallimanis G, Laoudi F, Papavasiliou E, Gabriel G. Endoscopic ultrasonography and computed tomography in preoperative (TNM) classification of oesophageal carcinoma [abstr]. *Endoscopy* 1992;**24**(suppl):653.

22. Tio TL, Cohen P, Coene PP, Udding J, den Hartog Jager FC, Tytgat GN. Endosonography and computed tomography of esophageal carcinoma: preoperative classification compared to the new (1987) TNM system. *Gastroenterology* 1989;**96**:1478–86.

23. Hasegawa N, Niwa Y, Arisawa T et al. Preoperative staging of superficial esophageal carcinoma: comparison of an ultra-sound probe and standard endoscopic ultrasonography. *Gastrointest Endosc* 1996;**44**:388–93.

24. Murata Y, Suzuki S, Ohta M et al. Small ultrasonic probes for determination of the depth of superficial esophageal cancer. *Gastrointest Endosc* 1996;**44**:23–8.

25. Catalano MF, Alcocer E, Chak A et al. Evaluation of metastatic celiac axis lymph nodes in patients with esophageal carcinoma: accuracy of EUS. *Gastrointest Endosc* 1999; **50**: 352–6.

26. Lightdale CJ, Kulkarni KG. Role of endoscopic ultrasonography in the staging and follow-up of esophageal cancer. *J Clin Oncol* 2005;**23**:4483–9.

27. Parmar KS, Zwischenberger JB, Reeves AL, Waxman I. Clinical impact of endoscopic ultrasound-guided fine needle aspiration of celiac axis lymph nodes (M1a disease) in esophageal cancer. *Ann Thorac Surg* 2002;**73**:916–20.

28. Puli SR, Reddy JB, Bechtold ML et al. Staging accuracy of esophageal cancer by endoscopic ultrasound: a meta-analysis and systematic review. *World J Gastroenterol* 2008;**14**(10):1479–90.

29. van Vliet EP, Heijenbrok-Kal MH, Hunink MG et al. Staging investigations for oesophageal cancer: a meta-analysis. *Br J Cancer* 2008; **98**(3):547–57.

30. Kato H, Miyazaki T, Nakajima M et al. The incremental effect of positron emission tomography on diagnostic accuracy in the initial staging of esophageal carcinoma. *Cancer* 2005;**103**(1):148–56.

31. Little SG, Rice TW, Bybel B et al. Is FDG-PET indicated for superficial esophageal cancer? *Eur J Cardiothorac Surg* 2007;**31**(5):791–6.

32. Kato H, Takita J, Miyazaki T et al. Glut-1 glucose transporter expression in esophageal squamous cell carcinoma is associated with tumor aggressiveness. *Anticancer Res* 2002;**22**(5):2635–9.

33. Kato H, Takita J, Miyazaki T et al. Correlation of 18-F-fluorodeoxyglucose (FDG) accumulation with glucose transporter (Glut-1) expression in esophageal squamous cell carcinoma. *Anticancer Res* 2003;**23**:3263–72.

34. Shenfine J, Barbour AP, Wong D et al. Prognostic value of maximum standardized uptake values from preoperative positron emission tomography in resectable adenocarcinoma of the esophagus treated by surgery alone. *Dis Esophagus* 2009;**22**(8):668–75.

35. Rizk N, Downey RJ, Akhurst T et al. Preoperative 18[F]-fluorodeoxyglucose positron emission tomography standardized uptake values predict survival after esophageal adenocarcinoma resection. *Ann Thorac Surg* 2006;**81**(3):1076–81.

36. van Westreenen HL, Westerterp M, Bossuyt PM et al. Systematic review of the staging performance of 18F-fluorodeoxyglucose positron emission tomography in esophageal cancer. *J Clin Oncol* 2004;**22**(18):3805–12.

37. Kato H, Kimura H, Nakajima M et al. The additional value of integrated PET/CT over PET in initial lymph node staging of esophageal cancer. *Oncol Rep* 2008;**20**(4):857–62.

38. Flamen P, Lerut A, Van Cutsem E et al. Utility of positron emission tomography for the staging of patients with potentially operable esophageal carcinoma. *J Clin Oncol* 2000;**18**:3202–10.

39. Block MI, Patterson GA, Sundaresan RS et al. Improvement in staging of esophageal cancer with the addition of positron emission tomography. *Ann*

*Thorac Surg* 1997;**64**(3):770–6; (discussion 776–7).

40. van Westreenen HL, Westerterp M, Sloof GW *et al.* Limited additional value of positron emission tomography in staging oesophageal cancer. *Br J Surg* 2007;**94**(12):1515–20.

41. Law SY, Fok M, Wong J. Pattern of recurrence after oesophageal resection for cancer: clinical implications. *Br J Surg* 1996;**83**(1):107–11.

42. Flamen P, Lerut A, Van Cutsem E *et al.* The utility of positron emission tomography for the diagnosis and staging of recurrent esophageal cancer. *J Thorac Cardiovasc Surg* 2000;**120**(6):1085–92.

43. Guo H, Zhu H, Xi Y *et al.* Diagnostic and prognostic value of 18F-FDG PET/CT for patients with suspected recurrence from squamous cell carcinoma of the esophagus. *J Nucl Med* 2007;**48**(8):1251–8.

44. Sun L, Su XH, Guan YS *et al.* Clinical usefulness of 18F-FDG PET/CT in the restaging of esophageal cancer after surgical resection and radiotherapy. *World J Gastroenterol* 2009;**15**:1836–42.

45. Sagar PM, Gauperaa T, Sue-Ling H *et al.* An audit of the treatment of cancer of the oesophagus. *Gut* 1994;**35**:941–5.

46. Hulscher JB, Tijssen JG, Obertop H *et al.* Transthoracic versus transhiatal resection for carcinoma of the esophagus: a meta-analysis. *Ann Thorac Surg* 2001;**72**:306–13.

47. Chung SC, Stuart RC, Li AK. Surgical therapy for squamous-cell carcinoma of the oesophagus. *Lancet* 1994;**343**:521–4.

48. Bosset JF, Gignoux M, Triboulet JP *et al.* Chemoradiotherapy followed by surgery compared with surgery alone in squamous-cell cancer of the esophagus. *N Engl J Med* 1997;**337**:161–7.

49. Swisher SG, Ajani JA, Komaki R *et al.* Long-term outcome of phase II trial evaluating chemotherapy, chemoradiotherapy, and surgery for locoregionally advanced esophageal cancer. *Int J Radiat Oncol Biol Phys* 2003;**57**:120–7.

50. Wolfman NT, Scharling ES, Chen MY. Esophageal squamous carcinoma. *Radiol Clin North Am* 1994;**32**:1183–201.

51. Van Dam J. Endosonographic evaluation of the patient with esophageal cancer. *Chest* 1997;**112** (suppl 4):184S–90S.

52. Zuccaro G Jr, Rice TW, Goldblum J *et al.* Endoscopic ultrasound cannot determine suitability for esophagectomy after aggressive chemoradiotherapy for esophageal cancer. *Am J Gastroenterol* 1999;**94**:906–12.

53. Jones DR, Parker LA, Detterbeck FC *et al.* Inadequacy of computed tomography in assessing patients with esophageal carcinoma after induction chemoradiotherapy. *Cancer* 1999;**85**:1026–32.

54. Rehman S, Jayson GC. Molecular imaging of antiangiogenic agents. *Oncologist* 2005;**10**:92–103.

55. Wieder HA, Brucher BL, Zimmermann F *et al.* Time course of tumor metabolic activity during chemoradiotherapy of esophageal squamous cell carcinoma and response to treatment. *J Clin Oncol* 2004;**22**:900–8.

56. Weber WA, Ott K, Becker K *et al.* Prediction of response to preoperative chemotherapy in adenocarcinomas of the esophagogastric junction by metabolic imaging. *J Clin Oncol* 2001;**19**:3058–65.

57. Brucher BL, Weber W, Bauer M *et al.* Neoadjuvant therapy of esophageal SCC: response evaluation by PET. *Ann Surg* 2001;**233**:300–9.

58. Flamen P, Van Cutsem E, Lerut A *et al.* Positron emission tomography for assessment of the response to induction radiochemotherapy in locally advanced oesophageal cancer. *Ann Oncol* 2002;**13**:361–8.

59. Downey RJ, Akhurst T, Ilson D *et al.* Whole body 18F-FDG-PET and the response of esophageal cancer to induction therapy: results of a prospective trial. *J Clin Oncol* 2003;**21**:428–32.

60. Swisher SG, Erasmus J, Maish M *et al.* 2-Fluoro-2-deoxy-D-glucose positron emission tomography imaging is predictive of pathologic response and survival after preoperative chemoradiation in patients with esophageal carcinoma. *Cancer* 2004;**101**:1776–85.

61. Song SY, Kim JH, Ryu JS *et al.* FDG PET in the prediction of pathologic response after neoadjuvant chemoradiotherapy in locally advanced resectable esophageal cancer. *Int J Radiat Oncol Biol Phys* 2005;**63**:1053–9.

62. Swisher SG, Maish M, Erasmus JJ *et al.* Utility of PET, CT, and EUS to identify pathologic responders in esophageal cancer. *Ann Thorac Surg* 2004;**78**:1152–60.

63. Kato H, Kuwano H, Nakajima M *et al.* Usefulness of PET for assessing the response of neoadjuvant chemoradiotherapy in patients with esophageal cancer. *Am J Surgery* 2002;**184**:279–83.

64. Brink I, Hentschel M, Bley TA *et al.* Effects of neoadjuvant radio-chemotherapy on 18F-FDG-PET in esophageal carcinoma. *Eur J Surg Oncol* 2004;**30**:544–50.

65. Arslan N, Miller TR, Dehdashti F *et al.* Evaluation of response to neoadjuvant therapy by quantitative FDG with PET in patients with esophageal cancer. *Mol Imag Biol* 2002;**4**;301–10.

66. Hoekstra CJ, Paglianiti I, Hoekstra OS *et al.* Monitoring response to therapy in cancer using (18F)-2-fluoro-2-deoxy-D-glucose and positron emission tomography: an overview of different analytical methods. *Eur J Nucl Med* 2000;**27**:731–43.

67. Mamede M, El Fakhri G, Abreu-e-Lima P *et al.* Pre-operative estimation of esophageal tumor metabolic length in FDG-PET images with surgical pathology confirmation. *Ann Nucl Med* 2007;**21**(10):553–62.

68. Mamede M, Abreu-E-Lima P, Oliva MR *et al.* FDG-PET/CT tumor segmentation-derived indices of metabolic activity to assess response to neoadjuvant therapy and progression-free survival in esophageal cancer: correlation with histopathology results. *Am J Clin Oncol.* 2007;**30** (4):377–88.

69. Lordick F, Ott K, Krause BJ *et al.* PET to assess early metabolic response and to guide treatment of adenocarcinoma of the oesophagogastric junction: the MUNICON phase II trial. *Lancet Oncol* 2007;**8**(9):797–805.

70. Meyer Zum Büschenfelde C, Herrmann K, Schuster T *et al.* 18F-FDG PET-guided salvage neoadjuvant radiochemotherapy of adenocarcinoma of the esophagogastric junction: *The MUNICON II Trial. J Nucl Med* 2011;**52** (8):1189–96.

71. Hautzel H, Muller-Gartner H. Early changes in fluorine-18-FDG uptake during radiotherapy. *J Nucl Med* 1997;**38**:1384–6.

A 61-year-old female with history of scleroderma and gradually worsening dysphagia for the past 12 months, was referred for a FDG-PET study to rule out malignancy.

## Acquisition and processing parameters

Whole-body PET was performed 60 min after the intravenous administration of 17.8 mCi of FDG in fasting condition. Plasma glucose levels at the time of FDG injection were 100 mg/dL. The patient was encouraged to void before scanning, and images were obtained from the head to the proximal thighs with a combined PET/CT scanner. The patient was imaged in the supine position, without any specific breath-holding instructions. The unenhanced CT scan was performed

first, from the patient's head to the proximal thighs, using the following acquisition parameters: 140 kVp, 75 mA, 0.8 s per CT rotation, pitch of 1.675 : 1, and a reconstructed slice thickness of 3.75 mm, for a total scanning time of 42.4 s. The CT data were reconstructed using a filtered back-projection algorithm and a 512 × 512 matrix, with a transaxial field of view of 50 cm. The CT images were used to generate the transmission maps for attenuation correction of the PET acquisitions and for anatomic localization.

Immediately after the CT scan, and without changing the patient's position, the tabletop moved automatically to the PET position. The emission scan was acquired starting at the mid-thighs toward the head, for six bed positions of 4 min each

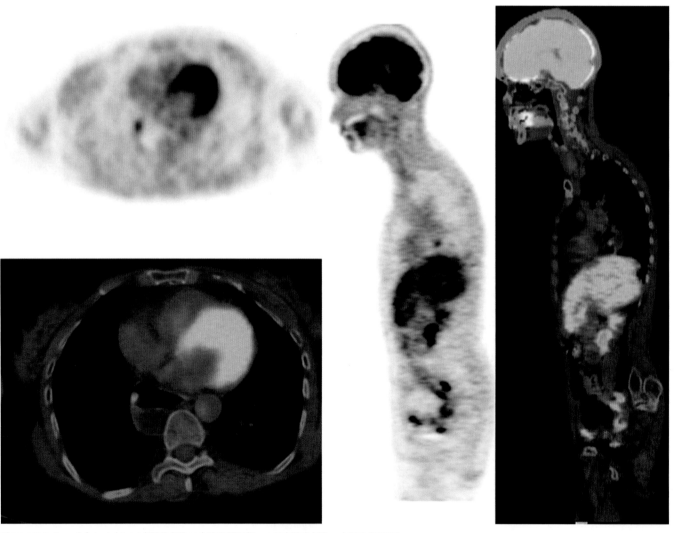

**Figure 8.1** From left to right: axial FDG-PET and FDG-PET/CT; sagittal FDG-PET and FDG-PET/CT.

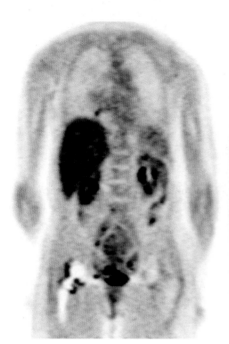 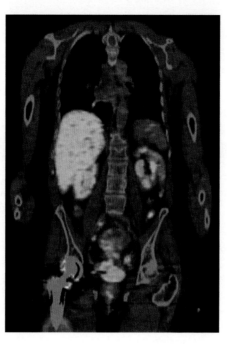

**Figure 8.2** Coronal FDG-PET and FDG-PET/CT.

(47 image planes/bed position, 15.7 cm longitudinal field of view). PET data were reconstructed using an ordered-subset expectation maximization iterative algorithm (30 subsets, 2 iterations).

## Findings and differential diagnosis

Axial and sagittal PET and PET/CT images (Figure 8.1) and coronal and fused PET/CT images (Figure 8.2) show that the esophagus is patulous and dilated with a small area of focal thickening in the right lateral wall of the distal esophagus with intense FDG uptake (SUVmax = 6). There are peripheral reticular opacities with honeycombing in both lung bases. There is no evidence of nodal or distant metastasis. There are no other sites of abnormal FDG avidity.

The finding of focal intense FDG uptake corresponding to an area of eccentric thickening is suspicious for early-stage esophageal cancer. The differential diagnosis would include esophagitis; however, its pattern tends to be linear rather than focal. Glycogenic acanthosis is included in the differential diagnosis as well. Interstitial abnormality in both lung bases represents non-specific interstitial pneumonitis in the setting of scleroderma. A patulous and dilated esophagus may be secondary to a motility disorder.

## Diagnosis and follow-up

An upper GI endoscopy revealed a small focus of intra-mucosal esophageal cancer in the distal esophagus, corresponding to the site of increased FDG uptake, which was biopsied and confirmed to be adenocarcinoma. The patient underwent three-hole esophagectomy for T1N0M0 esophageal cancer.

## Discussion and teaching points

FDG-PET is known to have higher sensitivity than CT in the detection of primary esophageal cancer (1). Focal moderate to intense endoluminal uptake raises concern for malignancy. As mentioned before, esophagitis and glycogenic acanthosis should be also considered in the differential diagnoses. Therefore, a focal area of moderate-to-intense FDG uptake with or without corresponding anatomical abnormality on CT warrants further evaluation with endoscopy and histopathological sampling to exclude esophageal cancer. Although PET and PET/CT offer little information regarding the depth of invasion, lesions' SUV values in patients with esophageal cancer tend to be quite high, and reflect the degree of metabolic activity of viable tumor cells, and can serve as a prognostic factor when stratifying survival (2). The two main histological cell types, squamous cell carcinoma and adenocarcinoma tend to have a significant difference in the SUV values. Squamous cell carcinomas tend to have higher SUV (2). Overexpression of glucose transporter 1 (GLUT-1) has been shown especially in squamous cell carcinoma and has been correlated with higher SUVs and a worse prognosis (3, 4). Higher pre-operative SUV values have been correlated with higher recurrence rates as well. Maximum SUV of 5.5 and T stage have been found to be significant prognostic predictors of disease-free survival in patients with squamous cell carcinoma lesions. Pre-operative FDG-PET SUVmax, especially in adenocarcinoma, has been correlated with outcome after esophageal adenocarcinoma resection, but remains less accurate than other post-operative prognostic variables. A high FDG-PET SUVmax could be used for risk stratification and identifying patients who are most likely to benefit from neoadjuvant therapies (5). Results from a retrospective study of 50 patients with confirmed adenocarcinoma of the esophagus, confirmed that SUVmax predicts overall survival as well (6). The investigators showed that FDG uptake in the primary lesion (in terms of SUVmax) may be used to subclassify anatomic stage into different prognostic groups based on metabolic malignancy, and as they stated: "SUVmax identifies patients who have a poor prognosis from a subset of patients that would otherwise be considered to have early-stage disease" (6).

## Take-home message

- It is essential to further evaluate any focal FDG uptake (especially those lesions that despite being small, are very hot) in the esophagus with direct visualization with endoscopy and biopsy.
- High pre-operative SUVmax of esophageal cancer lesions has been correlated with higher recurrence rates and has prognostic value.

## References

1. Block MI, Patterson GA, Sundaresan RS et al. Improvement in staging of esophageal cancer with the addition of positron emission tomography. *Ann Thorac Surg* 1997;**64**:770–7.

2. van Westreenen HL, Plukker JTM, Cobben DCP et al. Prognostic value of the standardized uptake value in esophageal cancer. *Am J Roentgenol* 2005; **185**:436–440.

3. Kato H, Takita J, Miyazaki T et al. Glut-1 glucose transporter expression in esophageal squamous cell carcinoma is associated with tumor aggressiveness. *Anticancer Res* 2002;**22**:2635–9.

4. Kato H, Takita J, Miyazaki T et al. Correlation of 18-F-fluorodeoxyglucose (FDG) accumulation with glucose transporter (Glut-1) expression in esophageal squamous cell carcinoma. *Anticancer Res* 2003;**23**:3263–72.

5. Shenfine J, Barbour AP, Wong D et al. Prognostic value of maximum standardized uptake values from preoperative positron emission tomography in resectable adenocarcinoma of the esophagus treated by surgery alone. *Dis Esophagus* 2009; **22**(8):668–75.

6. Rizk N, Downey RJ, Akhurst T et al. Preoperative 18[F]-fluorodeoxyglucose positron emission tomography standardized uptake values predict survival after esophageal adenocarcinoma resection. *Ann Thorac Surg* 2006;**81**(3):1076–81.

A 57-year-old male presented to his primary-care physician with vague sensation on swallowing in the area of the distal esophagus, but with no history of dysphagia or odynophagia. Routine laboratory values showed low ferritin level, prompting further evaluation with endoscopy. He was found to have Barrett's dysplasia in the lower esophagus and a fungating 3 cm mass at 40 cm. Biopsy revealed poorly differentiated adenocarcinoma. He was referred for a FDG-PET for staging and initial treatment strategy.

## Acquisition and processing parameters

Whole-body PET was performed 60 min after the intravenous administration of 21.7 mCi of FDG after fasting for 4 hours. Plasma glucose levels at the time of FDG injection were 96 mg/dL. The patient was encouraged to void before scanning, and images were obtained from the head to the proximal thighs with a combined PET/CT scanner. The patient was imaged in the supine position, without any specific breath-holding instructions. The unenhanced CT scan was performed first, from the patient's head to the proximal thighs, using the following acquisition parameters: 140 kVp, 75 mA, 0.8 s per CT rotation, pitch of 1.675 : 1, and a reconstructed slice thickness of 3.75 mm, for a total scanning time of 42.4 s. The CT data were reconstructed using a filtered back-projection algorithm and a 512 × 512 matrix, with a transaxial field of view of 50 cm. The CT images were used to generate the transmission maps for attenuation correction of the PET acquisitions and for anatomic localization.

Immediately after the CT scan, and without changing the patient's position, the tabletop moved automatically to the PET position. The emission scan was acquired starting at the mid-thighs toward the head, for six bed positions of 4 min each (47 image planes/bed position, 15.7 cm longitudinal field of view). PET data were reconstructed using an ordered-subset expectation maximization iterative algorithm (30 subsets, 2 iterations).

## Findings and differential diagnosis

PET and PET/CT images show intense FDG uptake corresponding to the thickening of the distal esophagus, which

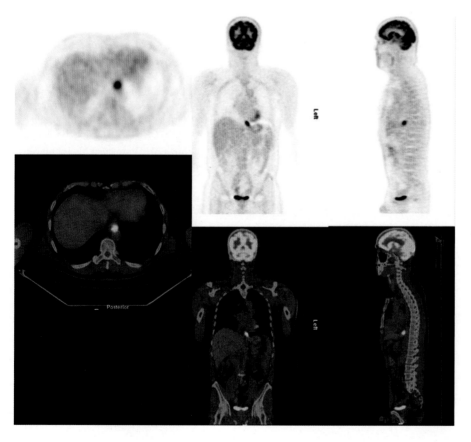

**Figure 8.3** Top row: axial, coronal, and sagittal FDG-PET. Bottom row: corresponding axial, coronal, and sagittal FDG-PET/CT fused images.

measures $2.4 \times 2.0$ cm and cranio-caudally extends from below the level of the left atrium to the gastric cardia. There is no anatomo-metabolic evidence of metastatic disease.

## Diagnosis and follow-up

The patient underwent endoscopic staging of his poorly differentiated adenocarcinoma and was staged as T2N1. In addition, one peri-esophageal lymph node was positive for adenocarcinoma metastasis, but did not have abnormal uptake on PET and was not enlarged by CT criteria. The patient was referred for neo-adjuvant chemoradiotherapy. Post-treatment FDG-PET (not shown) demonstrated interval decrease in FDG uptake in the distal esophagus, and no new sites of disease. He then underwent three-hole esophagectomy and a gastric pull-up.

## Discussion and teaching points

Barrett's esophagus is thought to be an adaptation to chronic acid exposure from reflux esophagitis (1). The progression of Barrett's metaplasia to adenocarcinoma correlates with changes in gene structure and expression, as well as structural protein changes (2). The most common somatic genetic changes include loss of p16 and p53 tumor suppressor genes, and also loss of APC, Rb and DCC, aneuploidy, and other cell-cycle abnormalities (2, 3). However, as it stands today, no single molecular marker can predict who will and who will not progress to cancer from Barrett's esophagus. The histology

of Barrett's esophagus is classified into four general categories: non-dysplastic, low-grade dysplasia, high-grade dysplasia, and frank carcinoma. High-grade dysplasia and frank carcinoma patients are recommended surgical treatment. Non-dysplastic and low-grade patients undergo annual observation with endoscopy (4). Ninety percent of patients initially presenting with Barrett's carcinoma have locally advanced disease on endoscopic surveillance (5). Pre-operative chemotherapy increases the chances of a curative resection in patients who respond to therapy. Barrett's esophagus presents as diffuse distal esophageal thickening on CT and moderate to intense focal or linear uptake on FDG-PET (6–8). Considering that Barrett's esophagitis is a pre-malignant condition, it is reasonable to recommend endoscopic correlation in patients with moderate to intense focal or linear esophageal uptake.

## Take-home message

- Linear uptake on FDG-PET is seen in esophagitis. However, since Barrett's esophagus is a pre-malignant condition, further evaluation with endoscopy is recommended for all patients presenting with linear or focal uptake with or without esophageal thickening on FDG-PET/CT.
- Endoscopic ultrasound is a strong adjunct to FDG-PET to stage Barrett's carcinoma, especially in those cases with normal size and metabolically negative nodes harboring tumor.

## References

1. Stein H, Siewert J. Barrett's esophagus: pathogenesis, epidemiology, functional abnormalities, malignant degeneration, and surgical management. *Dysphagia* 1993;**8**(3):276.

2. Dolan K, Garde J, Walker SJ et al. LOH at the sites of the DCC, APC, and TP53 tumor suppressor genes occurs in Barrett's metaplasia and dysplasia adjacent to adenocarcinoma of the esophagus. *Hum Pathol* 1999; **30**(12):1508–14.

3. Wijnhoven BP, Tilanus HW, Dinjens WN. Molecular biology of Barrett's adenocarcinoma. *Ann Surg* 2001; **233**(3):322–37.

4. Shaheen NJ, Richter JE. Barrett's oesophagus. *Lancet* 2009; **373**(9666):850–61.

5. Schauer M, Knoefel WT. Neoadjuvant chemotherapy in Barrett's carcinoma – prognosis and response prediction. *Anticancer Res* 2010;**30**(4):1065–70.

6. Bakheet SM, Amin T, Alia AG, Kuzo R, Powe J. F-18 FDG uptake in benign esophageal disease. *Clin Nucl Med* 1999;**24**(12):995–7.

7. Neto CA, Zhuang H, Ghesani N, Alavi A. Detection of Barrett's esophagus superimposed by esophageal cancer by FDG positron emission tomography. *Clin Nucl Med* 2001;**26**(12):1060.

8. Kamel EM, Thumshirn M, Truninger K et al. Significance of incidental 18F-FDG accumulations in the gastrointestinal tract in PET/CT: correlation with endoscopic and histopathologic results. *J Nucl Med* 2004;**45**(11):1804–10.

# Esophageal carcinoma with loco-regional metastasis

A 64-year-old male with a history of intermittent dysphagia for 10 years with progressive worsening over the last 12 months. Initial endoscopy showed a diffusely thickened lower esophagus and the biopsy was positive for malignant cells. Patient was referred for FDG-PET for initial treatment planning.

## Acquisition and processing parameters

Whole-body PET was performed 60 min after the intravenous administration of 19.7 mCi of FDG in fasting conditions. Plasma glucose levels at the time of FDG injection were 132 mg/dL. The patient was encouraged to void before scanning, and images were obtained from the head to the proximal thighs with a combined PET/CT scanner. The patient was imaged in the supine position, without any specific breath-holding instructions. The unenhanced CT scan was performed

first, from the patient's head to the proximal thighs, using the following acquisition parameters: 140 kVp, 75 mA, 0.8 s per CT rotation, pitch of 1.675 : 1, and a reconstructed slice thickness of 3.75 mm, for a total scanning time of 42.4 s. The CT data were reconstructed using a filtered back-projection algorithm and a 512 × 512 matrix, with a transaxial field of view of 50 cm. The CT images were used to generate the transmission maps for attenuation correction of the PET acquisitions and for anatomic localization.

Immediately after the CT scan, and without changing the patient's position, the tabletop moved automatically to the PET position. The emission scan was acquired starting at the mid-thighs toward the head, for six bed positions of 4 min each (47 image planes/bed position, 15.7 cm longitudinal field of view). PET data were reconstructed using an ordered-subset expectation maximization iterative algorithm (30 subsets, 2 iterations).

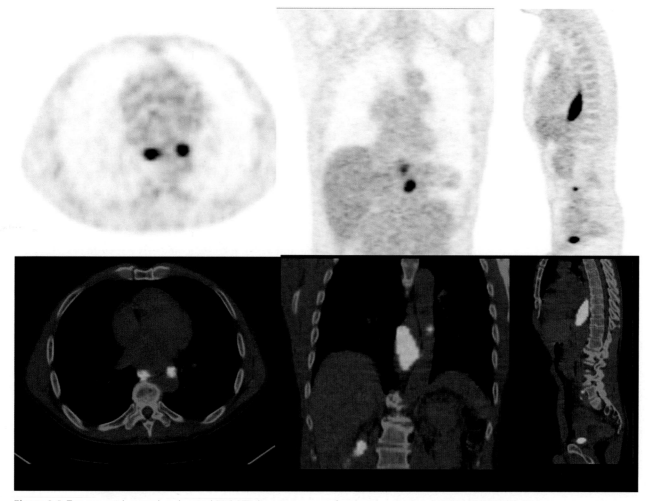

**Figure 8.4** Top row: axial, coronal, and sagittal FDG-PET slices. Bottom row: fused axial, coronal, and sagittal FDG-PET/CT slices.

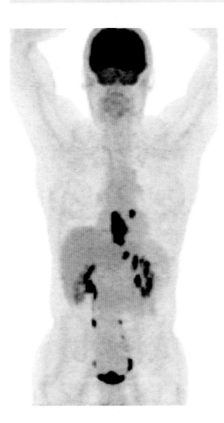

**Figure 8.5** Maximum intensity projection (MIP) image.

## Findings and differential diagnosis

PET, fused axial, sagittal and coronal PET/CT and MIP images (Figures 8.4 and 8.5) show diffuse thickening of the mid to distal esophagus (4.4 × 3.3 cm) with involvement of the EGJ with intense FDG avidity. A 1.3 cm gastrohepatic lymph node and a 1.1 cm periaortic lymph node are also FDG avid. There is no evidence of distant metastases. The lungs are clear without pulmonary nodules, consolidation, or pleural effusions. The findings are suggestive of esophageal carcinoma with metastases to gastrohepatic ligament and periaortic lymph nodes.

## Diagnosis and follow-up

Endoscopic ultrasound was used to confirm the PET findings and the malignancy was staged as T3N1M0. The patient was referred to the oncology department for neoadjuvant chemoradiation regimen. However, the patient's disease progressed and he was enrolled in a phase III sorafenib trial.

## Discussion and teaching points

The pooled sensitivity and specificity of PET for the detection of locoregional lymph node metastases is 51% and 84% respectively (1). The main limitation of PET for N staging is the number of false-negative and false-positive findings. Small nodes harboring tumor may not have increased FDG uptake or if they are too close to the primary lesion, it can be very difficult to distinguish their uptake from the adjacent tumor uptake, due to the lack of spatial resolution of PET (2, 3). Sometimes reactive nodes secondary to inflammation or esophagitis can have abnormal uptake, and yet not harbor malignant cells (2, 3). PET/CT can significantly improve the detection of loco-regional disease. Hybrid imaging with PET/CT can help overcome problems such as false-negatives secondary to small volume disease, poor spatial resolution, and motion artifacts, especially in the chest. Loco-regional nodes do not alter management and may be resected along with the primary tumor, however, it should be kept in mind that the number of metastatic nodes is one of the most important prognostic factors. Each additional node harboring metastasis increases risk. Lymph node ratio is no longer supported as a useful measure of metastatic burden.

## Take-home message

- The main limitation of PET for N staging is the number of false-negative and false-positive findings.
- Fused PET/CT images in at least two planes can help eliminate false-positives and false-negatives.
- Based on the 2010 revised AJCC staging system for esophageal cancer, regional nodes are now considered all nodes from peri-esophageal cervical nodes to celiac nodes.
- The number of metastatic nodes is one of the most important prognostic factors.
- Each additional node harboring metastasis increases risk.

## References

1. van Westreenen HL, Westerterp M, Bossuyt PM *et al.* Systematic review of the staging performance of 18F fluorodeoxyglucose positron emission tomography in esophageal cancer. *J Clin Oncol* 2004;**22**:3805–12.

2. Block MI, Patterson GA, Sundaresan RS *et al.* Improvement in staging of esophageal cancer with the addition of positron emission tomography. *Ann Thorac Surg* 1997;**64**:770–7.

3. Mamede M, Abreu-E-Lima P, Oliva MR *et al.* FDG-PET/CT tumor segmentation-derived indices of metabolic activity to assess response to neoadjuvant therapy and progression-free survival in esophageal cancer: correlation with histopathology results. *Am J Clin Oncol* 2007; **30**(4):377–88.

# Esophageal cancer with metastases to Virchow's lymph node (left supraclavicular node)

A 70-year-old male presenting to his primary-care physician with dysphagia, odynophagia, regurgitation, and hiccups. Endoscopy revealed a lobular polypoid mass in the distal esophagus, which was biopsied and was consistent with invasive adenocarcinoma. In addition a 4 mm lymph node was identified adjacent to the mass and positive for metastasis. Patient was referred for a pre-treatment FDG-PET/CT.

## Acquisition and processing parameters

Whole-body PET was performed 60 min after the intravenous administration of 20 mCi of FDG in fasting conditions. Plasma glucose levels at the time of FDG injection were 148 mg/dL. The patient was encouraged to void before scanning, and images were obtained from the head to the proximal thighs

with a combined PET/CT scanner. The patient was imaged in the supine position, without any specific breath-holding instructions. The unenhanced CT scan was performed first, from the patient's head to the proximal thighs, using the following acquisition parameters: 140 kVp, 75 mA, 0.8 s per CT rotation, pitch of 1.675 : 1, and a reconstructed slice thickness of 3.75 mm, for a total scanning time of 42.4 s. The CT data were reconstructed using a filtered back-projection algorithm and a 512 × 512 matrix, with a transaxial field of view of 50 cm. The CT images were used to generate the transmission maps for attenuation correction of the PET acquisitions and for anatomic localization.

Immediately after the CT scan, and without changing the patient's position, the tabletop moved automatically to the PET position. The emission scan was acquired starting at the

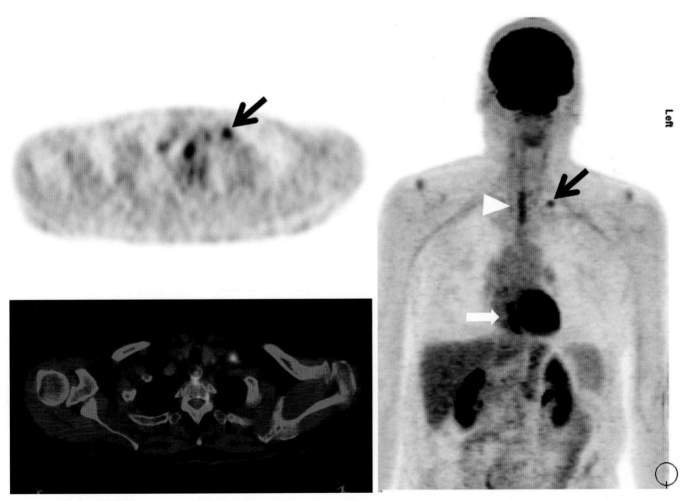

**Figure 8.6** Left: Axial FDG-PET and fused FDG-PET/CT; right: MIP image.

mid-thighs toward the head, for six bed positions of 4 min each (47 image planes/bed position, 15.7 cm longitudinal field of view). PET data were reconstructed using an ordered-subset expectation maximization iterative algorithm (30 subsets, 2 iterations).

## Findings and differential diagnosis

The images show intense FDG uptake in a moderately thickened distal esophagus and gastroesophageal junction consistent with the patient's known malignancy (white arrow). In addition, mild and linear uptake in a minimally thickened upper esophagus has uncertain etiology but is likely inflammatory esophagitis (white arrowhead). There is a small moderately intense focus in the left supraclavicular region, consistent with a 1.3 cm positive Virchow's node (black arrow). There is no abnormal uptake observed in the remainder of the thorax, or in the head, abdomen, or pelvis. The lungs are clear. There is no evidence of mediastinal lymphadenopathy. There are no pleural or pericardial effusions.

## Diagnosis and follow-up

The left supraclavicular node was biopsied and confirmed to be metastatic. The tumor was staged as T3, N1, and M1, and was referred for radiation therapy and weekly Taxol plus cisplatin therapy.

## Discussion and teaching points

The Virchow's node is a lymph node in the left supraclavicular fossa where the lymphatic drainage of most of the body (from the thoracic duct) enters the venous circulation via the left subclavian vein. The tumor cells block the thoracic duct leading to regurgitation into the surrounding nodes i.e., Virchow's node. It has also been conceptualized that the supraclavicular nodes represent the end node along the thoracic duct and hence the enlargement (1).

In order to estimate the accuracy of different radiologic criteria used to detect cervical lymph node metastasis, Van Den Berkel and colleagues (2) studied lymph node diameters, location, number, the presence of tumor, and the amount of necrosis and fatty metaplasia. The investigators found that a minimal diameter in the axial plane of 1 cm was the most accurate size criterion for predicting lymph node metastasis. In addition, three or more borderline nodes increased the sensitivity. Radiologically detectable necrosis ($\geq$ 3 mm) was characteristic of nodes harboring tumor cells and was present in 74% of positive nodes. On the other hand, nodal shape was not sensitive enough for the assessment of the cervical lymph node status (2).

The finding of an enlarged, hard node (also referred to as Troisier's sign) has long been regarded as strongly indicative of lymphatic spread from a gastrointestinal primary, and is sometimes referred to as the signal node or sentinel node. These patients have a significantly worse prognosis than patients with loco-regional metastases (3, 4). Although the revised staging system considers supraclavicular adenopathy as regional nodes, at our institution these patients are still managed as having unresectable disease, and they are treated with chemotherapy followed by chemoradiotherapy. Therefore, if the left supraclavicular lymph node is the only site of FDG-avid disease in the absence of loco-regional spread of tumor, further biopsy confirmation is recommended prior to treatment stratification.

## Take-home message

- The left supraclavicular group of lymph nodes have worse prognosis than other loco-regional adenopathy.
- Isolated FDG-avid supraclavicular nodes warrant histopathological confirmation, as there is significant difference in management if found to be positive for metastasis.

## References

1. Mizutani M, Nawata S, Hirai I, Murakami G, Kimura W. Anatomy and histology of Virchow's node. *Anat Sci Int* 2005;**80**(4):193–8.

2. Van Den Berkel M, Stel H, Castelijns J *et al.* Cervical lymph node metastases; assessment of radiology criteria. *Radiology* 1990; **177**:379–84.

3. Rice TW. Clinical staging of esophageal carcinoma. CT, EUS, and PET. *Chest Surg Clin North Am* 2000;**10**:471–85.

4. Eloubeidi MA, Wallace MB, Hoffman BJ *et al.* Predictors of survival for esophageal cancer patients with and without celiac axis lymphadenopathy: impact of staging endosonography. *Ann Thorac Surg* 2001;**72**:212–19.

## Esophageal cancer with distant metastases

A 71-year-old male presenting to his primary-care physician with progressive dysphagia. Endoscopy revealed a friable necrotic mass extending from 20–40 cm consistent with esophageal cancer. Endoscopic ultrasound staging was performed and the tumor was staged as T1N1 with a positive mediastinal node with malignant cells. FDG-PET/CT was performed for complete staging work-up.

## Acquisition and processing parameters

Whole-body PET was performed 60 min after the intravenous administration of 20 mCi of FDG in fasting conditions. Plasma glucose levels at the time of FDG injection were 122 mg/dL. The patient was encouraged to void before scanning, and images were obtained from the head to the proximal thighs

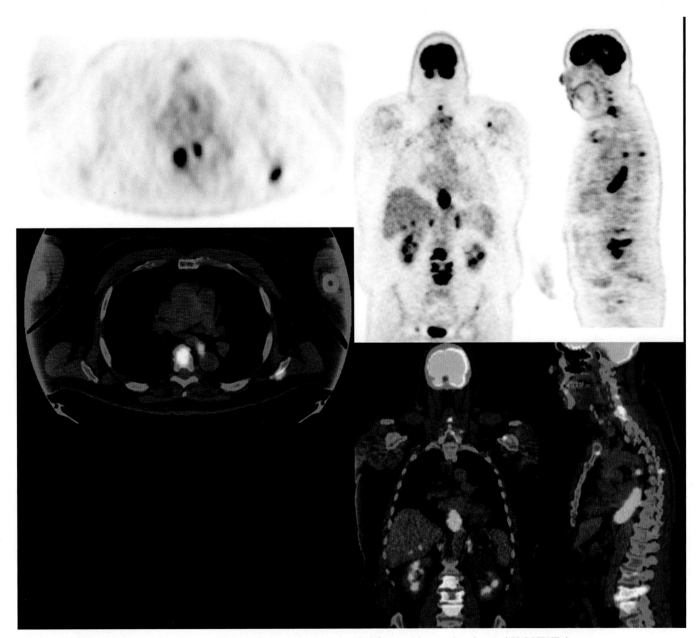

**Figure 8.7** Top row: axial, coronal, and sagittal FDG-PET; bottom row: corresponding fused axial, coronal, and sagittal FDG-PET/CT slices.

with a combined PET/CT scanner. The patient was imaged in the supine position, without any specific breath-holding instructions. The unenhanced CT scan was performed first, from the patient's head to the proximal thighs, using the following acquisition parameters: 140 kVp, 75 mA, 0.8 s per CT rotation, pitch of 1.675 : 1, and a reconstructed slice thickness of 3.75 mm, for a total scanning time of 42.4 s. The CT data were reconstructed using a filtered back-projection algorithm and a 512 × 512 matrix, with a transaxial field of view of 50 cm. The CT images were used to generate the transmission maps for attenuation correction of the PET acquisitions and for anatomic localization.

Immediately after the CT scan, and without changing the patient's position, the tabletop moved automatically to the PET position. The emission scan was acquired starting at the mid-thighs toward the head, for six bed positions of 4 minutes each (47 image planes/bed position, 15.7 cm longitudinal field of view). PET data were reconstructed using an ordered-subset expectation maximization iterative algorithm (30 subsets, 2 iterations).

## Findings and differential diagnosis

Images show long segment thickening involving the distal esophagus with intense FDG uptake corresponding to the known primary adenocarcinoma. There are intensely avid lymph nodes in the paraesophageal and right submandibular region. There are bilateral avid adrenal masses consistent with metastases, liver metastases, and extensive osseous lesions involving the axial and appendicular skeleton. Incidental note is made of bilateral renal cysts.

Intense FDG metabolism is seen along the course of a circumferentially thickened distal esophagus and in a para-esophageal node, which correlates with known primary esophageal adenocarcinoma. Disease is widely metastatic with intense soft tissue uptake in the right submandibular gland (7 mm), both adrenal glands (measuring 2.9 × 1.9 cm on the left and 1.3 × 1.3 cm on the right), and multiple separate areas in the right and left hepatic lobes. There are extensive osseous lesions involving the axial and appendicular skeleton highly FDG-avid in PET without obvious CT correlate.

## Diagnosis and follow-up

The patient was staged as stage IV as the FDG-PET/CT revealed widespread metastatic disease, and was referred to oncology for palliative chemoradiotherapy and Zometa for extensive osseous metastasis.

## Discussion and teaching points

Distant metastases have been reported in up to 30% of patients with esophageal cancer at initial presentation (1, 2). Patients with M1 disease are not candidates for curative resection. The most common sites of metastases are the liver, lungs,

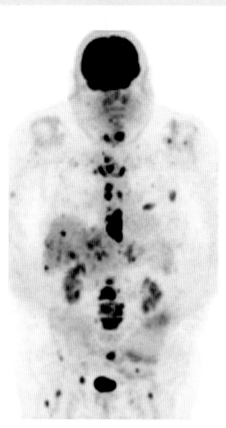

**Figure 8.8** Maximum intensity projection (MIP) image.

and bones in descending order (3). Other common sites include the adrenals and distant lymph nodes. Uncommon sites for distant metastases include the brain, skeletal muscle, subcutaneous tissues, thyroid gland, and pancreas (4). Synchronous neoplastic disease can be present in 1.5–5.5% of patients at initial presentation in the stomach, head and neck, and colon (4).

Pre-treatment FDG-PET is used for staging, restaging, and assessing response to therapy. van Westreenen *et al.* have reported a pooled sensitivity and specificity of 51% and 84%, respectively for the detection of loco-regional metastases. On the other hand, the accuracy is higher for distant metastases, with a pooled sensitivity and specificity of 67% and 97%, respectively (5).

A potential limitation of PET/CT is in the diagnosis of small hepatic metastases, as the unenhanced liver is very heterogeneous on both PET and CT, hence suspicious lesions in the liver should be confirmed with a dedicated CT abdomen with oral and intravenous contrast.

## Take-home message

- FDG-PET is the modality of choice for staging prior to treatment planning, and can help detect occult metastatic disease in patients thought to have localized tumors.
- FDG-PET is cost-effective as it helps prevent non-curative surgery by detecting metastases missed by other imaging modalities.

# References

1. Quint LE, Hepburn LM, Francis IR, Whyte RI, Orringer MB. Incidence and distribution of distant metastases from newly diagnosed esophageal carcinoma. *Cancer* 1995;**76**:1120–5.

2. Flanagan FL, Dehdashti F, Siegel BA *et al.* Staging of esophageal cancer with 18F-fluorodeoxy-glucose positron emission tomography. *Am J Roentgenol* 1997;**168**:417–24.

3. Quint LE, Hepburn LM, Francis IR, Whyte RI, Orringer MB. Incidence and distribution of distant metastases from newly diagnosed esophageal carcinoma. *Cancer* 1995;**76**:1120–5.

4. Bruzzi JF, Truong MT, Macapinlac H, Munden RF, Erasmus JJ. Integrated CT-PET imaging of esophageal cancer: unexpected and unusual distribution of distant organ metastases. *Curr Probl Diagn Radiol* 2007;**36**(1):21–9.

5. van Westreenen HL, Westerterp M, Bossuyt PM *et al.* Systematic review of the staging performance of 18F fluorodeoxyglucose positron emission tomography in esophageal cancer. *J Clin Oncol* 2004;**22**:3805–12.

# Esophageal cancer status post-esophagectomy and gastric pull-up

A 68-year-old male status post-esophagectomy and gastric pull-up with palpable neck nodes presents for a restaging PET/CT.

## Acquisition and processing parameters

Whole-body PET was performed 60 min after the intravenous administration of 22.7 mCi of FDG in fasting conditions. Plasma glucose levels at the time of FDG injection were 122 mg/dL. The patient was encouraged to void before scanning, and images were obtained from the head to the proximal thighs with a combined PET/CT scanner. The patient was imaged in the supine position, without any specific breath-holding instructions. The unenhanced CT scan was performed first, from the patient's head to the proximal thighs, using the following acquisition parameters: 140 kVp, 75 mA, 0.8 s per CT rotation, pitch of 1.675 : 1, and a reconstructed slice thickness of 3.75 mm, for a total scanning time of 42.4 s. The CT data were reconstructed using a filtered back-projection algorithm and a 512 × 512 matrix, with a transaxial field of view of 50 cm. The CT images were used to generate the transmission maps for attenuation correction of the PET acquisitions and for anatomic localization.

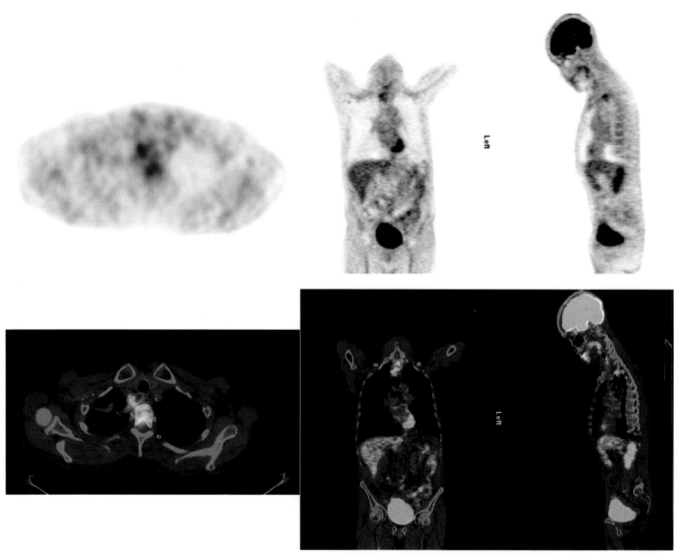

**Figure 8.9** Top row: axial, coronal, and sagittal FDG-PET slices; bottom row: corresponding fused axial, coronal, and sagittal FDG-PET/CT slices.

Immediately after the CT scan, and without changing the patient's position, the tabletop moved automatically to the PET position. The emission scan was acquired starting at the mid-thighs toward the head, for six bed positions of 4 min each (47 image planes/bed position, 15.7 cm longitudinal field of view). PET data were reconstructed using an ordered-subset expectation maximization iterative algorithm (30 subsets, 2 iterations).

## Findings and differential diagnosis

PET/CT images show focal and intense FDG uptake in a minimally thickened neo-esophagus in the upper mediastinum concerning for local recurrence. The differential diagnosis would include inflammation at the anastomotic site in the lower neck. There is a linear thickened parenchymal lesion in the right upper lobe of the lung that is not FDG avid.

## Diagnosis and follow-up

The left posterior neck nodes were biopsied and found to be consistent with metastases. Endoscopy also confirmed that there was evidence of local recurrence at the anastomotic site in the upper chest. The patient was referred for palliative chemotherapy.

## Discussion and teaching points

Little is known about the benefit of re-resection after loco-regional recurrence. Recurrence after transhiatal resection occurs early, approximately 11–24 months after surgery (1). Hulscher *et al.* (1) reported that approximately 23% of patients developed loco-regional recurrent disease, 15% patients had systemic recurrence, and 14% had both systemic and loco-regional recurrence. The authors also indicated that

8% of patients had only cervical lymph node metastases at restaging scans. Recurrence rates were related to post-operative lymph node status and the radicality of the operation, but it was not associated with localization or histologic type of the tumor.

Focal uptake at the anastomotic site 3 months post-surgery needs to be further evaluated with an endoscopy to exclude recurrence. Isolated anastomotic site recurrence is generally re-resected if the patient is able to undergo surgery. However, in general there are other sites of disease recurrence at the time of discovery of anastomotic recurrence. Pre-operative chemotherapy can decrease recurrence rates by 50% (2). More complete esophagectomy with greater than 5 cm resection margin in tumors involving the upper esophagus, and post-operative radiotherapy for patients with short resection margins, can help decrease the rate of local recurrence (3).

## Take-home message

- Leaving resection margins less than 5 cm especially in upper-third esophageal tumors is more likely to recur locally.
- Pre-operative chemotherapy can help prevent local recurrence, as well as post-operative radiation therapy when resection margins are less than 5 cm.
- Focal mild, moderate, or high uptake at the anastomotic site post-esophagectomy should be evaluated with endoscopy to exclude local recurrence. Beware of uptake in areas of resolving inflammation.
- Surgical resection of locally recurrent esophageal cancer may be considered if possible.

## References

1. Hulscher JB, van Sandick JW, Tijssen JG, Obertop H, van Lanschot JJ. The recurrence pattern of esophageal carcinoma after transhiatal resection. *J Am Coll Surg* 2000;**191**(2):143–8.

2. Law SYK, Fok M, Wong J. Pattern of recurrence after oesophageal resection for cancer: clinical implications. *Br J Surg* 1996; **83**:107–11.

3. Tam PC, Siu KF, Cheung HC, Ma L, Wong J. Local recurrences after subtotal esophagectomy for squamous cell carcinoma. *Ann Surg* 1987;**205**(2):189–94.

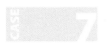

# Widespread recurrent distant metastases post-esophagectomy and gastric pull-up

A 46-year-old female, 4 months status post-esophagectomy and gastric pull-up had abdominal pain and found to have new liver lesions on ultrasound. She was referred for a FDG-PET/CT for further evaluation and restaging.

## Acquisition and processing parameters

Whole-body PET was performed 60 min after the intravenous administration of 21.5 mCi of FDG in fasting conditions. Plasma glucose levels at the time of FDG injection were 122 mg/dL. The patient was encouraged to void before scanning, and images were obtained from the head to the proximal thighs with a combined PET/CT scanner. The patient was imaged in the supine position, without any specific breath-holding instructions. The unenhanced CT scan was performed first, from the patient's head to the proximal thighs, using the following acquisition parameters: 140 kVp, 75 mA, 0.8 s per CT rotation, pitch of 1.675 : 1, and a reconstructed slice thickness of 3.75 mm, for a total scanning time of 42.4 s. The CT data were reconstructed using a filtered back-projection algorithm and a 512 × 512 matrix, with a transaxial field of view of 50 cm. The CT images were used to generate the transmission maps for attenuation correction of the PET acquisitions and for anatomic localization.

Immediately after the CT scan, and without changing the patient's position, the tabletop moved automatically to the PET position. The emission scan was acquired starting at the mid-thighs toward the head, for six bed positions of 4 minutes each (47 image planes/bed position, 15.7 cm longitudinal field of view). PET data were reconstructed using an ordered-subset expectation maximization iterative algorithm (30 subsets, 2 iterations).

## Findings and differential diagnosis

There are multiple FDG-avid liver metastases and diffuse osseous metastases involving the axial and appendicular skeleton. There is a new small left pleural effusion.

## Diagnosis and follow-up

The patient underwent liver biopsy, which confirmed metastatic esophageal adenocarcinoma. She was referred for palliative chemotherapy, however soon succumbed to her metastatic disease.

## Discussion and teaching points

In a study by Sugimachi et al. 33.3% patients in the curative resection group had distant recurrence, compared with 61.8% of those in the non-curative resection group (1). Extrathoracic recurrence was found in 41% of patients, and intrathoracic recurrence and systemic organ metastases in 25%. Law et al. (2) reported that up to 52% of patients who had undergone curative resection, had disease recurrence at a

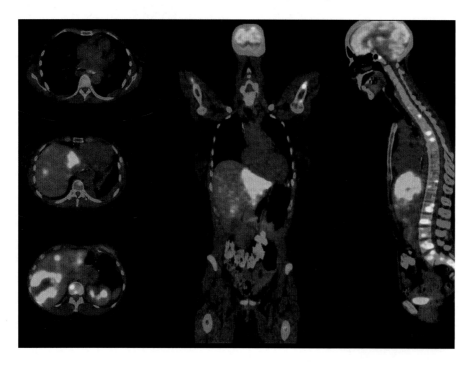

**Figure 8.10** Left: fused axial (at level of chest and liver), middle: coronal and right: sagittal FDG-PET/CT slices.

median follow-up of 20 months. The investigators indicated that hematopoietic recurrence was most commonly seen in instances of blood vessel invasion detected at the time of the surgery. On the other hand, lymph node recurrence was most frequent when there was lymphatic invasion or blood vessel invasion or both, and the post-operative survival time was double that of those with a hematologic recurrence (2).

## Take-home message

- Systemic recurrence following surgery for esophageal cancer is common.
- FDG-PET is the primary imaging modality for follow-up and can help identify the M stage more accurately.
- Hematological recurrence has worse prognosis than lymphatic-based failure.

## References

1.  Sugimachi K, Inokuchi K, Kuwano H *et al.* Patterns of recurrence after curative resection for carcinoma of the thoracic part of the esophagus. *Surg Gynecol Obstet* 1983;**157**(6): 537–40.

2.  Law SYK, Fok M, Wong J. Pattern of recurrence after oesophageal resection for cancer: clinical implications. *Br J Surg* 1996;**83**:107–11.

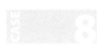 

A 53-year-old male with a stage IIIA adenocarcinoma of the esophageal-gastric junction. FDG-PET/CT imaging was ordered to monitor response to neoadjuvant chemoradiotherapy.

## Acquisition and processing parameters

Whole-body PET was performed at baseline, and after the second cycle of therapy (last day before the beginning of the third cycle). Images were obtained 60 min after the intravenous administration of 20 mCi of FDG in fasting conditions. Plasma glucose levels at the time of FDG injection were 99 mg/dL at baseline and 102 mg/dL after therapy. The patient was encouraged to void before scanning, and images were obtained from the head to the proximal thighs with a combined PET/CT scanner. The patient was imaged in the supine position, without any specific breath-holding instructions. The unenhanced CT scan was performed first, from the patient's head to the proximal thighs, using the following acquisition parameters: 140 kVp, 75 mA, 0.8 s per CT rotation, pitch of 1.675:1, and a reconstructed slice thickness of 3.75 mm, for a total scanning time of 42.4 s. The CT data were reconstructed using a filtered back-projection algorithm and a $512 \times 512$ matrix, with a transaxial field of view of 50 cm. The CT images were used to generate the transmission maps for attenuation correction of the PET acquisitions and for anatomic localization.

Immediately after the CT scan, and without changing the patient's position, the tabletop moved automatically to the PET position. The emission scans were acquired starting at the mid-thighs toward the head, for six bed positions of 4 minutes each (47 image planes/bed position, 15.7 cm longitudinal field of view). PET data were reconstructed using an ordered-subset expectation maximization iterative algorithm (30 subsets, 2 iterations).

## Findings and differential diagnosis

The baseline MIP image (Figure 8.11) shows an area of intense FDG uptake (SUVmax = 12) in the area of the esophageal-gastric junction corresponding to the patient's known esophageal malignancy. Post-therapeutic (after two cycles) MIP image (Figure 8.12) shows near-complete resolution of FDG uptake in the lesion (SUVmax = 2.7). Delta SUVmax was 77.5% estimated by using the following formula:

(Baseline SUVmax − Post-therapy SUVmax/Baseline SUVmax) × 100.

Both sets of images show normal FDG uptake in the kidneys, collecting systems, and bladder. No other areas of abnormal radiotracer uptake are seen.

## Diagnosis and follow-up

The patient completed a full course of treatment and underwent three-hole esophagectomy. The resected tumor specimen was examined by an experienced gastrointestinal pathologist to assess histopathologic response to therapy. The pathology results revealed the presence of fibrosis with areas of inflammation and necrosis without evidence of viable tumor cells, confirming complete response to therapy. The patient is presently doing well.

## Discussion and teaching points

Neoadjuvant therapy is used to control local and distant disease before esophageal cancer resection. The assessment of response to therapy in this population is of utmost importance to guide management and to obtain important prognostic information. Therefore, it is important to be able to accurately identify non-responders early during the course of treatment to minimize the cost and toxicity of unnecessary therapy. Furthermore, these patients have a poor prognosis (1, 2). On the other hand, those that respond to therapy tend to survive longer after esophagectomy. In this group of patients FDG-PET increases the sensitivity to detect residual disease.

Weber and colleagues (3) conducted a FDG-PET study in 40 esophageal cancer patients before and 2 weeks after the start of neoadjuvant chemotherapy. The gold standard was pathologic response assessed after esophagectomy. Using a 35% reduction in tumor SUV between the baseline and post-treatment scans, they reported a sensitivity and a specificity of 93% and 95%, respectively, to predict a pathologic response to therapy. The same group tested the accuracy of the 35% delta SUV threshold prospectively in 65 patients to discriminate between responding and non-responding esophageal tumors 14 days after the start of chemotherapy (4). The method had a sensitivity of 82% and a specificity of 78%, and again it was stressed that FDG-based metabolic response had prognostic value in their patient population.

Flamen et al. (5) studied the value of FDG-PET to assess response to chemoradiation therapy. They scanned their patients at baseline and 4–6 weeks after the completion of therapy. They reported a sensitivity of 71% and a specificity of 82%, with an accuracy of 78% to predict what the authors called a "major pathologic response" (which corresponded to more than 80% reduction of tumor-to-liver uptake ratio after therapy). The authors also stressed the prognostic value of the PET findings, indicating that PET major responders had a median survival after therapy of 16.3 months compared with 6.4 months for non-responders.

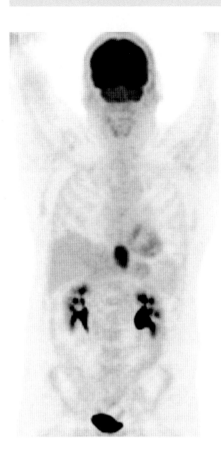

**Figure 8.11** Maximum intensity projection (MIP) image at baseline.

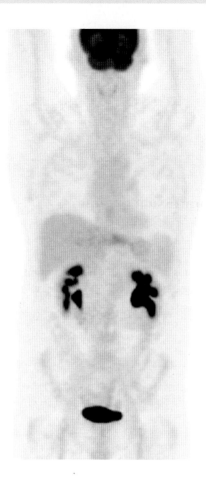

**Figure 8.12** Maximum intensity projection (MIP) image after two cycles of therapy.

The optimal timing of PET images is still the subject of ongoing research. According to the National Cancer Institute Consensus Recommendations for the use of PET to monitor therapy (6), the pre-treatment baseline scans should be acquired as close to start of therapy as possible (preferably < 2 weeks). Post-treatment scans should be acquired no sooner than 2 weeks after the end of chemotherapy to avoid transient variability of FDG uptake. PET scans after radiotherapy should not be acquired before 6–8 weeks from completion of treatment, in order to minimize false-positive FDG uptake in radiation-induced inflammation.

Assessment of response in PET images may be done visually by comparing lesion uptake with a reference standard, such as liver uptake (7). Using this criterion a complete metabolic response corresponds to tumoral FDG uptake that decreases to less or equal the activity levels observed in normal tissues or in the reference standard (e.g., liver). Thus, a complete response does not necessarily equal complete image normalization (as shown in this case), because the intensity of residual FDG uptake after treatment is in part due to the existing post-therapeutic inflammation and scar tissue present (8).

## Take-home message

- The aim of neoadjuvant treatment is to control both local and distant disease. Patients who respond to therapy have a better prognosis after surgery than those who do not.

- Treated malignant tissue may have reduced FDG activity because of both cell death and lower metabolism.

- For the most part there is a good correlation between FDG-PET-based response, histologic response, and improved overall survival.

- The best timing for response assessment is the one that allows for modification of treatment in non-responders minimizing the cost and toxicity of unnecessary therapy, and for the prompt initiation of salvage treatment.

- The sooner the normalization or reduction in tumoral FDG uptake occurs, the higher the probability that cure will be achieved, and therefore, the best indication of a favorable outcome.

- An important limitation of the technique is that it cannot resolve microscopic residual disease after treatment despite it being metabolically active. Thus, the duration of response cannot be predicted by the lack of uptake alone. Disease recurrence may arise from residual viable cells ($10^7$–$10^8$) that are undetectable by the resolution limits of PET. In addition, the intensity of lesion uptake observed after treatment is also influenced by the active inflammatory cells present, especially after radiotherapy.

# References

1. Lordick F, Ott K, Krause BJ *et al*. PET to assess early metabolic response and to guide treatment of adenocarcinoma of the oesophagogastric junction: the MUNICON phase II trial. *Lancet Oncol* 2007;**8**(9):797–805.

2. Meyer Zum Büschenfelde C, Herrmann K, Schuster T *et al*. 18F-FDG PET-guided salvage neoadjuvant radiochemotherapy ofadenocarcinoma of the esophagogastric junction: The MUNICON II Trial. *J Nucl Med* 2011; **52**(8):1189–96.

3. Weber WA, Ott K, Becker K *et al*. Prediction of response to preoperative chemotherapy in adenocarcinomas of the esophagogastric junction by metabolic imaging. *J Clin Oncol* 2001;**19**:3058–65.

4. Ott K, Weber WA, Lordick F *et al*. Metabolic imaging predicts response, survival, and recurrence in adenocarcinomas of the esophagogastric junction. *J Clin Oncol* 2006;**24**(29):4692–8.

5. Flamen P, Van Cutsem E, Lerut A *et al*. Positron emission tomography for assessment of the response to induction radiochemotherapy in locally advanced oesophageal cancer. *Ann Oncol* 2002;**13**:361–8.

6. Shankar LK, Hoffman JM, Bacharach S *et al*.; National Cancer Institute. Consensus recommendations for the use of 18F-FDG PET as an indicator of therapeutic response in patients in National Cancer Institute Trials. *J Nucl Med* 2006;**47**(6):1059–66.

7. MacManus MP, Hicks RJ, Matthews JP *et al*. Positron emission tomography is superior to computed tomography scanning for response-assessment after radical radiotherapy or chemoradiotherapy in patients with non-small-cell lung cancer. *J Clin Oncol* 2003;**21**(7):1285–92.

8. Mamede M, Abreu-E-Lima P, Oliva MR *et al*. FDG-PET/CT tumor segmentation-derived indices of metabolic activity to assess response to neoadjuvant therapy and progression-free survival in esophageal cancer: correlation with histopathology results. *Am J Clin Oncol* 2007;**30**(4): 377–88.

# Gastrointestinal tract

Christiaan Schiepers

## Introduction

In this chapter, the approach to gastrointestinal tumors will be discussed. Here we limit ourselves to colorectal cancer (CRC), stomach or gastric cancer, and GIST (gastrointestinal stromal tumor) sarcoma. Chapter 8 expands on esophageal cancer. Pancreas, liver, and biliary tract malignancies are discussed in Chapter 10.

Advances in diagnostic imaging technology have improved establishing the diagnosis, staging and restaging of disease, and monitoring response to therapy. Various imaging modalities are available for this purpose, including the anatomical, e.g., radiography, computed tomography (CT), sonography (US), magnetic resonance imaging (MRI), and functional modalities such as molecular imaging, radioimmuno- and receptor scintigraphy, and magnetic resonance spectroscopy.

Conventional diagnostic methods have limited accuracy in early detection of primary as well as recurrent CRC and gastric carcinoma. Assessment of disease extent or tumor burden is necessary for proper patient selection for surgery with curative intent, or stratification to chemotherapy and/or radiation treatment for patients with advanced disease. Appropriate non-invasive staging plays a pivotal role in patient management. Integrated modalities such as positron emission tomography/computed tomography (PET/CT) have changed the current work-up of patients with cancer (1). Some refer to these combined gantries as dual, multimodality or hybrid imaging systems.

## Colon and rectal cancer

Colorectal cancer is a common disease in the Western world, and together with lung, breast, and prostate cancer are the most frequently diagnosed neoplasms. In the USA, CRC frequency ranks third in men and second in women. Colorectal cancer is the third leading cause of cancer mortality because it has a better prognosis than the other common cancers (2–4). In 2009, a total of 146,970 new patients were estimated to be diagnosed with CRC, and 49,920 were expected to die from their disease (5). The incidence of CRC is slightly higher in

men than women (M/F ratio = 1.087), and the mortality rate is similar (M/F ratio = 1.023) (5). About three-quarters of patients have resectable disease, whereas only two-thirds can be cured by resection. In the remaining one-third, recurrence is diagnosed during the first 2 years after resection. A 5-year survival rate of approximately 60% is reported for the USA compared with approximately 40% for the European Union. The mortality rate of CRC is declining related to screening programs that are put in place, such as the hemoccult test and colonoscopy in asymptomatic individuals above age 50. Lifestyle changes contributed in part to its early detection with subsequent surgery.

## Historical perspective

[18]F-fluorodeoxyglucose (FDG) has been used most frequently as a tracer for metabolic imaging (6). FDG is able to measure changes in glucose utilization, which is enhanced in cancer. After the introduction of PET for body imaging (7), clinical studies have been aimed at staging CRC and evaluating the disease extent (8). Traditionally, three general regions of metastatic spread of CRC in the body are distinguished: local, hepatic, and extra-hepatic. Hypermetabolic foci in these regions are suspicious for primary tumor, recurrence or metastasis, and form the basis of metabolic imaging in oncology.

PET using FDG has not been studied systematically for primary CRC. Some studies (9) showed excellent sensitivity for PET, but poor specificity, whereas others did not find differences between primary and recurrent disease (10). Both CT and PET may miss involvement of local lymph nodes.

The role of PET using FDG for recurrent CRC has been investigated extensively and was approved for reimbursement in the late 1990s by Medicare. The meta-analysis of Huebner et al. (11) provided results as shown in Table 9.1 for the pooled data. They reviewed articles published during 1990–1999 that reported information on the use of new medical technology, and selected 11 studies fulfilling their strict guidelines. Sensitivity and specificity in the meta-analysis were all 95% or higher, except for the specificity at extra-hepatic sites, which

*A Case-Based Approach to PET/CT in Oncology*, ed. Victor H. Gerbaudo. Published by Cambridge University Press.
© Cambridge University Press 2012.

**Table 9.1** Clinical performance of FDG-PET in recurrent colorectal cancer.

| Body region | Patients | Sensitivity | Specificity |
|---|---|---|---|
| Local | 366 | 94.5% | 97.7% |
| Hepatic | 393 | 96.3% | 99.0% |
| Whole body | 281 | 97.0% | 75.6% |

Adapted from the meta-analysis of Huebner et al. (11).

revealed about 25% false-positive results. Studies included in the meta-analysis were from institutions in the USA, Europe, and Australia, and showed remarkable consistency of results. From the reported literature it is evident that FDG-PET has established a role in the work-up and staging of patients with recurrent CRC (12).

Serum carcinoembryonic antigen (CEA) is used clinically to monitor for possible recurrence. This technique has a reported sensitivity of 59% and specificity of 84% but cannot determine the location of recurrence (13). CT has been the conventional imaging modality used to localize recurrent disease with an accuracy of 25–73%. CT cannot reliably distinguish post-surgical changes from local recurrence, and is often equivocal (14–16). CT of the abdomen misses hepatic metastases in about 7% of patients and underestimates the number of lobes involved in one-third of patients. In addition, CT commonly misses metastases to the peritoneum, mesentery, and lymph nodes. Among the patients with negative CT, half will have non-resectable lesions at the time of exploratory laparotomy. The results for MR imaging are comparable to CT (17).

Sobhani et al. performed a prospective randomized trial enrolling 130 patients, in which two groups were compared after curative surgery (18). Final diagnosis was established by histology. One group had a conventional imaging follow-up and the other an FDG-PET examination. Recurrences were detected after a shorter time in the PET group (12.1 months) vs. the conventional group (15.4 months), and CRC recurrences were also more frequently cured by surgery, 10/25 in the PET group vs. 2/21 in the conventional group. They concluded that monitoring with FDG-PET during follow-up permits earlier detection of recurrence, and influences therapy strategy.

The results obtained with PET only using FDG, have been corroborated for PET/CT in several studies with sufficiently large patient groups. In addition to providing high-resolution CT images in all planes and projections, CT-based attenuation correction can be performed.

In a study comparing PET and PET/CT directly, Votrubova et al. (19) found the sensitivity, specificity, and accuracy of PET to be 80%, 69%, and 75%, compared with 89%, 92%, and 90% for PET/CT. PET/CT correctly detected 40/45 patients with recurrent CRC. False-negative PET/CT findings were related to microscopic recurrence and a miliary liver metastasis. False-positive PET/CT results were due to inflammatory foci. High glycolysis rates are found in many malignant tumor cells (20) and increased FDG uptake is usually associated with a high number of viable tumor cells and with high expression of glucose transporters (21). Abnormally increased FDG uptake is not specific for neoplasms (22). Inflammatory processes may show the same, and false-positive results have been reported for infections, e.g., pre-sacral abscess, diverticulitis, as well as inflammatory changes early after surgery, and from chemotherapy and radiation. Rosenbaum et al. (23) reported that an experienced nuclear medicine physician manages to differentiate malignant from non-malignant FDG uptake most of the time. Some findings may remain ambiguous, for which PET/CT improves the diagnostic accuracy by combining anatomic with metabolic information.

Kamel et al. published on the incidental uptake in the gastrointestinal tract (24). In their database of 3,281 patients who had a partial-body PET/CT scan, incidental FDG foci were described as associated with an abnormal soft-tissue density or wall thickening on CT. They found incidental lesions in 3% of patients, which were correlated with endoscopic and histopathologic results. They found 19% new cancers, 42% pre-cancerous lesions, 17% inflammatory lesions, 8% benign tumors, and 13% false-positive results. They concluded that although the frequency of incidental gastrointestinal tract lesions is low, they are associated with a substantial risk of an underlying cancerous or pre-cancerous lesion. The main lesson for the practicing physician is that a CT finding must be associated with the abnormal FDG focus, before it can be considered as a lesion. Gutman et al. (25) performed a study aimed at detection of colonic lesions, especially advanced neoplasms such as adenomas (villous or > 1 cm), and carcinomas. They reviewed 1,716 patients with various malignant diseases, except CRC, who had a PET/CT study using FDG and CT for attenuation correction only. Of 45 patients with an intense focus, 20 patients had colonoscopy. Histopathology revealed advanced neoplasms in 13/20 patients. They concluded that incidental focal colonic FDG uptake justifies a colonoscopy to detect premalignant lesions. PET/CT allows accurate localization and is useful to differentiate pathologic from physiologic FDG uptake.

The aim of the study of Kitajima et al. was to evaluate the accuracy of PET/CT using FDG and IV contrast for suspected recurrent CRC (26). PET/contrast-enhanced CT, PET/non-contrast-enhanced CT and enhanced CT were compared in 170 patients. Sensitivity, specificity, and accuracy of PET/contrast-enhanced CT were 93%, 96%, and 95%, those of PET/non-contrast-enhanced CT 89%, 95%, and 92%, and enhanced CT 80%, 94%, and 88%. Sensitivity and accuracy differed significantly. PET/contrast-enhanced CT resulted in a change of management in 38% of patients. Thus, the addition of CT, especially when using contrast, has increased the specificity of diagnostic imaging. Cantwell et al. compared the effect of CT with and without contrast, and correlated the results with Gd-enhanced MR imaging (27). The study was focused on detection and characterization of liver lesions in 33 CRC patients. The sensitivity, specificity, and accuracy for characterization of detected liver lesions on low-radiation dose PET/non-enhanced CT were 67%, 60%, and 66%, respectively; those on PET/enhanced-CT were 85%, 100%, and 86%, respectively; and those on MRI were 98%, 100%, and 98%, respectively. MR imaging turned out to be the best test for liver lesion characterization.

## Monitoring therapy response

A systematic review of the literature can be found in a review article from the group in Nijmegen, Netherlands (28). They reviewed studies on chemotherapy response in advanced CRC (five studies), after local ablative therapy (four studies) and pre-operative treatment response by radiation, chemotherapy, or combined therapy (19 studies). Metabolic imaging using FDG had a high predictive value in therapeutic management of CRC, and was a significant predictor of therapy outcome. The authors call for a systematic implementation of metabolic imaging with FDG in randomized trials (28).

Rosenberg et al. (29) investigated the value of PET/CT in predicting histopathological response of pre-operative radio-chemotherapy in 30 patients with rectal carcinoma at baseline, 14 days (early), and after completion (late) of therapy. The best differentiation of histopathological tumor response was achieved by a cut-off value of 35% reduction of initial FDG uptake at day 14 and 58% after completion of therapy. Using these figures, histopathological response was predicted with a sensitivity of 74% at day 14 and 79% at completion. The positive predictive value for early metabolic response was 82% and for late metabolic response was 83%. Negative predictive values were 58% at early and 64% at late time points. They concluded that PET/CT in rectal cancer can predict histopathological response. Peritumoral inflammatory cells caused false-negative results.

The available literature suggests that PET/CT using FDG and contrast enhancement is an accurate test for staging CRC and evaluating therapy response.

## Future outlook

The diagnostic information provided by metabolic imaging using FDG has improved management of patients with colorectal cancer. The biochemical and biological basis of the FDG-uptake mechanism has shifted the focus toward molecular biology and the interplay of transporters, enzymes, and genetic markers (30, 31). For an overview of some of the players in colon cancer the reader is referred to a review article of Jadvar et al. (32).

# Patient preparation and protocol

The body-imaging mode has become the standard for FDG-PET/CT in oncology (7, 33). After the FDG-uptake period, the patient is positioned in the scanner. Oral and intravenous contrast can be used to perform a helical CT of diagnostic quality. Thereafter, sequential acquisitions with the PET scanner are done along the length of the patient's body. The tissues cause varying degrees of attenuation and scatter and affect the final number of photons that reach the detectors. The CT can be used to correct for photon attenuation. With current multislice CT scanners, the duration of a scan of the torso is very short, especially when compared with the old-fashioned transmission scan. Statistical models are used to correct for scatter. High-quality images are generated by applying iterative reconstruction techniques.

The spatial resolution of the CT is better than that of the PET system. However, this is not the only determining factor in detecting abnormalities. The "contrast resolution" or difference between the lesion and its surroundings helps define an abnormality. The accuracy of anatomic images is limited by a lower lesion-to-background contrast. The target-to-background ratio is usually much higher for PET using FDG. Except for the lung, the high metabolic contrast predominates over anatomical contrast. Sensitivity of PET is also affected by lesion size, but metabolically active lesions as small as 5 mm have been detected.

Patients are studied in a prolonged fasting state to produce low insulin levels and induce low rates of glucose utilization by normal tissues. Malignant tissues are less dependent on hormone regulation, and thus will have higher uptake when compared with the surrounding normal tissues. A dose of 250–500 MBq (7–15 mCi) of FDG is the usual activity administered. After an uptake period of an hour, the patient is asked to void and positioned in the scanner.

The standard patient preparation for a PET or a CT study is also used for a routine PET/CT study. For PET, the fasting period for an FDG study, the dose administered, and the uptake period are the same. For CT, the settings of the kVp, mAs, and pitch are also the same as for standard equipment. There are two "modes" of CT operation: (1) low dose for attenuation correction and lesion localization; and (2) high dose for diagnostic quality, with and without contrast enhancement. In clinical practice, a diagnostic CT is required to localize and characterize abnormalities. Referring physicians also request a diagnostic CT as part of the examination. A PET scan of the upper body has a total acquisition time of 10–25 minutes. Patients are usually scanned from feet to head, taking advantage of the low bladder uptake after voiding at the beginning of acquisition.

From the patient's point of view, the dual-imaging modality is beneficial. Preparation such as fasting has to be done only once, and all imaging is performed in a single session in the imaging suite, greatly shortening the time spent. Such a scenario improves patient compliance and logistics.

At UCLA, oral contrast is given for the delineation of the bowel. A volume of 900 mL Ready-Cat® (2% barium sulfate, no glucose) is given orally in three portions at 60, 30, and 5 min before the acquisition starts. Our protocol comprises one CT acquisition of the chest during deep inspiration followed by one CT acquisition of torso, i.e., from the base of the skull to the mid-thigh level, after IV contrast enhancement. The CT acquisitions are followed by a PET scan of the same torso area, with the arms up. Currently, we have PET/CT systems consisting of 2, 6, 16, or 64-slice CT scanners combined with 15 or 22 cm axial field of view PET scanners.

The CT settings are such that diagnostic quality images can be generated: 120–140 kVp, variable tube current (120–170 mAs effective dose), pitch varying from 0.8 to 1.2, slice collimation 0.6–2 mm depending on the area of the body. The helical CT duration varies from 80 seconds to image the upper body for the 2-slice machine to 23 seconds for the 64-slice machine.

Intravenous contrast is routinely given. Non-ionic contrast (Omnipaque®) in a volume of 100–115 mL at a rate of 1.2 mL/s is administered. The IV contrast may cause regions of high attenuation that lead to typical CT-based attenuation artifacts, and pseudo FDG uptake (34, 35). The administered FDG dose is 7.8 MBq/kg (0.21 mCi/kg). The uptake interval between tracer administration and start of the PET acquisition is 1 hour. During the uptake period, the patient is comfortably resting in a chair with armrests, in a dimly lit room without radio or television to minimize brain stimulation. The patient is covered with blankets to prevent shivering and activation of brown adipose tissue. The bladder is emptied just before entering the imaging suite.

Our PET scanners have fast detectors (LSO: lutethium-ortho-silicate) allowing for 3-D imaging of 1–4 minutes per bed-position to accumulate the necessary counts. Patient body weight determines the imaging time, < 70 kg, 1 min/position, < 100 kg, 2 min/position, etc. (36). The overall PET acquisition takes 6–26 minutes. With this setup, a standard whole body PET/CT can be completed within 7–30 minutes.

In order to avoid misinterpretation of FDG images, it is critical to standardize the environment of the patient during the uptake period; to examine the patient for post-operative sites, tube placement, stoma, etc.; and to be aware of any invasive procedures or therapeutic interventions.

The contribution of breathing is less important for the abdomen than for the chest (37). Even the "mushroom" artifact caused by motion of the diaphragm and liver during CT acquisition does not seem to pose a real clinical problem in staging of cancers with liver involvement (see Chapter 1). Non-attenuation corrected tomograms and projection images are always available to check for possible artifacts induced by mis-registered PET/CT slices. Metal implants or contrast may also induce artifacts. Therefore, non-attenuation corrected images are routinely interpreted to eliminate possible imaging artifacts. In order to reduce bowel uptake, pharmacological interventions to inhibit secretion and motility have been proposed, but this does not seem necessary on a routine basis.

Evaluation of static PET images can be performed visually, or semi-quantitatively using the standardized uptake value (SUV) or a lesion-to-background ratio. The SUV is the measured activity in the lesion in Bq/mL divided by injected dose, expressed as kBq/kg of body weight. Strauss et al. (38) reported maximum SUVs of 1.1–4.2 for pelvic recurrences, and Takeuchi et al. (39) showed that an SUV cut-off of 2.8 diagnosed local recurrences with 100% accuracy. Abdel-Nabi et al. (9) found

SUVs of 2.8–14.5 for primary bowel cancers. Semi-quantitative evaluation offers a more objective way of reporting lesion uptake than visual image interpretation, and is useful for comparing lesion activity in consecutive studies obtained for treatment monitoring. Visual interpretation appears sufficient for clinical needs, and is equally effective for a one-time diagnosis.

## Clinical indications

In the late 1990s PET using FDG was approved for the following indications:

1. Evaluation of elevated serum CEA level with negative conventional imaging work-up.
2. Pre-operative staging of recurrent CRC.
3. Re-staging.

As of July 1, 2001 the CMS-approved indications for CRC are:

1. Diagnosis.
2. Staging.
3. Re-staging.

New modifiers were introduced by CMS for PET or PET/CT, which are effective for dates of services on or after April 6, 2009, and these are:

**PI** –PET or PET/CT to inform the initial treatment strategy of tumors that are biopsy proven or strongly suspected of being cancerous based on other diagnostic testing. Short descriptor: **PET tumor init tx strat**.

**PS** – PET or PET/CT to inform the subsequent treatment strategy of cancerous tumors when the beneficiary's treating physician determines that the PET study is needed to inform subsequent anti-tumor strategy. Short descriptor: **PET tumor subsq tx strategy**.

## Therapy monitoring

Accurate information about the effectiveness of radiotherapy and/or chemotherapy for colorectal cancer is important for continuation of the selected therapeutic regimen, or switching to an alternative regimen. The number of studies in which PET has been used successfully for monitoring therapy is relatively small, but monitoring chemotherapy in advanced colorectal cancer appears promising. Strauss and Conti (40) studied the response to therapy with PET for various tracers. Findlay et al. (41) evaluated the metabolism of liver metastases from CRC before and after treatment. The findings were compared with change in size on CT, and results were expressed as a tumor-to-liver uptake ratio. They were able to differentiate eventual responders from non-responders, both on a lesion-by-lesion and patient-based analysis. The Sloan-Kettering group also found good correlation between the response of hepatic metastasis to chemotherapy and FDG uptake (42). Their most promising finding was the positive correlation between PET findings at 4 weeks and CT findings at 12 weeks, while the MR imaging at 4 weeks did not show a change in tumor volume.

Results of the CELIM trial were reported recently in the *Lancet* (43). This phase II randomized trial investigated the response to neoadjuvant therapy with cetuximab in patients with unresectable liver metastases from CRC. The study showed that cetuximab yielded high response rates compared with historical controls. Resectability rates increased from 32% at baseline to 60% after chemotherapy.

Assessing response to radiation therapy (RT) was evaluated by Haberkorn *et al.* (44). Reduction in FDG uptake was found in half of the patients, and correlated with the palliative benefit. These investigators found that FDG uptake immediately following radiation may be due to inflammatory changes without residual tumor (44). They recommended a post-radiation interval of 6 months before evaluating response. The time course of FDG uptake post-radiation has not been studied systematically; but an interval of 4–6 months between RT and PET is recommended to assess presence of complete response.

Although the inflammatory response is real and may hamper image interpretation, early PET/CT scanning has a role to determine whether the tumor is sensitive to treatment. For assessing complete response, sufficient time needs to have elapsed, otherwise remaining FDG uptake may be incorrectly interpreted as residual or recurrent tumor. Schiepers *et al.* (45) investigated the effect of radiation after 10 fractionated doses of 3 Gy on primary rectal cancer (total dose 30 Gy). All cancers showed an effect of irradiation 2 weeks after finishing therapy, and one tumor was no longer detectable in the resected, irradiated specimen.

As a rule of thumb, assessing tumor response with FDG can be performed 3 months after completion of RT and 1 month after chemotherapy.

The European Organization for Research and Treatment of Cancer (EORTC) published a position paper on the use of FDG-PET for the measurement of tumor response in 1999 (46). The EORTC-PET study group formulated standard criteria for reporting alterations in FDG uptake to assess clinical and sub-clinical response to therapy. Although there was wide variation in the methodology between the PET centers surveyed, assessment of FDG uptake was thought to be a satisfactory method to monitor response to treatment. The group made initial recommendations on: (1) patient preparation, (2) timing of PET scans, (3) methods to measure FDG uptake with SUV, and (4) definition of FDG tumor response. Similar guidelines from the National Cancer Institute Trials were published as "Consensus Recommendations" in 2006 (47). Procedure guidelines for imaging with FDG were published by the Society of Nuclear Medicine in 2006 (48). No numerical criteria were given to distinguish responders from non-responders, or to differentiate complete from partial response, versus stable or progressive disease.

## Conclusion

Metabolic imaging with PET/CT using FDG is indicated as the initial test for staging of newly diagnosed and recurrent CRC.

In addition, it is indicated for pre-operative staging of known recurrence that is considered to be surgically resectable. The evidence suggests that CT contrast enhancement improves the accuracy by increasing specificity. PET/CT is valuable for distinguishing post-treatment changes from recurrent tumor, differentiation of benign from malignant lymph nodes, and for monitoring therapy. PET/CT reduces overall treatment cost by accurately distinguishing patients who will benefit from surgery from those who will not.

PET/CT is evolving as a molecular imaging modality, with further development of new radiopharmaceuticals, and probes for assessing the efficacy of drugs.

## Stomach cancer

Stomach cancer is not common in the Western world, and is more prevalent in Asia. Some of this difference has been linked to the diet, e.g., fish and seafood; other investigators relate it to higher mercury levels. In the USA, stomach cancer has a 25% higher prevalence than esophageal cancer but 15% lower mortality rate. It is about half as frequent as pancreas carcinoma (2–4). In 2009, a total of 21,130 new patients were estimated to be diagnosed with gastric carcinoma, and 10,620 were expected to die from their disease (5). The incidence of stomach cancer is higher in men than women (M/F ratio = 1.543), as is the mortality rate (M/F ratio = 1.470) (5). A 5-year survival rate of approximately 60% is reported for the USA compared with approximately 40% for the European Union.

The diagnosis of stomach cancer is established by endoscopy and biopsy. The role of endoscopic ultrasound (EUS) is directed toward evaluating local extent of disease, whereas abdominal US and CT are geared toward metastatic workup. A relationship has been found with the phenotype, whereby the intestinal growth type has higher FDG uptake than the diffuse growth type (49, 50). This translates in higher sensitivity of FDG for the detection of intestinal type gastric cancer.

Sun *et al.* (51) investigated the role of PET/CT in **gastric cancer recurrence** after initial surgical resection in 23 patients. The final diagnosis was confirmed by histology. Overall accuracy was 83% and the PPV 86%. Although the studied population is too small for meaningful conclusions, their results suggest that true recurrence can be diagnosed effectively. Sim *et al.* (52) investigated gastric cancer recurrence in a similar scenario and found that the addition of contrast-enhanced CT to FDG-PET did not increase sensitivity significantly, except for the detection of peritoneal seeding. Contrast-enhanced CT appeared superior to PET/CT for lymph node staging in the publication of Kim *et al.* (53), otherwise the two modalities performed comparably.

In patients with gastric carcinoma, the **lymph node status** is crucial in determining treatment planning and prognosis. A systematic literature search on the role of imaging was reported by Kwee and Kwee in 2009 (54), who found 54 studies using six different imaging modalities. EUS was over-represented

(30 studies) whereas FDG-PET was under-represented (five studies). The included studies were of "moderate methodological quality." The sensitivity was uniformly low ranging from 12% to 95%, with CT being the best with a median sensitivity of 80%. The specificity was better, varying from 50% to 100%, with FDG-PET being more specific at 93%. The authors concluded that anatomic imaging and PET-only cannot reliably be used to confirm or exclude lymph-node metastasis. The performance of PET/CT and functional MRI still has to be determined. Both CT and PET appear to have relatively low sensitivity for detection of regional lymph node metastases. Hence, the role of PET/CT in nodal staging is rather limited. The sensitivity improves somewhat from N1 to N3 disease. The specificity, on the other hand, hovers in the 90s and Dassen *et al.* (49) reported a median specificity of 96%, which seems adequate for clinical applications and patient management.

The literature suggests that the role of PET/CT in nodal staging of gastric carcinoma is still being investigated. The specificity appears sufficient, but the sensitivity is probably too low.

**Monitoring therapy response** is not used routinely, but appears very promising in categorizing tumor phenotype, i.e., gastric cancers without FDG uptake have poor outcome, and in differentiating responders from non-responders to therapy. Randomized trials have shown that pre-operative chemotherapy does not improve survival (55). Several studies have found that patients who have an objective response have a favorable prognosis, which is better than surgery alone. Unfortunately, only 30–40% of patients are responders to chemotherapy, and FDG-PET is able to stratify this subgroup. Ott *et al.* showed that the 2-year survival was 90% in responders vs. 25% in non-responders (55). They showed that FDG-PET after 2 weeks of therapy could correctly predict histopathologic response after 3 months. This study prospectively demonstrated that in patients with gastric cancer, response to pre-operative chemotherapy could be predicted by FDG-PET early during the course of therapy. By avoiding the morbidity and costs of ineffective therapy, FDG-PET imaging facilitates the use of pre-operative chemotherapy.

In their 2008 study, Ott *et al.* (56) tested the chemosensitivity of locally advanced gastric cancer. In patients with FDG-avid tumors, therapy response and survival could be predicted, and they were able to associate metabolic responders with a high histopathologic response rate. The tumors that were not

FDG-avid had a poorer prognosis. Thus, lack of FDG uptake may be used for therapy modification early on.

The literature suggests that there will be a role of PET/CT in gastric carcinoma by stratifying patients for neoadjuvant therapy and monitoring treatment response.

## Gastrointestinal stromal tumor

Gastrointestinal stromal tumor (GIST) is a sarcoma; it is an uncommon tumor with an incidence of 16–20 per million in the USA; they comprise 3% of all GI malignancies and 6% of all sarcomas. Approximately 80–95% of tumors have a mutation in the *c-kit* gene and produce the KIT protein. These tumors are derived from GI mesenchymal cells, and most of them express the CD117 and/or CD34 antigen. Approximately 65% of GIST sarcomas are found in the stomach.

The interest in this type of tumor relates to the availability of treatment with relatively few side effects. Tyrosine kinase inhibitors such as imatinib mesylate (Gleevec®) are extremely effective and dramatic metabolic responses have been seen. Approximately 15% of patients do not respond to imatinib mesylate, therefore, it is important to assess the response of the tumor to this type of therapy. FDG-PET/CT is ideal to monitor this.

GIST sarcomas have been reviewed by several investigators (57–59). For the surgical approach the reader is referred to the article of Pisters and Patel (60) and for the imaging approach to Antoch *et al.* (59). The initial studies by Van den Abbeele and her co-workers have been quoted widely. Her view from the oncologist's viewpoint and the role of FDG-PET/CT can be found in the *Oncologist* (61).

The role of FDG-PET/CT centers on the evaluation of the tumor's sensitivity to therapy, i.e., type of tyrosine kinase inhibitor, and surveillance of therapy. Over time, many patients become resistant to imatinib mesylate, and a newer generation of tyrosine kinase inhibitors has been developed for second-line treatment.

The most important role of FDG-PET/CT is to document treatment effectiveness. Within 24 hours a dramatic response may be seen in tumors that are sensitive. Restaging PET/CT can be done to demonstrate whether the patient is a complete or partial responder, in order to be able to change patient management. Relapse of disease can easily be demonstrated with molecular imaging using FDG.

# References

1. Schiepers C. PET/CT in colorectal cancer. *J Nucl Med* 2003;**44**(11):1804–5.

2. Landis SH, Murray T, Bolden S, Wingo PA. Cancer statistics, 1999. *CA Cancer J Clin* 1999;**V49**(N1):8–31.

3. Wingo PA, Ries LAG, Rosenberg HM, Miller DS, Edwards BK. Cancer incidence and mortality, 1973–1995: a report card for the U.S. *Cancer* 1998;**V82**(N6):1197–207.

4. Jemal A, Tiwari RC, Murray T *et al.* Cancer statistics, 2004. *CA Cancer J Clin* 2004;**54**(1):8–29.

5. Jemal A, Siegel R, Ward E *et al.* Cancer statistics, 2009. *CA Cancer J Clin* 2009;**59**(4):225–49.

6. Coleman RE. FDG imaging. *Nucl Med Biol* 2000;**27**(7):689–90.

7. Dahlbom M, Hoffman EJ, Hoh CK *et al.* Whole-body positron emission tomography. 1. methods and performance characteristics. *J Nucl Med* 1992;**33**(6):1191–9.

8. Schiepers C, Hoh CK. Positron emission tomography as a diagnostic tool in oncology. *Eur Radiol* 1998;**8**(8):1481–94.

9. Abdel-Nabi H, Doerr RJ, Lamonica DM *et al.* Staging of primary colorectal carcinomas with fluorine-18 fluorodeoxyglucose whole-body PET:

correlation with histopathologic and CT findings. *Radiology* 1998; **206**(3):755–60.

10. Ruhlmann J, Schomburg A, Bender H *et al.* Fluorodeoxyglucose whole-body positron emission tomography in colorectal cancer patients studied in routine daily practice. *Diseas Colon Rectum* 1997;**40**(10):1195–204.

11. Huebner RH, Park KC, Shepherd JE *et al.* A meta-analysis of the literature for whole-body FDG PET detection of recurrent colorectal cancer. *J Nucl Med* 2000;**41**(7):1177–89.

12. Schiepers C, Penninckx F, De Vadder N *et al.* Contribution of PET in the diagnosis of recurrent colorectal cancer: comparison with conventional imaging. *Eur J Surg Oncol* 1995;**21**(5):517–22.

13. Moertel CG, Fleming TR, MacDonald JS *et al.* An evaluation of the carcinoembryonic antigen (CEA) test for monitoring patients with resected colon cancer. *J Am Med Assoc* 1993; **270**(8):943–7.

14. Charnley RM. Imaging of colorectal carcinoma. *Radiology* 1990;**V174** (N1):283.

15. Steele G, Bleday R, Mayer RJ *et al.* A prospective evaluation of hepatic resection for colorectal carcinoma metastases to the liver – Gastrointestinal-Tumor-Study-Group Protocol-6584. *J Clin Oncol* 1991;**V9**(N7):1105–12.

16. McDaniel KP, Charnsangavej C, Dubrow RA *et al.* Pathways of nodal metastasis in carcinomas of the cecum, ascending colon, and transverse colon – CT demonstration. *Am J Roentgenol* 1993;**V161**(N1):61–4.

17. Nelson RC, Chezmar JL, Sugarbaker PH, Bernardino ME. Hepatic tumors-comparison of CT during arterial portography, delayed CT, and MR imaging for preoperative evaluation. *Radiology* 1989;**V172**(N1):27–34.

18. Sobhani I, Tiret E, Lebtahi R *et al.* Early detection of recurrence by 18FDG-PET in the follow-up of patients with colorectal cancer. *Br J Cancer* 2008; **98**(5):875–80.

19. Votrubova J, Belohlavek O, Jaruskova M *et al.* The role of FDG-PET/CT in the detection of recurrent colorectal cancer. *Eur J Nucl Med Mol Imaging* 2006;**33**(7):779–84.

20. Warburg O. On the origin of cancer cells. *Science* 1956;**123**:309–14.

21. Wahl RL. Targeting glucose transporters for tumor imaging – sweet idea, sour result. *J Nucl Med* 1996; **V37**(N6):1038–41.

22. Strauss LG. Fluorine-18 deoxyglucose and false-positive results: a major problem in the diagnostics of oncological patients. *EurJ Nucl Med* 1996;**23**(10):1409–15.

23. Rosenbaum SJ, Lind T, Antoch G, Bockisch A. False-positive FDG PET uptake – the role of PET/CT. *Eur Radiol* 2006;**16**(5):1054–65.

24. Kamel EM, Thumshirn M, Truninger K *et al.* Significance of incidental 18F-FDG accumulations in the gastrointestinal tract in PET/CT: correlation with endoscopic and histopathologic results. *J Nucl Med* 2004;**45**(11):1804–10.

25. Gutman F, Alberini JL, Wartski M *et al.* Incidental colonic focal lesions detected by FDG PET/CT. *Am J Roentgenol* 2005;**185**(2):495–500.

26. Kitajima K, Murakami K, Yamasaki E *et al.* Performance of integrated FDG PET/contrast-enhanced CT in the diagnosis of recurrent colorectal cancer: comparison with integrated FDG PET/non-contrast-enhanced CT and enhanced CT. *Eur J Nucl Med Mol Imaging* 2009;**36**(9):1388–96.

27. Cantwell CP, Setty BN, Holalkere N *et al.* Liver lesion detection and characterization in patients with colorectal cancer: a comparison of low radiation dose non-enhanced PET/CT, contrast-enhanced PET/CT, and liver MRI. *J Comput Assist Tomogr.* 2008;**32**(5):738–44.

28. de Geus-Oei LF, Vriens D, van Laarhoven HW, van der Graaf WT, Oyen WJ. Monitoring and predicting response to therapy with 18F-FDG PET in colorectal cancer: a systematic review. *J Nucl Med* 2009;**50**(Suppl 1): 43S–54S.

29. Rosenberg R, Herrmann K, Gertler R *et al.* The predictive value of metabolic response to preoperative radiochemotherapy in locally advanced rectal cancer measured by PET/CT. *Int J Colorectal Dis* 2009; **24**(2):191–200.

30. Phelps ME. Inaugural article: positron emission tomography provides molecular imaging of biological processes. *Proc Natl Acad Sci US A* 2000;**97**(16):9226–33.

31. Phelps ME. PET: the merging of biology and imaging into molecular imaging. *J Nucl Med* 2000; **41**(4):661–81.

32. Jadvar H, Alavi A, Gambhir SS. 18F-FDG uptake in lung, breast, and colon cancers: molecular biology correlates and disease characterization. *J Nucl Med* 2009;**50**(11):1820–7.

33. Hoh CK, Schiepers C, Seltzer MA *et al.* PET in oncology: will it replace the other modalities? *Semin Nucl Med* 1997;**27**(2):94–106.

34. Goerres GW, Hany TF, Kamel E, von Schulthess GK, Buck A. Head and neck imaging with PET and PET/CT: artefacts from dental metallic implants. *Eur J Nucl Med Mol Imaging* 2002; **29**(3):367–70.

35. Halpern BS, Dahlbom M, Waldherr C *et al.* Cardiac pacemakers and central venous lines can induce focal artifacts on CT-corrected PET images. *J Nucl Med* 2004;**45**(2):290–3.

36. Halpern BS, Dahlbom M, Quon A *et al.* Impact of patient weight and emission scan duration on PET/CT image quality and lesion detectability. *J Nucl Med* 2004;**45**(5):797–801.

37. Goerres GW, Burger C, Schwitter MW *et al.* PET/CT of the abdomen: optimizing the patient breathing pattern. *Eur Radiol* 2003;**13**(4):734–9.

38. Strauss LG, Clorius JH, Schlag P *et al.* Recurrence of colorectal tumors: PET evaluation. *Radiology* 1989; **170**(2):329–32.

39. Takeuchi O, Saito N, Koda K, Sarashina H, Nakajima N. Clinical assessment of positron emission tomography for the diagnosis of local recurrence in colorectal cancer. *Br J Surg* 1999; **86**(7):932–7.

40. Strauss LG, Conti PS. The applications of PET in clinical oncology. *J Nucl Med* 1991;**V32**(N4):623–48.

41. Findlay M, Young H, Cunningham D *et al.* Noninvasive monitoring of tumor metabolism using fluorodeoxyglucose and positron emission tomography in colorectal cancer liver metastases: correlation with tumor response to fluorouracil [see comments]. *J Clin Oncol* 1996;**14**(3):700–8.

42. Akhurst T, Larson SM. Positron emission tomography imaging of colorectal cancer. *Semin Oncol* 1999; **26**(5):577–83.

43. Folprecht G, Gruenberger T, Bechstein WO *et al.* Tumour response and secondary resectability of colorectal liver metastases following neoadjuvant chemotherapy with cetuximab: the CELIM randomised phase 2 trial. *Lancet Oncol.* 2010;**11**(1):38–47.

44. Haberkorn U, Strauss LG, Dimitrakopoulou A *et al.* PET studies of fluorodeoxyglucose metabolism in patients with recurrent colorectal tumors receiving radiotherapy. *J Nucl Med* 1991;**32**(8):1485–90.

45. Schiepers C, Haustermans K, Geboes K *et al.* The effect of preoperative radiation therapy on glucose utilization and cell kinetics in patients with primary rectal carcinoma. *Cancer* 1999;**85**(4):803–11.

46. Young H, Baum R, Cremerius U *et al.* Measurement of clinical and subclinical tumour response using [F-18]-fluorodeoxyglucose and positron emission tomography: review and 1999 EORTC recommendations. *Eur J Cancer* 1999;**V35**(N13):1773–82.

47. Shankar LK, Hoffman JM, Bacharach S *et al.* Consensus recommendations for the use of 18F-FDG PET as an indicator of therapeutic response in patients in National Cancer Institute Trials. *J Nucl Med* 2006;**47**(6):1059–66.

48. Delbeke D, Coleman RE, Guiberteau MJ *et al.* Procedure guideline for tumor imaging with 18F-FDG PET/CT 1.0. *J Nucl Med* 2006;**47**(5):885–95.

49. Dassen AE, Lips DJ, Hoekstra CJ, Pruijt JF, Bosscha K. FDG-PET has no definite role in preoperative imaging in gastric cancer. *Eur J Surg Oncol* 2009;**35**(5):449–55.

50. Stahl A, Ott K, Weber WA *et al.* FDG PET imaging of locally advanced gastric carcinomas: correlation with endoscopic and histopathological findings. *Eur J Nucl Med Mol Imaging* 2003;**30**(2):288–95.

51. Sun L, Su XH, Guan YS *et al.* Clinical role of 18F-fluorodeoxyglucose positron emission tomography/computed tomography in post-operative follow up of gastric cancer: initial results. *World J Gastroenterol* 2008; **14**(29):4627–32.

52. Sim SH, Kim YJ, Oh DY *et al.* The role of PET/CT in detection of gastric cancer recurrence. *BMC Cancer* 2009;**9**:73.

53. Kim EY Lee WJ, Choi D *et al.* The value of PET/CT for preoperative staging of advanced gastric cancer: comparison with contrast-enhanced CT. *Eur J Radiol* 2011;**79**(2):183–8.

54. Kwee RM, Kwee TC. Imaging in assessing lymph node status in gastric cancer. *Gastric Cancer* 2009;**12**(1):6–22.

55. Ott K, Fink U, Becker K *et al.* Prediction of response to preoperative chemotherapy in gastric carcinoma by metabolic imaging: results of a prospective trial. *J Clin Oncol* 2003; **21**(24):4604–10.

56. Ott K, Herrmann K, Lordick F *et al.* Early metabolic response evaluation by fluorine-18 fluorodeoxyglucose positron emission tomography allows in vivo testing of chemosensitivity in gastric cancer: long-term results of a prospective study. *Clin Cancer Res* 2008; **14**(7):2012–18.

57. Esteves FP, Schuster DM, Halkar RK. Gastrointestinal tract malignancies and positron emission tomography: an overview. *Semin Nucl Med* 2006;**36**(2):169–81.

58. Goerres GW, Stupp R, Barghouth G *et al.* The value of PET, CT and in-line PET/CT in patients with gastrointestinal stromal tumours: long-term outcome of treatment with imatinib mesylate. *Eur J Nucl Med Mol Imaging* 2005;**32**(2):153–62.

59. Antoch G, Kanja J, Bauer S *et al.* Comparison of PET, CT, and dual-modality PET/CT imaging for monitoring of imatinib (STI571) therapy in patients with gastrointestinal stromal tumors. *J Nucl Med* 2004;**45**(3):357–65.

60. Pisters PW, Patel SR. Gastrointestinal stromal tumors: current management. *J Surg Oncol* 2010; **102**:530–8.

61. Van den Abbeele AD. The lessons of GIST – PET and PET/CT: a new paradigm for imaging. *Oncologist* 2008;**13**(Suppl 2):8–13.

A 66-year-old female with adenocarcinoma of the sigmoid colon. Status post-resection; stage III (pT3N2). Subsequent chemotherapy (FOLFOX) was given for 6 months. An FDG-PET/CT was ordered to plan the subsequent treatment strategy, 2 months after finishing chemotherapy.

## Acquisition and processing parameters

| Equipment | PET/CT system |
|---|---|
| CT | 16-slice, 120 kVp, 114 mA (effective dose), 0.8 s/rotation, pitch 0.6, collimation 3 mm |
| Reconstruction | Filtered back-projection, convolution kernel B31f |
| PET | LSO, 3-D, 16 cm axial FOV, 81 slices, six bed positions from base skull to proximal femur |
| Reconstruction | OSEM-2-D, 2 iterations, 8 subsets, convolution kernel Gaussian 5 mm |
| Patient preparation | Fasting for 6 hours |
| | Serum glucose level 107 mg/dL; Serum creatinine 0.7 mg/dL |
| Dose | 13.1 mCi of FDG |
| Oral contrast | ReadiCat 3 portions of 300 mL at −55, −30 and 0 minutes before FDG injection |
| IV contrast | 115 mL Omnipaque-350 at a rate of 1.2 mL/s |
| Uptake interval | 60 min |

## Findings and differential diagnosis

No focus of abnormal uptake in the pelvis. Normal liver appearance. Abnormally increased uptake in the neck bilaterally, retrocrural areas, and peri-renal regions. No associated lesions on CT. The differential diagnoses include brown adipose tissue or a normal variant.

A

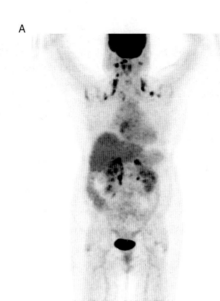

**Figure 9.1A** Anterior projection of an MIP FDG-PET image.

## Diagnosis and teaching points

CRC does not often metastasize to the neck, but it is possible. Here, the abnormal neck uptake is asymmetric, so detailed inspection is necessary on all three planes, axial, coronal and sagittal, with careful attention to CT to discriminate fat versus muscle or lymph node. The axial cuts in Figure 9.1B show uptake outside the kidneys that correlates with fat density on CT. The coronal cuts demonstrate that this is not related to the crus of the diaphragm.

## Take-home message

- Not all increased activity is related to neoplastic disease (1, 2).
- The observed abnormal activity is not in areas where CRC spreads.
- Inspection of CT shows that the density of the tissues with increased FDG uptake is related to fat.
- Muscles can exhibit increased uptake as well (1, 2).

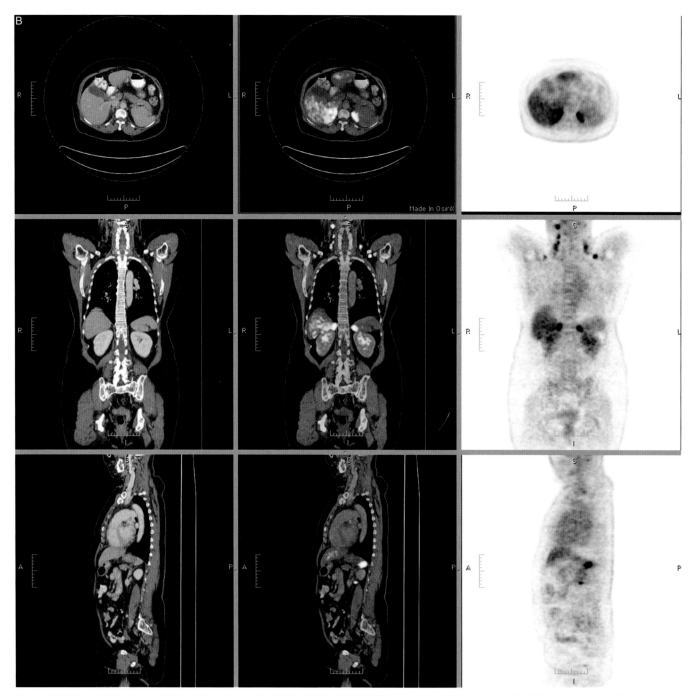

**Figure 9.1B** Transaxial and coronal slices of a representative CT slice (left) and FDG-PET slice (right) and the fused FDG-PET/CT image in the middle.

# References

1.  Strauss LG. Fluorine-18 deoxyglucose and false-positive results: a major problem in the diagnostics of oncological patients. *Eur J Nucl Med* 1996;**23**(10):1409–15.

2.  Rosenbaum SJ, Lind T, Antoch G, Bockisch A. False-positive FDG PET uptake – the role of PET/CT. *Eur Radiol* 2006;**16**(5):1054–65.

A 50-year-old female with a multi-lobulated polyp on the mucosal surface of the ileocecal valve measuring 3–4 cm, which was discovered on colonoscopy. Histopathology revealed that this tubulovillous adenoma contained adenocarcinoma, without lymphovascular invasion.

FDG-PET/CT was obtained to stage for initial treatment strategy.

## Acquisition and processing parameters

| Equipment | PET/CT system |
|---|---|
| CT | 64-slice, 120 kVp, 80 mA (effective dose), 0.5 s/ rotation, pitch 0.8, collimation 1.2 mm |
| Reconstruction | Filtered back-projection, convolution kernel B31f |
| PET | LSO, 3-D, 22 cm axial FOV, 109 slices, five bed positions from base skull to proximal femur |
| Reconstruction | OSEM-2-D, 2 iterations, 8 subsets, convolution kernel Gaussian 5 mm |
| Patient preparation | Fasting for 6 hours |
| | Serum glucose level 77 mg/dL |
| Dose | 11.3 mCi FDG |
| Oral contrast | None |
| IV contrast | None |
| Uptake interval | 59 min |

## Findings and differential diagnosis

Figure 9.2A shows cecal wall thickening with abnormally increased activity in the right lower quadrant, corresponding to the known primary. Abnormal uptake in a right paracaval lymph node is highly suspicious for metastasis. Note the uptake left of the midline that corresponds to excreted FDG in the left ureter. Figure 9.2B shows abnormal density in the liver segment IVa, with abnormally increased activity, suspicious for liver metastasis. In this case the differentials include primary tumor of the cecum. Abnormal lymph node, and liver lesion that could represent metastases or another primary neoplasm.

## Diagnosis and follow-up

The patient underwent sub-total abdominal colectomy, with resection of the lymph node and a partial hepatectomy of segment 2 and 3. Histopathology of the primary tumor revealed a moderately differentiated, adenocarcinoma of the cecum of 5.9 cm in size, arising from an adenovillous adenoma, and negative surgical margins. Liver and lymph node pathology revealed metastatic colonic adenocarcinoma. Subsequently she had six cycles of chemotherapy (FOLFOX6-avastin), and 2 weeks after completion of treatment, she had another PET/CT study. Results are shown in Case 2 – part II (Figures 9.2C, D).

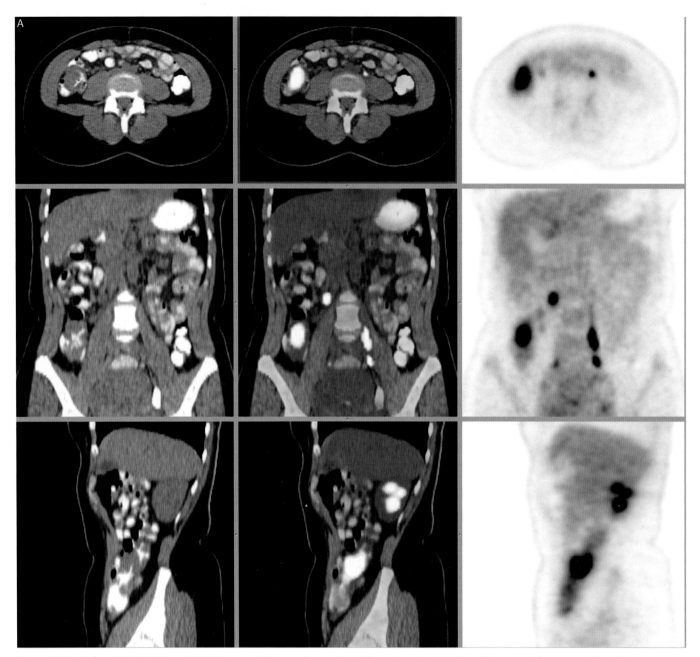

**Figure 9.2A** CT, fused FDG-PET/CT, and FDG-PET, transaxial (top row), coronal (middle row), and sagittal slices (bottom row) focusing on the right lower abdominal quadrant.

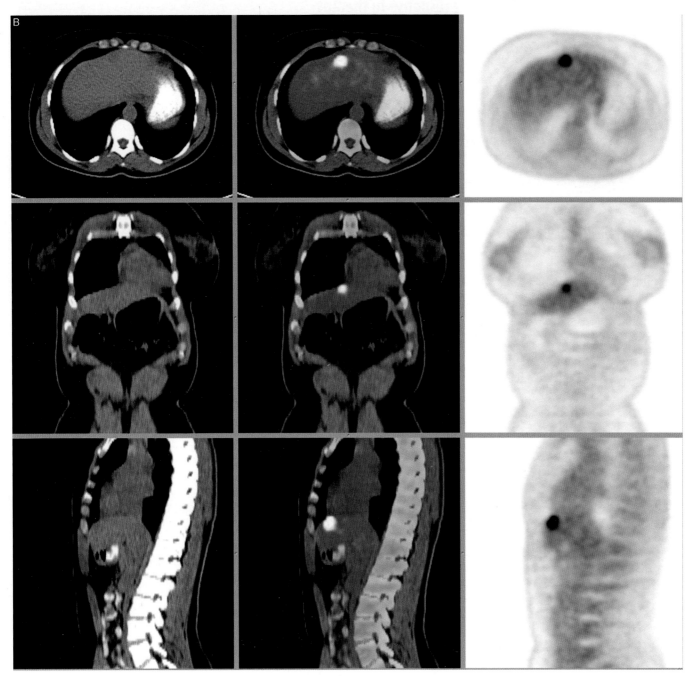

**Figure 9.2B** CT, fused FDG-PET/CT, and FDG-PET, transaxial (top row), coronal (middle row), and sagittal slices (bottom row) focused on the liver.

A 50-year-old female with adenocarcinoma of the cecum. Status post-resection of primary cancer and metastasis to a lymph node and the liver. Status post six cycles of chemotherapy (see Figures 9.2 A, B for initial staging). An FDG-PET/CT was ordered to plan subsequent treatment strategy.

## Acquisition and processing parameters

| | |
|---|---|
| Equipment | PET/CT system |
| CT | 64-slice, 120 kVp, 119 mA (effective dose), 0.5 s/rotation, pitch 0.8, collimation 3 mm |
| Reconstruction | Filtered back-projection, convolution kernel B31f |
| PET | LSO, 3-D, 16 cm axial FOV, 81 slices, six bed positions from base skull to proximal femur |
| Reconstruction | OSEM-2-D, 2 iterations, 8 subsets, convolution kernel Gaussian 5 mm |
| Patient preparation | Fasting for 6 hours |
| | Serum glucose level 99 mg/dL; Serum creatinine 0.7 mg/dL |
| Dose | 16.8 mCi FDG |
| Oral contrast | ReadiCat 900 mL |
| IV contrast | 115 mL Omnipaque-350 at a rate of 1.2 mL/s |
| Uptake interval | 58 min |

## Findings and differential diagnosis

Cecum primary and the lymph node are no longer seen, status post-resection. The axial CT slice in Figure 9.2C shows the suture line, without any abnormal foci. The lesion in the liver was also resected and a photopenic area is now seen in Figure 9.2D.

## Discussion and teaching points

The initial FDG-PET/CT scan revealed that this patient had stage IV disease and needed major surgery. Subsequently she had chemotherapy because of the advanced stage of her disease. The second PET/CT scan revealed that she is a complete responder to the instituted therapy, i.e., surgery plus adjuvant chemotherapy.

### Take-home message

- The tubulovillous adenoma discovered on routine colonoscopy turned out to be the harbinger of far more advanced disease.
- Accurate staging of disease is mandatory (1). In this manner the appropriate strategy for intervention and patient management can be planned, e.g., neo-adjuvant therapy vs. immediate surgery. Other strategies, i.e., surgical vs. medical vs. radiation therapy or a combination of these can be chosen accordingly.
- The clinical stage of disease has prognostic value and the patient can be informed what to expect if the usual course of events is anticipated (1, 2).
- The follow-up period for this patient is too short to predict final outcome, but the favorable FDG-PET/CT response puts this patient in a category for which a longer survival is expected (2, 3).

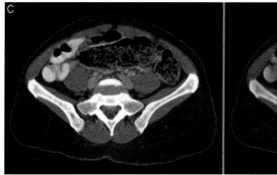
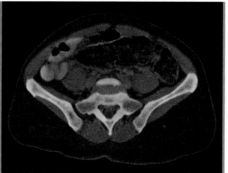
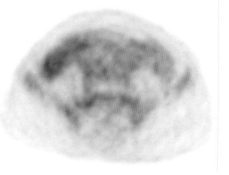

**Figure 9.2C** CT, fused FDG-PET/CT, and FDG-PET, transaxial slices at the level of the anastomosis.

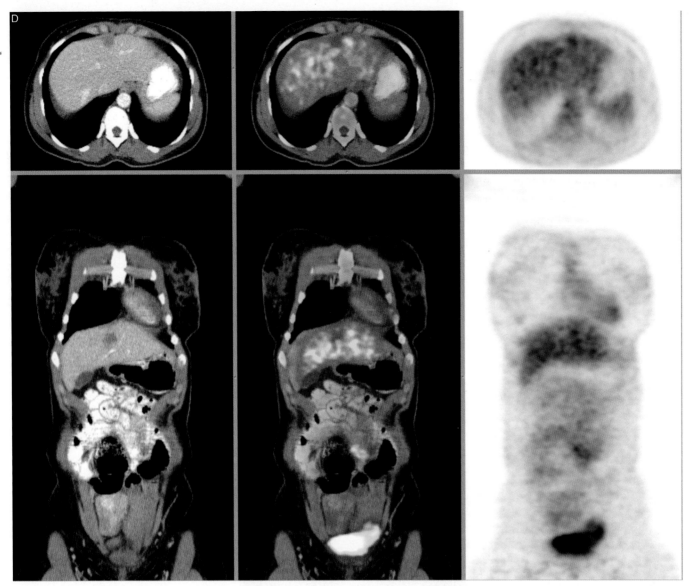

**Figure 9.2D** CT, fused FDG-PET/CT, and FDG-PET, transaxial (top) and coronal slices (bottom), focused on the liver.

# References

1. Abdel-Nabi H, Doerr RJ, Lamonica DM *et al.* Staging of primary colorectal carcinomas with fluorine-18 fluorodeoxyglucose whole-body PET: correlation with histopathologic and CT findings. *Radiology* 1998;**206**(3):755–60.

2. Shankar LK, Hoffman JM, Bacharach S *et al.* Consensus recommendations for the use of 18F-FDG PET as an indicator of therapeutic response in patients in National Cancer Institute Trials. *J Nucl Med* 2006; **47**(6):1059–66.

3. De Geus-Oei LF, Vriens D, van Laarhoven HW, van der Graaf WT, Oyen WJ. Monitoring and predicting response to therapy with 18F-FDG PET in colorectal cancer: a systematic review. *J Nucl Med* 2009;**50**(Suppl 1): 43S–54S.

A 41-year-old male with rectal cancer, staged as uT3N0 by endoscopic ultrasound. An FDG-PET/CT was done for staging before pre-operative radiation therapy (initial treatment strategy).

## Acquisition and processing parameters

| | |
|---|---|
| Equipment | PET/CT system |
| CT | 64-slice, 120 kVp, 162 mA (effective dose), 0.5 s/rotation, pitch 0.8, collimation 3 mm |
| Reconstruction | Filtered back-projection, convolution kernel B31f |
| PET | LSO, 3-D, 22 cm axial FOV, 109 slices, six bed positions |
| Reconstruction | OSEM-2-D, 2 iterations, 8 subsets, convolution kernel Gaussian 5 mm |

| | |
|---|---|
| Patient preparation | Fasting for 6 hours |
| | Serum glucose level 79 mg/dL; Serum creatinine 0.7 mg/dL |
| | The patient is in the prone position, in preparation for CT simulation and IMRT planning |
| Dose | 13.7 mCi FDG |
| Oral contrast | ReadiCat 3 portions of 300 mL at −55, −30 and 0 minutes before FDG injection |
| IV contrast | 115 mL Omnipaque-350 at a rate of 1.2 mL/s |
| Uptake interval | 92 min |

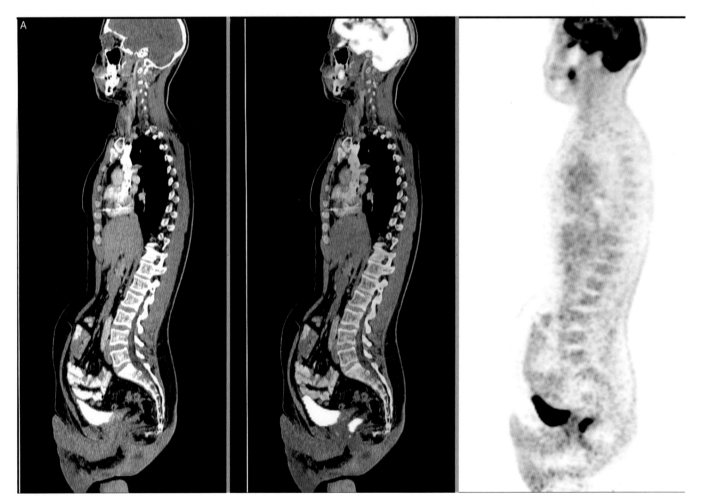

**Figure 9.3A** Sagittal CT, fused FDG-PET/CT, and FDG-PET slices.

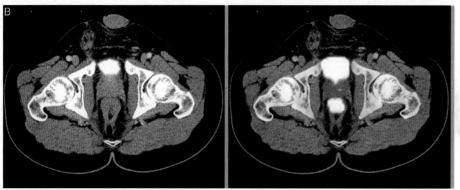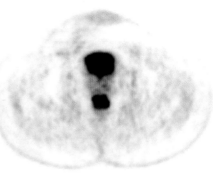

**Figure 9.3B** Transaxial CT, fused FDG/PET/CT, and FDG-PET slices.

## Findings and differential diagnosis

Intense FDG uptake in the known rectal primary. No evidence for regional metastasis or distant metastatic disease.

## Clinical follow-up

Patient received 5040 cGy in 28 fractionated doses over 39 days to the rectum. Patient tolerated the treatment well and had no side effects. The patient was scheduled to undergo FDG-PET/CT to monitor response to radiation therapy before surgery. See Case 3 – part II.

A 41-year-old male with rectal cancer, and pre-operative radiation treatment, undergoing PET/CT imaging for subsequent treatment strategy planning.

## Acquisition and processing parameters

| | |
|---|---|
| Equipment | PET/CT system |
| CT | 64-slice, 120 kVp, 138 mA (effective dose), 0.5 s/rotation, pitch 0.8, collimation 3 mm |
| Reconstruction | Filtered back-projection, convolution kernel B31f |
| PET | LSO, 3-D, 22 cm axial FOV with 109 slices, six bed positions |
| Reconstruction | OSEM-2-D, 2 iterations, 8 subsets, convolution kernel Gaussian 5 mm |
| Patient preparation | Fasting for 6 hours |
| | Serum glucose level 98 mg/dL |
| | Serum creatinine 0.7 mg/dL |
| Dose | 12.9 mCi FDG |
| Oral contrast | ReadiCat 900 mL |
| IV contrast | 115 mL Omnipaque-350 |
| Uptake interval | 64 min |

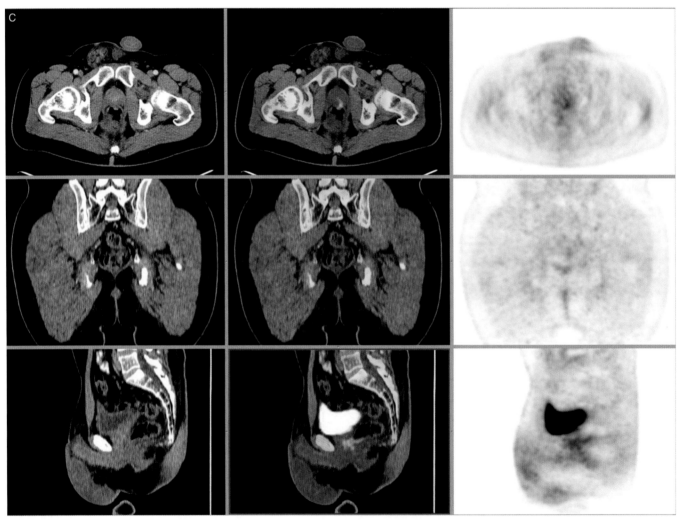

**Figure 9.3C** FDG-PET/CT post-radiation therapy: transaxial (top row), coronal (middle row) and sagittal (lower row), CT, fused FDG-PET/CT, and FDG-PET slices, respectively.

## Findings

The retro-vesicular mass in the rectum with intense uptake is no longer seen. Some non-specific FDG uptake is seen in the prostate bed and bowel wall. No evidence of distant metastasis. The patient is categorized as having a complete response to radiation therapy.

## Clinical follow-up

One month later the patient had a low anterior resection, coloanal anastomosis and diverting iliostomy. Pathology revealed an adenocarcinoma of the rectum; pT2N0Mx.

A 41-year-old male with rectal cancer, uT3N0 by endoscopic ultrasound. Status post neoadjuvant radiation with complete response (Figure 9.3C). No distant metastasis by imaging. Status post low anterior resection, coloanal anastomosis and diverting iliostomy. Pathology revealed an adenocarcinoma of the rectum; pT2N0Mx. An FDG-PET/CT was performed 5 months after surgery.

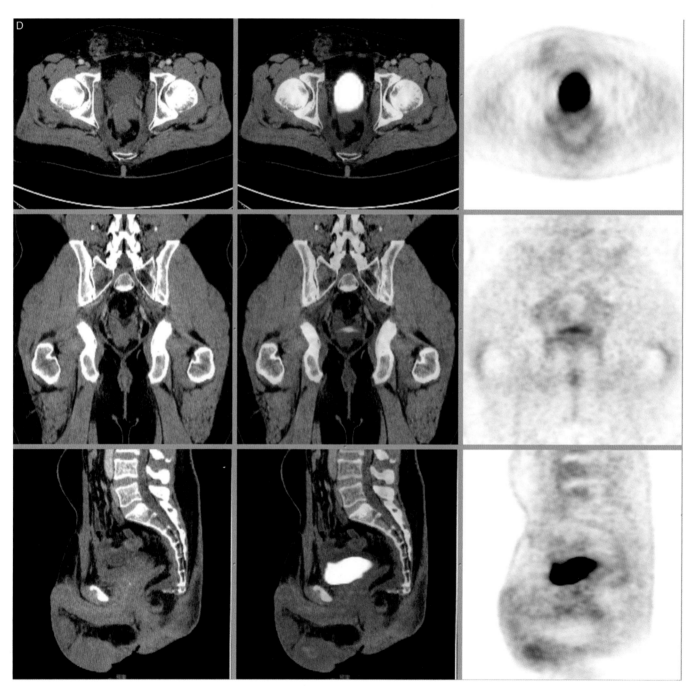

**Figure 9.3D** Five-month post-surgical FDG-PET/CT: transaxial (top row), coronal (middle row) and sagittal (lower row), CT, fused FDG-PET/CT, and FDG-PET slices, respectively.

## Acquisition and processing parameters

| | |
|---|---|
| Equipment | PET/CT system |
| CT | 16-slice, 120 kVp, 118 mA (effective dose), 0.8 s/rotation, pitch 0.6, collimation 3 mm |
| Reconstruction | Filtered back-projection, convolution kernel B31f |
| PET | LSO, 3-D, 16 cm axial FOV, 81 slices, six bed positions from base skull to proximal femur |
| Reconstruction | OSEM-2-D, 2 iterations, 8 subsets, convolution kernel Gaussian 5 mm |
| Patient preparation | Fasting for 6 hours |
| | Serum glucose level 97 mg/dL Serum creatinine 0.8 mg/dL |
| Dose | 10.5 mCi FDG |
| Oral contrast | None |
| IV contrast | 115 mL Omnipaque-350 at a rate of 1.2 mL/s |
| Uptake interval | 76 min |

## Findings

Again, there is no abnormal FDG uptake in the pelvis. No changes are noted when compared with the PET/CT in Figure 9.3C.

## Reference

1. Schiepers C, Haustermans K, Geboes K *et al.* The effect of preoperative radiation therapy on glucose utilization and cell kinetics in patients with primary rectal carcinoma. *Cancer* 1999;**85**(4):803–11.

## Clinical follow-up

One month after this FDG-PET/CT scan the patient had closure and take down of his enterostomy.

## Discussion and teaching points

The initial PET/CT scan revealed that this patient had local disease only. After radiation therapy no metabolically active tumor was found. The patient was scheduled for resection, had no complications, and the temporary enterostomy was closed after 6 months.

## Take-home message

- Accurate staging of disease is necessary to institute proper management (1).
- FDG-PET/CT confirmed the presence of local disease.
- Neoadjuvant therapy for rectal cancer is indicated for T3 disease to improve overall survival (1).
- This patient turned out to be a complete responder, as confirmed by FDG-PET/CT. The routine post-operative care was provided and there were no complications.

A 73-year-old female with episodes of rectal bleeding described as bright red blood in the stool; query rectal versus anal cancer. Biopsy at 4 cm of the anal verge revealed squamous cell carcinoma. FDG-PET/CT was performed for staging before therapy.

## Acquisition and processing parameters

| Equipment | PET/CT system |
| --- | --- |
| CT | 64-slice, 120 kVp, 85 mA (effective dose), 0.5 s/rotation, pitch 0.8, collimation 3 mm |
| Reconstruction | Filtered back-projection, convolution kernel B31f |
| PET | LSO, 3-D, 22 cm axial FOV with 109 slices, six bed positions |
| Reconstruction | OSEM-2-D, 2 iterations, 8 subsets, convolution kernel Gaussian 5 mm |

| Patient preparation | Fasting for 6 hours |
| --- | --- |
| | Serum glucose level 119 mg/dL; Serum creatinine 0.6 mg/dL |
| Dose | 12 mCi FDG |
| Oral contrast | ReadiCat 900 mL |
| IV contrast | 115 mL Omnipaque-350 |
| Uptake interval | 118 min |

## Findings and clinical follow-up

Focus of intensely increased FDG uptake (SUV 6.4) in the distal rectum, consistent with the known primary squamous cell carcinoma. Subsequently the patient was treated with concurrent chemoradiotherapy (see Case 4 – part II).

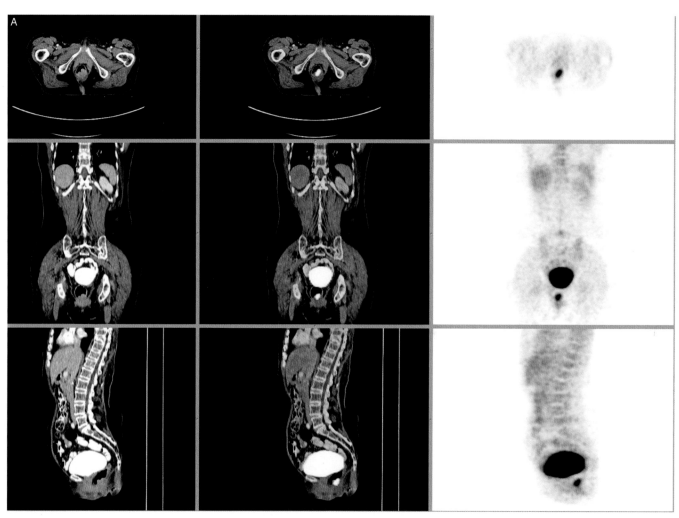

**Figure 9.4A** FDG-PET/CT: transaxial (top row), coronal (middle row) and sagittal (lower row), CT, fused FDG-PET/CT, and FDG-PET slices, respectively.

A 73-year-old female with rectal cancer. FDG-PET/CT was performed after completion of radiation therapy, 4,500 cGy to the pelvis and a boost of 1,500 cGy to the rectum. She also had two cycles of chemotherapy. The following post-therapy FDG-PET/CT study was done 4 months after the initial staging PET/CT, for subsequent treatment strategy.

## Acquisition and processing parameters

| Equipment | PET/CT system |
| --- | --- |
| CT | 64-slice, 120 kVp, 78 mA (effective dose), 0.5 s/rotation, pitch 0.8, collimation 3 mm |
| Reconstruction | Filtered back-projection, convolution kernel B31f |
| PET | LSO, 3-D, 22 cm axial FOV with 109 slices, six bed positions |

| Reconstruction | OSEM-2-D, 2 iterations, 8 subsets, convolution kernel Gaussian 5 mm |
| --- | --- |
| Patient preparation | Fasting for 6 hours |
| | Serum glucose level 99 mg/dL; serum creatinine 0.6 mg/dL |
| Dose | 10.7 mCi FDG |
| Oral contrast | ReadiCat 900 mL |
| IV contrast | 115 mL Omnipaque-350 |
| Uptake interval | 69 min |

## Findings

Linear area of increased uptake in the distal rectum. The maximum SUV has decreased from 6.4 (Figure 9.4A) to 3.5, and the findings were interpreted as inflammatory response to therapy.

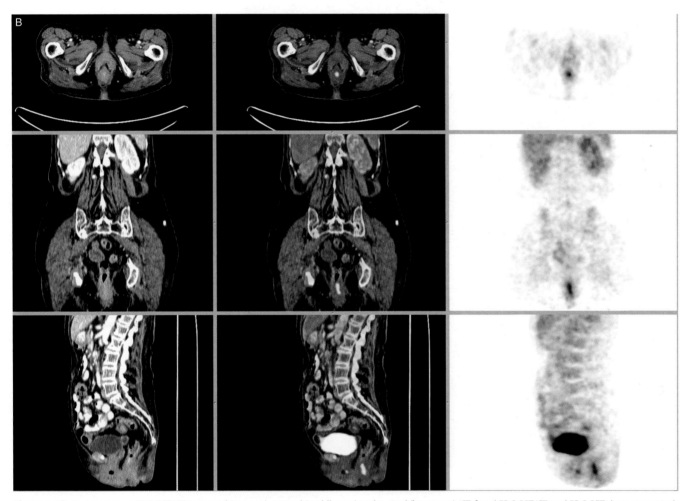

**Figure 9.4B** Post-treatment FDG/PET/CT: transaxial (top row), coronal (middle row) and sagittal (lower row), CT, fused FDG-PET/CT, and FDG-PET slices, respectively.

A 73-year-old female with rectal cancer. The following repeat FDG-PET/CT was performed 3 months after the post-therapy scan (Figure 9.4C), to evaluate the status of FDG uptake in the area previously interpreted as inflammatory changes following treatment, in order to exclude the possibility of residual tumor.

## Acquisition and processing parameters

| Equipment | PET/CT system |
| --- | --- |
| CT | 64-slice, 120 kVp, 110 mA (effective dose), 0.5 s/rotation, pitch 0.8, collimation 3 mm |
| Reconstruction | Filtered back-projection, convolution kernel B31f |

| PET | LSO, 3-D, 22 cm axial FOV with 109 slices, six bed positions |
| --- | --- |
| Reconstruction | OSEM-2-D, 2 iterations, 8 subsets, convolution kernel Gaussian 5 mm |
| Patient preparation | Fasting for 6 hours |
| | Serum glucose level 91 mg/dL, Serum creatinine 0.5 mg/dL |
| Dose | 11.6 mCi FDG |
| Oral contrast | ReadiCat 900 mL |
| IV contrast | 115 mL Omnipaque-350 |
| Uptake interval | 85 min |

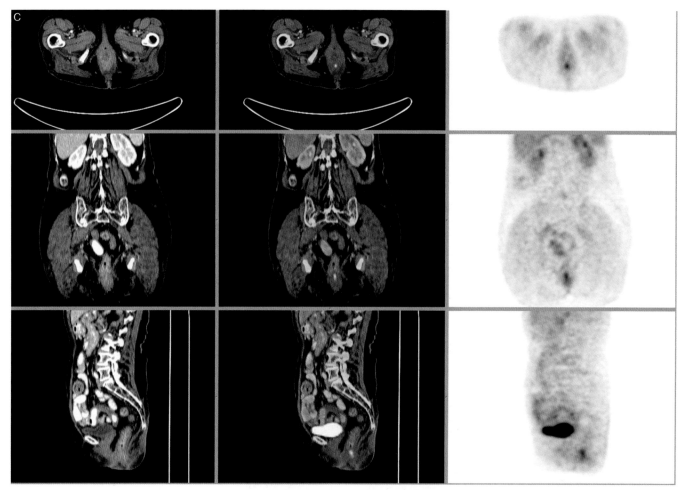

**Figure 9.4C** Second post-treatment FDG-PET/CT: transaxial (top row), coronal (middle row) and sagittal (lower row), CT, fused FDG-PET/CT, and FDG-PET slices, respectively.

## Findings

Again seen is the focus of increased uptake in the distal rectum (Figure 9.4C). The area seems smaller on PET and similar on CT when compared with Figure 9.4B. The maximum SUV appears stable at 3.7 and the scan was interpreted as not significant change from prior, with the uptake related to post-therapy changes. No evidence for local recurrence.

## Diagnosis and clinical follow-up

Clinical evaluation 8 months after this FDG-PET/CT showed no evidence for recurrence or metastatic disease.

## Discussion and teaching points

This patient had a squamous cell carcinoma, which was treated with chemo-radiation. The initial FDG-PET/CT scan revealed only local disease. After therapy, there was still metabolic activity seen in the distal rectum and anal area. This was interpreted as inflammatory changes after therapy, which was confirmed in a subsequent FDG-PET/CT scan. The last scan excluded tumor recurrence.

## Take-home message

- Accurate staging of disease is important and necessary.
- In patients with a different histology, surgery may not be the first approach.
- The FDG-PET/CT showed local disease only. This patient turned out to be a responder with a metabolic activity that dropped about 50%.
- Subsequent imaging confirmed a stable situation with some uptake that was likely physiologic.
- Maximum SUV of the tumor measured about 1 hour after tracer administration may be used as a marker for therapy response (1, 2).

## References

1. Young H, Baum R, Cremerius U et al. Measurement of clinical and subclinical tumour response using [F-18]-fluorodeoxyglucose and positron emission tomography: Review and 1999 EORTC recommendations. *Eur J Cancer* 1999;**V35**(N13):1773–82.

2. Shankar LK, Hoffman JM, Bacharach S et al. Consensus recommendations for the use of 18F-FDG PET as an indicator of therapeutic response in patients in National Cancer Institute Trials. *J Nucl Med* 2006; 47(6):1059–66.

A 41-year-old female with newly diagnosed sigmoid cancer, with the tumor extending 9 cm from the anal verge by rigid sigmoidoscopy. EUS stage was uT3N1. FDG-PET/CT was performed for initial staging, before pre-operative radiation therapy.

## Acquisition and processing parameters

| | |
|---|---|
| Equipment | PET/CT system |
| CT | 64-slice, 120 kVp, 148 mA (effective dose), 0.5 s/rotation, pitch 0.8, collimation 3 mm |
| Reconstruction | Filtered back-projection, convolution kernel B31f |
| PET | LSO, 3-D, 22 cm axial FOV with 109 slices, six bed positions |
| Reconstruction | OSEM-2-D, 2 iterations, 8 subsets, convolution kernel Gaussian 5 mm |
| Positioning | Prone, in preparation of CT simulation and IMRT planning |
| Patient preparation | Fasting for 6 hours |
| | Serum glucose level 77 mg/dL; Serum creatinine 0.8 mg/dL |
| Dose | 11.3 mCi FDG |
| Oral contrast | ReadiCat 900 mL |
| IV contrast | 115 mL Omnipaque-350 |
| Uptake interval | 108 min |

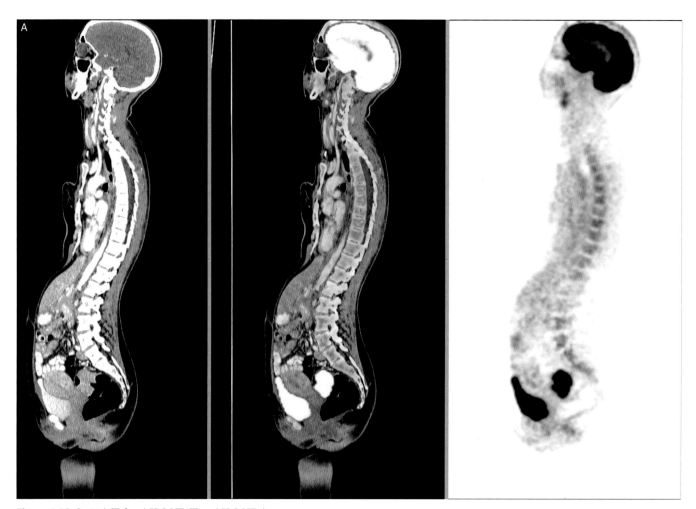

**Figure 9.5A** Sagittal CT, fused FDG-PET/CT, and FDG-PET slices.

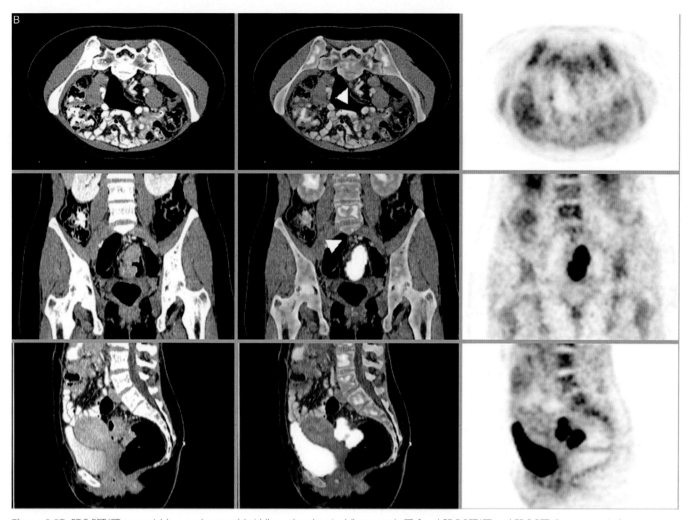

**Figure 9.5B** FDG-PET/CT: transaxial (top row), coronal (middle row) and sagittal (lower row), CT, fused FDG-PET/CT, and FDG-PET slices, respectively.

## Findings

Highly FDG-avid presacral mass consistent with the known primary in the sigmoid colon (Figures 9.5A and B). One sub-centimeter pre-vertebral lymph node had mild-to-moderate uptake (Figure 9.5B, white arrowhead on fused transaxial and coronal images). Intense FDG activity is seen in the bladder on the sagittal slices. There is no evidence of distant metastatic disease.

## Diagnosis and clinical follow-up

Patient received 4,500 cGy of IMRT in 25 fractions over 34 days to the pelvis with a 540 cGy boost in 3 fractions over 3 days to the recto-sigmoid colon. Three months after completion of therapy, the FDG-PET/CT was repeated and showed decreased FDG uptake in the primary, and resolution of uptake in the node. One week later, the patient was brought to the operating room and the tumor was resected. Sixteen lymph nodes were removed. Pathology revealed adenocarcinoma, stage pT3a/bN0Mx with all nodes free of disease. No K-ras mutation in codons 12 or 13 was detected.

## Discussion and teaching points

The initial FDG-PET/CT scan revealed a fairly large local tumor with small nodes on CT of which one was FDG avid. Three months after radiation therapy, the metabolic activity of the primary tumor had decreased significantly and the node was no longer metabolically active. At resection an adenocarcinoma was found that had penetrated the mucosa, with all of the 16 resected lymph nodes negative for metastasis.

## Take-home message

- Accurate staging of disease is necessary for proper planning of therapy (1, 2). Here the initial scan was suspicious for lymph node involvement. After IMRT the nodes turned out negative at pathology. It is not possible to conclude that the nodes were never involved with tumor or that they originally had micrometastases that responded to radiation treatment.
- This case shows that FDG-PET/CT can be used to accurately stage disease and monitor radiation treatment alone (1, 2). This patient did not receive neo-adjuvant chemotherapy and was not scheduled for additional chemotherapy after surgery.

# References

1.  De Geus-Oei LF, Vriens D, van Laarhoven HW, van der Graaf WT, Oyen WJ. Monitoring and predicting response to therapy with 18F-FDG PET in colorectal cancer: a systematic review. *J Nucl Med* 2009;**50**(Suppl 1): 43S–54S.

2.  Schiepers C, Haustermans K, Geboes K *et al.* The effect of preoperative radiation therapy on glucose utilization and cell kinetics in patients with primary rectal carcinoma. *Cancer* 1999;**85**(4):803–11.

A 45-year-old female, generally healthy, who was diagnosed with iron-deficiency anemia. She responded well to iron supplement medication. A few months after IUD placement, she started to have crampy abdominal pain and bloating. She had no nausea, vomiting, black or red stools, and no weight loss. Her primary-care physician ordered a CT of the abdomen and pelvis, which revealed peri-appendicular fluid, cecal wall thickening and a liver mass. An FDG-PET/CT was ordered for staging and initial treatment strategy planning.

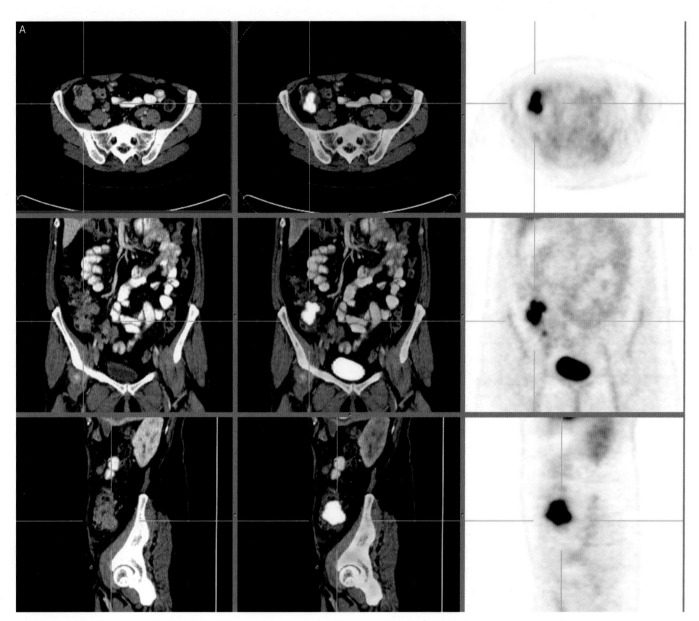

**Figure 9.6A** FDG-PET/CT: transaxial (top row), coronal (middle row) and sagittal (lower row), CT, fused FDG-PET/CT, and FDG-PET slices, respectively at the level of the cecum.

## Acquisition and processing parameters

| | |
|---|---|
| Equipment | PET/CT system |
| CT | 16-slice, 120 kVp, 121 mA (effective dose), 0.8 s/rotation, pitch 1, collimation 3 mm |
| Reconstruction | Filtered back-projection, convolution kernel B31f |
| PET | LSO, 3-D, 16 cm axial FOV, 81 slices, six bed positions from base skull to the proximal femur |
| Reconstruction | OSEM-2-D, 2 iterations, 8 subsets, convolution kernel Gaussian 5 mm |
| Patient preparation | Fasting for 6 hours |
| | Serum glucose level 104 mg/dL, Serum creatinine 0.9 mg/dL |
| Dose | 15.8 mCi FDG |

| | |
|---|---|
| Oral contrast | ReadiCat 3 portions of 300 mL at −55, −30 and 0 minutes before FDG injection |
| IV contrast | 115 mL Omnipaque-350 at a rate of 1.2 mL/s |
| Uptake interval | 63 min |

## Findings and differential diagnosis

Cecal mass with abnormally increased FDG uptake in the right lower quadrant, consistent with a primary tumor. The mass extends into the ileocecal valve with occlusion of the appendix. The abnormal uptake in the dilated appendix suggests subacute inflammatory process. Abnormal uptake is seen in large complex liver mass, consistent with metastases. Differential diagnoses include primary cecal cancer with metastases; primary hepatic cancer; appendicitis.

## Clinical follow-up

Patient had surgery to resect the cecal mass.

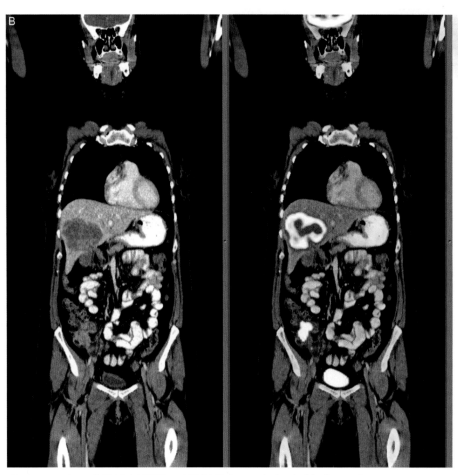
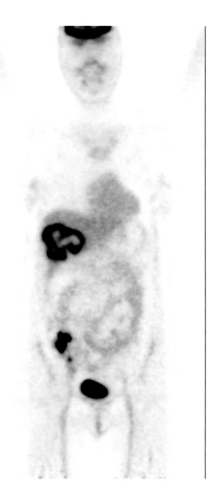

**Figure 9.6B** Coronal CT, FDG-PET/CT, and FDG-PET slices at the level of the liver and cecum.

A 45-year-old female, referred to surgery for resection of primary cancer in the cecum with metastasis to the liver (see Figures 9.6A and B for initial staging). Status post-resection of the proximal colon and ileum. Pathology revealed an adeno-carcinoma of the cecum, moderately differentiated, 6.0 cm in size with local extension; 1/25 lymph nodes were positive for metastases. The assigned stage was pT4aN1aM1 based on liver metastasis detected on PET/CT. No K-ras mutation was detected in codons 12 or 13. The appendix contained a mucoid, tan fluid and showed signs of perforation. The patient was started on chemotherapy (FOLFOX6-avastin) and was referred to have an FDG-PET/CT for restaging after six cycles of treatment.

## Acquisition and processing parameters

| | |
|---|---|
| Equipment | PET/CT system |
| CT | 16-slice, 120 kVp, 112 mA (effective dose), 0.8 s/rotation, pitch 1, collimation 3 mm |
| Reconstruction | Filtered back-projection, convolution kernel B31f |
| PET | LSO, 3-D, 16 cm axial FOV, 81 slices, six bed positions from base skull to proximal femur |
| Reconstruction | OSEM-2-D, 2 iterations, 8 subsets, convolution kernel Gaussian 5 mm |
| Patient preparation | Fasting for 6 hours |
| | Serum glucose level 97 mg/dL; Serum creatinine 0.6 mg/dL |
| Dose | 16.4 mCi FDG |
| Oral contrast | ReadiCat 900 mL |
| IV contrast | 115 mL Omnipaque-350 |
| Uptake interval | 56 min |

## Findings

The cecal mass and the abnormal uptake in the appendix are no longer seen, status post-resection (Figure 9.6C). The uptake in the liver has significantly decreased compared with Figure 9.6B indicative of response to therapy. At the medial and inferior margins of the complex mass, there is still increased FDG uptake. This is consistent with residual tumor versus inflammatory response. Patient was classified as having partial response and additional radiofrequency (RF) ablation is being contemplated at the time of writing.

## Diagnosis and clinical follow-up

Adenocarcinoma of the cecum with regional and hepatic metastases. Appendicitis.

## Discussion and teaching points

This patient presented initially with anemia and subsequently with appendicitis although the signs and symptoms were not typical. Initial anatomic imaging suggested metastatic colon cancer. The presence of more advanced disease was diagnosed by the FDG-PET/CT scan performed for initial staging. Findings were confirmed at surgery. The liver metastasis was complex and was treated with chemotherapy. Although the patient was a responder, the re-staging scan suggested areas of residual tumor. Radiofrequency ablation will be initiated for local control.

## Take-home message

- Patients and their disease may present in very different ways. This unfortunate woman presented with anemia that responded to medical therapy. Later symptoms were associated with placement of an IUD. Clinical symptoms and signs do not always guide the physician in the right direction. Although some of this patient's complaints could be related to appendicitis, there was no evidence of a Murphy sign or leukocytosis. Despite the paucity of traditionally taught symptoms and signs, a perforated appendix was found coincidentally at surgery. The suspected clinical diagnosis of appendicitis, which could not be confirmed with typical findings on physical exam and labs, was confirmed at surgery.
- The classic hallmarks of cancer, wasting and weight loss, were not present in this patient. The first sign that this patient's symptoms were related to a malignancy came from anatomic imaging with CT ordered by the patient's physician. Thereafter, the usual work-up for colorectal cancer was initiated and the suspected clinical diagnosis was confirmed.
- Anatomic and molecular imaging revealed that the patient had advanced disease (stage IV). This means that there is no indication for neo-adjuvant therapy. After the surgical intervention, chemotherapy was started and the early re-staging PET/CT scan revealed a favorable response. She was not a complete responder and further therapy with radiofrequency ablation will be initiated.
- Physicians should approach every patient with an open mind and try to explain all symptoms and signs verbalized by the patient. The power of anatomic and molecular imaging is elegantly demonstrated here in arriving at the correct diagnosis, and the findings were nicely confirmed at surgery and histopathology (1–3).

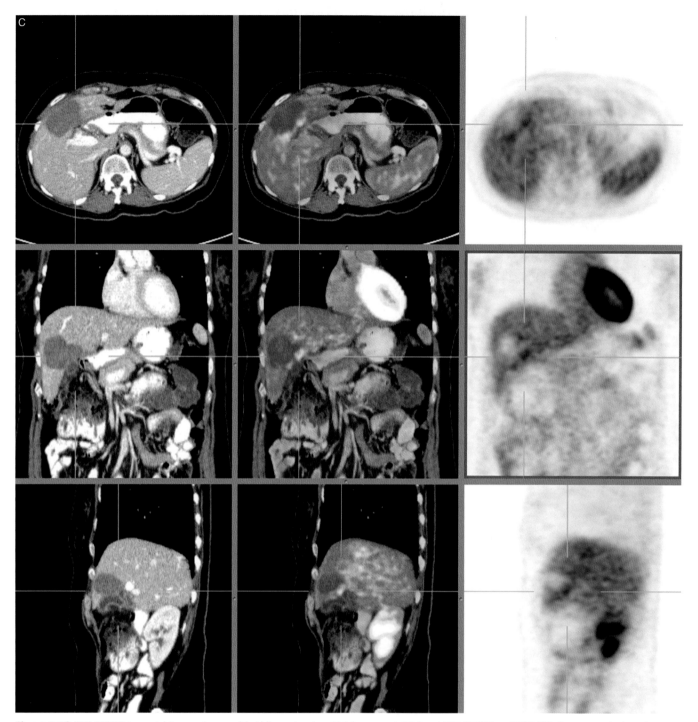

**Figure 9.6C** FDG-PET/CT: transaxial (top row), coronal (middle row) and sagittal (lower row), CT, fused FDG-PET/CT, and FDG-PET slices, respectively at the level of the liver mass.

# References

1. Akhurst T, Larson SM. Positron emission tomography imaging of colorectal cancer. *Semin Oncol* 1999;**26**(5):577–83.

2. Young H, Baum R, Cremerius U *et al.* Measurement of clinical and subclinical tumour response using [F-18]-fluorodeoxyglucose and positron emission tomography: review and 1999 EORTC recommendations. *Eur J Cancer* 1999;**V35**(N13):1773–82.

3. Folprecht G, Gruenberger T, Bechstein WO *et al.* Tumour response and secondary resectability of colorectal liver metastases following neoadjuvant chemotherapy with cetuximab: the CELIM randomised phase 2 trial. *Lancet Oncol* 2010; **11**(1):38–47.

A 79-year-old female with osteoarthritis requiring NSAID presents with tarry stools and symptomatic anemia. She has also a history of GERD and hypertension. Admitting diagnosis is upper GI bleed from chronic NSAID use versus peptic ulcer disease. During endoscopy a bleeding gastric mass is found. FDG-PET/CT was ordered for staging and initial treatment strategy planning.

## Acquisition and processing parameters

| Equipment | PET/CT system |
| --- | --- |
| CT | 2-slice, 130 kVp, 130 mA, 1 s/rotation, pitch 1.25, collimation 5 mm |
| Reconstruction | Filtered back-projection, convolution kernel B31f |

| | |
| --- | --- |
| PET | LSO, 3-D, 16 cm axial FOV, 59 slices, six bed positions from base skull to proximal femur |
| Reconstruction | OSEM-2-D, 2 iterations, 8 subsets, convolution kernel Gaussian 5 mm |
| Patient preparation | Fasting for 6 hours |
| | Serum glucose level 104 mg/dL; Serum creatinine 1.1 mg/dL |
| Dose | 13.1 mCi FDG |
| Oral contrast | ReadiCat 900 mL |
| IV contrast | 120 mL Omnipaque-350 at a rate of 1 mL/s |
| Uptake interval | 83 min |

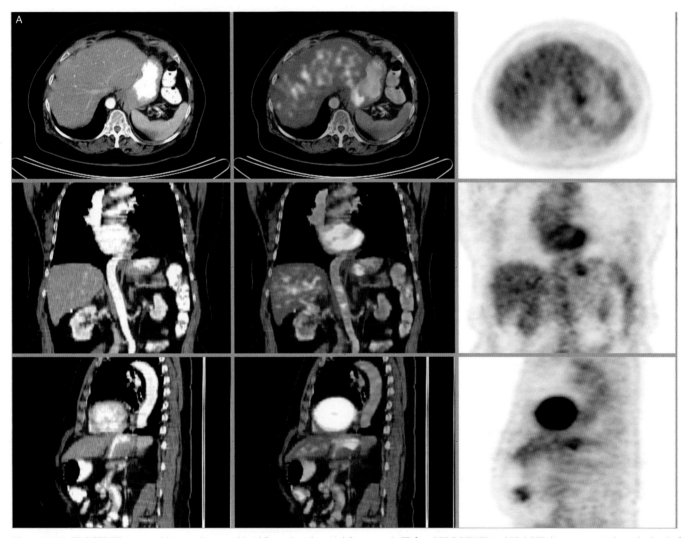

**Figure 9.7A** FDG-PET/CT: transaxial (top row), coronal (middle row) and sagittal (lower row), CT, fused FDG-PET/CT, and FDG-PET slices, respectively, at the level of the thorax and upper abdomen.

## Findings and differential diagnosis

An FDG-avid mass is found in the proximal stomach. There is no FDG-avid lymphadenopathy.

Differential diagnoses include gastroesophageal reflux with bleed, peptic ulcer disease, and gastric cancer.

## Diagnosis and clinical follow-up

Biopsy revealed a moderately differentiated adenocarcinoma. The EUS stage was µT2N1.

A proximal gastrectomy, esophago-gastrostomy, and pyloroplasty were performed. Pathology revealed a 4.5 cm moderately differentiated adenocarcinoma, and 11 regional and six lower esophageal nodes were all negative for metastasis. Stage pT2N0Mx.

A 83-year-old female, status post partial gastrectomy for gastric cancer (see Figure 9.7A for initial staging). The patient had chemotherapy after surgery but no radiation therapy. She was referred to nuclear medicine for restaging 4 years after the initial diagnosis.

## Acquisition and processing parameters

| Equipment | PET/CT system |
|---|---|
| CT | 64-slice, 120 kVp, 80 mA (effective dose), 0.5 s/rotation, pitch 0.8, collimation 3 mm |
| Reconstruction | Filtered back-projection, convolution kernel B31f |

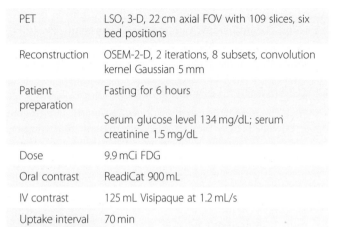

| PET | LSO, 3-D, 22 cm axial FOV with 109 slices, six bed positions |
|---|---|
| Reconstruction | OSEM-2-D, 2 iterations, 8 subsets, convolution kernel Gaussian 5 mm |
| Patient preparation | Fasting for 6 hours |
|  | Serum glucose level 134 mg/dL; serum creatinine 1.5 mg/dL |
| Dose | 9.9 mCi FDG |
| Oral contrast | ReadiCat 900 mL |
| IV contrast | 125 mL Visipaque at 1.2 mL/s |
| Uptake interval | 70 min |

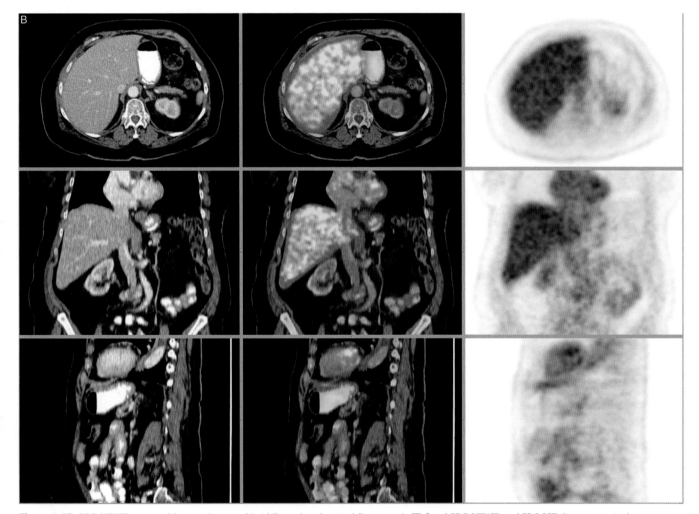

**Figure 9.7B** FDG-PET/CT: transaxial (top row), coronal (middle row) and sagittal (lower row), CT, fused FDG-PET/CT, and FDG-PET slices, respectively, at the level of the upper abdomen.

## Findings

Note the suture line at the posterior end of the remainder of the stomach. There is no PET/CT evidence of a mass or adenopathy; there are no abnormal FDG foci.

## Diagnosis and clinical follow-up

Adenocarcinoma of the stomach, status post partial gastrectomy and chemotherapy 4 years ago. The present FDG-PET/CT study shows no evidence of disease recurrence, regional or distant metastatic disease.

## Discussion and teaching points

This patient presented initially with symptomatic anemia and upper GI bleed. EUS found a bleeding mass in the stomach, and biopsy revealed a uT2N1 adenocarcinoma. Initial anatomic imaging suggested limited disease to the proximal stomach, and partial gastrectomy was performed.

## Take-home message

- Gastric cancer generally has a dismal prognosis (1).
- Metastatic spread to the lymph nodes is a poor prognostic sign (2).
- The current case was diagnosed by EUS as N1 disease. FDG-PET/CT did not confirm this and suggested N0 disease, which was confirmed by pathology. This downstages the patient into a more favorable category (3).
- Restaging at 4 years showed that she was still free of disease, i.e., a complete responder to therapy.

## References

1. Stahl A, Ott K, Weber WA *et al.* FDG PET imaging of locally advanced gastric carcinomas: correlation with endoscopic and histopathological findings. *Eur J Nucl Med Mol Imaging* 2003;**30**(2):288–95.

2. Kwee RM, Kwee TC. Imaging in assessing lymph node status in gastric cancer. *Gastric Cancer* 2009;**12**(1): 6–22.

3. Kim EY, Lee JW, Choi D *et al.* The value of PET/CT for preoperative staging of advanced gastric cancer: comparison with contrast-enhanced CT. *Eur J Radiol* 2011;**79**:183–8.

A 71-year-old female presenting with abdominal discomfort and weight loss. She underwent upper endoscopy, and biopsy revealed a CD117 positive gastrointestinal stromal tumor (GIST) sarcoma. FLT-PET/CT was ordered to stage the disease and to plan the initial treatment strategy

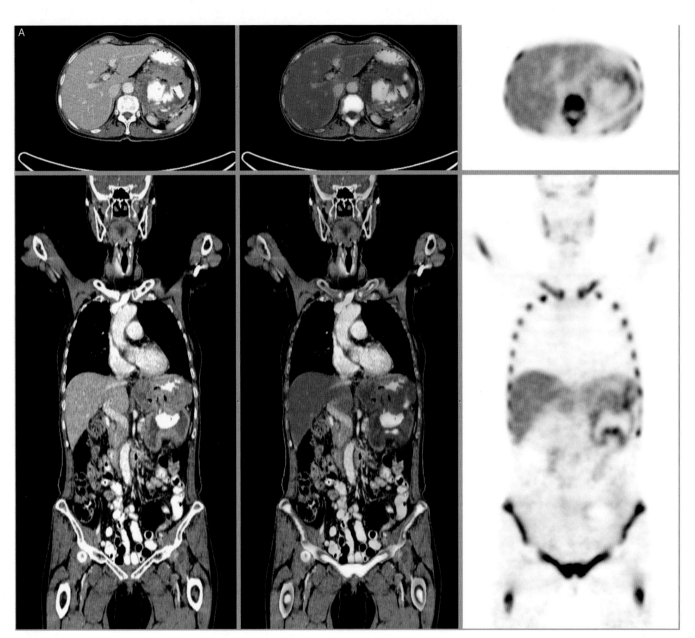

**Figure 9.8A** Baseline FLT-PET/CT: transaxial (top row) and coronal (lower row) CT, fused FDG-PET/CT, and FDG-PET slices, respectively.

## Acquisition and processing parameters

| | |
|---|---|
| Equipment | PET/CT system |
| CT | 64-slice, 120 kVp, 87 mA (effective dose), 0.5 s/rotation, pitch 0.8, collimation 3 mm |
| Reconstruction | Filtered back-projection, convolution kernel B31f |
| PET | LSO, 3-D, 22 cm axial FOV with 109 slices, five bed positions |
| Reconstruction | OSEM-2-D, 2 iterations, 8 subsets, convolution kernel Gaussian 5 mm |
| Patient preparation | Fasting for 6 hours |
| | Serum glucose level 104 mg/dL; serum creatinine 0.5 mg/dL |
| Dose | 5.9 mCi FLT (3″-deoxy-3″-18F-fluorothymidine) |
| Oral contrast | ReadiCat 900 mL |
| IV contrast | 120 mL Omnipaque-350 at a rate of 1.2 mL/s |
| Uptake interval | 80 min |

## Findings

A complex mass is seen on CT in the left upper quadrant surrounding the oral contrast in the stomach (Figure 9.8A). There are nodular areas of increased FLT uptake suggestive of locally increased cellular proliferation. Note that there is no brain uptake of FLT, since it does not cross the blood–brain barrier.

## Diagnosis and clinical follow-up

GIST sarcoma of the stomach. The patient was put on imatinib mesylate (Gleevec®) 400 mg once a day.

A 71-year-female, with GIST sarcoma of the stomach; 1 month on Gleevec® therapy.

FDG-PET/CT was ordered for subsequent treatment strategy planning after 1 month of therapy.

## Acquisition and processing parameters

| Equipment | PET/CT scanner |
|---|---|
| CT | 2-slice, 130 kVp, 130 mA, 1 s/rotation, pitch 1.25, collimation 4 mm |
| Reconstruction | Filtered back-projection, kernel B30s |
| PET | LSO, 3-D, 158 mm axial FOV, 47 slices, seven bed positions |
| Reconstruction | OSEM-2-D with 2 iterations, 8 subsets, convolution kernel Gaussian 5 mm |

| Patient preparation | Fasting for 6 hours |
|---|---|
|  | Serum glucose level 78 mg/dL; serum creatinine 0.6 mg/dL |
| Dose | 12.9 mCi FDG |
| Oral contrast | ReadiCat 900 mL |
| IV contrast | 120 mL Omnipaque at 1.0 mL/s |
| Uptake interval | 70 min |

## Findings

There is an FDG avid mass in the stomach (Figure 9.8B). Compared with the baseline CT scan (Figure 9.8A) the mass is smaller in size.

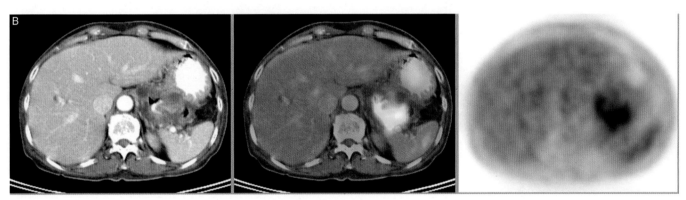

**Figure 9.8B** Transaxial CT, fused FDG-PET/CT and FDG-PET slices after 1 month of therapy.

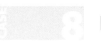

## Part III

## Clinical follow-up

A 71-year-old female with GIST sarcoma of the stomach; 3 months on daily imatinib mesylate therapy. FDG-PET/CT was performed to monitor response to therapy

## Findings

The previously seen mass (in Figure 9.8B) has further decreased in size on CT, and is no longer FDG-avid (Figure 9.8C). Patient is classified as having a complete metabolic response.

## Diagnosis and clinical follow-up

One week after the FDG-PET/CT scan, the patient had surgery. She underwent radical resection of the tumor with en-bloc resection of the GE-junction, posterior proximal stomach, distal pancreatectomy, and splenectomy. Pyloroplasty was also performed. Pathology revealed a 5.6 cm GIST sarcoma at the GE junction (CD117 (+), CD34 (+), and (+) for mutation in KIT gene exon 11). The tumor invaded the perigastric fat. Sixteen reactive lymph nodes were resected and found to be negative for GIST sarcoma. Surgical margins were negative. Treatment effect was estimated at 90%.

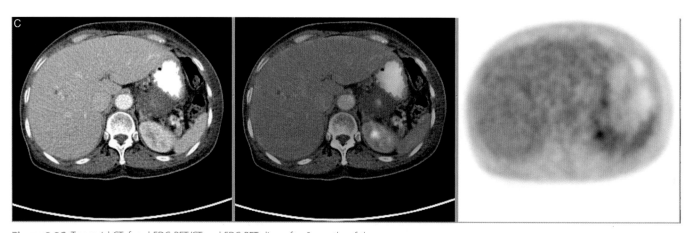

**Figure 9.8C** Transaxial CT, fused FDG-PET/CT and FDG-PET slices after 3 months of therapy.

A 71-year-old female with GIST sarcoma of the stomach; 4 months after resection.

## Findings

Note the staples at the medial aspect of the remainder of the stomach. There is no FDG-avid mass or adenopathy; there are no abnormal foci of uptake (Figure 9.8D). The FDG-avid focus on the left kidney is related to excreted FDG in the urine.

## Diagnosis and clinical follow-up

GIST sarcoma of the stomach with favorable response to imatinib mesylate therapy, status post partial gastrectomy. There is no FDG-PET/CT evidence of active disease recurrence, regional or distant metastasis.

## Discussion and teaching points

The initial scan showed areas of increased cell proliferation on the FLT-PET scan. These areas are best suited for biopsy and subsequent flow cytometry, measurement of the proliferation index, and antigen detection. After one month of imatinib therapy, there was good response, and after 3 months the abnormal metabolic activity had resolved. The tumor was still seen on CT.

Subsequently the patient was treated with en-bloc resection of the GIST sarcoma, proximal posterior part of the stomach, tail of the pancreas, and spleen. Four months after surgery, the FDG-PET/CT was negative in the upper abdomen. Clinical follow-up 2 months later did not reveal recurrence of disease.

## Take-home message

- PET/CT using FDG is the method of choice to monitor treatment response of GIST sarcoma (1–4).
- The combination of tyrosine kinase inhibitors followed by surgery, cured the patient of the disease as assessed at 6 months follow-up (5).

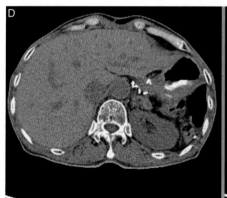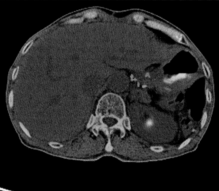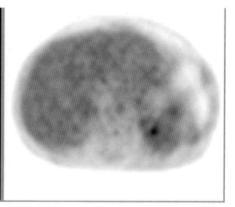

**Figure 9.8D** Transaxial CT, fused FDG-PET/CT and FDG-PET slices 4 months after surgery.

## References

1. Pisters PW, Patel SR. Gastrointestinal stromal tumors: current management. *J Surg Oncol* 2010;**102**:530–8.

2. Van den Abbeele AD. The lessons of GIST – PET and PET/CT: a new paradigm for imaging. *Oncologist* 2008;13(Suppl 2):8–13.

3. Goerres GW, Stupp R, Barghouth G *et al*. The value of PET, CT and in-line PET/CT in patients with gastrointestinal stromal tumors: long-term outcome of treatment with imatinib mesylate. *Eur J Nucl Med Mol Imaging* 2005;**32**(2):153–62.

4. Antoch G, Kanja J, Bauer S *et al*. Comparison of PET, CT, and dual-modality PET/CT imaging for monitoring of imatinib (STI571) therapy in patients with gastrointestinal stromal tumors. *J Nucl Med* 2004;**45**(3):357–65.

5. Gan HK, Seruga B, Knox JJ. Sunitinib in solid tumors. *Expert Opin Investig Drugs* 2009;**18**(6):821–34.

# Pancreas and liver

Aaron C. Jessop and Dominique Delbeke

## Pancreatic cancer

### General concepts and epidemiology

According to the American Cancer Society, it is estimated that 43,140 Americans will be diagnosed with pancreatic carcinoma in 2010 with an estimated 36,800 deaths. This represents the 10th most commonly diagnosed malignancy, but the fourth leading cause of cancer-related death (1). Pancreatic adenocarcinoma is one of the most lethal of all malignancies with a 1-year survival of 20–25% and a 5-year survival rate of approximately 5% (2). Survival for pancreatic adenocarcinoma remains dismally low despite advances in diagnostic and therapeutic development over the past several years. Currently, the only potentially curative treatment is surgical resection, which is only an option for 15–20% of patients. For those who are surgical candidates, 5-year survival following pancreaticoduodenectomy remains low at 25–30% in patients with no nodal involvement.

Tumors arising from the pancreas can be exocrine or endocrine in origin. The most common type of **exocrine tumor** of the pancreas is ductal adenocarcinoma. Adenosquamous, squamous, and giant cell tumors are much less common. Acinar cell carcinomas are rare and have a similar prognosis as for ductal carcinoma. Pancreatic **neuroendocrine tumors** such as insulinoma, glucagonoma, and gastrinoma are uncommon and are often associated with other endocrine abnormalities. Pancreatic endocrine tumors are usually slow growing and are typically found in the body or tail of the pancreas. Benign cysts, pseudocysts, and cystadenomas may occur within the pancreas, although malignant cystic neoplasms may also occur.

Pancreatic adenocarcinoma arises primarily from the pancreatic ducts, most commonly in the head of the pancreas. Early in the course of the disease, patients are often asymptomatic, leading to a delay in diagnosis. The advanced stage at diagnosis is one of the reasons for such a high mortality rate. At the time of diagnosis, 7% of patients have localized disease, 26% have regional disease, and 52% have distant metastasis (1). When symptoms occur, they are usually related to bile duct obstruction from compression or invasion of the bile ducts. Symptoms include epigastric pain, weight loss, and jaundice.

### Staging of pancreatic ductal adenocarcinoma

Accurate staging of pancreatic adenocarcinoma is essential, as the treatment and prognosis differ greatly based on the stage at the time of diagnosis. The goal of staging is essentially to categorize patients into three groups, which are approached differently from a therapeutic standpoint. As surgery is the only curative approach, it is important to first identify the patients who are considered to have surgically resectable disease (stages I and II). The second group consists of patients with locally advanced disease, but no evidence of distant metastasis (stage III). Although not considered surgically resectable, these patients may benefit from external-beam radiation along with chemotherapy. The third group includes patients with metastasis (stage IV) who, given the short survival, would benefit most from chemotherapy and palliative measures as indicated.

Staging of pancreatic cancer based on the TNM (tumor, node, metastasis) system is outlined in Tables 10.1 and 10.2 (3). While stages I and II are generally considered resectable, and stages III and IV are considered non-resectable, there are certain tumors that fit into a "borderline resectable" category. Although there is not a clear consensus as to what constitutes resectability, the National Comprehensive Cancer Network (NCCN) considers borderline resectable tumors those with severe unilateral or bilateral SMV/portal impingement, less than 180° tumor abutment of the SMA, abutment or encasement of hepatic artery, SMV occlusion (if of a short segment and reconstruction is possible), and for tumors in the tail of the pancreas, SMA or celiac encasement of less than 180° (4).

As tumor resectability depends greatly on extension to major arterial structures and whether involvement or occlusion of major venous structures is present, detailed anatomical evaluation is of the utmost importance during staging. Various imaging modalities are available to aid in the staging of pancreatic cancer, all of which have advantages and disadvantages. Along with conventional imaging modalities, FDG-PET/CT

**Table 10.1** Tumor, node, metastasis (TNM) classification for staging of pancreatic adenocarcinoma (3).

| T (Primary tumor) | N (Regional lymph nodes) | M (Distant metastasis) |
|---|---|---|
| T0: No evidence of primary | N0: No nodal metastasis | M0: No distant metastasis |
| Tis: *In situ* | N1: Regional lymph node metastasis | M1: Distant metastasis |
| T1: Limited to pancreas $\leq 2\,cm$ | | |
| T2: Limited to pancreas $> 2\,cm$ | | |
| T3: Extends beyond pancreas, no involvement of celiac axis or superior mesenteric artery | | |
| T4: Involves celiac axis or superior mesenteric artery | | |

**Table 10.2** Anatomic staging of pancreatic adenocarcinoma (3).

| Stage | TNM description | Summary |
|---|---|---|
| 0 | Tis: N0 M0 | *In situ* disease |
| I | IA: T1 N0 M0 | Potentially resectable disease confined to the pancreas |
| | IB: T2 N0 M0 | |
| II | IIA: T3 N0 M0 | Usually resectable; may involve venous structures, adjacent organs, nodes, or hepatic artery, but not celiac axis or superior mesenteric artery |
| | IIB: T1–3 N1 M0 | |
| III | T4 N0–1 M0 | Locally advanced disease; unresectable due to celiac axis or superior mesenteric artery involvement |
| IV | T1–4 N0–1 M1 | Metastatic; unresectable due to distant metastasis |

can provide valuable information to guide therapy in patients with diagnosed or suspected pancreatic cancer. The role of PET/CT is discussed later in this chapter.

Contrast-enhanced CT is currently the method of choice for initial evaluation of pancreatic cancer (5). The strength of CT is not only in detecting the pancreatic mass, but also in assessing involvement of adjacent organs and vascular invasion. The reported diagnostic accuracy of CT for both detection of pancreatic cancer and establishing the resectability status ranges between 85%–95% (6, 7). Given the high recurrence rate of pancreatic cancer, however, this may be an overestimate in actual performance of CT for assessment of true resectability. Limitations of CT include the detection of small peritoneal and hepatic metastases. Furthermore, evaluation of the pancreas on CT may be challenging in the setting of pancreatitis or other equivocal findings such as enlargement of the pancreatic head without detection of a distinct lesion (8). Endoscopic ultrasonography (EUS) has higher sensitivity than CT for detection of pancreatic carcinoma and performs similarly for nodal staging and resectability (7). EUS has the advantage of allowing fine needle aspiration for tissue

diagnosis. Relative to CT, disadvantages of EUS include operator dependency and the inability to evaluate for liver metastasis.

Endoscopic retrograde cholangiopancreatography (ERCP) allows for high-resolution anatomical assessment of the biliary tree with the injection of contrast material. Tissue sampling and interventional procedures, such as stent placement, can also be performed at the time of ERCP. Despite a high sensitivity for detection of pancreatic carcinoma, ERCP is an invasive procedure and may be complicated by iatrogenic pancreatitis. Given the high accuracy of other non-invasive techniques, the role of ERCP is limited to cases where pancreatic cancer is suspected, but there is no identifiable tumor on CT. It may also be used for decompression of patients with non-resectable disease or in the setting of chronic pancreatitis (9, 10).

Gadolinium-enhanced MRI has been increasingly used for evaluation of the pancreas and performs similar to CT, with some studies showing a higher sensitivity for detection of pancreatic masses (11). MRI also has similar sensitivity to CT for detection of focal hepatic lesions, although this requires a multitude of pulse sequences. MR cholangiopancreatography (MRCP) is a non-invasive technique that can be performed at the same time as MRI. MRCP utilizes T2-weighted images to visualize fluid-containing structures and permits visualization of the biliary tree without administration of contrast agents. Although MRCP does not provide the resolution ERCP, it can demonstrate intraluminal filling defects and luminal narrowing (12).

## Treatment overview

The only potentially curative treatment for pancreatic cancer is surgical resection. Unfortunately, only a minority of patients are candidates for resection due to the often advanced stage at presentation. The Whipple pancreaticoduodenectomy is the most common surgical procedure performed, and consists of removal of the distal portion of the stomach, gallbladder, pancreatic head, and a large portion of the duodenum. Extensive retroperitoneal lymphadenectomy has been advocated by some, but has not been shown to increase survival, and is associated with increased morbidity (13). Patients who are not surgical candidates may benefit from palliative procedures to relieve jaundice or duodenal obstruction.

Historic data are conflicting as to the role of adjuvant chemoradiation in the treatment of surgically resectable pancreatic cancer. NCCN guidelines currently support the use of either adjuvant chemoradiation or chemotherapy alone, although an optimal regimen has not been established and patients are encouraged to enter clinical trials to establish the efficacy of adjuvant therapy regimens. Patients with locally advanced disease who are considered unresectable, but without distant spread, may benefit from radiation therapy. Although chemotherapy is never curative for patients with metastatic pancreatic cancer, disease-related symptoms and survival may be improved by the use of monotherapy with gemcitabine, or gemcitabine-based combined therapy (4).

## The role of FDG-PET/CT in evaluation of pancreatic carcinoma

FDG-PET/CT is a power adjunct to conventional anatomical imaging modalities for evaluation of patients with pancreatic cancer (14). Like many malignancies, pancreatic adenocarcinoma demonstrates increased metabolic activity and glucose utilization. This is due to an increase in glucose transporter (GLUT) proteins as well as an increase in hexokinase activity (15–17). FDG enters cells in a similar manner to glucose and is trapped due to phosphorylation by hexokinase, but does not continue in metabolic pathways as glucose would. Because of this, FDG accumulates within malignant tissue at a higher concentration than adjacent benign tissues.

## Diagnosis

In addition to conventional anatomic imaging, metabolic evaluation with FDG-PET can improve the pre-operative diagnosis of pancreatic cancer (18–19). The average sensitivity and specificity of FDG-PET for differentiation of benign from malignant lesions has been reported as 94% and 90% respectively in a summary of the literature in 2001 (20). In many of the included studies, the accuracy of FDG-PET was superior to that of CT, which was found to have weighted averages of sensitivity and specificity of 82% and 75%. Rose et al. reported similar results with sensitivity and specificity of 92% and 85% for FDG-PET compared with 65% and 62% for CT (21). In this study, the sensitivity of PET was found to be less dependent on lesion size, while the sensitivity of CT was found to improve with increase in lesion size (21).

FDG-PET has also been shown to have prognostic value in patients with pancreatic cancer. A higher degree of FDG uptake within pancreatic tumors correlates with a worse prognosis. For example, Nakata et al. noted an inverse relationship between standard uptake value (SUV) and survival in 24 patients with unresectable pancreatic adenocarcinoma (22). In a multivariate analysis of 52 patients performed by Zimny et al., patients with higher SUV values had a shorter median survival (5 months for SUV above 6.1) compared with those with lower SUV values (9 months for SUV below 6.1) (23).

FDG-PET/CT has been shown to be helpful in the evaluation of cystic pancreatic neoplasms. Although data are limited, studies have shown FDG-PET to be superior to CT in distinguishing benign from malignant pancreatic cystic lesions. In a prospective study of 50 patients with pancreatic cystic lesions, FDG-PET was found to be a useful adjunct to diagnostic CT in identifying malignant pancreatic cystic lesions. The sensitivity, specificity, positive and negative predictive value, and accuracy of FDG-PET in detecting malignant tumors were 94%, 94%, 89%, 97%, and 94% respectively, as compared with 65%, 88%, 73%, 83%, and 80% for CT (24).

## Initial staging

As described earlier, staging of pancreatic adenocarcinoma is performed by the TNM system. Anatomical imaging modalities such as diagnostic CT or EUS are necessary for accurate T staging. Metabolic imaging with FDG-PET does not yield enough anatomical detail to demonstrate the relationship of tumor with adjacent organs and vascular structures and, therefore, cannot accurately assess local tumor resectability. N staging is a challenge for all imaging modalities, including PET/CT, due to the close proximity of regional lymph nodes to the primary tumor. FDG-PET is not superior to CT for N staging, but has been found to be more accurate than CT for M staging (25).

FDG-PET/CT has been shown to have a significant impact on patient management. In a study by Delbeke et al. (25), FDG-PET in addition to diagnostic CT, altered the surgical management of 43% in a series of 65 patients. Of these, 27% were found to have CT-occult pancreatic carcinoma, and 14% were found to have unsuspected distant metastases. FDG-PET was also helpful in the clarification of benign pancreatic lesions that were felt to be equivocal on CT. The degree to which FDG-PET/CT alters management does depend, in part, on the therapeutic philosophy of the surgeon. In one series of 59 patients, FDG-PET/CT changed management in 16% of patients who were previously presumed resectable based on conventional pre-operative assessment, and was found to be a cost-effective modality by improving patient selection for surgery (26).

## Restaging

Following therapy, FDG-PET is a useful modality for detection of recurrent pancreatic cancer. In particular, PET/CT is helpful for evaluation of equivocal CT abnormalities in the resection bed, to restage patients with rising tumor markers and a negative conventional work-up, and to evaluate new hepatic lesions that are too small to biopsy. In one study of 31 patients with suspected recurrence after surgery, FDG-PET outperformed CT and MRI for detection of local recurrence. CT and MRI were more sensitive for the detection of hepatic metastases. Of 25 patients with local recurrences upon follow-up, initial imaging suggested relapse in 23 patients. Of these, FDG-PET detected 96% (22/23) and CT/MRI 39% (9/23). Among 12 liver metastases, FDG-PET detected only 42% (5/12), while CT/MRI detected 92% (11/12). Seven out of nine abdominal lesions were malignant upon follow-up, all of which were detected by FDG-PET, but none were detected with CT/MRI. FDG-PET also detected extra-abdominal metastases in two patients (27).

One recent study evaluated the performance of FDG-PET/CT with intravenous contrast as compared with PET/non-contrasted CT and CT alone for recurrent pancreatic cancer. PET/CT with contrast performed superior to both PET/CT without contrast and diagnostic CT alone. Patient-based analysis showed that sensitivity, specificity, and accuracy of PET/contrast-enhanced CT were 91.7%, 95.2%, and 93.3%, respectively, whereas those of PET/non-enhanced CT were 83.3%, 90.5%, and 86.7%, and those of enhanced CT alone were 66.7%, 85.7%, and 75.6% (28).

### Monitoring response to therapy

Multiple small series of patients have indicated that FDG-PET may be useful for assessing response to neoadjuvant therapy (29, 30). For example, in a pilot study by Rose et al. of nine patients who underwent FDG-PET before and after neoadjuvant chemoradiation, four had evidence of tumor regression by PET, three showed stable disease, and two showed tumor progression (21). CT was unable to detect any response to neoadjuvant therapy in this group. Eight patients had FDG-PET performed to evaluate for suspected recurrent disease after resection. Four were noted to have new regions of uptake in the resection bed; four had evidence of new hepatic metastases. All proved to have metastatic pancreatic adenocarcinoma.

## Hepatobiliary malignancies
### Hepatocellular carcinoma

Primary liver cancer is the fifth most common malignancy in men and the eighth in women worldwide, with a worldwide 5-year survival rate of 6.5% (31). Hepatocellular carcinomas (HCC) arise from malignant transformation of hepatocytes and represent the majority of primary hepatic malignancies. Chronic hepatic diseases, such as cirrhosis and viral hepatitis, are often encountered in association with HCC. HCC is becoming increasingly common within the USA, which is likely due to the hepatitis C epidemic (32, 33). Other primary hepatic malignancies such as angiosarcoma, epithelioid angioendothelioma, and primary lymphoma of the liver are relatively rare.

Cirrhosis is the primary risk factor for HCC. The ongoing process of hepatocellular injury, inflammation, regeneration, and repair characteristic of cirrhosis is thought to favor carcinogenesis (34). Once cirrhosis is present, HCC occurs in 1–4% of patients yearly (35). Low-grade HCC and hepatic adenoma can be difficult to distinguish, even with core biopsy. A capsule is frequently present in small HCCs, but is rarely found in large tumors. While invasion of the portal vein is common with large HCCs, inferior vena cava and hepatic vein

involvement is uncommon, occurring in only 5% of cases. Metastatic spread of HCC occurs primarily to regional lymph nodes, lungs, and skeleton. HCC is often associated with elevated serum levels of α-fetoprotein.

HCC lesions typically demonstrate arterial hypervascularity, which is due to the hepatic arterial blood supply of HCC, unlike the surrounding liver that receives the majority of its blood supply from the portal vein. The diagnosis of HCC can be made without tissue sampling in cirrhotic patients with an arterially enhancing nodule greater than 2 cm in diameter and an α-fetoprotein level greater than 200 ng/mL (36, 37). For lesions smaller than 2 cm, biopsy is recommended as conventional imaging techniques are less accurate for distinguishing HCC from other benign or malignant hepatic lesions of this size.

The sensitivity of ultrasound for detection of HCC varies significantly in the literature (35% to 84%) (38). The variability is likely because ultrasound is dependent on patient size and operator skill. Multiphase, contrast-enhanced CT takes advantage of the early arterial enhancement of HCC and is the conventional modality for the evaluation of the liver in many institutions. In a literature review by Fung et al. (39), the sensitivity of CT for detection of HCC in non-explanted livers was 80–95%. MRI permits lesion characterization based on the enhancement pattern as well as T1 and T2 signal characteristics. MRI showed sensitivities of 75–94% in the same literature review (39).

## FDG-PET/CT for evaluation of hepatocellular carcinoma

The accumulation of FDG in HCC shows significant variability due to varying degrees of glucose-6-phosphatase activity within these tumors (40, 41). Because of this, three patterns of FDG uptake may be seen in HCC: activity greater than, equal to, or less than background hepatic uptake. The phosphorylation kinetic constant ($k3$) has been shown to be elevated in virtually all malignant tumors, including HCC. FDG accumulates within many malignant tumors due to the elevated $k3$ and a low dephosphorylation kinetic constant ($k4$). In HCC, however, $k4$ may be similar to $k3$, causing egress of FDG from malignant cells and a lack of increased FDG accumulation relative to normal hepatocytes. A correlation does exist between the degree of FDG uptake, $k3$, and the grade of malignancy (42). Higher levels of FDG uptake are associated with more poorly differentiated HCC and with higher levels of α-fetoprotein. Because of this, FDG-PET may have a prognostic significance in the evaluation of HCC (43, 44).

Due to the metabolic characteristics outlined above, FDG-PET is only able to detect 50–70% of HCCs, but has a sensitivity of greater than 90% for other malignant primary and metastatic liver lesions (45, 46). Benign hepatic tumors, such as focal nodular hyperplasia, adenoma, and regenerating nodules, demonstrate FDG uptake similar in intensity in comparison to the normal liver. Rare exceptions to this include abscesses with granulomatous inflammation. FDG-PET is of limited value for the assessment of patients with chronic hepatitis C and focal hepatic lesions, because of both the low sensitivity of FDG-PET for detection of HCC, and the high prevalence of HCC in this patient population (47).

In patients with HCC that do show increased FDG uptake, PET can be an accurate modality for detection of unsuspected regional and distant metastases. In some cases, FDG-PET is the only imaging modality to demonstrate the primary lesion and its metastases (46). In one series of 91 patients, FDG-PET was found to have a sensitivity of 64% for detection of HCC. Despite the relatively low sensitivity, PET had a significant impact in the management of 28% of patients by detecting unsuspected metastases (including liver transplant candidates), guiding high-yield biopsy sites, detecting recurrent disease, and monitoring response to chemoembolization (48). FDG-PET has also been shown to be useful in previously treated patients with rising $\alpha$-fetoprotein levels and no evidence of recurrence by anatomical imaging modalities. In one series of 26 patients with elevated $\alpha$-fetoprotein, FDG-PET was found to have a sensitivity, specificity, and accuracy of 73%, 100%, and 74% respectively for detection of otherwise occult recurrent disease. FDG-PET was able to detect both intra- and extrahepatic lesions (49).

### $^{11}$C-acetate PET/CT for evaluation of hepatocellular carcinoma

$^{11}$C-acetate is a promising radiopharmaceutical for evaluation of malignancies such as HCC, which demonstrate limited avidity for FDG. There are multiple possible biochemical pathways that may lead to the accumulation of $^{11}$C-acetate within tumors. Of the various metabolic pathways, participation in free fatty acid (lipid) synthesis is felt to be the dominant pathway for incorporation into HCC.

Multiple studies have demonstrated the complementary role of both FDG and $^{11}$C-acetate PET in the evaluation of HCC (50–53). In a study by Ho *et al.* (51) of 57 patients with various hepatobiliary tumors, the sensitivities of FDG and $^{11}$C-acetate for detection of HCC were 47% and 87% respectively, with a combined sensitivity of 100%. In general, well-differentiated tumors showed higher avidity for $^{11}$C-acetate, while poorly differentiated tumors were more likely to be FDG avid. In a later series of 121 patients with metastatic HCC, dual-tracer PET/CT was found to have a sensitivity, specificity, and accuracy of 98%, 86%, and 96% respectively on a patient basis for detection of HCC metastasis (52).

## Cholangiocarcinoma

Cholangiocarcinomas arise from epithelial cells of the intra- and extrahepatic bile ducts. These tumors account for approximately 3% of gastrointestinal malignancies and 10–15% of all primary hepatic malignancies (54). The most important predisposing factor for the development of cholangiocarcinoma in Western countries is primary sclerosing cholangitis, with an approximately 10% lifetime risk of developing malignancy (55).

Other predisposing factors include ulcerative colitis, parasitic liver infections (liver fluke *Clonorchis sinensis*), congenital biliary cystic disease, intrahepatic biliary stones, and liver cirrhosis. Although rare, these tumors can be highly lethal, because they are often advanced at the time of diagnosis.

Cholangiocarcinomas can be classified by location as intrahepatic, perihilar, or distal (56). Cholangiocarcinomas can also be divided into three morphologic subtypes: polypoid intraluminal masses, exophytic lesions, and infiltrating sclerosing lesions (most common). Peripheral intrahepatic cholangiocarcinomas arise from the interlobular biliary ducts. Klatskin tumors are perihilar cholangiocarcinomas that arise at the confluence of the left and right hepatic ducts. Perihilar malignancies often have a worse prognosis, as they are difficult to resect due to the proximity to vascular structures as well as the potential for hepatic spread of tumor. Distal cholangiocarcinomas are often diagnosed earlier because of biliary obstruction.

Cholangiocarcinomas can be difficult to detect on CT due to their small size and isodensity in comparison to normal liver parenchyma. Typical CT features of mass-forming cholangiocarcinomas include a homogeneous attenuation mass with irregular peripheral enhancement and gradual centripetal enhancement. On MRI, cholangiocarcinomas usually have high signal intensity on T2-weighted images and low signal intensity on T1-weighted images with a similar enhancement pattern as seen with CT. Imaging characteristics can vary greatly, however, depending on the morphologic type of the tumor (57).

MRCP is a useful adjunct to conventional MRI, and may be helpful in evaluating the extension of perihilar tumors. ERCP and percutaneous transhepatic cholangiography (PTC) are not usually indicated for peripheral intrahepatic tumors, but are useful in most perihilar cholangiocarcinomas for evaluation of the intraductal extent of the tumor. ERCP/PTC is the modality of choice for evaluation of the infiltrating sclerosing morphologic subtype. Malignant biliary strictures typically taper irregularly and are associated with proximal ductal dilatation, although this can be difficult to distinguish from sclerosing cholangitis. Biliary drainage may also be performed at the time of ERCP/PTC.

## FDG-PET/CT for evaluation of cholangiocarcinoma

Multiple studies have confirmed the utility of FDG-PET for the evaluation of cholangiocarcinomas. In one study by Anderson *et al.* (58), FDG-PET was performed on 36 consecutive patients with suspected cholangiocarcinoma due to either a nodular mass larger than 1 cm in diameter or the presence of a suspicious infiltrating lesions. In lesions with nodular morphologic subtype, the sensitivity of FDG-PET for detection of the primary lesion was 85%. For the infiltrating lesions, however, the sensitivity was only 18%. The low sensitivity for detection of the latter may be related to the low cellular density of this subtype. FDG-PET had a significant impact on patient care, resulting in change in surgical management in 30% of patients, primarily due to the detection of unsuspected distant metastases. The overall sensitivity for detection of metastases was 65%, with three false-negatives found to have carcinomatosis at surgery. FDG-PET successfully detected all extra-abdominal metastases.

Apart from the morphologic pattern, the usefulness of FDG-PET in the differential diagnosis of cholangiocarcinoma is also dependent on the primary site of disease. While FDG-PET has been shown to be helpful in intrahepatic and common bile duct lesions, PET is less optimal for evaluation of perihilar cholangiocarcinomas (59, 60). FDG-PET has been shown to be of significant value in detection of unsuspected distant metastases. In another series of 126 patients, FDG-PET changed management in 24% of patients by detection of additional unsuspected disease (61). In this series, the sensitivity for detection of metastatic disease was 96% with a specificity of 89%. FDG-PET was also shown to be useful in detecting recurrent disease, with a reported sensitivity and specificity of 89% and 100% respectively (61).

## Gallbladder carcinoma

Carcinoma of the gallbladder is the most common type of biliary cancer and the sixth most common type of gastrointestinal malignancy (62). The most common histologic cell type is adenocarcinoma, accounting for greater than 90% of gallbladder carcinomas. Other less common cell types include squamous, adenosquamous, carcinoid, malignant gastrointestinal stromal tumors, and small cell carcinomas (63). The incidence of gallbladder carcinoma is approximately three times higher in women than in men. Associated risk factors include cholelithiasis, obesity, and chronic gallbladder infections (64). Patients are often asymptomatic early in the course of the disease and diagnosis does not often occur until an advanced stage. As venous drainage of the gallbladder is directly to the liver, invasion of hepatic parenchyma is not uncommon. Regional lymph node spread may also occur. Perforation of the gallbladder may lead to peritoneal spread of tumor.

## FDG-PET/CT for evaluation of gallbladder carcinoma

As gallbladder carcinoma is often found incidentally at cholecystectomy, FDG-PET is not often performed for primary evaluation of suspected lesions (65). FDG-PET is more often used for staging following cholecystectomy or for restaging in the setting of a suspected recurrence. FDG has been shown to accumulate within gallbladder carcinoma (66) and has been shown to be useful in distinguishing scar tissue from malignant recurrence at the surgical incision site when CT findings were equivocal (67).

FDG-PET/CT has not been evaluated in many large series of patients, primarily due to the rarity of the disease. The sensitivity of FDG-PET for detection of gallbladder carcinoma has been reported to be between 78–86% (58, 61, 68). In one study of 99 patients with either gallbladder carcinoma or cholangiocarcinoma, FDG-PET/CT did not perform significantly better than CT in diagnosis of primary tumors. PET/CT did have a significantly higher sensitivity for detection of distant metastases when compared with CT (94.7% for PET/CT and 63.2% for CT) (69). The sensitivity for detection of extrahepatic metastases has been reported as low as 50% in one small series, with false negative findings primarily due to carcinomatosis (58).

## Summary

FDG-PET/CT is a powerful metabolic adjunct to conventional anatomical imaging for evaluation of pancreatic carcinoma. In particular, FDG-PET is useful for pre-operative diagnosis of pancreatic carcinoma when CT fails to identify a discrete tumor mass or when FNA is non-diagnostic. FDG-PET imaging is useful for M staging as well as restaging by detecting CT occult metastatic disease, which allows avoidance of non-curative surgical resection in this group of patients. FDG-PET is also helpful in distinguishing post-therapy changes from tumor recurrence and holds promise for assessing response to neoadjuvant chemoradiation therapy. It should be noted, however, that therapeutic options for non-responders or patients with recurrent pancreatic carcinoma are limited.

Most benign hepatic lesions show a similar degree of FDG uptake in comparison to normal liver uptake. FDG-PET/CT can help differentiate malignant from benign hepatic lesions, although false-negative results may occur with HCC and infiltrating cholangiocarcinoma. Due to varying degrees of uptake within HCC, FDG-PET/CT is of limited diagnostic utility for the detection of HCC in patients with hepatitis C and/or cirrhosis and regenerating nodules. In patients with primary malignant hepatic tumors that accumulate FDG, PET/CT can identify unexpected distant metastases. Although unlikely to become widely available because of the short half-life of Carbon-11 (20 minutes), $^{11}$C-acetate PET/CT does play a complementary role with FDG-PET/CT for the evaluation of HCC, with a high combined sensitivity for detection of primary and metastatic lesions.

## References

1. Jemal A, Siegel R, Xu J, Ward E. Cancer statistics, 2010. *CA Cancer J Clin* 2010;**60**(5):277–300.

2. Horner MJ, Ries LAG, Krapcho M *et al.* (eds). SEER Cancer Statistics Review, 1975–2006. Bethesda, MD: National Cancer Institute. [http://seer.cancer.gov/csr/1975_2006/, based on November 2008 SEER data submission, posted to the SEER web site, 2009].

3. Katz MH, Hwang R, Fleming JB, Evans DB. Tumor-node-metastasis staging of pancreatic adenocarcinoma. *CA Cancer J Clin* 2008;**58**:111–25.

4. NCCN (National Comprehensive Cancer Network) Guidelines. [Available online at http://www.nccn.org/professionals/physician_gls/f_guidelines.asp] [Accessed 1.17.2010].

5. Ichikawa T, Erturk SM, Sou H *et al.* MDCT of pancreatic adenocarcinoma: optimal imaging phases and multiplanar reformatted imaging. *Am J Roentgenol* 2006;**187**:1513–20.

6. Vargas R, Nino-Murcia M, Trueblood W, Jeffrey RB, Jr. MDCT in pancreatic adenocarcinoma: prediction of vascular invasion and resectability using a multiphasic technique with curved planar reformations. *Am J Roentgenol* 2004;**182**:419–25.

7. DeWitt J, Devereaux B, Chriswell M *et al.* Comparison of endoscopic ultrasonography and multidetector computed tomography for detecting and staging pancreatic cancer. *Ann Intern Med* 2004;**141**:753–63.

8. Lammer J, Herlinger H, Zalaudek G, Hofler H. Pseudotumorous pancreatitis. *Gastrointest Radiol* 1985;**10**:59–67.

9. NIH state-of-the-science statement on endoscopic retrograde cholangiopancreatography (ERCP) for diagnosis and therapy. *NIH Consens State Sci Statements* 2002;**19**:1–26.

10. Erickson RA. ERCP and pancreatic cancer. *Ann Surg Oncol* 2004;**11**:555–7.

11. Ichikawa T, Haradome H, Hachiya J *et al.* Pancreatic ductal adenocarcinoma: preoperative assessment with helical CT versus dynamic MR imaging. *Radiology* 1997;**202**:655–62.

12. Lopez Hanninen E, Amthauer H, Hosten N *et al.* Prospective evaluation of pancreatic tumors: accuracy of MR imaging with MR cholangiopancreatography and MR angiography. *Radiology* 2002;**224**:34–41.

13. Yeo CJ, Cameron JL, Lillemoe KD *et al.* Pancreaticoduodenectomy with or without distal gastrectomy and extended retroperitoneal lymphadenectomy for periampullary adenocarcinoma, part 2: randomized controlled trial evaluating survival, morbidity, and mortality. *Ann Surg* 2002;**236**:355–66; discussion 66–8.

14. Delbeke D, Martin WH. PET and PET/CT for pancreatic malignancies. *Surg Oncol Clin N Am* 2010;**19**:235–54.

15. Monakhov NK, Neistadt EL, Shavlovskii MM, Shvartsman AL, Neifakh SA. Physicochemical properties and isoenzyme composition of hexokinase from normal and malignant human tissues. *J Natl Cancer Inst* 1978;**61**:27–34.

16. Higashi T, Tamaki N, Honda T *et al.* Expression of glucose transporters in human pancreatic tumors compared with increased FDG accumulation in PET study. *J Nucl Med* 1997;**38**:1337–44.

17. Reske SN, Grillenberger KG, Glatting G *et al.* Overexpression of glucose transporter 1 and increased FDG uptake in pancreatic carcinoma. *J Nucl Med* 1997;**38**:1344–8.

18. Delbeke D, Pinson CW. Pancreatic tumors: role of imaging in the diagnosis, staging, and treatment. *J Hepatobiliary Pancreat Surg* 2004;**11**:4–10.

19. Kauhanen SP, Komar G, Seppanen MP *et al.* A prospective diagnostic accuracy study of 18F-fluorodeoxyglucose positron emission tomography/computed tomography, multidetector row computed tomography, and magnetic resonance imaging in primary diagnosis and staging of pancreatic cancer. *Ann Surg* 2009;**250**:957–63.

20. Gambhir SS, Czernin J, Schwimmer J *et al.* A tabulated summary of the FDG PET literature. *J Nucl Med* 2001;**42**:1S–93S.

21. Rose DM, Delbeke D, Beauchamp RD *et al.* 18Fluorodeoxyglucose-positron emission tomography in the management of patients with suspected pancreatic cancer. *Ann Surg* 1999;**229**:729–37; discussion 37–8.

22. Nakata B, Nishimura S, Ishikawa T *et al.* Prognostic predictive value of 18F-fluorodeoxyglucose positron emission tomography for patients with pancreatic cancer. *Int J Oncol* 2001;**19**:53–8.

23. Zimny M, Fass J, Bares R *et al.* Fluorodeoxyglucose positron emission tomography and the prognosis of pancreatic carcinoma. *Scand J Gastroenterol* 2000;**35**:883–8.

24. Sperti C, Pasquali C, Decet G *et al.* F-18-fluorodeoxyglucose positron emission tomography in differentiating malignant from benign pancreatic cysts: a prospective study. *J Gastrointest Surg* 2005;**9**:22–8; discussion 8–9.

25. Delbeke D, Rose DM, Chapman WC *et al.* Optimal interpretation of FDG PET in the diagnosis, staging and management of pancreatic carcinoma. *J Nucl Med* 1999;**40**:1784–91.

26. Heinrich S, Goerres GW, Schafer M *et al.* Positron emission tomography/computed tomography influences on the management of resectable pancreatic cancer and its cost-effectiveness. *Ann Surg* 2005;**242**:235–43.

27. Ruf J, Lopez Hanninen E, Oettle H *et al.* Detection of recurrent pancreatic cancer: comparison of FDG-PET with CT/MRI. *Pancreatology* 2005;**5**:266–72.

28. Kitajima K, Murakami K, Yamasaki E *et al.* Performance of integrated FDG-PET/contrast-enhanced CT in the diagnosis of recurrent pancreatic cancer: comparison with integrated FDG-PET/non-contrast-enhanced CT and enhanced CT. *Mol Imaging Biol* 2010;**12**:452–9.

29. Bang S, Chung HW, Park SW *et al.* The clinical usefulness of 18-fluorodeoxyglucose positron emission tomography in the differential diagnosis, staging, and response evaluation after concurrent chemoradiotherapy for pancreatic cancer. *J Clin Gastroenterol* 2006;**40**:923–9.

30. Kuwatani M, Kawakami H, Eto K *et al.* Modalities for evaluating chemotherapeutic efficacy and survival time in patients with advanced pancreatic cancer: comparison between FDG-PET, CT, and serum tumor markers. *Intern Med* 2009;**48**:867–75.

31. Bosch FX, Ribes J, Diaz M, Cleries R. Primary liver cancer: worldwide incidence and trends. *Gastroenterology* 2004;**127**:S5–S16.

32. El-Serag HB, Davila JA, Petersen NJ, McGlynn KA. The continuing increase in the incidence of hepatocellular carcinoma in the United States: an update. *Ann Intern Med* 2003;**139**:817–23.

33. Russo MW, Wei JT, Thiny MT *et al.* Digestive and liver diseases statistics, 2004. *Gastroenterology* 2004;**126**:1448–53.

34. McCaughan GW, Koorey DJ, Strasser SI. Hepatocellular carcinoma: current approaches to diagnosis and management. *Intern Med J* 2002;**32**:394–400.

35. Fattovich G, Giustina G, Degos F *et al.* Morbidity and mortality in compensated cirrhosis type C: a retrospective follow-up study of 384

patients. *Gastroenterology* 1997;**112**:463–72.

36. Levy I, Greig PD, Gallinger S, Langer B, Sherman M. Resection of hepatocellular carcinoma without preoperative tumor biopsy. *Ann Surg* 2001;**234**:206–9.

37. Torzilli G, Minagawa M, Takayama T *et al.* Accurate preoperative evaluation of liver mass lesions without fine-needle biopsy. *Hepatology* 1999;**30**:889–93.

38. Koteish A, Thuluvath PJ. Screening for hepatocellular carcinoma. *J Vasc Interv Radiol* 2002;**13**:S185–90.

39. Fung KT, Li FT, Raimondo ML *et al.* Systematic review of radiological imaging for hepatocellular carcinoma in cirrhotic patients. *Br J Radiol* 2004;**77**:633–40.

40. Weber G, Cantero A. Glucose-6-phosphatase activity in normal, pre-cancerous, and neoplastic tissues. *Cancer Res* 1955;**15**:105–8.

41. Weber G, Morris HP. Comparative biochemistry of hepatomas. III. Carbohydrate enzymes in liver tumors of different growth rates. *Cancer Res* 1963;**23**:987–94.

42. Torizuka T, Tamaki N, Inokuma T *et al.* In vivo assessment of glucose metabolism in hepatocellular carcinoma with FDG-PET. *J Nucl Med* 1995;**36**:1811–17.

43. Trojan J, Schroeder O, Raedle J *et al.* Fluorine-18 FDG positron emission tomography for imaging of hepatocellular carcinoma. *Am J Gastroenterol* 1999;**94**:3314–19.

44. Iwata Y, Shiomi S, Sasaki N *et al.* Clinical usefulness of positron emission tomography with fluorine-18-fluorodeoxyglucose in the diagnosis of liver tumors. *Ann Nucl Med* 2000;**14**:121–6.

45. Delbeke D, Martin WH, Sandler MP *et al.* Evaluation of benign vs malignant hepatic lesions with positron emission tomography. *Arch Surg* 1998;**133**:510–15; discussion 5–6.

46. Khan MA, Combs CS, Brunt EM *et al.* Positron emission tomography scanning in the evaluation of hepatocellular carcinoma. *J Hepatol* 2000;**32**:792–7.

47. Liangpunsakul S, Agarwal D, Horlander JC, Kieff B, Chalasani N. Positron emission tomography for detecting occult hepatocellular carcinoma in hepatitis C cirrhotics awaiting for liver transplantation. *Transplant Proc* 2003;**35**:2995–7.

48. Wudel LJ, Jr., Delbeke D, Morris D *et al.* The role of [18F] fluorodeoxyglucose positron emission tomography imaging in the evaluation of hepatocellular carcinoma. *Am Surg* 2003;**69**:117–24; discussion 24–6.

49. Chen YK, Hsieh DS, Liao CS *et al.* Utility of FDG-PET for investigating unexplained serum AFP elevation in patients with suspected hepatocellular carcinoma recurrence. *Anticancer Res* 2005;**25**:4719–25.

50. Delbeke D, Pinson CW. 11C-acetate: a new tracer for the evaluation of hepatocellular carcinoma. *J Nucl Med* 2003;**44**:222–3.

51. Ho CL, Yu SC, Yeung DW. 11C-acetate PET imaging in hepatocellular carcinoma and other liver masses. *J Nucl Med* 2003;**44**:213–21.

52. Ho CL, Chen S, Yeung DW, Cheng TK. Dual-tracer PET/CT imaging in evaluation of metastatic hepatocellular carcinoma. *J Nucl Med* 2007;**48**:902–9.

53. Park JW, Kim JH, Kim SK *et al.* A prospective evaluation of 18F-FDG and 11C-acetate PET/CT for detection of primary and metastatic hepatocellular carcinoma. *J Nucl Med* 2008;**49**:1912–21.

54. Aljiffry M, Abdulelah A, Walsh M *et al.* Evidence-based approach to cholangiocarcinoma: a systematic review of the current literature. *J Am Coll Surg* 2009;**208**:134–47.

55. de Groen PC, Gores GJ, LaRusso NF, Gunderson LL, Nagorney DM. Biliary tract cancers. *N Engl J Med* 1999;**341**:1368–78.

56. Nakeeb A, Pitt HA, Sohn TA *et al.* Cholangiocarcinoma. A spectrum of intrahepatic, perihilar, and distal tumors. *Ann Surg* 1996;**224**:463–73; discussion 73–5.

57. Chung YE, Kim MJ, Park YN *et al.* Varying appearances of cholangiocarcinoma: radiologic-pathologic correlation. *Radiographics* 2009;**29**:683–700.

58. Anderson CD, Rice MH, Pinson CW *et al.* Fluorodeoxyglucose PET imaging in the evaluation of gallbladder carcinoma and cholangiocarcinoma. *J Gastrointest Surg* 2004;**8**:90–7.

59. Moon CM, Bang S, Chung JB *et al.* Usefulness of 18F-fluorodeoxyglucose positron emission tomography in differential diagnosis and staging of cholangiocarcinomas. *J Gastroenterol Hepatol* 2008;**23**:759–65.

60. Kim YJ, Yun M, Lee WJ, Kim KS, Lee JD. Usefulness of 18F-FDG PET in intrahepatic cholangiocarcinoma. *Eur J Nucl Med Mol Imaging* 2003;**30**:1467–72.

61. Corvera CU, Blumgart LH, Akhurst T *et al.* 18F-fluorodeoxyglucose positron emission tomography influences management decisions in patients with biliary cancer. *J Am Coll Surg* 2008;**206**:57–65.

62. Donohue JH, Stewart AK, Menck HR. The National Cancer Data Base report on carcinoma of the gallbladder, 1989–1995. *Cancer* 1998;**83**:2618–28.

63. Goldin RD, Roa JC. Gallbladder cancer: a morphological and molecular update. *Histopathology* 2009;**55**:218–29.

64. Lazcano-Ponce EC, Miquel JF, Munoz N *et al.* Epidemiology and molecular pathology of gallbladder cancer. *CA Cancer J Clin* 2001;**51**:349–64.

65. Duffy A, Capanu M, Abou-Alfa GK *et al.* Gallbladder cancer (GBC): 10-year experience at Memorial Sloan-Kettering Cancer Centre (MSKCC). *J Surg Oncol* 2008;**98**:485–9.

66. Hoh CK, Hawkins RA, Glaspy JA *et al.* Cancer detection with whole-body PET using 2-[18F]fluoro-2-deoxy-D-glucose. *J Comput Assist Tomogr* 1993; **17**:582–9.

67. Lomis KD, Vitola JV, Delbeke D *et al.* Recurrent gallbladder carcinoma at laparoscopy port sites diagnosed by positron emission tomography: implications for primary and radical second operations. *Am Surg* 1997;**63**:341–5.

68. Rodriguez-Fernandez A, Gomez-Rio M, Llamas-Elvira JM *et al.* Positron-emission tomography with fluorine-18-fluoro-2-deoxy-D-glucose for gallbladder cancer diagnosis. *Am J Surg* 2004;**188**:171–5.

69. Lee SW, Kim HJ, Park JH *et al.* Clinical usefulness of 18F-FDG PET-CT for patients with gallbladder cancer and cholangiocarcinoma. *J Gastroenterol* 2010;**45**:560–6.

A 62-year-old male presented with three weeks of abdominal pain. Diagnostic CT of the abdomen revealed extensive retroperitoneal adenopathy and hepatic steatosis. FDG-PET/CT was requested for further evaluation.

## Acquisition and processing parameters

The fasting blood glucose level was 184 mg/dL. FDG (22.4 mCi) was administered intravenously via a right-hand IV. The patient voided prior to imaging. Following a 67-min distribution time, PET/CT images were acquired from the head to the proximal thighs in a supine position with the arms positioned above the head. Transmission images were acquired using a low-dose CT scan from head to proximal thigh without intravenous contrast. The CT data were reconstructed using a filtered back-projection algorithm and a $512 \times 512$ matrix, with a transaxial field of view of 70 cm and a reconstructed slice thickness of 3.75 mm. CT images were used for attenuation correction and anatomical localization. Immediately following the transmission CT acquisition, emission images were acquired with a dedicated full-ring PET tomograph from the head to the proximal thighs over the same field of view as the transmission scan. PET data were reconstructed using an ordered-subset expectation maximization iterative algorithm (20 subsets, 2 iterations).

## Findings and differential diagnosis

Coronal PET, CT, fused PET/CT and MIP images (Figure 10.1) and axial CT, PET, and fused PET/CT images at multiple levels (Figure 10.2) demonstrate intense uptake within a large mass in the head of the pancreas measuring 8.5 cm in its greatest axial dimension. Intense uptake is seen diffusely throughout the liver, most prominently in the left hepatic lobe. There is intense uptake corresponding to subcarinal/right peribronchial and extensive retroperitoneal adenopathy. Mild uptake is seen along the peritoneal surface and within free intraperitoneal fluid. Additional transmission CT findings include a 0.9 cm non-calcified pulmonary nodule in the anterior aspect of the right middle lobe without associated FDG uptake (Figure 10.2 top row). Additional subcentimeter non-calcified pulmonary nodules (not shown) were identified in the lower lung fields bilaterally.

The findings are most consistent with primary pancreatic cancer with extensive hepatic and nodal metastasis. Accumulation of FDG along the peritoneal lining and within peritoneal

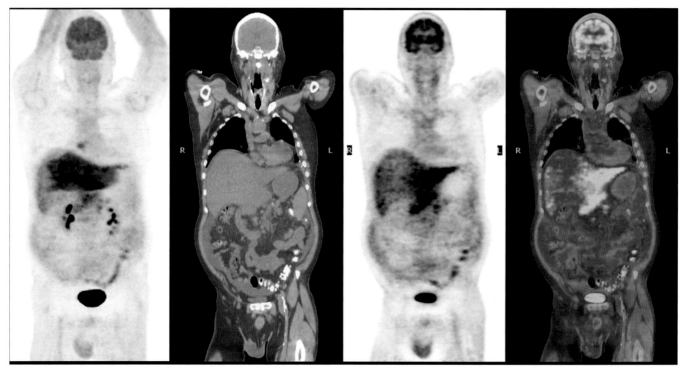

**Figure 10.1** From left to right: MIP, coronal CT, FDG-PET, and fused FDG-PET/CT images.

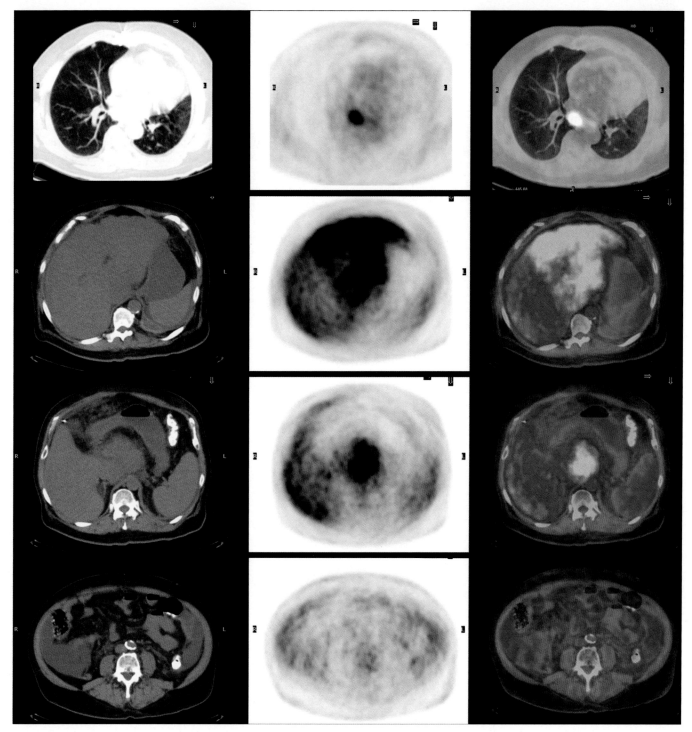

**Figure 10.2** Chest and abdomen: from left to right: axial CT, FDG-PET, and fused FDG-PET/CT.

fluid likely represents peritoneal carcinomatosis with malignant ascites. Differential considerations include peritonitis, although this is less likely given the clinical scenario. The subcentimeter pulmonary nodules are below the PET resolution, but are highly suggestive of pulmonary metastases despite the lack of FDG uptake.

## Diagnosis and clinical follow-up

CT-guided biopsy of a retroperitoneal lymph node revealed poorly differentiated adenocarcinoma of pancreatic origin. Given the advanced stage, palliative measures were instituted. The patient died 8 days following the PET/CT.

## Discussion and teaching points

This case demonstrates the utility of FDG-PET/CT for whole body staging of pancreatic adenocarcinoma. The diagnostic CT of the abdomen and pelvis acquired prior to the PET/CT underestimated the extent of disease. The pancreatic head mass was initially felt to represent extension of the extensive retroperitoneal adenopathy, which was also present. FDG-PET/CT was able to clarify the presence of the pancreatic mass in addition to metastatic retroperitoneal adenopathy. The diffusely decreased attenuation in the liver seen on the diagnostic CT was initially felt to be due to hepatic steatosis with some areas of fatty sparing. The intense uptake on FDG was able to clarify diffuse tumor infiltration of the liver. A recent study of 23 patients with diffuse low attenuation in the liver showed that there is no effect on SUV values by hepatic steatosis alone (1).

The small pulmonary nodules and subcarinal lymph node were not detected on CT due to the limited field of view. The pulmonary nodules were not identifiable on the PET images, but were clearly seen on the transmission CT images of the thorax. As lesions smaller than 1.0 cm are detected with less sensitivity by PET, it is essential to carefully interpret the CT images in addition to the PET and fused PET/CT images. In one series of 321 patients who underwent FDG-PET/CT, 84% were found to have abnormalities that were not FDG avid, including patients with multiple pulmonary metastases (2).

As seen in this case, FDG-PET/CT can have a significant impact on the management of patients with pancreatic adenocarcinoma, particularly with detection of unsuspected metastases and clarification of equivocal findings on CT. In one study, FDG-PET altered the management in 28 of 65 patients (43%) with pancreatic carcinoma. Metastases were detected both on CT and FDG-PET in 10 of 21 patients with stage IV disease, but PET demonstrated hepatic metastases not identified or equivocal on CT, and/or distant metastases unsuspected clinically in seven additional patients (33%). In four patients (19%), neither CT nor PET imaging showed evidence of metastases, but surgical exploration revealed carcinomatosis in three patients and a small liver metastasis in one patient (3). Mild diffuse peritoneal uptake, as in this case, has been described as a pattern of uptake in patients with peritoneal carcinomatosis (4).

## Take-home message

- FDG-PET/CT is a powerful metabolic modality for assessing the extent of metastatic disease that may be occult on anatomic imaging.
- It is essential to carefully interpret the CT component of PET/CT as not all lesions are detected by PET alone.

## References

1. Abele JT, Fung CI. Effect of hepatic steatosis on liver FDG uptake measured in mean standard uptake values. *Radiology* 2010;**254**:917–24.

2. Bruzzi JF, Truong MT, Marom EM *et al.* Incidental findings on integrated PET/CT that do not accumulate 18F-FDG. *AJR Am J Roentgenol* 2006;**187**:1116–23.

3. Delbeke D, Rose DM, Chapman WC *et al.* Optimal interpretation of FDG PET in the diagnosis, staging and management of pancreatic carcinoma. *J Nucl Med* 1999;**40**:1784–91.

4. Turlakow A, Yeung HW, Salmon AS, Macapinlac HA, Larson SM. Peritoneal carcinomatosis: role of (18)F-FDG PET. *J Nucl Med* 2003;**44**:1407–12.

A 71-year-old male with locally advanced pancreatic adenocarcinoma felt to be borderline resectable based on CT findings (Figure 10.3) due to involvement of the superior mesenteric vein and abutment of the superior mesenteric artery. He underwent neoadjuvant radiation and chemotherapy and was referred for restaging with FDG-PET/CT (Figure 10.4) prior to surgical resection.

## Acquisition and processing parameters

The fasting blood glucose level was 97 mg/dL. FDG (11.7 mCi) was administered intravenously via a right antecubital IV. The patient voided prior to imaging. Following a 60-min distribution time, PET/CT images were acquired from the head to the proximal thighs in a supine position with the arms positioned above the head. First, transmission images were acquired using a low-dose CT scan from head to proximal thigh without intravenous contrast. The CT data were reconstructed using a filtered back-projection algorithm and a $512 \times 512$ matrix, with a transaxial field of view of 70 cm and reconstructed slice thickness of 3.75 mm. CT images were used for attenuation correction and anatomical localization. Immediately following the transmission CT acquisition, emission images were acquired with a dedicated full-ring PET tomograph from the proximal thighs to the head over the same field of view as the transmission scan. PET data were reconstructed using an ordered-subset expectation maximization iterative algorithm (20 subsets, 2 iterations).

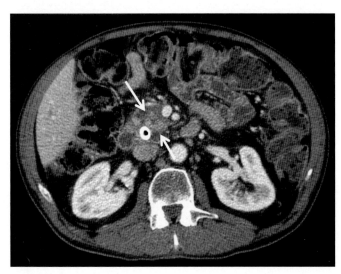

**Figure 10.3** Axial abdominal CT with contrast.

## Findings and differential diagnosis

MIP PET as well as axial PET and fused PET/CT images at multiple levels (Figure 10.4) demonstrate mild to moderate uptake corresponding to a 3.3 cm mass in the pancreatic head (bottom row). The low degree of uptake may be due to partially treated disease, although no baseline PET/CT was performed prior to neoadjuvant therapy to assess the FDG avidity of the primary tumor. At the right lateral aspect of the mass, there is focal intense uptake associated with a stent in the common bile duct. This is non-specific and may be due to inflammation or viable tumor. A 2.1 cm low-density lesion near the dome of the liver (middle row) shows intense uptake, consistent with hepatic metastasis. A 1.0 cm subcarinal lymph node (top row) shows intense uptake, likely metastastic despite the small size.

## Diagnosis and clinical follow-up

Due to the presence of the FDG-avid hepatic and mediastinal nodal metastasis, the patient was considered to have stage IV pancreatic adenocarcinoma. Surgery was cancelled and chemotherapy continued.

## Discussion and teaching points

This case illustrates the usefulness of FDG-PET/CT in reassessing patients with pancreatic adenocarcinoma following therapy. Initially, the patient was considered borderline resectable with locally advanced disease due to involvement of the superior mesenteric vein and abutment of the superior mesenteric artery. An aggressive surgical approach was considered. FDG-PET/CT following neoadjuvant radiation and chemotherapy was able to detect an unsuspected hepatic metastasis, obviating the need for surgical resection, which would have been associated with significant morbidity without affecting survival.

Data suggest that FDG-PET is a useful modality to assess tumor response to neoadjuvant therapy, and to diagnose recurrent disease following surgery (1, 2). In this case, the pancreatic mass, apart from the biliary stent, showed low levels of FDG uptake. This may have been due to a local response to radiation therapy. The FDG-avid hepatic and subcarinal lesions, however, were unknown and would not have been included in the radiation port. Other roles for FDG-PET/CT in the post-therapy setting include the evaluation of equivocal CT abnormalities in the resection bed that are difficult to differentiate from radiation-induced fibrosis, for the evaluation of new hepatic lesions that are equivocal on CT and too small to biopsy, and for restaging of patients with rising serum tumor marker levels and a negative conventional work-up.

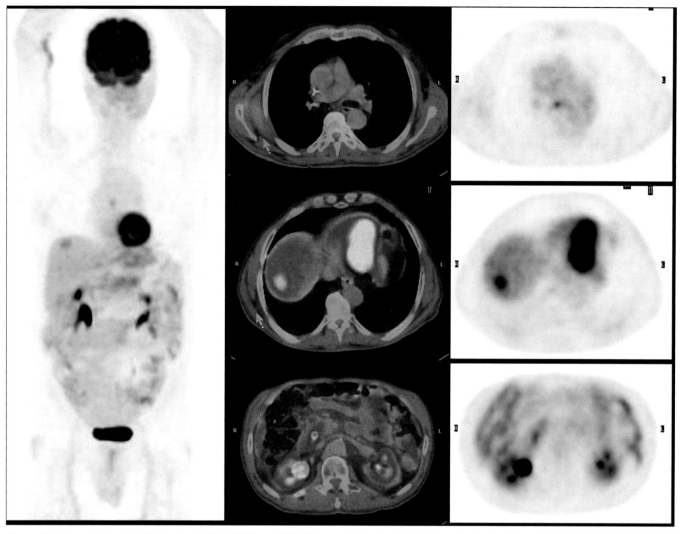

**Figure 10.4** From left to right: MIP, fused axial FDG-PET/CT, and FDG-PET images of the chest and abdomen.

Patients with pancreatic cancer often undergo placement of biliary stents in order to relieve obstructive jaundice. Increased FDG uptake associated with biliary stents is not an uncommon finding and has been described in the absence of malignancy or cholangitis (3, 4). This is felt to represent local inflammatory changes in the tissues adjacent to the stent. In patients with known pancreatic or biliary tract cancer, this does interfere with interpretation, as inflammatory uptake cannot be distinguished from viable FDG-avid tumor based on PET/CT alone. It is important, however, to be familiar with sources of potential false-positive findings.

## Take-home message

- FDG-PET/CT is a useful modality for the assessment of tumor response to neoadjuvant therapy prior to surgical resection.
- One of the strengths of PET/CT is the ability to detect unsuspected distant metastases and to characterize the nature of equivocal findings on CT.
- Inflammatory uptake associated with biliary stents is common and can be difficult to distinguish from uptake due to malignancy.

## References

1. Rose DM, Delbeke D, Beauchamp RD et al. 18Fluorodeoxyglucose-positron emission tomography in the management of patients with suspected pancreatic cancer. *Ann Surg* 1999;**229**:729–37; discussion 37–8.

2. Bang S, Chung HW, Park SW et al. The clinical usefulness of 18-fluorodeoxyglucose positron emission tomography in the differential diagnosis, staging, and response evaluation after concurrent chemoradiotherapy for pancreatic cancer. *J Clin Gastroenterol* 2006;**40**:923–9.

3. Lin EC, Studley M. Biliary tract FDG uptake secondary to stent placement. *Clin Nucl Med* 2003;**28**:318–19.

4. Shreve PD, Anzai Y, Wahl RL. Pitfalls in oncologic diagnosis with FDG PET imaging: physiologic and benign variants. *Radiographics* 1999;**19**:61–77; quiz 150–1.

A 70-year-old female with known carcinoid of the pancreas. She underwent resection of a mass in the head of the pancreas several years previously. An additional mass in the tail of the pancreas has been slowly increasing in size on serial CT examinations. Due to an abrupt increase in size, she was referred for FDG-PET/CT.

## Acquisition and processing parameters

The fasting blood glucose level was 97 mg/dL. FDG (11.3 mCi) was administered intravenously via a right PICC line. The patient voided prior to imaging. Following a 65-min distribution time, PET/CT images were acquired from the head to the proximal thighs in a supine position with the arms positioned above the head. Transmission images were acquired using a low-dose CT scan from head to proximal thighs without intravenous contrast. The CT data were reconstructed using a filtered back-projection algorithm and a $512 \times 512$ matrix, with a transaxial field of view of 70 cm and a reconstructed

slice thickness of 3.75 mm. CT images were used for attenuation correction and anatomical localization. Immediately following the transmission CT acquisition, emission images were acquired with a dedicated full-ring PET tomograph from the proximal thighs to the head over the same field of view as the transmission scan. PET data were reconstructed using an ordered-subset expectation maximization iterative algorithm (20 subsets, 2 iterations).

## Findings and differential diagnosis

Axial unenhanced CT, PET, and PET/CT fused images through the thorax (Figure 10.5) demonstrate moderate FDG uptake corresponding to a 1.1 cm round, non-calcified pulmonary nodule in the base of the left lower lobe. Axial and coronal CT, PET, and PET/CT fused images through the abdomen (Figure 10.6) show moderate uptake (similar to liver) within a $4.7 \times 4.2$ cm soft tissue mass in the tail of the pancreas, anterior to the upper pole of the left kidney. Activity

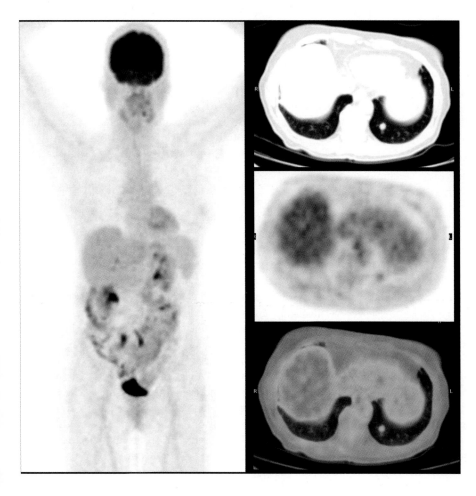

**Figure 10.5** Maximum intensity projection (MIP) image and axial unenhanced CT, FDG-PET, and FDG-PET/CT fused images through the thorax.

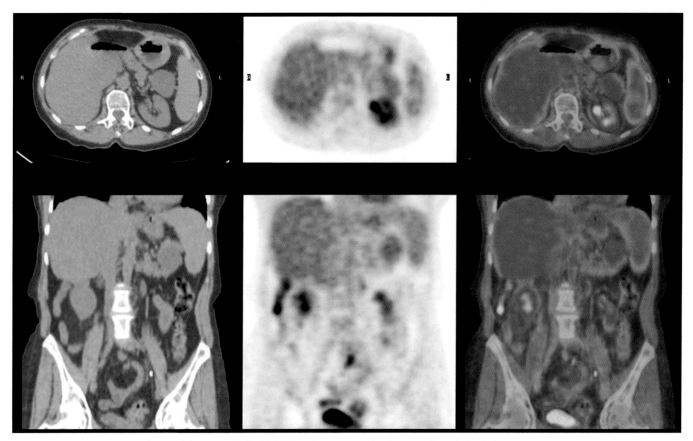

**Figure 10.6** Axial (top row) and coronal (bottom row) CT, FDG-PET, and FDG-PET/CT fused images through the abdomen.

within the gastrointestinal and genitourinary tracts is otherwise within physiologic limits.

The findings are most consistent with a pancreatic neuroendocrine tumor with pulmonary metastasis.

## Diagnosis and clinical follow-up

The patient has known biopsy-proven pancreatic carcinoid and underwent resection of a pancreatic head mass and liver metastases several years prior to the FDG-PET/CT examination. The pancreatic tail mass had been slowly growing over a period of years, but not resected due to the morbidity associated with complete pancreatectomy as well as other comorbidities. Given the findings on PET/CT, surgery was recommended, but the patient elected conservative management.

## Discussion and teaching points

Pancreatic neuroendocrine tumors make up a small fraction of all pancreatic neoplasms. These are often located in the body and tail of the pancreas and are usually slow-growing tumors. Most neuroendocrine tumors, including carcinoid, islet cell tumors, and paragangliomas express somatostatin receptors (SSR) and can be imaged effectively with somatostatin analogs, such as [111]In-pentetreotide (1). The expression of SSRs is heterogeneous, however, which is likely related to the degree

of differentiation of the tumor. Well-differentiated SSR-positive tumors may be false-negative on FDG-PET and are more reliably detected with somatostatin receptor imaging. On the other hand, more aggressive tumors may show less uptake with [111]In-pentetreotide and have increased uptake on FDG-PET (2). Studies have shown that even within the same patient, there may be some lesions that have high [111]In-pentetreotide/low FDG uptake and others with high FDG uptake/low [111]In-pentetreotide uptake. Tumors that show increased uptake in FDG-PET have been associated with a poorer prognosis (3).

This patient did undergo [111]In-pentetreotide scintigraphy 3 years before, which showed no abnormal uptake in the region of the pancreatic mass (Figure 10.7). On FDG-PET/CT the primary pancreatic mass and pulmonary metastasis are readily visible, although the degree of uptake is moderate. As the degree of uptake is similar to that of liver, the sensitivity for detection of hepatic metastases may be diminished in this patient.

[68]Ga-labeled somatostatin analogs, such as [68]Ga-DOTA-TOC and [68]Ga-DOTA-TATE are showing great promise for evaluation of neuroendocrine tumors. One of the benefits of using [68]Ga is that it is generator produced and not dependent on an on-site cyclotron. In a prospective study of 84 patients, [68]Ga-DOTATOC had a sensitivity, specificity, and accuracy of 97%, 92%, and 96% respectively on a per-patient basis for detection of neuroendocrine tumors. This was

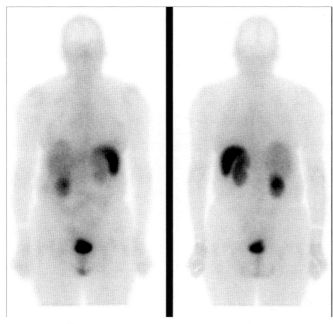

superior to both CT at 61%, 71%, 73%, and SPECT (either [99m]Tc-HYNIC-TOC or [111]In-DOTA-TOC) at 52%, 92%, and 58% respectively (4). [68]Ga-labeled somatostatin analogs have performed superior to FDG for the evaluation of well-differentiated neuroendocrine tumors, although FDG may play a complementary role in the evaluation of high-grade neuroendocrine tumors (5).

## Take-home message

- Pancreatic neuroendocrine tumors are rare, slow-growing tumors often arising in the body or tail of the pancreas.
- Well-differentiated neuroendocrine tumors may be false-negative on FDG-PET/CT. Poorly differentiated neuroendocrine tumors tend to have higher FDG uptake and less uptake of [111]In-pentetreotide.
- New positron-emitting radiopharmaceuticals, such as [68]Ga-labeled somatostatin analogs, are showing great promise for the evaluation of neuroendocrine tumors.

**Figure 10.7** [111]In-pentetreotide whole-body scan (left: anterior; right: posterior).

## References

1. Kaltsas G, Rockall A, Papadogias D, Reznek R, Grossman AB. Recent advances in radiological and radionuclide imaging and therapy of neuroendocrine tumours. *Eur J Endocrinol* 2004;**151**:15–27.

2. Adams S, Baum R, Rink T *et al.* Limited value of fluorine-18 fluorodeoxyglucose positron emission tomography for the imaging of neuroendocrine tumours. *Eur J Nucl Med* 1998;**25**:79–83.

3. Pasquali C, Rubello D, Sperti C *et al.* Neuroendocrine tumor imaging: can 18F-fluorodeoxyglucose positron emission tomography detect tumors with poor prognosis and aggressive behavior? *World J Surg* 1998;**22**:588–92.

4. Gabriel M, Decristoforo C, Kendler D *et al.* 68Ga-DOTA-Tyr3-octreotide PET in neuroendocrine tumors: comparison with somatostatin receptor scintigraphy and CT. *J Nucl Med* 2007;**48**:508–18.

5. Kayani I, Bomanji JB, Groves A *et al.* Functional imaging of neuroendocrine tumors with combined PET/CT using 68Ga-DOTATATE (DOTA-DPhe1, Tyr3-octreotate) and 18F-FDG. *Cancer* 2008;**112**:2447–55.

# Pancreatitis

A 64-year-old female with nausea, weakness, diarrhea, and hyperbilirubinemia was found to have a low density, peripherally enhancing mass in the pancreatic head on CT (Figure 10.8A) causing obstruction of the common bile duct with proximal ductal dilatation (Figure 10.8B). The patient underwent endoscopic ultrasound (EUS) and biopsy the next day confirming pancreatic adenocarcinoma. The day following EUS-guided biopsy, she underwent FDG-PET/CT for staging. Whole-body MIP and axial PET, PET/CT fused, and transmission CT images are provided (Figure 10.9).

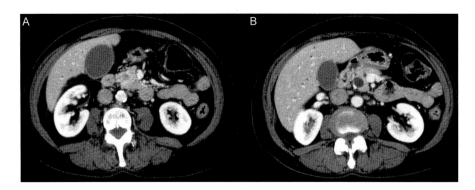

**Figure 10.8** Axial contrast CT slices through the abdomen.

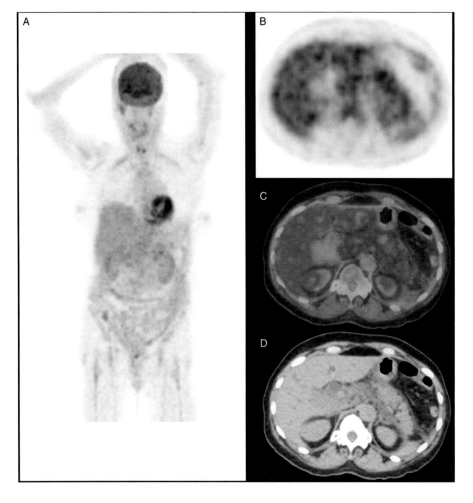

**Figure 10.9** (A) Maximum intensity projection (MIP); (B) axial FDG-PET; (C) axial fused FDG-PET/CT slice; (D) axial unenhanced CT.

## Acquisition and processing parameters

The fasting blood glucose level was 131 mg/dL. FDG (14 mCi) was administered intravenously via a right antecubital IV. The patient voided prior to imaging. Following a 75-min distribution time, PET/CT images were acquired from the head to the proximal thighs in a supine position with the arms positioned above the head. First, transmission images were acquired using a low-dose CT scan from head to proximal thigh without intravenous contrast. The CT data were reconstructed using a filtered back-projection algorithm and a $512 \times 512$ matrix, with a transaxial field of view of 70 cm and a reconstructed slice thickness of 3.75 mm. CT images were used for attenuation correction and anatomical localization. Immediately following the transmission CT acquisition, emission images were acquired with a dedicated full-ring PET tomograph from the proximal thighs to the head over the same field of view as the transmission scan. PET data were reconstructed using an ordered-subset expectation maximization iterative algorithm (20 subsets, 2 iterations).

## Findings and differential diagnosis

FDG-PET/CT images demonstrate diffusely increased uptake throughout the body and tail of an enlarged pancreas. Transmission CT images (Figure 10.9C) demonstrate stranding in the peripancreatic fat with associated mild FDG uptake (Figures 10.9A and 10.9B). The anatomical findings are new since the contrasted CT performed 2 days before. Due to diffuse background uptake, the mass in the pancreatic head is not distinguishable from the remainder of the inflamed pancreas with regard to FDG uptake. No distant FDG-avid metastases are identified.

## Diagnosis and clinical follow-up

The FDG-PET/CT findings were correlated with amylase and lipase the same day, which were markedly elevated, supporting the diagnosis of acute pancreatitis. She went on to have ERCP with biliary stent placement in order to relieve biliary obstruction, followed by a rapid decline in bilirubin levels. Surgery was delayed due to acute inflammation, but she eventually underwent a successful Whipple procedure following neoadjuvant chemotherapy with gemcitabine.

## Discussion and teaching points

Inflammatory processes, such as acute pancreatitis, can lead to increased accumulation of FDG within the affected organ. Both glucose and FDG are substrates for cellular mediators of inflammation. Chronic and acute pancreatitis, with or without associated abscess formation, can result in false-positive interpretations on FDG-PET (1, 2). Alternatively, FDG uptake due to inflammation may mask malignant findings. In this case, the known primary pancreatic head lesion was masked by the diffuse uptake in the remainder of the inflamed pancreas. Due to local inflammatory changes, evaluation for regional nodal metastasis is also limited. Even in the presence of local inflammation, however, FDG-PET/CT can be helpful for evaluation of distant metastasis.

The etiology of the patient's acute pancreatitis may have been due to mechanical obstruction of the common duct due to the pancreatic head mass. The timing of the inflammatory changes, shortly following EUS-guided fine needle aspiration, may suggest an iatrogenic cause. Acute pancreatitis is a rare complication of EUS-guided biopsy of pancreatic masses, occurring in approximately 0.29% of cases (3). For patients undergoing ERCP, however, pancreatitis is the most common serious complication. The incidence of post-ERCP pancreatitis is as high as 5.4%, depending on risk factors and whether ERCP was diagnostic or therapeutic (4).

## Take-home message

- Inflammation due to pancreatitis leads to accumulation of FDG within the pancreas.
- FDG uptake due to inflammation may mask underlying malignant findings.
- Inflammatory lesions such as acute or chronic pancreatitis may lead to false-positive interpretations of FDG-PET/CT.
- Acute pancreatitis is a rare complication of EUS-guided biopsy and the most common serious complication of ERCP.

## References

1. Zimny M, Buell U, Diederichs CG, Reske SN. False-positive FDG PET in patients with pancreatic masses: an issue of proper patient selection? *Eur J Nucl Med* 1998;**25**:1352.

2. Shreve PD. Focal fluorine-18 fluorodeoxyglucose accumulation in inflammatory pancreatic disease. *Eur J Nucl Med* 1998; **25**:259–64.

3. Eloubeidi MA, Gress FG, Savides TJ *et al.* Acute pancreatitis after EUS-guided FNA of solid pancreatic masses: a pooled analysis from EUS centers in the United States. *Gastrointest Endosc* 2004;**60**:385–9.

4. Arata S, Takada T, Hirata K *et al.* Post-ERCP pancreatitis. *J Hepatobiliary Pancreat Sci* 2010;**17**:70–8.

# Gallbladder carcinoma

A 70-year-old male underwent an attempted cholecystectomy for presumed cholecystitis, which was aborted due to findings suspicious for gallbladder carcinoma. He underwent gastrojejunostomy due to duodenal obstruction from tumor involvement. FDG-PET/CT was requested for staging.

## Acquisition and processing parameters

The fasting blood glucose level was 136 mg/dL. FDG (12.6 mCi) was administered intravenously via a right antecubital IV. The patient voided prior to imaging. Following a 90-min distribution time, PET/CT images were acquired from the head to the proximal thighs in a supine position with the arms positioned above the head. First, transmission images were acquired using a low-dose CT scan from head to proximal thigh without contrast. The CT data were reconstructed using a filtered back-projection algorithm and a 512 × 512 matrix, with a transaxial field of view of 70 cm and slice thickness of 3.75 mm. CT images were used for attenuation correction and anatomical localization. Immediately following the transmission CT acquisition, emission images were acquired with a dedicated full-ring PET tomograph from the proximal thighs to the head over the same field of view as the transmission scan. PET data were reconstructed using an ordered-subset expectation maximization iterative algorithm (20 subsets, 2 iterations).

## Findings and differential diagnosis

Whole-body MIP and three fused PET/CT slices through the upper abdomen (Figure 10.10) demonstrate intense FDG uptake within a gallbladder mass (Figure 10.10D). There is also intense uptake within the adjacent hepatic parenchyma in the region of the gallbladder fossa (Figure 10.10B). A focus

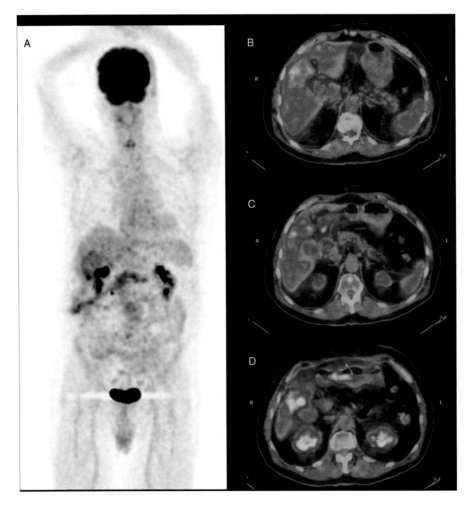

**Figure 10.10** (A) Whole-body MIP image; (B–D) fused FDG-PET/CT slices through the upper abdomen.

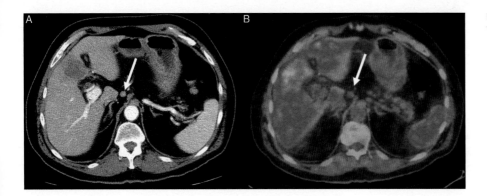

**Figure 10.11** (A) axial contrast CT image; (B) Axial fused FDG-PET/CT through the abdomen.

of intense uptake is seen in the posterior aspect of the proximal portion of the duodenum (Figure 10.10C). A 1.0 cm periportal lymph node shows moderate uptake (Figure 10.10B). Intense uptake anteriorly in the upper mid-abdomen corresponds to suture material at the gastrojejunostomy site (Figure 10.10D).

The findings are consistent with FDG-avid primary gallbladder carcinoma with metastasis to the adjacent hepatic parenchyma and duodenum. The small periportal lymph node is seen on diagnostic CT images, but does not meet size criteria for pathogenicity (Figure 10.11, arrow). Given the PET/CT findings, the lymph node is likely metastatic despite the small size, although this was not histologically confirmed. Differential considerations include increased uptake within an inflammatory lymph node in view of recent surgery. Intense activity at the gastrojejunostomy site is likely due to post-surgical inflammation.

## Diagnosis and clinical follow-up

A biopsy of the liver confirmed well-differentiated adenocarcinoma. Based on the findings on FDG-PET/CT and diagnostic CT, the patient was considered to have stage IV gallbladder carcinoma due to the extent of liver involvement and adjacent organ invasion (duodenum). Due to the advanced stage at presentation, intensive chemotherapy was elected rather than an extensive surgical procedure that would unlikely result in a cure and would be associated with significant morbidity.

## Discussion and teaching points

Unfortunately, as in this case, patients are often asymptomatic early in the course of gallbladder cancer and diagnosis does not often occur until an advanced stage. Presenting symptoms, such as nausea, weight loss, anorexia, and right upper quadrant pain, are non-specific and similar to symptoms of benign gallbladder

pathology. With advanced disease, patients may develop common bile duct obstruction with associated jaundice. In this case, the patient was diagnosed during an attempted cholecystectomy for suspected cholecystitis. Gastrojejunostomy was performed due to duodenal obstruction from tumor invasion.

Risk factors for gallbladder carcinoma include cholelithiasis, obesity, and chronic gallbladder infections (1). The incidence of gallbladder cancer varies widely geographically and is higher in areas with an increased prevalence of gallstones. Historically, porcelain gallbladder was felt to have a strong association with gallbladder carcinoma, although more recent studies suggest the relationship may be weaker than once thought (2, 3).

FDG-PET has been shown to be a useful modality in evaluation of carcinoma of the gallbladder, particularly when ultrasound and/or CT findings are inconclusive (4). Due to the rarity of the disease, FDG-PET/CT has not been evaluated in many large series of patients. In one study of 99 patients with either gallbladder carcinoma or cholangiocarcinoma, FDG-PET/CT did not perform significantly better than CT in diagnosis of the primary tumor. PET/CT did, however, have a significantly higher positive predictive value than CT for diagnosis of regional lymph node metastasis (94.1% for PET/CT and 77.5% for CT). PET/CT also had a significantly higher sensitivity for detection of distant metastases than CT (94.7% for PET/CT and 63.2% for CT) (5).

## Take-home message

- Gallbladder carcinoma is a rare malignancy that often presents at an advanced stage due to lack of symptoms early in the course of the disease.
- FDG-PET/CT can be useful in staging patients with gallbladder carcinoma, particularly in evaluating nodal and distant metastasis.

## References

1. Lazcano-Ponce EC, Miquel JF, Munoz N et al. Epidemiology and molecular pathology of gallbladder cancer. *CA Cancer J Clin* 2001;**51**:349–64.

2. Towfigh S, McFadden DW, Cortina GR et al. Porcelain gallbladder is not associated with gallbladder carcinoma. *Am Surg* 2001;**67**:7–10.

3. Stephen AE, Berger DL. Carcinoma in the porcelain gallbladder: a relationship revisited. *Surgery* 2001;**129**:699–703.

4. Rodriguez-Fernandez A, Gomez-Rio M, Llamas-Elvira JM et al. Positron-emission tomography with fluorine-18-fluoro-2-deoxy-D-glucose for gallbladder cancer diagnosis. *Am J Surg* 2004;**188**:171–5.

5. Lee SW, Kim HJ, Park JH et al. Clinical usefulness of 18F-FDG PET-CT for patients with gallbladder cancer and cholangiocarcinoma. *J Gastroenterol* 2010;**45**:560–6.

A 78-year-old male underwent percutaneous transhepatic cholangiography (PTC) and biopsy of an intrahepatic biliary mass revealing cholangiocarcinoma. At the time of PTC, a drain was placed to relieve biliary obstruction. FDG-PET/CT was requested for initial staging.

## Acquisition and processing parameters

The fasting blood glucose level was 89 mg/dL. FDG (11.2 mCi) was administered intravenously via a right hand IV. The patient voided prior to imaging. Following a 65-min distribution time, PET/CT images were acquired from the head to the proximal thighs in a supine position with the arms positioned above the head. First, transmission images were acquired using a low-dose CT scan from head to proximal thigh without intravenous contrast. The CT data were reconstructed using a filtered back-projection algorithm and a $512 \times 512$ matrix, with a transaxial field of view of 70 cm and a reconstructed slice thickness of 3.75 mm. CT images were used for attenuation correction and anatomical localization. Immediately following the transmission CT acquisition, emission images were acquired with a dedicated full-ring PET tomograph from the proximal thighs to the head over the same field of view as the transmission scan. PET data were reconstructed using an ordered-subset expectation maximization iterative algorithm (20 subsets, 2 iterations).

## Findings and differential diagnosis

Whole-body PET MIP and axial unenhanced CT, PET, and fused PET/CT images through the abdomen (Figure 10.12) show intense uptake corresponding to a 3.9 cm low-density mass in the region of the porta hepatis. A small focus of intense uptake is also seen along the course of an internal/ external biliary drain as it exits the liver and courses near the stomach. No distant FDG-avid metastases are identified.

The intensely FDG-avid porta hepatis mass is most consistent with the patient's known primary cholangiocarcinoma.

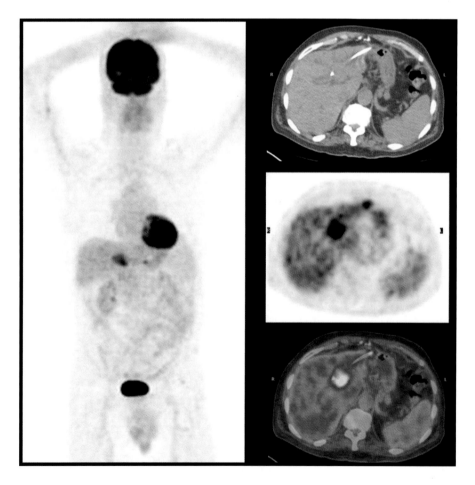

**Figure 10.12** Whole-body FDG-PET MIP and axial unenhanced CT, FDG-PET, and fused FDG-PET/CT images through the abdomen.

The focal activity along the biliary drain is likely due to local inflammatory changes. Malignancy is less likely in this location, but remains a possibility.

## Diagnosis and clinical follow-up

Given the lack of FDG-avid distant metastases on PET/CT, the patient was considered for local resection. Unfortunately, the patient also underwent CT angiography, which revealed encasement of the main hepatic artery and occlusion of the left portal vein, rendering the mass unresectable. The patient was referred to medical oncology for chemotherapy.

## Discussion and teaching points

Cholangiocarcinomas are rare tumors that arise from the biliary tract and account for 10–15% of all hepatic malignancies (1). These tumors develop from epithelial cells in the intrahepatic or extrahepatic bile ducts. Intrahepatic cholangiocarcinomas can be either perihilar or peripheral. Perihilar tumors can be surgically challenging due to potential for extension of tumor along the hepatic ducts as well as the proximity to the major vessels, as seen in this case.

FDG-PET/CT was requested in this case to better define the extent of the primary tumor and to assess for the presence of unsuspected distant metastases. Cholangiocarcinomas are sometimes difficult to evaluate with CT because they may be isodense with the normal liver parenchyma. The location of the tumor can be implied by the point at which intrahepatic ductal dilatation begins or where hepatic atrophy is identified. Cholangiocarcinomas typically demonstrate markedly delayed enhancement on both CT and MRI.

In contrast to HCC, which may have varying degrees of FDG uptake due to variable glucose-6-phosphatase activity,

many cholangiocarcinomas are FDG avid. Not all of the morphological subtypes accumulate FDG, however, and there may be false-negative results because of the diffuse infiltrating pattern of these tumors. The sensitivity of FDG-PET for the detection of cholangiocarcinomas with a nodular morphology is 85%, but only 18% for infiltrating tumors (2). False-negative studies with FDG may also occur with peritoneal carcinomatosis. Increased uptake due to inflammatory changes along a biliary stent may lead to false-positive findings. In this case, focal uptake was seen along the internal/external biliary drain. Cholangitis may also be a source of false-positive findings. There is evidence, however, that FDG-PET can be of value in evaluating patients with sclerosing cholangitis and suspected cholangiocarcinoma (3). Despite the above-mentioned limitations, FDG-PET can have a significant impact on patient care and has been reported to change surgical management in 24–30% of cases due to detection of occult metastases (2, 4).

## Take-home message

- FDG avidity of cholangiocarcinoma varies within different morphological subtypes. FDG accumulates readily in the nodular subtype with a sensitivity of 85%, but sensitivity is only 18% for infiltrating tumors.
- It is essential to be familiar with causes of potential false-positive findings (cholangitis and inflammation due to biliary stents) and of false-negative findings (peritoneal carcinomatosis and infiltrating tumors) to give meaningful interpretations of FDG-PET/CT of cholangiocarcinoma.
- FDG-PET/CT has a significant effect on patient management, primarily due to detection of occult metastases.

## References

1. Aljiffry M, Abdulelah A, Walsh M et al. Evidence-based approach to cholangiocarcinoma: a systematic review of the current literature. *J Am Coll Surg* 2009;**208**:134–47.

2. Anderson CD, Rice MH, Pinson CW et al. Fluorodeoxyglucose PET imaging in the evaluation of gallbladder carcinoma and cholangiocarcinoma. *J Gastrointest Surg* 2004;**8**:90–7.

3. Keiding S, Hansen SB, Rasmussen HH et al. Detection of cholangiocarcinoma in primary sclerosing cholangitis by positron emission tomography. *Hepatology* 1998;**28**:700–6.

4. Corvera CU, Blumgart LH, Akhurst T et al. 18F-fluorodeoxyglucose positron emission tomography influences management decisions in patients with biliary cancer. *J Am Coll Surg* 2008;**206**:57–65.

A 56-year-old male with a large liver mass and α-fetoprotein of greater than 17 000 ng/mL. Biopsy revealed moderately differentiated hepatocellular carcinoma (HCC). He underwent PET/CT with [11]C-acetate (Figure 10.13 right) and FDG (Figure 10.13 left) on the same day.

## Acquisition and processing parameters

[11]C-acetate (34.8 mCi) was administered intravenously via a left antecubital IV. Following a 20-min distribution interval, [11]C-acetate PET/CT images were acquired from the head to the proximal thighs in a supine position with the arms along the sides.

Later that same day, the patient underwent FDG-PET/CT. The fasting blood glucose level was 72 mg/dL. FDG (10.2 mCi) was administered intravenously via a left antecubital IV. The patient voided prior to imaging. Following a 75-min distribution time, FDG-PET/CT images were acquired from the head to the proximal thighs in a supine position with the arms along the sides.

For both FDG and [11]C-acetate PET/CT, transmission images were acquired using a low-dose CT scan from head to proximal thigh without intravenous contrast. The CT data were reconstructed using a filtered back-projection algorithm and a $512 \times 512$ matrix, with a transaxial field of view of 70 cm and a reconstructed slice thickness of 3.75 mm. CT images were used for attenuation correction and anatomical localization. Immediately following the transmission CT acquisition, emission images were acquired with a dedicated full-ring PET tomograph from the proximal thighs to the head over the same field of view as the transmission scan. PET data were reconstructed using an ordered-subset expectation maximization iterative algorithm (20 subsets, 2 iterations).

## Findings and differential diagnosis

The [11]C-acetate images demonstrate physiologic activity in the liver and spleen. There is no significant physiologic uptake in

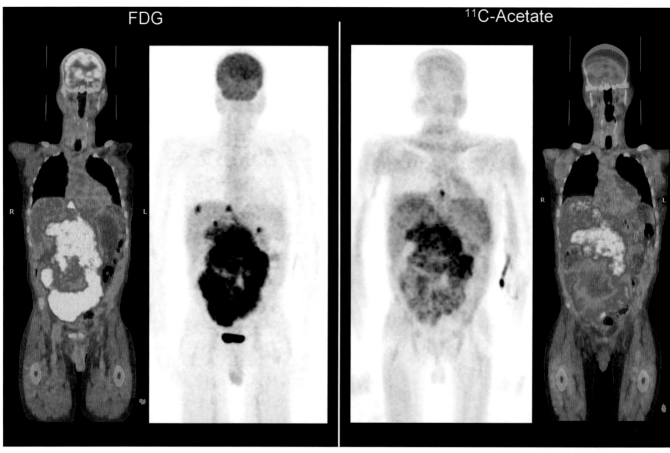

**Figure 10.13** From left to right: coronal fused FDG-PET/CT, FDG-PET, coronal [11]C-acetate-PET, and fused [11]C-acetate-PET/CT.

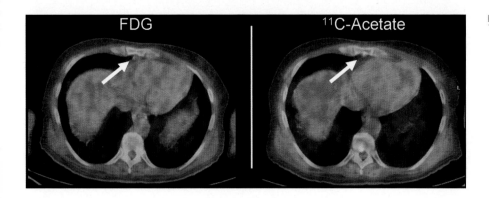

**Figure 10.14** Axial fused FDG-PET/CT, and fused [11]C-acetate-PET/CT.

the pancreas. The FDG images demonstrate physiologic activity in the brain, myocardium, liver, spleen, intestines, and renal collecting system.

On both the FDG and [11]C-acetate images, there is intense uptake within an 18 × 12 cm mass within the left hepatic lobe, which extends inferiorly to the level of the pelvis along the anterior aspect of the abdomen. Central photopenia is noted within the mass. Of note, FDG uptake appears more intense than [11]C-acetate uptake, particularly along the inferior portion of the mass. There are two foci of intense FDG uptake near the dome of the liver, one in subsegment 8 and the other likely in subsegment 4A, which are not [11]C-acetate avid. A 1.0 cm right pericardiophrenic lymph node (Figure 10.14) shows intense [11]C-acetate uptake, but does not demonstrate significant FDG avidity.

The combined FDG and [11]C-acetate PET/CT findings are most consistent with HCC involving a large, partially necrotic mass with satellite metastatic foci in the liver and a pericardiophrenic node. The primary mass and metastatic lesions demonstrate variable degrees of FDG and [11]C-acetate uptake in a complementary fashion.

## Diagnosis and clinical follow-up

Metastatic HCC. Given the size of the mass and the extent of metastasis, he was not eligible for liver transplantation. He was offered medical therapy and died 2 months following the PET/CT.

## Discussion and teaching points

This case demonstrates the complementary role of FDG and [11]C-acetate for evaluation of HCC (1). [11]C-acetate was first used to assess the oxidative metabolism of the myocardium. Among the possible metabolic pathways, participation in free fatty acid (lipid) synthesis is believed to be the dominant method of incorporation into tumors. Radiolabeled acetate accumulates in tissues with high levels of anabolic metabolism, such as the pancreas, although this was not observed in this patient.

FDG accumulation is variable in HCC due to differing amounts of glucose-6-phosphatase present within these tumors. FDG uptake is greater in HCC than in normal hepatic parenchyma in approximately 50–70% of patients. High levels of FDG accumulation have been associated with tumors that are poorly differentiated as well as higher levels of α-fetoprotein. On the other hand, [11]C-acetate tends to show greater accumulation in well-differentiated HCC. As demonstrated in this case, HCCs are heterogeneous tumors, with different portions of tumors being either FDG- or [11]C-acetate-avid, according to their level of differentiation. Metastatic lesions also show different levels of avidity for either FDG or [11]C-acetate, hence the utility of a combined approach for evaluation of HCC with PET/CT (2, 3). As seen in this case, some lesions are detected by both FDG and [11]C-acetate, while others are only detected by one or the other, even in the same patient.

In one study of dual-tracer PET/CT for the evaluation of metastatic HCC, a positive correlation was found between the specific tracer avidity of the primary tumor and metastases within the same patient. Some metastases, however, were seen with only one of the tracers. Clinically significant changes in management were found in patients with true-positive metastasis, of whom 19% were detected by [11]C-acetate alone. Dual-tracer PET/CT was found to be more effective than single tracer PET/CT in identifying patients for curative therapy. Both tracers were found to be complementary and have incremental value compared with either alone. The combined sensitivity for detection of metastatic HCC using both tracers was greater than 95% (4).

## Take-home message

- PET/CT with FDG and [11]C-acetate are complementary in the evaluation of HCC.
- Due to tumor biology, HCC shows variable uptake with FDG and [11]C-acetate. FDG uptake is generally higher in poorly differentiated tumors while [11]C-acetate tends to show higher uptake in well-differentiated tumors.
- Uptake with both tracers can be variable within individual tumors and within separate metastatic lesions in the same patient.

# References

1.  Delbeke D, Pinson CW. 11C-acetate: a new tracer for the evaluation of hepatocellular carcinoma. *J Nucl Med* 2003;**44**:222–3.

2.  Ho CL, Yu SC, Yeung DW. 11C-acetate PET imaging in hepatocellular carcinoma and other liver masses. *J Nucl Med* 2003;**44**:213–21.

3.  Park JW, Kim JH, Kim SK, *et al.* A prospective evaluation of 18F-FDG and 11C-acetate PET/CT for detection of primary and metastatic hepatocellular carcinoma. *J Nucl Med* 2008;**49**:1912–21.

4.  Ho CL, Chen S, Yeung DW, Cheng TK. Dual-tracer PET/CT imaging in evaluation of metastatic hepatocellular carcinoma. *J Nucl Med* 2007;**48**:902–9.

## Chapter 11

# Breast

Muhammad A. Chaudhry and Richard L. Wahl

## Introduction

Breast cancer is the most common type of cancer and is the second leading cause of cancer mortality in women. It was estimated that 207,090 women would be diagnosed with and 39,840 women would die of cancer of the breast in 2010 in the USA. There is a rising incidence of breast cancer; however, on the brighter side, there has been a decline in mortality over the last several years (1). These changes are attributed to both early diagnosis and more effective treatment. Risk factors for breast cancer include age, family history and genetics, a later first pregnancy, and obesity.

Infiltrating or invasive ductal cancer is the most common histological type of breast cancer and comprises 70–80% of all cases. Other types of breast cancer include DCIS (ductal carcinoma in situ), LCIS (lobular carcinoma in situ), and inflammatory and invasive lobular carcinoma. Tumors involving the nipple are classified as Paget's disease (intraductal and invasive ductal).

Initial disease staging is a crucial step in optimizing the management of breast cancer patients. Increasingly, molecular phenotyping of breast cancer is applied to help ascertain whether the cancer is likely to respond to chemotherapy or immunotherapy. A variety of factors influence the choice of treatment options including but not limited to age, menopausal status, local disease status (e.g., size and extent of the mass), axillary nodal disease involvement, hormone receptor status (estrogen/progesterone receptor expression), and Human Epidermal Growth Factor Receptor 2 (HER2/neu) expression.

The status of the axillary lymph nodes remains the single most important prognostic variable in the staging of early breast cancer, although molecular phenotyping provides complementary information. The 10-year survival rate in patients with histologically negative axillary nodes ranges from 65–80% versus 38–63% in those with involvement of 1 to 3 nodes, and 13–27% in those with more than 3 positive axillary nodes. The likelihood of axillary nodal involvement is directly related to the size of the primary tumor at diagnosis (2).

The American Joint Committee (AJCC) criteria for cancer staging are shown in Table 11.1.

Currently, the diagnosis of breast cancer is based on breast self-examination, physical examination by trained personnel, mammography supplemented as necessary by ultrasonography and MRI, and histological examination of identified breast lesions. Breast examination has low specificity and is not very sensitive for detection of small lesions, but is useful for detection of palpable breast masses.

Mammography has a relatively high sensitivity, ranging from 54% to 81% depending on age, breast density, and menopausal status (3). The use of a computer-aided detection system (CAD) with mammography has resulted in an increase in the rate of cancer detection in some studies (4). In randomized clinical trials, screening mammography has resulted in a reduction of breast cancer mortality by about 25–45% in women over the age of 40 (5).

Although mammography has a high sensitivity for detecting breast cancer in fatty breasts, it is of limited value in several situations, such as detection of malignancy in dense breasts or post-surgical breasts (e.g., after breast augmentation, lumpectomy, or breast-conserving therapy for breast cancer), early detection of tumor recurrence after surgery, and monitoring response to therapy (6, 7).

## Treatment

### Surgical

Over the years, surgical management of local disease has evolved from radical mastectomy to more localized excisions supplemented by radiation and/or chemotherapy. At present, nearly one-third of women with breast cancer in the USA are managed by lumpectomy. Breast-conserving surgery followed by radiation therapy has become accepted as an alternative to mastectomy for most patients with ductal carcinoma in situ or early-stage invasive breast cancer.

The use of pre-operative chemotherapy has made it possible to downstage disease to make it more amenable to less

*A Case-Based Approach to PET/CT in Oncology*, ed. Victor H. Gerbaudo. Published by Cambridge University Press.
© Cambridge University Press 2012.

**Table 11.1** American Joint Committee on Cancer (AJCC) breast cancer staging.

| Tumor (T) | | Regional lymph node (N) | | Distant metastases (M) | |
|---|---|---|---|---|---|
| T0 | No primary tumor found | N0 | No regional nodal metastases | M0 | No distant metastases |
| Tis | Carcinoma in situ | N1 | Metastases in mobile ipsilateral axillary lymph nodes | M1 | Distant metastases |
| T1 | Invasive cancer < 2 cm in greatest dimension | N2a | Metastases to fixed ipsilateral axillary lymph nodes | | |
| T1mic | Tumor ≤ 0.1 cm in greatest dimension | N2b | Metastases to ipsilateral internal mammary lymph nodes with an absence of ipsilateral axillary lymph node metastases | | |
| T1a | Tumor > 0.1 cm but ≤ 0.5 cm in greatest dimension | N3 | Metastases in ipsilateral infraclavicular (level III axillary) lymph node(s) with or without level I, II axillary lymph node involvement; or in clinically detected ipsilateral internal mammary lymph node(s) with clinically evident level I, II axillary lymph node metastases; or metastases in ipsilateral supraclavicular lymph node(s) with or without axillary or internal mammary lymph node involvement | | |
| T1b | Tumor > 0.5 cm but ≤ 1 cm in greatest dimension | N3a | Metastases in ipsilateral infraclavicular lymph node(s) | | |
| T1c | Tumor > 1 cm but ≤ 2 cm in greatest dimension | N3b | Metastases in ipsilateral internal mammary lymph node(s) and axillary lymph node(s) | | |
| T2 | Tumor > 2 cm but ≤ 5 cm in greatest dimension | N3c | Metastases in ipsilateral supraclavicular lymph node(s | | |
| T3 | Tumor > 5 cm in greatest dimension | | | | |
| T4 | Tumor of any size with direct extension to chest wall or skin | | | | |

radical surgical management. Sentinel node imaging and/or mapping have allowed surgeons to avoid standard axillary lymph node dissection and its associated complications in women with local or early-stage breast carcinoma (8).

## Radiation therapy

Radiation therapy is an essential tool in the management of women with breast carcinoma. It is an important part of breast-conserving therapy in early-stage invasive disease. It has been shown that women with DCIS who received post-operative radiation therapy following a wide surgical excision had a lower recurrence rate in the ipsilateral breast along with a significantly reduced risk of invasive recurrence (9). This trend persisted in a follow-up report by the same group (10). Women who present with an advanced stage of disease have a

higher risk of recurrence. Radiation therapy has shown promising results in women receiving radiation following mastectomy and receiving radiation following neoadjuvant chemotherapy. It also plays a role in alleviating symptoms of metastatic disease, especially when it involves bony structures.

## Hormonal therapy

Hormonal therapies are directed at either reducing the synthesis of estrogen or blocking estrogen receptors in hormone-dependent tumors. Women with a positive estrogen-receptor to progesterone-receptor ratio (ER/PR) have a significantly higher response rate of approximately 50% compared with 10% in women with absence of ER/PR receptors. A number of therapies are used as palliative treatment for patients with hormone-sensitive metastatic disease and as adjuvant

**Table 11.2** Diagnostic performance of FDG-PET in suspicious breast lesions.

| Authors | PET or PET/CT | N | Lesions | Sensitivity | Specificity | PPV | NPV | Accuracy |
|---------|--------------|-----|---------|-------------|-------------|-------|-------|----------|
| Walter et al. (34) | PET | 40 | 42 | 63 | 74 | na | na | na |
| Avril et al. (35) | PET | 144 | 185 | 64–80 | 76–94 | 89–87 | 52–61 | 73–79 |
| Adler et al. (36) | PET | 28 | 35 | 96 | 100 | 100 | 89 | 97 |
| Avril et al. (37) | PET | 51 | 72 | 83 | 84 | 87 | 79 | 83 |
| Scheidhauer et al. (38) | PET | 30 | 30 | 91 | 86 | 95 | 75 | 90 |
| Dehdashti et al. (39) | PET | 32 | 32 | 88 | 100 | 100 | 73 | 91 |
| Palmedo et al. (40) | PET | 20 | 22 | 92 | 86 | 92 | 67 | 82 |
| Nitzsche et al. (41) | PET | 37 | 20 | 94 | 100 | 100 | 80 | 95 |
| Schirrmeister et al. (22) | PET | 117 | 117 | 93 | 75 | 92 | 78 | 89 |
| Heinisch et al. (42) | PET | 36 | 40 | 68 | 73 | 81 | 58 | 70 |
| Hoh et al. (20) | PET | 17 | 17 | 88 | | | | |
| Yutani et al. (52) | PET | 38 | 38 | 79 | | | | |
| Wahl et al. (44) | PET | 10 | 10 | 100 | | | | |

treatment for hormone-sensitive early breast cancer. Hormonal therapies have been shown to decrease the risk of breast cancer in patients at high risk for breast cancer (9, 11). Aromatase inhibitors which diminish intracellular estrogen production are playing a growing role in breast cancer therapy in addition to estrogen-receptor blocking agents.

## Immunotherapy

Expression of HER2/neu is associated with an increased risk of relapse. It is expressed in approximately 30% of all breast cancers. Studies have demonstrated that treatment with humanized monoclonal antibody against HER2/neu can reduce the risk of recurrence by 50% when given either following completion of adjuvant chemotherapy or concurrently and after taxane therapy in women with HER2/neu positive disease (12, 13). Recently, antibody-only therapy has shown efficacy in advanced breast cancer in a limited subset of patients.

## Chemotherapy

Different chemotherapy regimens are in use in neoadjuvant and adjuvant settings. The use of systemic therapy after local management of breast cancer substantially improves survival. In terms of patient survival, anthracycline-containing regimens are superior to those not containing anthracyclines, and regimens containing both an anthracycline and a taxane are superior to regimens containing an anthracycline alone (14).

## Role of FDG-PET and PET/CT

## Diagnosis

FDG uptake is considerably higher in malignant tumors than in normal tissues. Several studies have demonstrated that

FDG-PET has high sensitivity (64–96%) and specificity (80–100%) for detection of primary breast cancer and for differentiating breast cancer from benign lesions. The accuracy of PET for primary diagnosis is variable depending on lesion size. Small primary tumors can fail to be detected, while larger tumors are detected quite consistently with whole-body PET imaging. The use of whole-body PET to exclude cancer in subcentimeter breast cancers is not recommended. By contrast, dedicated high-resolution positron emission mammography systems can detect smaller primary lesions, but are not yet widely deployed.

False-positive results have been reported in infectious and inflammatory lesions, including hemorrhagic inflammation after biopsy or surgery, due to accumulation of FDG in inflammatory cells (15). However, these conditions often can be easily recognized clinically. Table 11.2 summarizes the results of studies done over the years evaluating FDG-PET in suspicious breast lesions. Limited studies have been done evaluating the role of FDG-PET/CT in suspicious breast lesions (16). Table 11.3 summarizes results of a few studies done to evaluate comparative performance of FDG-PET versus MRI in diagnosis, staging, and restaging of primary breast lesions. In general, MRI is a more sensitive technique, but PET is more specific for breast cancer.

## Initial staging
## Locoregional staging

Axillary nodal disease involvement remains a significant adverse prognostic marker in the management of breast cancer. Over the years, studies have reported sensitivities ranging from 20% to 100% and specificities from 65% to 100%. Wahl et al. analyzed the performance of FDG-PET in

**Table 11.3** Diagnostic performance of FDG-PET and PET/CT in comparison with MRI.

| Authors | Number of patients (no. of lesions) | FDG-PET or PET/CT | Staging/ Restaging | Sensitivity | Specificity | MRI | Sensitivity | Specificity |
|---|---|---|---|---|---|---|---|---|
| Walter et al. (34) | 40 (42) | PET | Staging | 63 | 74 | MRI | 89 | 91 |
| Igaaru et al. (45) | 21 | PET/CT | Staging | 75 | 92.3 | MRI | 85.7 | 85.7 |
| Goerres et al. (46) | 32 | PET | Restaging | 79 | 94 | MRI | 100 | 72 |
| Heinisch et al. (47) | 36 (40) | PET | Diagnosis | 68 | 73.3 | MRI | 92 | 73.3 |
| Heusner et al. (23) | 40 | PET/CT | Diagnosis | 95 | 79 | MRI | 100 | 73 |

**Table 11.4** Diagnostic performance of FDG-PET/CT in axillary nodal disease assessment.

| Authors | Number of patients | Follow-up | Sensitivity | Specificity | Accuracy |
|---|---|---|---|---|---|
| Chae et al. (26) | 108 | Histopathology | 48.5 | 84 | 73.2 |
| Taira et al. (48) | 90 (92 axillae) | Histopathology | 48 | 92 | 79 |
| Monzawa et al. (49) | 50 | Histopathology | 20 | 97 | 74 |
| Heusner et al. (50) | 61 | Histopathology | 58 | 92 | 79 |
| Fuster et al. (51) | 52 | Histopathology and/or 1 year follow-up | 70 | 100 | 89 |
| Ueda et al. (52) | 183 (visual assessment) | Histopathology | 58 | 95 | 83 |
| Yutani et al. (43) | 38 | Histopathology | 50 | | |
| Wahl et al. (44) | 9 | Histopathology | 89 | | |
| Wahl et al. (17) | 360 | Histopathology | 61 | 80 | |
| Utech et al. (53) | 124 | Histopathology | 100 | 75 | 84 |

over 300 patients presenting with newly diagnosed breast cancer. The PET results were compared with those of pathologic analysis of axillary lymph nodes. Overall, FDG-PET was 61% sensitive and 80% specific for detecting axillary metastases, with a positive predictive value of 62% and a negative predictive value of 79%; receiver operating characteristic curve analysis showed that FDG-PET had high specificity for nodal disease when a standardized uptake with a threshold value of 1.8 was used, though with lower sensitivity of only 25%. The authors concluded that "FDG PET should not be routinely recommended for axillary staging" in women with breast cancer (17). Similarly, other studies have shown a moderate sensitivity for assessment of axillary nodal disease and FDG-PET/CT does not replace the current standard practice of sentinel node mapping followed by biopsy. Table 11.4 summarizes results of studies evaluating the performance of FDG-PET in axillary nodal disease assessment.

In untreated primary breast cancer, FDG uptake has been correlated with known prognostic factors by several investigators. The prognostic information provided by FDG-PET may offer insight about the expected behavior of the tumor and guide the aggressiveness of the therapy. Strong positive correlations were found between FDG uptake (SUV) and several tumor characteristics, including histologic grade, cell proliferation indices, histologic type (with greater uptake in ductal cancers by comparison with lobular cancers), microvessel density, and the number of tumor cells in a given volume (18, 19).

Currently, conventional or limited axillary nodal dissection, guided by lymphatic mapping using the sentinel lymph node technique, represents the standard of care in patients with invasive breast cancer. False-negative results with PET occur chiefly in patients with small tumor deposits (typically < 1 cm).

Based on the current data, a positive FDG-PET may alleviate the need for a complete axillary nodal dissection, or may eliminate the need for a sentinel node procedure, because of its high specificity; however, a negative FDG-PET does not preclude axillary nodal sampling or dissection given the high false-negative rate. In addition to detection of axillary nodal involvement, FDG-PET has the potential to detect involvement of other nodal groups, including the internal mammary and supraclavicular nodes. Involvement of the internal mammary nodes in the absence of axillary nodal involvement is uncommon (approximately 10%) and the prognosis of such patients does not differ significantly from that of patients with metastases only to the axillary nodes (2). However, a poorer prognosis has been reported when both axillary and internal mammary nodal groups are involved.

## Systemic staging

Breast cancer can metastasize to many organs, including bone, liver, lung, and brain. Whole-body PET and PET/CT imaging plays a major role in documenting the systemic extent of malignant disease as it can detect not only the primary tumor and nodal metastases, but also skeletal and visceral metastases in a single study.

Several clinical studies have shown that FDG-PET is more sensitive than other currently utilized non-invasive techniques for demonstrating the true extent of metastatic disease and will quite often reveal unsuspected metastatic disease (20–23). A recent study by Heusner et al. compared the diagnostic value of diffusion-weighted MRI (DWI-MRI) to FDG-PET/CT for staging breast cancer. DWI-MRI showed a significantly higher false-positive rate of 82% compared with 11% for PET/CT (24). In a study by Mahner et al. FDG-PET was found to be superior to conventional imaging procedures (CT, chest radiography, abdominal ultrasound, bone scintigraphy) in detecting distant metastases (25).

FDG-PET is more sensitive to detect osteolytic metastatic disease compared with osteoblastic disease as shown by Cook et al. in 23 patients with documented osseous metastatic breast cancer (26). FDG-PET detected more osteolytic lesions than bone scintigraphy (mean of 14.1 vs. 7.8 lesions) compared with osteoblastic lesions where FDG-PET detected significantly fewer lesions than bone scintigraphy ($P < 0.05$) (22). [18]F-sodium fluoride (NaF)-PET may add sensitivity to the detection of osteoblastic metastases.

## Restaging

Locoregional recurrence occurs in 7–30% of patients with breast cancer. Clinical detection of locoregional recurrence is limited as post-therapy changes may present with signs and symptoms similar to those of locoregional recurrence. Anatomical imaging may not be able to reliably distinguish post-therapy changes from recurrent disease in patients with a prior history of surgical and/or radiation treatment.

Studies have shown that FDG-PET is a useful adjunct to conventional imaging techniques in evaluating patients with suspected locoregional or distant recurrent disease (27, 28). Bender et al. studied 75 patients with suspected recurrent breast cancer and demonstrated that FDG-PET is a useful adjunct to MRI and/or CT in the detection of recurrent disease involving lymph nodes and visceral organs (28). For lymph node involvement, the sensitivity and specificity were 97% and 91%, respectively for FDG-PET and 74% and 95%, respectively for CT/MRI. For detection of recurrent disease in visceral organs, the sensitivity was 96% for FDG-PET and 57% for CT and/or MRI. Overall sensitivity, specificity, accuracy, positive- and negative-predictive values of FDG-PET were 81%, 100%, 87%, 100%, and 50%, respectively.

## Response to treatment

Early and prompt evaluation of the response to treatment is crucial in management of breast cancer patients in order to avoid futile, expensive therapies and related comorbidity. Changes in metabolism precede changes in size and FDG-PET has the ability to monitor glucose metabolism in tumors. In a prospective study, Wahl et al. demonstrated an early and significant decrease in tumor glucose metabolism (both semiquantitatively and quantitatively) 8 days after institution of effective chemohormonotherapy in 8 patients with locally advanced breast carcinoma; the reduction in tumor metabolism antedated changes in tumor size (29). No significant decline in tumor FDG uptake was noted in three non-responders.

In another study to assess the value of FDG-PET in predicting response to therapy, Schelling et al. studied 22 patients undergoing chemotherapy for locally advanced breast cancer and showed that after the first course of therapy, all responders (defined as pathologic complete response or minimal residual disease) were identified using a decline in tumor SUV to a level below 55% of baseline [100% (3/3) sensitivity and 85% (11/13) specificity]. After the second course of therapy using the same threshold, all but one of the responders was identified [91% (5/6) sensitivity and 94% (15/16) specificity]. Similar results have been reported by others in patients with advanced breast cancer (30).

Assessment of response to therapy in osseous metastatic disease is difficult with conventional imaging, bone scintigraphy, plain radiography, CT, or MRI, as changes indicative of response to therapy occur slowly. In addition, the issue of scintigraphic "flare reaction" that often occurs early in the course of therapy on bone scans may mistakenly lead to discontinuation of therapy. Stafford et al. have used serial FDG-PET in patients with breast cancer being treated for osseous metastatic disease (31). The investigators found that changes in FDG uptake with therapy correlate well with the overall clinical assessment of response. The percentage change in FDG uptake with therapy showed a strong correlation with the percentage change in the values of tumor marker.

## Positron emission mammography (PEM)

More recently, dedicated positron emission mammography (PEM) units have been developed to overcome the limitations of whole-body PET imaging system in detecting smaller lesions. Preliminary data have suggested that PEM has high diagnostic accuracy and has higher specificity compared with MRI, which potentially could lead to fewer false-positive findings for PEM (32). Similarly, in a recent study by Schilling et al., PEM and MRI showed similar sensitivity of 92.8% (33). PEM is a promising technological advancement and will help to overcome the limitations of whole-body PET imaging.

# References

1. American Cancer Society. Breast Cancer Facts & Figures 2009–2010. [www.cancer.org]

2. Hellman S, Harris JR. Natural history of breast cancer. In JR Harris, ME Lippman, M Marrow, CK Osborne (Eds.), *Diseases of the Breast.* 2nd edn. Philadelphia: Lippincott Williams and Wilkins, 2000, pp. 407–23.

3. Whitman GJ. The role of mammography in breast cancer prevention. *Curr Opin Oncol* 1999;**11**:414–18.

4. Dean JC, Ilvento CC. Improved cancer detection using computer-aided detection with diagnostic and screening mammography: prospective study of 104 cancers. *Am J Roentgenol* 2006;**187**:20–8.

5. Feig SA. Role and evaluation of mammography and other imaging methods for breast cancer detection, diagnosis, and staging. *Semin Nucl Med* 1999;**29**:3–15.

6. Sickles EA. Mammographic features of early breast cancer. *Am J Roentgenol* 1984;**143**:461–4.

7. Moskowitz M. The predictive value of certain mammographic signs in screening for breast cancer. *Cancer* 1983;**51**:1007–11.

8. Waljee DF, Newman LA. Neoadjuvant systemic therapy and the surgical managnent of breast cancer. *Surg Clin N Am* 2007;**87**(20):399–415.

9. Fisher B, Dignam K, Wolmark N *et al.* Lumpectomy and radiation therapy for the treatment of intraductal breast cancer: findings from national surgical adjuvant breast and bowel project B-17. *J Clin Oncol* 1998;**16**:441–52.

10. Fisher B, Anderson S, Brynat J *et al.* Twenty-year follow-up of a randomized trial comparing total mastectomy, lumpectomy, and lumpectomy plus irradiation for the treatment of invasive breast cancer. *N Engl J Med* 2002; **347**(16):1233–41.

11. Pindar MC, Buzdar AU. Endocrine therapy for breast cancer. In RS Freedman, AU Buzdar (Series Eds.), *Breast Cancer*, 2nd edn. *MD Anderson Cancer Care Series*. Houston, TX: MD Anderson Cancer Care Center, 2008, pp. 411–34.

12. Slamon DJ, Godolphin W, Jones LA *et al.* Studies of HER2/neu proto-oncogene in human breast and ovarian cancer. *Science* 1989;**12**(244):707–12.

13. Slamon DJ, Eirmann NR, Pienkowski MM *et al.* Phase III Randomized trial comparing doxorubicin and cyclophosphamide followed by docetaxel (AC-> T) with doxorubicin and cyclophosphamide followed by docetaxel and trastuzumab (AC-> TH) with docetaxel, carboplatin and trastuzumab (TCH) in HER2 positive early breast cancer patients: BCIRG 006 study [abstract 1]. *Breast Cancer Res Treat* 2005;**94**:S5.

14. Buzdar AU, Singletary SE, Valero V *et al.* Evaluation of paclitaxel in adjuvant chemotherapy for patients with operable breast cancer: preliminary data of a prospective randomized trial. *Clin Cancer Res* 2002;**8**(5):1073–9.

15. Bakheet SM, Powe J, Kandil A *et al.* F-18 FDG uptake in breast infection and inflammation. *Clin Nucl Med* 2000;**25**:100–3.

16. Tatsumi M, Cohade C, Mourtzikos KA, Fishman EK, Wahl RL. Initial experience with FDG-PET/CT in the evaluation of breast cancer. *Eur J Nucl Med Mol Imaging* 2006;**33**(3):254–62.

17. Wahl RL, Siegel BA, Coleman RE *et al.* PET Study Group. Prospective multicenter study of axillary nodal staging by positron emission tomography in breast cancer: a report of the Staging Breast Cancer with PET Study Group. *J Clin Oncol* 2004;**22** (2):277–85.

18. Bos R, van Der Hoeven JJ, van Der Wall E *et al.* Biologic correlates of (18) fluorodeoxyglucose uptake in human breast cancer measured by positron emission tomography. *J Clin Oncol* 2002;**20**:379–87.

19. Crippa F, Seregni E, Agresti R *et al.* Association between [18F] fluorodeoxyglucose uptake and postoperative histopathology, hormone receptor status, thymidine labelling index and p53 in primary breast cancer: a preliminary observation. *Eur J Nucl Med* 1998;**25**:1429–1434.

20. Hoh CK, Hawkins RA, Glaspy JA *et al.* Cancer detection with whole-body PET using 2-[18F]fluoro-2-deoxy-D-glucose. *J Comput Assist Tomogr* 1993;**17**:582–9.

21. Cook GJ, Houston S, Rubens R, Maisey MN, Fogelman I. Detection of bone metastases in breast cancer by 18FDG PET: differing metabolic activity in osteoblastic and osteolytic lesions. *J Clin Oncol* 1998;**16**:3375–9.

22. Schirrmeister H, Kuhn T, Guhlmann A *et al.* Fluorin-18 2-deoxy-2-fluoror-D-glucose PET in the preoperative staging of breast cancer: comparison with the standard staging procedure. *Eur J Nucl Med* 2001;**28**(3):351–8.

23. Heusner TA, Kuemmel S, Umutlu L *et al.* Breast cancer staging in a single session: whole-body PET/CT mammography. *J Nucl Med* 2008;**49** (8):1215–22.

24. Heusner, Kuemmel S, Koeninger A *et al.* Diagnostic value of diffusion-weighted magnetic resonance imaging (DWI) compared to FDG PET/CT for whole-body breast cancer staging. *Eur J Nucl Med Mol Imaging* 2010;**37** (6):1077–86.

25. Mahner S, Schirrmacher S, Brenner W *et al.* Comparison between positron emission tomography using 2-[fluorine-18]fluoro-2-deoxy-D-glucose, conventional imaging and computed tomography for staging of breast cancer. *Ann Oncol* 2008;**19**(7): 1249–54.

26. Chae BJ, Bae JS, Kang BJ *et al.* Positron emission tomography-computed tomography in the detection of axillary lymph node metastasis in patients with early breast cancer. *Jpn J Clin Oncol* 2009;**39**(5):284–9.

27. Moon DH, Maddahi J, Silerman DH *et al.* Accuracy of whole body fluorine-18-FDG PET for the detection of recurrent or metastatic breast carcinoma. *J Nucl Med* 1998;**39**(3): 431–5.

28. Bender H, Kirst J, Palmedo H *et al.* Value of 18fluoro-deoxyglucose positron emission tomography in the staging of recurrent breast carcinoma. *Anticancer Res* 1997;**17**:1687–92.

29. Wahl RL, Zasadny K, Helvie M *et al.* Metabolic monitoring of breast cancer chemohormonotherapy using positron emission tomography: initial evaluation. *J Clin Oncol* 1993;**11**: 2101–11.

30. Schelling M, Avril N, Nahrig J *et al.* Positron emission tomography using [(18)F]Fluorodeoxyglucose for monitoring primary chemotherapy in breast cancer. *J Clin Oncol* 2000;**18**:1689–95.

31. Stafford SE, Gralow JR, Schubert EK *et al.* Use of serial FDG PET to measure the response of bone-dominant breast cancer to therapy. *Acad Radiol* 2002;**9**:913–21.

32. Berg WA, Madsen KS, Schilling K *et al.* Breast cancer: comparative effectiveness of positron emission mammography and MR imaging in presurgical planning for the ipsilateral breast. *Radiology* 2011;**258**(1):59–72.

33. Schilling K, Narayanan D, Kalinyak JE *et al.* Positron emission mammography in breast cancer presurgical planning: comparison with magnetic resonance imaging. *Eur J Nucl Med Mol Imaging* 2011;**38**(1):23–36.

33. Taira N, Ohsumi S, Takabatake D *et al.* Determination of indication for sentinel lymph node biopsy in clinical node-negative breast cancer using preoperative 18F-FDG positron emission tomography/computed tomography fusion imaging. *Jpn J Clin Oncol* 2009;**39**(1):16–21.

34. Walter C, Scheidhauer K, Scharl A *et al.* Clinical and diagnostic value of preoperative MRI mammography and FDG-PET in suspicious breast lesions. *Eur J Radiol* 2003;**13**(7):1651–6.

35. Avril N, Rosé CA, Schelling M *et al.* Breast imaging with poriston emission tomography and fluorine-18 fluorodeoxyglucose: use and limitations. *J Clin Oncol* 2000;**18**(20):3495.

36. Adler LP, Crowe JP, al-Kaisi NK, Sunshine JL. Evaluation of breast masses and axillary lymph nodes with [F-18] 2-deoxy-2-fluoro-D-glucose PET. *Radiology* 1993;**187**:743–50.

37. Avril N, Dose J, Janicke F *et al.* Metabolic characterization of breast tumors with positron emission tomography using F-18 fluorodeoxyglucose. *J Clin Oncol* 1996;**14**:1848–57.

38. Scheidhauer K, Scharl A, Pietrzyk U *et al.* Qualitative 18F-FDG positron emission tomography in primary breast cancer; clinical relevance and practicability. *Eur J Nucl Med* 1996;**23**(6):618–23.

39. Dehdashti F, Mortimer JE, Siegel BA *et al.* Positron tomographic assessment of estrogen receptors in breast cancer: comparison with FDG-PET and in vitro receptor assays. *J Nucl Med* 1995;**36**(10):1766–74.

40. Palmedo H, Bender H, Grünwald F *et al.* Comparison of fluorine-18fluorodeoxyglucose positron emission tomography and technetium-99m methoxyisobutylisonitrile scintimammography in the detection of breast tumours. *Eur J Nucl Med.* 1997;**24**(9):1138–45.

41. Nitzsche EU, Hoh CK, Dalbohm NM *et al.* Whole body positron emission tomography in breast cancer. *Rofo Fortschr Geb Rontgenstr* 1993;**158**(4):293–8.

42. Heinisch M, Gallowitsch HJ, Mikosch P *et al.* Comparison of FDG-PET and dynamic contrast enhanced MRI in the evaluation of suggestive of breast lesions. *Breast* 2003;**12**(1):17–22.

43. Yutani K, Shiba E, Kusuoka H *et al.* Comparison of FDG-PET with MIBI_SPECT in the detection of breast cancer and axillary lymph node metastasis. *J Comput Assist Tomogr* 2000;**24**(2):274–80.

44. Wahl RL, Cody RL, Hutchins GD, Mudgett EE. Primary and metastatic breast carcinoma: initial clinical evaluation with PET with the radiolabeled glucose analogue 2-[F-18]-fluoro-2-deoxy-D-glucose. *Radiology* 1991;**179**:765–70.

45. Iagaru A, Masamed R, Keesara S *et al.* Breast MRI and 18F-FDG PET/CT in the management of breast cancer. *Ann Nucl Med* 2007;**21**(1):33–8.

46. Goerres GW, Michel SC, Fehr MK *et al.* Follow-up of women with breast cancer: comparison between MRI and FDG-PET. *Eur Radiol* 2003;**13**(7):1635–44.

47. Heinisch M, Gallowitsch HJ, Mikosch P *et al.* Comparison of FDG-PET and dynamic contrast enhanced RM in the evaluation of suggestive of breast lesions. *Breast* 2003;**12**(1):17–22.

49. Monzawa S, Adachi S, Suzuki K *et al.* Diagnostic performance of fluorodeoxyglucose-positron emission tomography/computer tomography of breast cancer in detecting axillary lymph node metastasis: comparison with ultrasonography and contrast-enhanced CT. *Ann Nucl Med* 2009;**23**(10):855–61.

50. Heusner TA, Kuemmel S, Hahn S *et al.* Diagnostic value of full-dose FDG PET/CT for axillary lymph node staging in breast cancer patients. *Eur J Nucl Med Mol Imaging* 2009;**36**(10):1543–50.

51. Fuster D, Duch J, Paredes P *et al.* Preoperative staging of large primary breast cancer with 18F-Fluorodeoxyglucose positron emission/computed tomography compared with conventional procedures. *J Clin Oncol* 2008;**26**(29);4746–51.

52. Ueda, Tsuda H, Asakawa H *et al.* Utility of 18F-Fluoro-deoxyglucose emission tomography/computed tomography fusion imaging (18F-FDG PET/CT) in combination with ultrasonography for axillary staging in primary breast cancer. *BMC Cancer* 2008;**8**:165

53. Utech CI, Young CS, Winter PF. Prospective evaluation of FDG-PET in breast cancer for staging of the axilla related to surgery and immunocytochemistry. *Eur J Nucl Med* 1996;**23**(12):1588–93.

# Diagnosis

A 39-year-old female presented with a palpable left breast mass. An initial mammogram showed a 2 cm mass in the left inner breast. An additional suspicious mass with microcalcifications was seen in the upper central right breast. Subsequent MRI showed a 2.5 cm spiculated mass in the 9 o'clock position of the left breast, and a 1.3 cm suspicious mass in the 12 o'clock position of the right breast. A Breast Imaging Reporting and Data System (BIRADS) category 5 (highly suggestive of malignancy) was assigned to both breasts.

## Acquisition and processing parameters

At our institution the PET imaging protocol requires that the plasma glucose level be lower than 200 mg/dL and that the patient should be fasted for at least 4 hours prior to the administered dose of 8.1 MBq of FDG per kilogram. In this case the time from injection to initiation of imaging was 60 min. Images were acquired on a GE DVCT LySO-crystal 64-slice scanner. Immediately before the start of scanning, the patient was given the opportunity to void. The CT study occurred immediately before the PET study and involved data acquisition under shallow-breathing conditions. CT parameters were as follows: 140 kVP, 20–200 mA (modulated), pitch 0.984 : 1, rotation time 0.5 s. Images were reconstructed with filtered back projection. Whole-body PET data acquisition started at a level just below the pelvis and ended at the skull base. PET parameters were as follows: acquisition mode 3-D, 255 s scan time/bed position, with a bed position overlap of 11 slices. Images were reconstructed with an ordered-subsets expectation maximization (OSEM) algorithm using the following parameters: 2 iterations, 21 subsets, a 3.0-mm post-reconstruction Gaussian filter, and 4.7-mm pixels.

## Findings and differential diagnosis

Coronal whole-body FDG-PET/CT images (Figure 11.1A) demonstrate a focus of intense FDG uptake fusing to a left medial breast mass at approximately the 9 o'clock position. The mass measured 22 × 13 mm and has a SUV lbm (lean body mass) max of 6.2. Multiple left axillary nodes are seen with the largest measuring approximately 13 × 10 mm with an SUV lbm max of 3.2, highly suspicious for nodal metastases (shown on transverse images, Figures 11.1D1, 11.1D2).

Axial (Figure 11.1B) images show no definite evidence of FDG uptake in the right breast parenchyma especially in the region of the suspicious abnormality observed on the MRI. This is suggestive of a less aggressive histology and/or benign etiology (Figures 11.1A, 11.1B).

Mild to moderate FDG uptake is seen in the lower cervical, bilateral supraclavicular and superior axillae, corresponding to adipose tissue on CT images (Figures 11.1C, 11.1D). This represents physiological FDG uptake in activated brown adipose tissue.

## Diagnosis and clinical follow-up

Fine needle aspiration of the left breast mass showed moderately differentiated infiltrating ductal carcinoma. Immunohistochemical analysis showed the presence of estrogen and progesterone receptors (ER+/PR+) with a proliferation index (Ki 67) of 10%. The HER2/neu ratio was negative. Fine needle aspiration (FNA) of a left axillary lymph node revealed metastatic adenocarcinoma (not shown). Core biopsy of the right breast mass proved to be a fibroadenoma.

## Discussion and teaching points

FDG-PET/CT can be a useful adjunct to conventional imaging to assess the presence of disease. FDG uptake reflects glucose metabolism by tumors and the level of uptake may to some extent correspond with the aggressiveness of the disease. Prior to treatment, FDG-PET/CT plays a complementary role to conventional anatomical imaging. It helps differentiate between benign and malignant etiologies, helps direct biopsies and to assess overall tumor burden. In this case, the fibroadenoma did not have significant FDG uptake, but in some fibroadenoma uptake can be substantial.

In younger patients, care should be taken when evaluating FDG uptake. Physiological radiotracer uptake in brown adipose tissue is relatively common. This may complicate assessment of nodal disease. Correlation with anatomical imaging (e.g., CT) should be made to corroborate the presence of nodal disease. Different maneuvers including pharmacological methods have been applied to overcome this potential pitfall.

## Take-home message

- FDG-PET/CT can be used as an adjunct to conventional anatomical imaging to help distinguish between benign and malignant breast lesions if lesion size is sufficiently large. However, it is not a substitute for biopsy. The intense FDG uptake in an enlarged axillary node is consistent with axillary metastases and suggests proceeding directly to surgery as opposed to sentinel node biopsy to be an appropriate strategy.

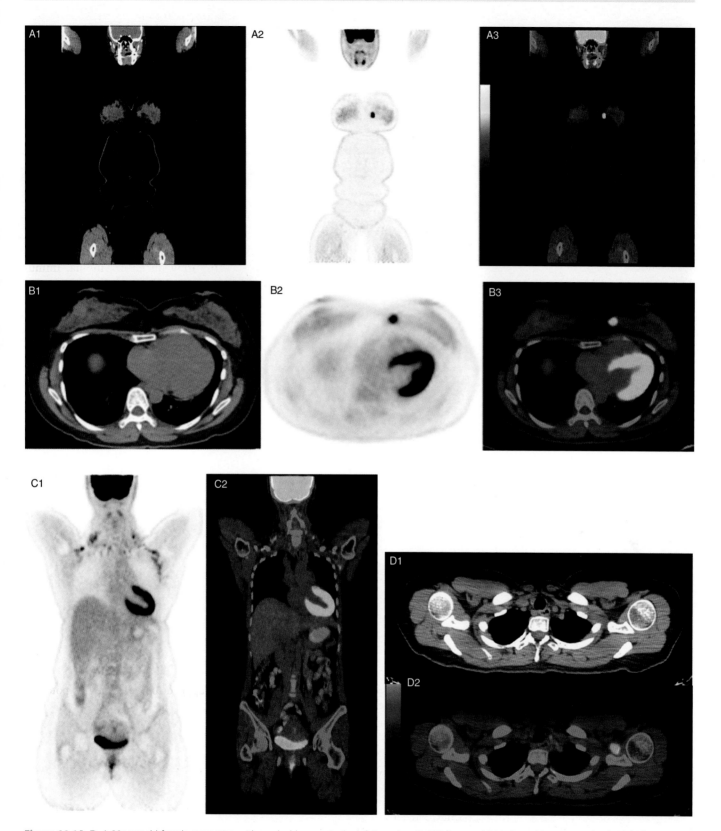

**Figure 11.1A–D** A 39-year-old female presenting with a palpable mass in the left inner breast. MRI shows additional suspicious masses in the right breast. Coronal images (A) show a focus of FDG uptake in the left inner breast. There is no evidence of abnormal FDG uptake in the right breast. Mild diffuse FDG uptake is seen in the right breast parenchyma. This is physiological in a pre-menopausal female. (B) Axial images show an intensely FDG-avid mass in the left inner breast. There is no evidence of abnormal FDG uptake in the right breast. (C, D) Coronal and axial images show mild to moderate FDG uptake bilaterally in the lower neck, supraclavicular fossae, upper mediastinum, and superior axillae. These correspond to adipose tissue on the CT images (C2, D2).

# References

1. Brown RS, Wahl RL. Overexpression of Glut-1 glucose transporter in human breast cancer. An immunohistochemical study. *Cancer* 1993;**72**(10):2979–85.

2. Scheidhauer K, Walter C, Seemann MD. FDG PET and other imaging modalities in the primary diagnosis of suspicious breast lesions. *Eur J Nucl Med Mol Imaging* 2004;**31**(Suppl 1): S70–9.

3. Cochade C, Osman M, Pannu HK, Wahl RL. Uptake in supraclavicular area ("USA-Fat");description on 18F-FDG PET/CT. *J Nucl Med* 2003; **44**(2):170–6.

4. Aukema TS, Vogel WV, Heofnagel CA *et al.* Prevention of brown adipose tissue activation in 18F-FDG PET/CT of breast cancer patients receiving neoadjuvant systemic therapy. *J Nucl Med Technol* 2010; **38**(1):24–7.

46-year-old female with a newly diagnosed right breast infiltrating poorly differentiated ductal carcinoma.

## Acquisition and processing parameters

After a 4-hour fast and serum glucose measurement, the patient received 8.1 MBq of FDG per kilogram. Her blood glucose was 103 mg/dL prior to FDG administration. Time from injection to initiation of images was 62 min. Images were acquired on a GE Discovery LS BGO 4-slice scanner. Immediately before the start of scanning, patients were given the opportunity to void. The CT study occurred immediately before the PET study and involved data acquisition under shallow-breathing conditions. CT parameters were as follows: 140 kVP, 20–200 mA (modulated), pitch 1.5, rotation time 0.8 s. Images were reconstructed with filtered back projection. Whole-body PET data acquisition commenced at a level just below the pelvis. PET parameters were as follows: acquisition mode 2-D, scan time/bed position 300 s, bed position overlap 3 slices. Images were reconstructed with ordered-subsets expectation maximization algorithm using the following parameters: 2 iterations, 28 subsets, a 5.5-mm post-reconstruction Gaussian filter, and 3.9-mm pixels.

## Findings and differential diagnosis

FDG-PET/CT demonstrates mild focal FDG uptake in the inferior aspect of the right breast, SUVmax (lean body mass) 2.5 (Figure 11.2A, arrow). Multiple FDG-avid enlarged axillary and a subpectoral lymph nodes are seen, the largest measures 2.6 × 2.3 cm with a SUVmax (lbm) of 6.2. Multiple FDG-avid

lytic lesions involve the right proximal humerus, T6 and L3 vertebral bodies, bilateral iliac bones, and the right ischium.

## Diagnosis and clinical follow-up

The patient's bilateral mammogram prior to FDG PET/CT showed two areas of calcifications in the inferolateral right breast. No abnormalities were noted in the left breast. She had sonographic evaluation of the right breast, which demonstrated two foci in right inferolateral breast at the 9 o'clock position. The largest measured 2.4 cm at 2 cm from the nipple, while the second lesion measured 2.1 cm at 8 cm from the nipple.

Subsequent biopsy of her right breast lesions revealed infiltrating poorly differentiated ductal carcinoma. Metastatic disease was also found in axillary lymph nodes. Subsequent to PET/CT she underwent CT-guided fine needle aspiration of left iliac bone, which revealed metastatic carcinoma. Tumor markers were positive for breast carcinoma.

## Discussion and teaching points

Whole body FDG-PET/CT can potentially play a crucial role in staging breast cancer. FDG-PET has been shown to have high diagnostic specificity in detecting nodal disease. However, in patients with negative axillae on whole-body imaging, further evaluation with sentinel node biopsy should be performed to rule out disease involvement in other nodes. When systemic metastases are present at presentation, axillary nodal status is less relevant and may not be determined

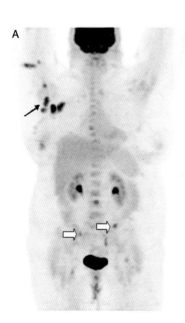

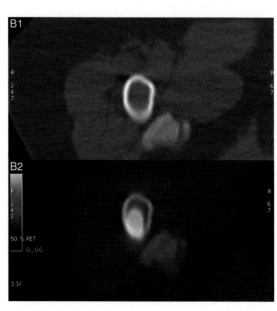

**Figure 11.2A–D** A 46-year-old female with newly diagnosed poorly differentiated infiltrating ductal carcinoma of the right breast was referred for a staging FDG-PET/CT. The MIP image of whole-body FDG-PET/CT (A) reveals disease in the right axillary lymph nodes (arrow) and additional disease foci are seen in osseous structures (thick arrows). Axial images (B, C, D) reveal FDG-avid foci in right proximal humerus (B), right iliac bone (C) and left iliac bone (D). Lytic changes are seen on the accompanying CT images.

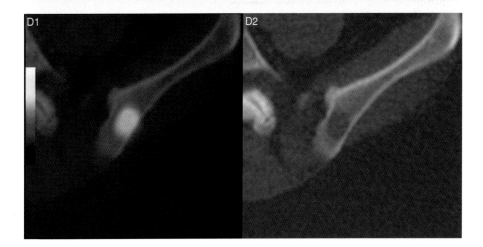

**Figure 11.2A–D** (cont.)

pathologically, choosing rather to focus on the distant disease status.

Skeletal metastases are the most common site of distant disease in breast cancer, accounting for up to 90% of all metastatic disease. The current standard of care is to perform bone scintigraphy to survey the skeleton. Although FDG-PET/CT has been shown to be superior to standard bone scintigraphy in identifying lytic and intramedullary metastases, FDG-PET has limited sensitivity in detecting blastic lesions. The increasing utilization of hybrid PET/CT imaging will lead to increased diagnostic accuracy and confidence. Recent studies have shown FDG-PET/CT and bone scintigraphy to be equally effective with FDG-PET typically detecting more active metastases than a bone scan. With NaF-PET now more widely available, there is an excellent PET method for detecting blastic disease.

## Take-home message

- Whole-body FDG-PET/CT can be helpful as an adjunct to conventional anatomical imaging in revealing sites of metastatic disease. It may be useful to detect sites of occult metastases in patients when a higher grade or stage of the disease is suspected. In this case, intense FDG uptake in lytic metastases indicated advanced disease and indicated systemic therapy was essential.

## References

1. Tatsumi M, Cohade C, Mourtzikos KA *et al*. Initial experience with FDG PET/CT in the evaluation of breast cancer. *Eur J Nucl Med Mol Imaging* 2006;**333**(**93**):254–62.

2. Morris PG, Lynch C, Feeney JN *et al*. Integrated positron emission tomography/computed tomography may render bone scintigraphy unnecessary to investigate suspected metastatic breast cancer. *J Clin Oncol* 2010;**28**(19):3154–9.

## Restaging/treatment response

A 48-year-old female had a history of in-situ and infiltrating ductal adenocarcinoma involving the right breast. She was status post modified radical mastectomy with metastatic involvement of ipsilateral lymph nodes. She was being evaluated for systemic metastatic disease.

## Acquisition and processing parameters

After a 4-h fast and serum glucose measurement, the patient was administered 8.1 MBq of FDG per kilogram. Her blood glucose was 79 mg/dL prior to FDG administration. Time from injection to initiation of images was 60 minutes. Images were acquired on a GE Discovery LS BGO 4-slice scanner. Immediately before the start of scanning, the patients was given the opportunity to void. The CT study was acquired immediately before the PET study and involved data acquisition under shallow-breathing conditions. CT parameters were as follows: 140 kVP, 20–200 mA (modulated), and pitch 1.5, rotation time 0.8 s. Images were reconstructed with filtered back projection. Whole-body PET data acquisition commenced at a level just below the pelvis. PET parameters were as follows: acquisition mode: 2-D, scan time/bed position 300 s, bed position overlap 3 slices. Images were reconstructed with ordered-subsets expectation maximization algorithm with the following parameters: 2 iterations, 28 subsets, a 5.5-mm post-reconstruction Gaussian filter, and 3.9-mm pixels.

## Findings and differential diagnosis

The staging PET (Figure 11.3A) shows post-operative changes in the right breast. The MIP images (Figure 11.3A1) show multiple mild to moderately FDG-avid lesions involving the spine, ribs, pelvis, and right scapula. Pre-treatment axial images through pelvis (Figures 11.3B1, 11.3B2) show an intensely FDG-avid lytic lesion involving the right iliac wing and the L5 pedicle on the left side. Similarly at T10 vertebral level, FDG-avid lesion is noted (Figures 11.3C1, 11.3C2). Without PET images, lesions are difficult to discern on CT images alone. Post-treatment images through pelvis (Figures 11.3B3, 11.3B4) and T10 vertebral level (Figures 11.3C3, 11.3C4) show multiple sclerotic foci throughout the vertebral bodies and bilateral iliac bones. PET/CT images show an interval decrease in FDG uptake.

## Diagnosis and clinical follow-up

A 48-year-old woman with a history of right breast infiltrating ductal adenocarcinoma, and ipsilateral nodal disease. Her post-surgery PET/CT showed FDG-avid osseous metastases involving the spine, ribs, pelvis, and right scapula. Subsequent bone marrow biopsy showed small deposits of metastatic carcinoma morphologically similar to patient's primary breast carcinoma. She was started on hormonal therapy and was re-assessed with FDG-PET/CT 3 months later. Her whole body PET/CT while on treatment shows (Figures 11.3A2, 11.3B3, 11.3B4, 11.3C3, 11.3C4) significant reduction in FDG-avidity in the osseous lesions.

## Discussion and teaching points

Osseous metastases are seen in approximately 25–80% of patients with breast cancer. Evaluation of the response of bone metastases to treatment is a complex process for oncologists. Bone metastases can be osteoblastic or osteolytic. This complicates an accurate assessment of disease burden as well as assessment of treatment response. Bone scintigraphy continues to be an excellent tool for the detection of osteoblastic bone metastases, but it is problematic for osteolytic lesions because there is no significant bone reaction to be detected on a bone scan. Changes in the bone scan significantly lag behind the response of bone metastases and may even transiently worsen or "flare" in response to successful therapy.

The flare phenomenon has been attributed to an increased uptake of diphosphonates that accompanies healing of the surrounding bone as the tumor is successfully treated. This is particularly true for most lytic metastases. Stafford *et al.* showed that changes in FDG uptake correlated with the clinical assessment of response in bone-dominant metastatic breast cancer. The changes in FDG uptake also correlated with changes in breast cancer tumor markers, which are used clinically to assess the response of treated bone metastases (1). A follow-up report showed that changes in FDG uptake predicted time to progression, a more robust clinical endpoint than response, and that the level of FDG predicted the likelihood of a skeletal event (2). Studies using FDG-PET/CT showed similar findings and also showed that correlative changes in CT – in particular, increased sclerosis associated with response to treatment – could provide important complementary information to PET.

A study by Tateishi *et al.* also showed that both metabolic and structural changes on FDG-PET/CT predicted time to progression of bone metastases (3). When interpreting FDG-PET studies to evaluate the response of bone metastases, it is important to recognize that although an absence of FDG uptake after therapy of a previously FDG-positive metastasis indicates a good response to treatment and a favorable

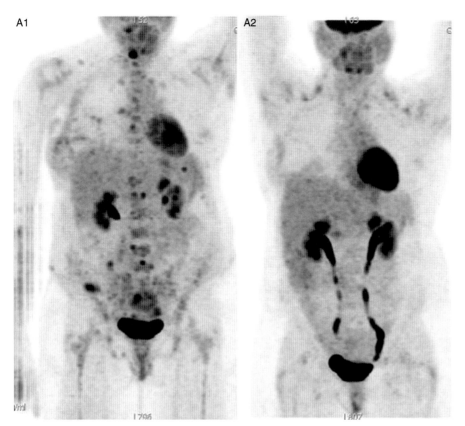

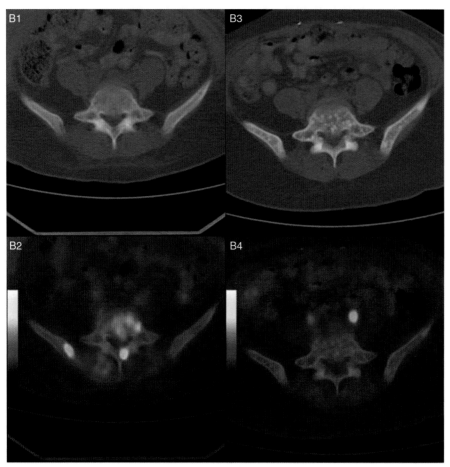

**Figure 11.3A–C** A 54-year-old female had a history of infiltrating ductal adenocarcinoma involving the right breast. Pre-treatment MIP images (A1) and post-hormonal therapy (A2) scans show resolution of FDG-avid foci in the bones. Post-surgical inflammatory changes (A1) have resolved on the post-treatment scan (A2). Axial images (B) through iliac bone show pre-treatment (B1, 2) and post-treatment (B3, 4) changes. FDG uptake is resolved and CT images show sclerotic changes on the post-treatment images (right) indicating response to treatment. Similarly, axial images through a T10 vertebral body (C) show a lytic lesion on the pre-treatment (C1, 2) images with multiple sclerotic lesions on the post-treatment images (C3, 4).

**Figure 11.3A–C** (cont.)

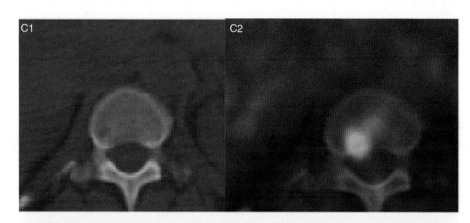

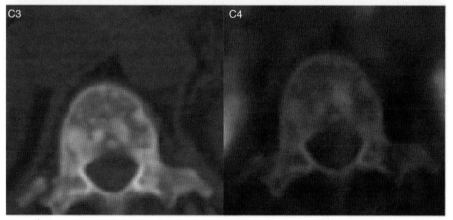

prediction for time to progression, it does not necessarily indicate an absence of disease.

## Take-home message

- FDG-PET and PET/CT can often play a significant role in the assessment of osseous involvement along with evaluation of response to treatment in patients with breast cancer. In

cases with bone metastases, careful knowledge of the treatment history is essential. Markedly abnormal CT scans with sclerosis can occur after successful therapy and these should not be confused with active disease. In addition, active metastases can be invisible on CT scans, so absence of a CT abnormality in the presence of a positive PET image should not be taken as reflective of a false-positive PET.

## References

1. Stafford SE, Gralow JR, Schubert EK *et al.* Use of serial FDG PET to measure the response of bone-dominant breast cancer to therapy. *Acad Radiol* 2002;**9**:913–21.

2. Specht JM, Tam SL, Kurland BF *et al.* Serial 2-[18F] fluoro-2-deoxy-D-

glucose positron emission tomography (FDG-PET) to monitor treatment of bone dominant metastatic breast cancer predicts time to progression (TTP). *Breast Cancer Res Treat* 2007;**105**:87–94.

3. Tateishi U, Gamez C, Dawood S *et al.* Bone metastases in patients with

metastatic breast cancer: morphologic and metabolic monitoring of response to systemic therapy with integrated PET/CT. *Radiology* 2008;**247**(1): 189–96.

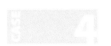

A 53-year-old woman with an initial diagnosis of stage IV left breast cancer with osseous metastases. She is status post radiation treatment to her spine and is being maintained on tamoxifen.

## Acquisition and processing parameters

The patient's blood glucose level prior to FDG administration was 95 mg/dL. Time from injection to initiation of image acquisition was 68 min. Images were acquired on a GE LS BGO-crystal 16-slice PET/CT scanner. The patient received two bottles of oral contrast for this study. After a 4-hour fast and serum glucose measurement, the patient received 8.1 MBq of FDG per kilogram intravenously. Her blood glucose was 97 mg/dL prior to FDG administration. Images were acquired on a GE DVCT LySO-crystal 64-slice scanner. Immediately before the start of scanning, the patient was given the opportunity to void. The CT study occurred immediately before the PET study and involved data acquisition under shallow-breathing conditions. CT parameters were as follows: 140 kVP, 20–200 mA (modulated), pitch 0.984 : 1, rotation time 0.5 s. Images were reconstructed with filtered back projection. Whole-body PET data acquisition commenced at a level just below the pelvis. PET parameters were as follows: acquisition mode: 3-D, scan time/bed position 255 s, bed position overlap 11 slices. Images were reconstructed with ordered-subsets expectation maximization algorithm with the following parameters: 2 iterations, 21 subsets, a 3.0-mm post-reconstruction Gaussian filter, and 4.7-mm pixels.

## Findings and differential diagnosis

Overall there is evidence of disease progression with multiple foci of FDG activity fusing to bones throughout the axial and appendicular skeleton. The FDG activity appears to be encroaching into the spinal canal at the level of the T7 vertebral body. No definite abnormality was seen on CT.

## Diagnosis and clinical follow-up

The patient underwent additional imaging with MRI, which revealed extensive metastatic disease.

## Discussion and teaching points

A significant percentage of women with breast cancer will develop recurrent disease. Current ASCO guidelines recommend careful history taking, physical examination, and regular mammography for appropriate detection of breast cancer recurrence. Since assessment of biomarkers alone may be false-negative, it is usually supplanted by conventional imaging. Despite the accuracy of these imaging modalities, they are not always able to localize the disease, especially in cases of relapse in an already treated patient in whom the distinction between post-surgical changes and recurrence may be very difficult.

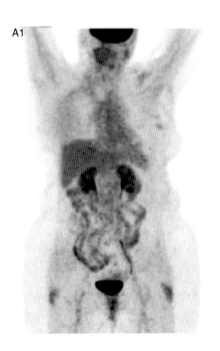
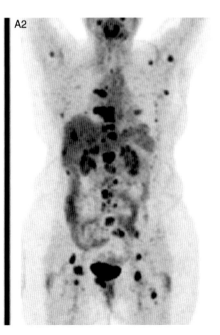

**Figure 11.4A–C** A 53-year-old female with a known history of stage IV breast cancer was being maintained on hormonal therapy. The MIP scan (A1) shows her last negative FDG-PET; a follow-up FDG-PET shows disease recurrence (A2). Axial CT images through a vertebral body (B1, B2) show no evidence of disease, but the presence of disease is appreciated mainly on FDG-PET images (B4) with minimal changes on the accompanying CT images (B2). Similarly, no evidence of disease is seen in the right pubic bone (C1, C3). Subsequent images (C4) show FDG-avid disease involving the right pubic bone with minimal changes on accompanying CT images (C2).

Figure 11.4A–C (cont.)

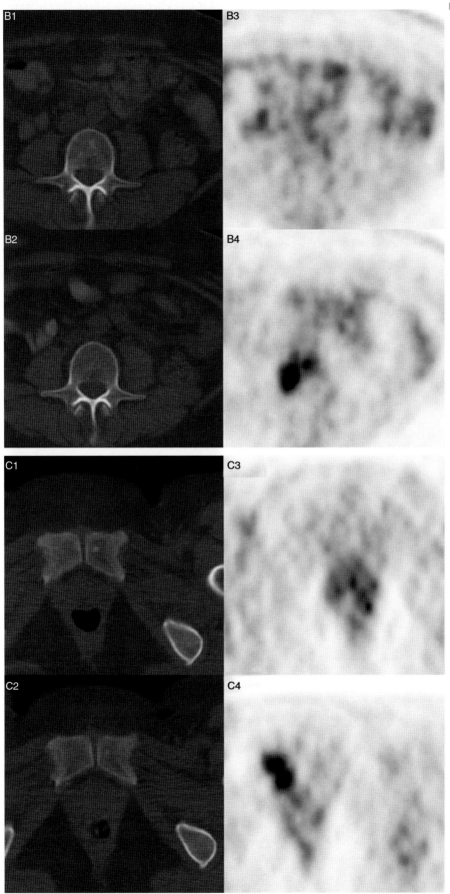

FDG-PET/CT is useful in select conditions of biochemical recurrence or when conventional imaging is negative.

Kamel *et al.* compared FDG-PET findings to tumor marker levels (CA 15.3) in 60 patients. In a lesion-based analysis, a total of 50 lesions were validated by histology, conventional imaging, and follow-up. PET was true-positive in 28 lesions, true-negative in 16, false-positive in 3 and false-negative in 3 cases (1). Similarly, Grassetto and colleagues reported the value of FDG-PET/CT in woman with rising biomarkers and found disease in 40/89 (45%) women (2).

Serum biomarkers are not perfect indicators of disease status and provide no localizing information as to disease site. Thus, PET/CT complements biomarkers in assessing possible metastatic disease to bone.

## Take-home message

- FDG-PET/CT is helpful in the detection of occult recurrent disease in women with rising biomarkers and negative conventional morphological imaging.

## References

1. Kamel EM, Wyss MT, Fehr MK *et al.* [18F]-fluorodeoxyglucose positron emission tomography in patients with suspected breast cancer. *J Cancer Res Clin Oncol* 2003;**129**:147–53.

2. Grassetto G, Fornasiero A, Otello D *et al.* 18F-FDG PET/CT in patients with breast cancer and rising Ca 15.3 with negative conventional imaging: a multicentre study. *Eur J Radiol* 2011; **80**(3):828–33.

A 46-year-old female with a history of moderately differentiated triple positive right breast ductal carcinoma [ER (+), PR (+), and Her2 (+)]. She presented for re-evaluation during neoadjuvant treatment with chemotherapy and herceptin.

## Acquisition and processing parameters

The patient's blood glucose level prior to FDG administration was 102 mg/dL. Time from injection to initiation of image acquisition was 58 min. Oral contrast was administered. Images were acquired on a GE LS BGO-crystal 4-slice PET/CT scanner. After a 4-hour fast and serum glucose measurement, the patient was administered 8.1 MBq of FDG per kilogram. Her blood glucose was 97 mg/dL prior to FDG administration. Time from injection to initiation of images was 64 min. Images were acquired on a GE DVCT LySO-crystal 64-slice scanner. Immediately before the start of scanning, the patient was given the opportunity to void. The CT study occurred immediately before the PET study and involved data acquisition under shallow-breathing conditions. CT parameters were as follows: 140 kVP, 20–200 mA (modulated), pitch 0.984:1, rotation time 0.5 s. Images were reconstructed with filtered back projection. Whole-body PET data acquisition commenced at a level just below the pelvis. PET parameters were as follows: acquisition mode: 3-D, scan time/bed position 255 s, bed position overlap 11 slices. Images were reconstructed with ordered-subsets expectation maximization algorithm with the following parameters: 2 iterations, 21 subsets, a 3.0-mm post-reconstruction Gaussian filter, and 4.7-mm pixels.

## Findings and differential diagnosis

Staging FDG-PET/CT (Figure 11.5A1, MIP images) reveals intensely FDG-avid disease involving the right breast mass (SUVmax 9.6) along with metastatic involvement of the axillary lymph nodes (SUVmax 6.8). Her staging PET/CT (Figure 11.5A1, arrow) showed a suspicious contralateral left supraclavicular lymph node (SUVmax 2.1).

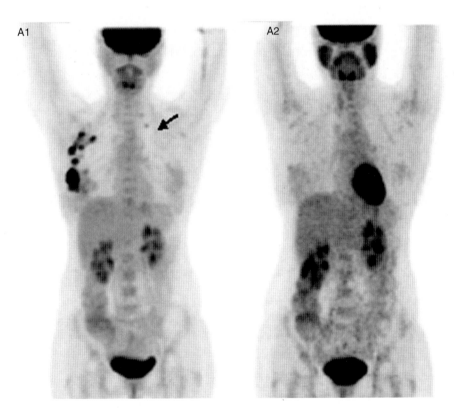

**Figure 11.5A–B** A 46-year-old female presented with a history of triple positive breast cancer. Her staging FDG-PET (A1, B1, and B3) shows involvement of the right breast and there is also involvement of ipsilateral lymph nodes. This staging FDG-PET/CT also revealed a left supraclavicular lymph node (A1, arrow) and a subsequent biopsy confirmed metastatic disease. Her mid-treatment whole-body (A2) and the fused FDG-PET/CT scan (B4) demonstrate a near-complete metabolic response to therapy. Mild residual asymmetry is seen in the mass in the right breast compared with the left (A2, B4). A small amount of fat stranding remains surrounding normalized right axillary lymph nodes (B2, B4). FDG uptake in the left supraclavicular lymph node has resolved (A2).

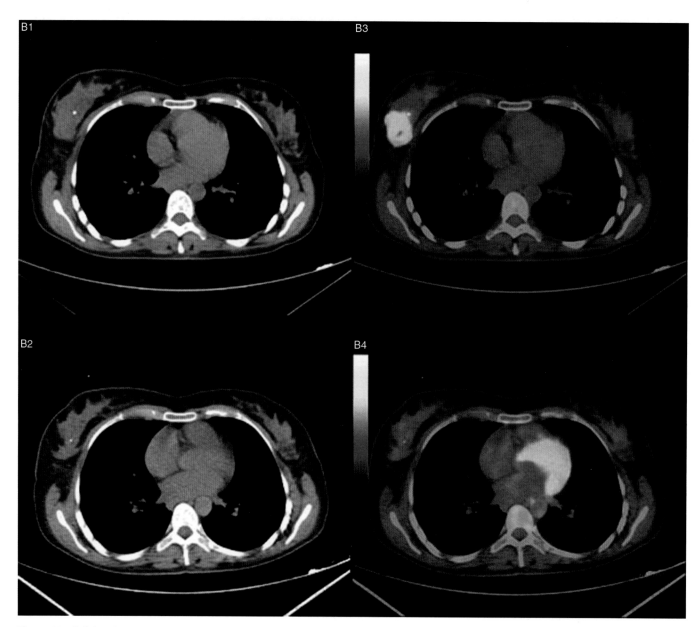

**Figure 11.5A–B** (cont.)

She underwent neoadjuvant treatment with chemotherapy and herceptin. Her mid-treatment whole-body FDG-PET/CT scan (Figure 11.5A2) demonstrates a near-complete metabolic response to therapy. Mild residual asymmetry is seen in the mass in the right breast compared with the left. A small amount of fat stranding remains surrounding normalized right axillary lymph nodes. FDG uptake in the left supraclavicular lymph node has resolved.

## Diagnosis and clinical follow-up

Her baseline biopsy had shown infiltrative moderately differentiated ductal carcinoma involving the right breast. Metastatic carcinoma also involved right axillary lymph nodes. Her staging PET/CT (Figure 11.5A1) showed a left supraclavicular lymph node which proved to be metastatic disease on subsequent tissue

sampling. She was considered to have locally advanced disease and was started on neoadjuvant treatment. Her mid-treatment FDG-PET/CT (Figures 11.5B2, 11.5B4) showed a near-complete metabolic response. She underwent a right radical modified mastectomy two months after the PET/CT scan. Her right breast mass showed a pathological response and no invasive carcinoma was identified. Her lymph nodes showed post-treatment changes.

## Discussion and teaching points

One of the earliest studies of FDG-PET to monitor response to breast cancer treatment was performed by Wahl et al. and showed significant quantitative differences in the FDG uptake measured before and after 2 months of therapy for responders versus non-responders (1). Almost all of the subsequent studies reported similar findings and found that if a primary tumor showed a decline in FDG uptake by approximately 50% or more this was predictive of a good response. Other studies have demonstrated that the extent of residual breast and axillary disease after treatment is prognostic for both disease-free survival and overall survival (2). Similar studies have shown that the use of FDG-PET and PET/CT early in the course of treatment lead to an accurate prediction of response.

## Take-home message

- FDG-PET/CT plays a significant role in the evaluation of early treatment response and influences the subsequent management of disease in breast cancer patients. Earlier assessment of response during treatment can lead to decreased morbidity and mortality and avoid futile treatments.

## References

1. Wahl RL, Zasadny K, Helvie M *et al.* Metabolic monitoring of breast cancer chemohormonotherapy using positron emission tomography: initial evaluation. *J Clin Oncol* 1993;**11**:2101–11.

2. Bassa P, Kim EE, Inoue T *et al.* Evaluation of preoperative chemotherapy using PET with fluorine-18-fluorodeoxyglucose in breast cancer. *J Nucl Med* 1996;**37**:931–8.

A 59-year-old female, recently diagnosed with triple negative poorly differentiated ductal carcinoma in the right breast, was referred for a whole-body PET/CT scan to stage her disease.

## Acquisition and processing parameters

The patient's blood glucose level prior to FDG administration was 92 mg/dL. After a 4-hour fast and serum glucose measurement, the patient received 8.1 MBq of FDG per kilogram intravenously. Her blood glucose was 97 mg/dL prior to FDG administration. Time from injection to initiation of images was 55 min. Images were acquired on a GE DVCT LySO-crystal 64-slice scanner. Immediately before the start of scanning, the patient was given the opportunity to void. The CT study occurred immediately before the PET study and involved data acquisition under shallow-breathing conditions. CT parameters were as follows: 140 kVP, 20–200 mA (modulated), pitch 0.984 : 1, rotation time 0.5 s. Images were reconstructed with filtered back projection. Whole-body PET data acquisition commenced at a level just below the pelvis. PET parameters were as follows: acquisition mode 3-D, scan time/bed position 255 s, bed position overlap 11 slices. Images were reconstructed with ordered-subsets expectation maximization algorithm using the following parameters: 2 iterations, 21 subsets, a 3.0-mm post-reconstruction Gaussian filter, and 4.7-mm pixels.

## Findings and differential diagnosis

MIP image from FDG-PET/CT demonstrates diffuse metastatic disease ranging from the neck to the pelvis. Areas involved include the left neck lymph nodes, mediastinum, left thyroid lobe, liver, retroperitoneal and intraperitoneal lymph nodes, the C7 vertebral body, and perirectal lymph nodes. An intensely FDG-avid centrally necrotic mass involving the left adrenal gland is suspicious for malignant involvement (Figures 11.6B1–11.6B4). Note that MIP images do not provide precise lesion localization as they do not show clearly the depth of the lesions in the patient. Thus, 3-D images including transverse, coronal, and sagittal slices are needed. There are intensely FDG-avid nodules in the left and right upper lobes of the lungs, also suspicious for metastatic disease. The intensely FDG-avid right breast mass with ipsilateral axillary lymphadenopathy is consistent with the patient's recent biopsy-proven ductal carcinoma (Figures 11.6A, 11.6B1, 11.6B2).

## Diagnosis and clinical follow-up

Biopsy-proven ductal carcinoma.

## Discussion and teaching points

Triple negative breast cancer comprises approximately 15–20% of all breast cancers. About two-thirds of these are high-grade (grade III) at diagnosis, compared with less than one-third of other breast cancers. A significantly higher percentage is found in Jewish (Ashkenazi) and possibly Hispanic women. These women are also more likely to have BRCA1 mutations. The overall prognosis of this subclass of patients is poor due to aggressive disease and the lack of available targeted therapies. They have a higher relapse rate due to their high-grade disease.

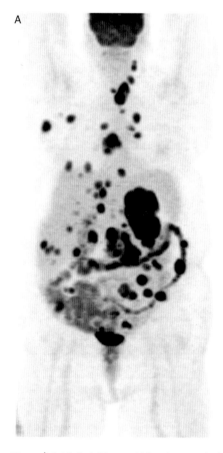

**Figure 11.6A–B** A 59-year-old female, recently diagnosed with triple negative poorly differentiated ductal carcinoma in the right breast. (A) MIP image from FDG-PET/CT demonstrates diffuse metastatic disease ranging from the neck to the pelvis. (B1-B2) Coronal CT and fused FDG-PET/CT slices. (B3, B4) Axial CT and fused FDG-PET/CT images.

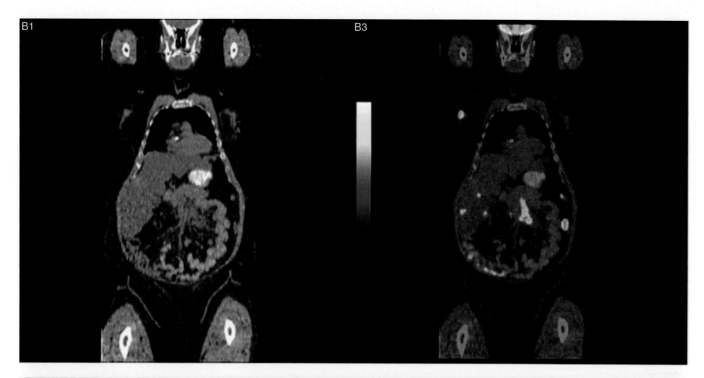

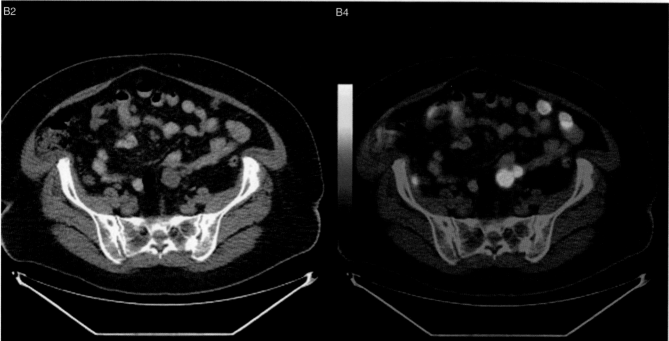

**Figure 11.6A–B** (cont.)

Recent studies have shown that triple negative cancers have higher FDG uptake compared with non-triple negative breast cancer (1, 2). It has also been shown that SUVmax correlates with the proliferation index of triple negative breast cancer, which has a higher proliferation index as measured by Ki67 compared with non-triple negative breast cancers (3).

## Take-home message

- FDG uptake correlates with biological factors in breast cancer. High levels of FDG uptake are seen in patients with aggressive biology such as triple negative (ER/PR/HER2) disease. These lesions can be staged systemically with whole-body FDG-PET/CT.

# References

1. Basu S, Chen W, Tchou J *et al.* Comparison of triple-negative and estrogen receptor-positive/progesterone receptor-positive/HER2-negative breast carcinoma using quantitative fluorine-18 fluorodeoxyglucose/positron emission tomography imaging parameters: a potentially useful method for disease characterization. *Cancer* 2008; **112**(5):995–1000.

2. Groheux D, Giacchetti S, Moretti JL *et al.* Correlation of high (18) F-FDG uptake to clinical, pathological and biological prognostic factors in breast cancer. *Eur J Nucl Med Mol Imag* 2011;**38**:426–35.

3. Tchou J, Sonnad S, Bergey M *et al.* Degree of tumor FDG uptake correlates with proliferation index in triple negative breast cancer. *Mol Imag Biol* 2010,**12**:657–62.

A 48-year-old female with history of endometrial carcinoma underwent a whole-body FDG-PET/CT scan for restaging.

## Acquisition and processing parameters

After a 4-hour fast and serum glucose measurement, patients were administered 8.1 MBq of FDG per kilogram. Her blood glucose was 79 mg/dL prior to FDG administration. Time from injection to initiation of images was 62 min. Images were acquired on a GE Discovery LS BGO 4-slice scanner. Immediately before the start of scanning, the patient was given the opportunity to void. The CT study occurred immediately before the PET study and involved data acquisition under shallow-breathing conditions. CT parameters were as follows: 140 kVP, 20–200 mA (modulated), and pitch 1.5, rotation time 0.8 s. Images were reconstructed with filtered back projection. Whole-body PET data acquisition commenced at a level just below the pelvis. PET parameters were as follows: acquisition mode 2-D, scan time/bed position 300 s, bed position overlap 3 slices. Images were reconstructed with ordered-subsets expectation maximization algorithm with the following parameters: 2 iterations, 28 subsets, a 5.5-mm post-reconstruction Gaussian filter, and 3.9-mm pixels.

## Findings and differential diagnosis

Whole-body images reveal a focus of moderate FDG uptake in the left breast (Figures 11.7A, 11.7B1, 11.7B3, arrows). The presence of intensely FDG-avid disease is also seen in the vaginal cuff in the pelvis (Figures 11.7B2, 11.7B4). The differential diagnosis for the breast lesion includes primary breast cancer, inflammatory changes, and less commonly metastases. The pelvic finding is very concerning for recurrent endometrial cancer.

## Diagnosis and clinical follow-up

The patient underwent fine needle aspiration of the left breast mass, which revealed a primary invasive ductal carcinoma of the breast.

## Discussion and teaching points

A standard oncology FDG-PET/CT exam covers most of the body areas extending from base of skull to mid-thighs. The brain is often excluded as the normal brain has intense FDG uptake which can make detecting metastases quite difficult. Whole-body PET/CT provides assessment of local disease as well as distant sites of disease. This helps to accurately estimate the overall disease burden and optimize management. Additional sites of related or unrelated disease involvement are discovered during imaging. A retrospective analysis of bone scans by Beatty et al. found a second primary malignancy in 31% (n = 41), benign disease in 47% (n = 62), and metastatic disease from their known malignancy in 23% (n = 30) of patients (1). Similarly, focal FDG uptake in the thyroid gland has been reported with approximately one-third of the lesions turning out to be malignant (2).

In a recent study by Chung et al., 163/45,000 patients had breast findings unrelated to a primary malignancy. It included physiological and pathological uptake (3). Ishimori reported that at least 1.2% of PET/CT scans in cancer patients find an unexpected second malignancy (4).

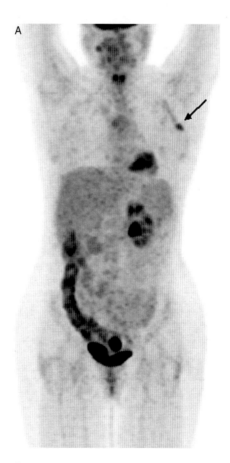

**Figure 11.7A–B** A 48-year-old female with history of endometrial carcinoma. (A) MIP and axial fused FDG-PET/CT and FDG-PET images reveal a focus of mild to moderate FDG uptake in the left breast (A, B1, B3 arrows). Intense focus of FDG-avid disease present in the vaginal cuff in the pelvis (B2, B4).

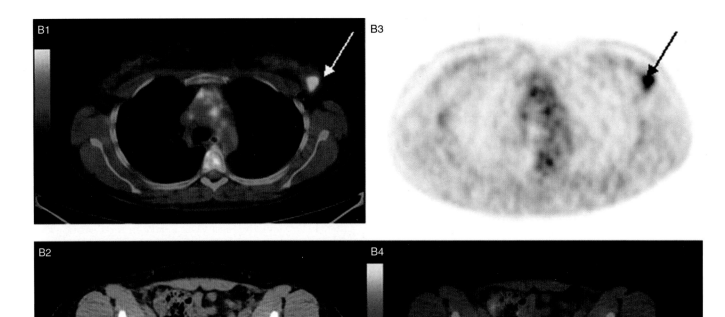

**Figure 11.7A–B** (cont.)

## Take-home message

- Incidental findings on a whole-body FDG-PET/CT study should be investigated further to rule out the presence of malignancy as they are not infrequent. Intense focal FDG uptake in the breast must be investigated as breast primary cancers represent one of the most common incidental cancers seen on PET/CT.

## References

1. Beatty JS, Williams HT, Aldridge BA *et al.* Incidental PET/CT findings in the cancer patient: how should they be managed? *Surgery* 2009;**146**(2):274–81.

2. Eloy JA, Brett EM, Fatterpekar G *et al.* The significance and management of incidental [18F]fluorodeoxyglucose-positron-emission tomography uptake in the thyroid gland in patients with cancer. *Am J Neuroradiol* 2009;**30**(7):1431–4.

3. Chung A, Schoder J, Sampson M *et al.* Incidental lesions identified by 18F-fluorordeoxyglucose-positron emission tomography. *Ann Surg Oncol* 2010;**17**(8):2119–25.

4. Ishimori T, Patel PV, Wahl RL. Detection of unexpected primary malignancies with PET/CT. *J Nucl Med* 2005;**46**(5):752–7.

# Cervix, uterus, and ovary

Scott Britz-Cunningham

## Introduction

The female genital tract has a complex embryologic origin, tying together elements of the paramesonephric ducts, coelomic epithelium, mesenchyme, and primordial germ cells in an equally intricate physiology, characterized by dramatic changes in function not only over a woman's full life cycle (menarche, pregnancy, and menopause), but with her rapid monthly rhythm of ovulation and menstruation. It should not be surprising that the pathology of this organ system is similarly complex. Tumors of the female pelvis are not only common, but exceedingly varied, including epithelial carcinomas, stromal tumors, sarcomas, and hybrids such as carcinosarcomas. Since these tumors may differ markedly as to FDG avidity, aggressiveness, and route of spread, facile generalizations should be avoided. PET/CT imaging needs to be rigorously correlated with all available clinical and histopathologic information, and with an intimate understanding of the biology of the type of tumor(s) under consideration. The astute PET/CT interpreter also needs to have a clear idea of the clinical purpose of the scan. Is it being performed for initial diagnosis and staging, for therapy planning, or for detection of recurrence? The utility and predictive value of PET may differ in each of these settings, as will be explained in more detail in the case discussions below.

The objectives of this chapter are to furnish the reader with a basic understanding of the range of tumor types affecting each organ, and of the established or emerging role of PET/CT within each clinical context, thus enabling him to derive the maximum amount of information from a given scan. It goes without saying that these principles are to be enlarged from the reader's own fund of experience and personal observation.

## Staging

Beyond the simple task of identifying the presence of malignant or potentially malignant tissue, the PET/CT reader should attempt to give a comprehensive picture of the extent of spread of disease, in order to guide subsequent patient management. While a detailed discussion of staging is beyond the scope of this chapter (readers are referred to the indispensable *AJCC Cancer Staging Manual* (1)), the PET/CT interpreter should be on the lookout for bellwether findings that may upstage the patient and affect the treatment regimen. In particular:

- Which organ appears to be the primary site of malignancy?
- How big is the tumor? (CT measurement of both long and short axes should always be included.)
- Does the primary tumor extend beyond the anatomic boundaries of its organ of origin? (For example, does a cervical cancer extend into the vagina or endometrial cavity, and, if so, how far?)
- Does the tumor extend to, or beyond, a serosal surface?
- Does the tumor, either visibly or potentially, involve adjacent organs, such as rectum, bladder, ureters, urethra, or bone?
- Does the tumor extend into the parametrium or a supporting ligament, such as the broad ligament or mesovarium? (Such ligaments are rich in lymphatic and venous effluents, and can be jumping-off points for metastatic spread.)
- Does the tumor extend into the presacral pelvic nervous plexus? (Not only can tumors travel for significant distances along nerve trunks, but involvement of nerves may limit the surgical approach, and can cause significant morbidity, in terms of pain and loss of bowel and bladder function.)
- Is there evidence of nodal spread? (The PET/CT reader should form the habit of systematically scrutinizing each nodal station, particularly including femoral; inguinal; external, internal, and common iliac; pelvic sidewall/ obturator; periaortic; retrocrural; and left supraclavicular nodes, which are all in the direct path of drainage for many pelvic malignancies. Upper abdominal and mediastinal

*A Case-Based Approach to PET/CT in Oncology*, ed. Victor H. Gerbaudo. Published by Cambridge University Press.

nodes should be examined as well, especially if there is evidence of nodal spread elsewhere.)

- Is the omentum or mesentery involved? (This may be difficult to distinguish from physiologic bowel activity, and CT features, such as thickening or stranding, may be necessary to make the diagnosis.)
- Are there distant metastases to organs such as bone, liver, adrenal, lung, stomach or brain?
- Does any part of the tumor appear to be necrotic?
- Is the primary tumor multifocal?
- Is ascites present? Is there a pleural effusion? (Whether there is FDG activity in the ascites fluid is probably irrelevant, as it is neither a sensitive nor a specific sign of malignancy) (2).
- What is the maximum intensity of FDG uptake? (In some cases, this has been shown to have independent prognostic value.)
- Is the tumor causing compressive obstruction of ureter, urethra or bowel?
- Are there optimal sites for biopsy?

## Technical issues

Interpreting FDG-PET/CT of the pelvis can be difficult, due to physiologic uptake from bladder, ureters, urinary contamination of skin and vulva, bowel, anorectal canal, and even muscular activity. Furthermore, gross misregistration errors can occur, due to time-lapse-related differences in bladder filling during the CT and PET portions of the scan. Familiarity with pelvic anatomy and normal uptake patterns is essential, if mistakes are to be avoided. In viewing the PET image, careful correlation must be made to the CT. In particular, the ureters should be traced along as much of their length as is practicable, to avoid misidentification of focal urinary activity as a metastatic lymph node. All three axes should be examined, particularly the sagittal plane, which offers the best differentiation of the uterus or cervix from adjacent bladder and rectum. Activity in the bladder or in a bladder diverticulum is usually much higher than is possible in tumors (with SUV in the range of 20–40 or even higher), which aids in identification. However, more modest uptake in a tumor immediately adjacent to the bladder can be obscured by scattering ("blooming") of this intense activity. Down-windowing the images can sometimes help to minimize this scattering effect.

Catheterization for decompression of the bladder has been recommended to minimize background activity. Vesselle *et al.* (3) have described a technically rigorous protocol, involving IV hydration, diuresis with furosemide, bladder catheterization and saline irrigation, as well as an isosomotic bowel prep to minimize intestinal activity. While these methods may help to provide a "cleaner" scan, they are laborious and have yet to be shown to significantly increase the diagnostic accuracy of experienced readers.

## Physiologic uptake

In premenopausal women, the female reproductive organs themselves can have significant FDG uptake, which fluctuates with the ovulatory cycle. Uptake in the endometrium appears as an inverted cone-shaped pattern, which peaks twice in the cycle: in early menstruation (SUV around 5) (4), and again during ovulation (SUV around 3.7). Similar peaks can also be seen outside the uterus, in focal areas of endometriosis. Increased uterine and vaginal uptake can also be observed in a post-partum setting (see Figure 12.3 below).

The fallopian tubes have also been reported to show increased uptake at mid-cycle.

Ovarian uptake has a single peak at ovulation, and is typically ovoid or focal, corresponding to a ruptured follicle. More persistent uptake can be seen in a corpus luteum. It should be noted that uptake related to ovarian cycling will still be observed in a pre-menopausal woman who has had a hysterectomy, but not oophorectomy. These cases can be especially difficult, because it is difficult to determine where the patient is in her monthly cycle.

Physiologic uptake can be difficult to distinguish from a true neoplasm. Often the clinical context can help to resolve any diagnostic issues. This necessitates a detailed gynecologic history, including pregnancy status, parturition, breastfeeding, spontaneous abortion, dilation and curettage or other surgical procedure, use of oral contraceptives or other hormonal supplements, and the date of the last menstrual period. If needed, focal ovarian uptake can be investigated by bringing the patient back in 2 weeks, at which time uptake related to a ruptured follicle or corpus luteum will have resolved (see Figure 12.2 below). When this is not possible, an SUV of 7.9 has been suggested as a cutoff between benign and malignant ovarian lesions (4).

In a post-menopausal woman not undergoing hormone replacement therapy, ovarian or endometrial uptake is abnormal, and should always elicit further investigation, with ultrasound as an immediate next step. Physiologic endometrial uptake has been reported in patients taking estrogenic supplements, however, imaging findings alone cannot distinguish this from atypical endometrial hyperplasia. Gynecologic consultation is prudent in such cases.

# Normal/benign variants
## Menstrual uptake

A

B

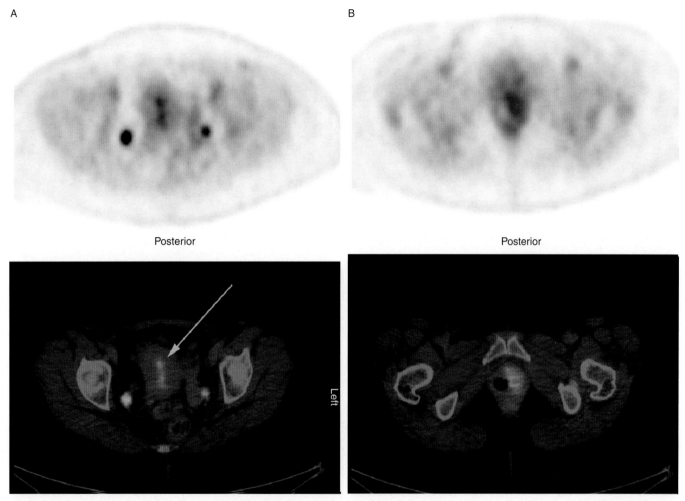

Posterior

Posterior

Left

**Figure 12.1** This 46-year-old premenopausal female was evaluated for multiple lung nodules. (A) Increased uptake is seen in the endometrial cavity (blue arrow), which correlated with patient's report of menstrual activity. (B) This was corroborated by the presence of a tampon (white arrow) within the vagina.

## Ovulation

A

B

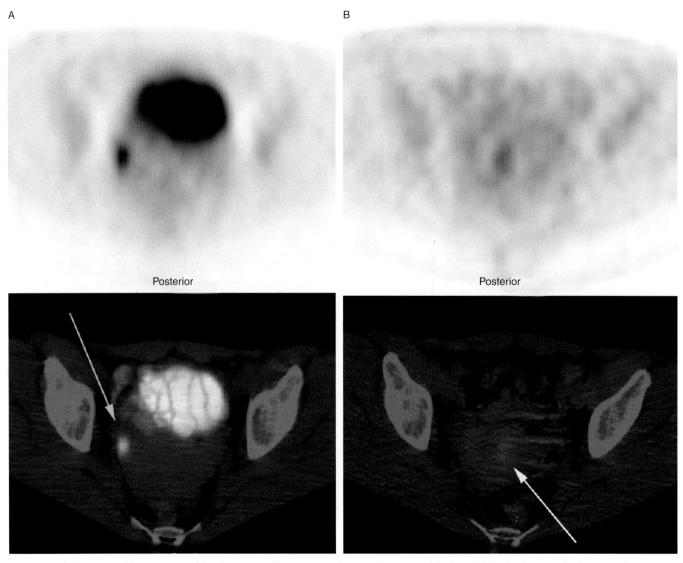

**Figure 12.2** This 41-year-old premenopausal female presented for restaging of a synovial sarcoma of the lung. (A) On the first scan, focal FDG uptake is seen in the right ovary (blue arrow). (B) Sixteen days later, a repeat FDG-PET/CT shows complete resolution of the ovarian uptake, indicating that this was due to ovulation rather than metastasis. New uptake is seen in the uterine cavity (white arrow), consistent with menstruation.

**Parturition**

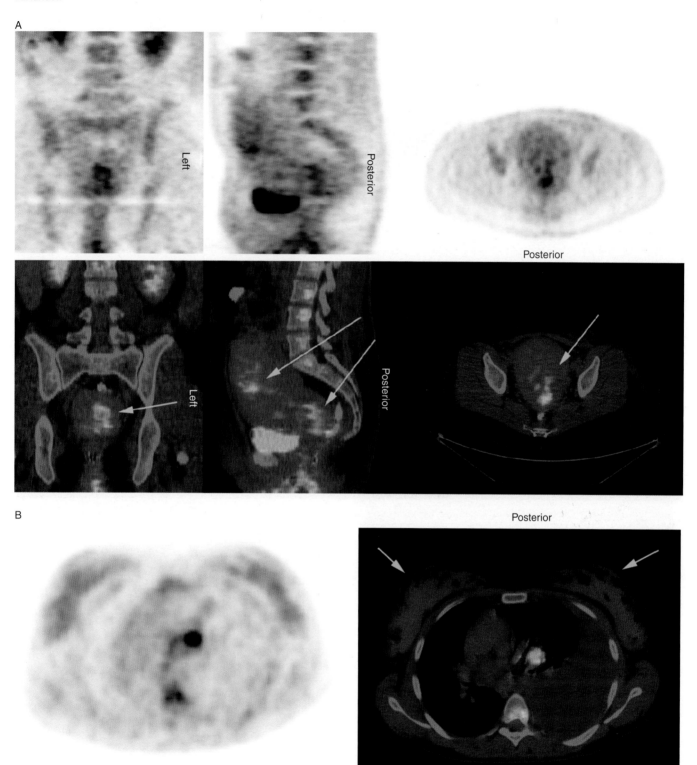

**Figure 12.3** This 35-year-old female was evaluated for pulmonary adenocarcinoma. She had given birth to a daughter by vaginal delivery three days before the scan. (A) Moderate FDG avidity is seen in the cavity of the markedly enlarged uterus (blue arrow), consistent with post-partum endometritis. (B) Lactation is evidenced by glandular hypertrophy and mild FDG avidity within the breasts (blue arrows). A large left pleural effusion is present, displacing the left lung and mediastinum rightward. This was related to the patient's intensely FDG-avid pulmonary tumor.

## Intrauterine contraceptive device

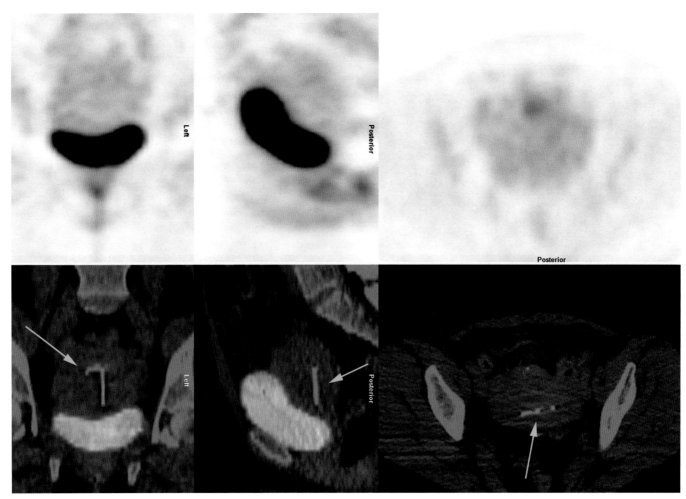

**Figure 12.4** This 61-year-old postmenopausal female was being followed for a desmoid tumor of the neck. A T-shaped intrauterine device (IUD) (blue arrow) is clearly visible within the cavity of the uterus, which is irregularly enlarged due to partially calcified fibroids. Note that IUDs can occasionally be seen in postmenopausal women, as delivery agents for hormonal therapy.

## Pessary

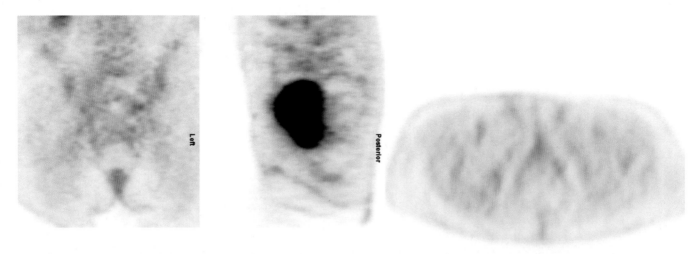

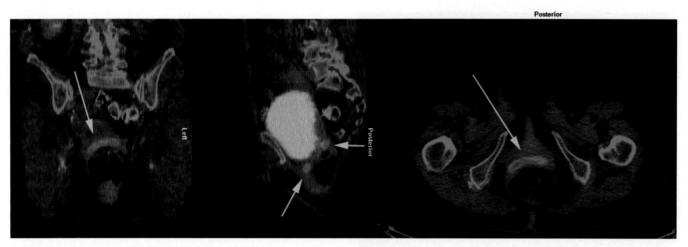

**Figure 12.5** This 86-year-old female with a history of breast cancer underwent FDG-PET/CT to evaluate pulmonary nodules. A ring-shaped pessary (blue arrows) is present in the upper vagina. Despite this, significant pelvic floor prolapse is seen.

### Bartholin's cyst

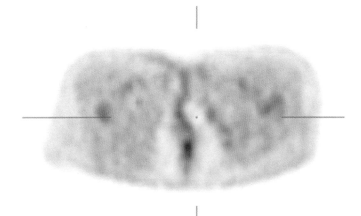

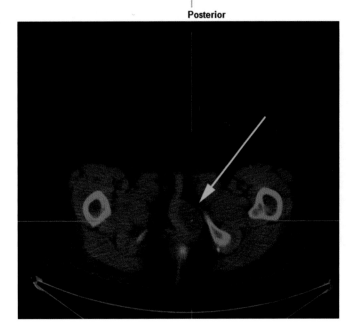

**Figure 12.6** This 46-year-old premenopausal female was being restaged for lung cancer. A 4.8 × 3.0 cm low-density mass is seen on the left side of the labia, displacing the midline structures toward the right. On FDG-PET, it appears photopenic, suggesting a predominantly acellular composition. This is a typical appearance for a Bartholin's cyst. If the cyst ruptures or becomes inflamed, mild-to-moderate FDG uptake may become apparent at the rim.

## Uterine fibroid

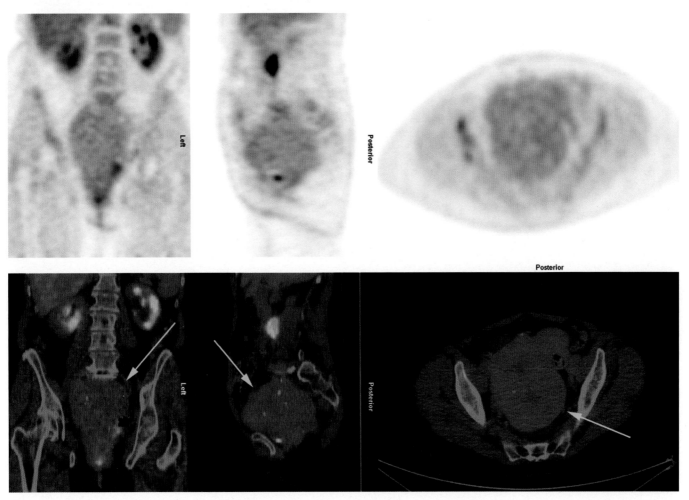

**Figure 12.7** This 75-year-old female with a history of breast cancer underwent a FDG-PET/CT exam to investigate an enlarging lung nodule. The uterus is markedly enlarged for the patient's age, with a lobulated appearance due to the presence of multiple large fibroids. These are speckled with small calcifications, visible in all three planes. The FDG uptake in the fibroids is slightly heterogeneous, but maximally is less than that seen in the liver and bone marrow. In a degenerating fibroid, uptake can be higher than this; however, suspicion should arise whenever there is focally intense uptake or necrosis. In such cases, the possibility of a leiomyosarcoma should be considered (see Case 5).

# References

1. American Joint Committee on Cancer. *AJCC Cancer Staging Manual: Seventh Edition*. New York, NY: Springer, 2010.

2. McAuley G, Ghesani S, Britz-Cunningham S. FDG uptake does not distinguish malignant from benign pleural effusions. *J Nucl Med* 2010;**51**(Suppl 2):258.

3. Vesselle HJ, Miraldi FD. FDG PET of the retroperitoneum: normal anatomy, variants, pathologic conditions, and strategies to avoid diagnostic pitfalls. *Radiographics* 1998;**18**(4):805–23; discussion 823–4.

4. Lerman H, Metser U, Grisaru D *et al.* Normal and abnormal 18F-FDG endometrial and ovarian uptake in pre- and postmenopausal patients: assessment by PET/CT. *J Nucl Med* 2004;**45**(2):266–71.

# Vulvar cancer

A 65-year-old female presented with vulvar and vaginal itching. After biopsy showed well-differentiated invasive squamous cell carcinoma, she underwent a radical right vulvectomy and right inguinal node dissection. No metastatic nodes were found. Surgical margins were positive for VIN2, but no residual invasive carcinoma was noted. Follow-up chemotherapy and radiation therapy was performed. She did well for the next 10 years, after which she returned to clinic with periclitoral itching and burning. Recurrent squamous cell carcinoma was diagnosed, and a radical resection performed. One year later, she presented with a draining vulvar and inguinal mass, which was initially thought to be an abscess. A FDG-PET/CT scan was performed (Figure 12.8A). The inguinal lesion was biopsied, and found to be recurrent squamous cell carcinoma. Following neoadjuvant external-beam radiation therapy and radiosensitizing chemotherapy with cisplatin and 5-fluorouracil, the mass was resected. Except for persistent left leg lymphedema, she did well for the next 4 years, when she returned to clinic complaining of vaginal burning, exacerbated by urination. A second FDG-PET/CT was performed (Figure 12.8B).

## Acquisition and processing parameters

For Case 1 and for all other cases in this chapter, the patient was injected intravenously with $777 \pm 111$ MBq ($21 \pm 3$ mCi) of FDG after fasting for 4–6 hours, and whole-body images were acquired on a Discovery ST PET/CT scanner (General Electric, Milwaukee, WI, USA), $83 \pm 22$ min after tracer administration. The unenhanced CT scan was performed first, from the patient's head to the proximal thighs, using the following acquisition parameters: 140 kVp, 75–120 mA (varying according to the patient's weight), 0.8 s per CT rotation, pitch of 1.675 : 1, with a reconstructed slice thickness of 3.75 mm, for a total scanning time of 42.4 s. The CT data were reconstructed using a filtered back-projection algorithm and a $512 \times 512$ matrix, with a transaxial field of view of 50 cm. Immediately after the CT scan, the emission scan was acquired in 2-D mode starting at the mid-thighs toward the head, for 6–7 bed positions of 4 min each (47 image planes/bed position, 15.4 cm longitudinal field of view). CT images were used to generate the transmission maps for attenuation correction of the PET acquisitions. PET data were reconstructed using an ordered-subset expectation maximization iterative algorithm (30 subsets, 2 iterations), yielding a volume of 47 slices.

## Findings and differential diagnosis

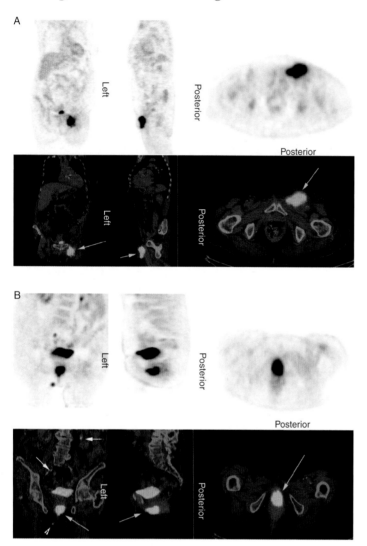

**Figure 12.8** (A) shows a 5.6 × 3.3 cm lobulated intensely FDG-avid soft tissue mass (blue arrow) seen in the left inguinal region, abutting the lower abdominal musculature and close to the left femoral vessels, consistent with metastasis. (B) FDG-PET/CT obtained 4 years later, shows that the left inguinal uptake has resolved, reflecting interval resection of the metastasis. A new, intensely FDG-avid mass is now seen in the perineum, consistent with local recurrence (blue arrow). Left mid abdominal and right mid pelvic small foci of FDG uptake (white arrows) correspond to physiologic FDG uptake in the ureters. Focal area of uptake on vulvar skin (arrowhead) corresponds to radioactive urine contamination.

## Diagnosis and clinical follow-up

(a) Squamous cell carcinoma of the vulva (metastatic to left inguinal lymph node). (b) Squamous cell carcinoma of the vulva (locally recurrent). The lesion was treated with external beam irradiation and interstitial brachytherapy, with concomitant carboplatin chemotherapy. No further recurrences were noted within a 7-month follow-up period. The patient complained of urinary incontinence, a common side-effect of pelvic irradiation. Due to distortion of urethral anatomy, a suprapubic catheter was placed.

## Discussion and teaching points

### Clinical background

Vulvar carcinoma is predominantly a disease of older women (age peak 65–75 years). The overwhelming majority of cases (86%) are of squamous cell origin. Significant associations are seen with HPV infection (particularly in the rare younger patient) and with syphilis. Malignant melanoma (5%) is occasionally seen, most commonly on the labia minora or clitoris. Rare tumor types include sarcoma (prognosis depends mainly upon histologic grade); basal cell carcinoma (typically found on the labia majority; rarely metastasizes); and Bartholin gland adenocarcinoma (an enlarged Bartholin gland in a post-menopausal woman should be presumed cancerous until proven otherwise.)

Regardless of histologic type, spread is typically via lymphatics. Either ipsilateral or contralateral superficial femoral nodes are first affected, with subsequent passage to deep femoral and then iliac nodes. The clitoris may drain directly to obturator nodes in the pelvis. Given this orderly sequence, sentinel node staging might be expected to be useful (the relapse rate is 0.3% for patients with negative inguinal nodes), however, it has not yet come into universal practice. Nodal metastases are more frequent in patients with larger tumors (> 3 cm), deeper invasion (> 5 mm), poorer differentiation, or lymphovascular involvement on histological examination.

Treatment is primarily surgical. The standard approach has been a radical vulvectomy with bilateral inguinal node dissection; an ipsilateral pelvic node dissection is added if positive inguinal nodes are found. This may be combined with radiation therapy to the pelvic nodes, although irradiation of the primary tumor is usually avoided, due to the risk of severe vulvitis. Adjuvant chemotherapy, typically with cisplatin and 5-fluorouracil, has also seen use.

Prognosis is highly dependent upon nodal status. Five-year survival is 96% if no nodes are present. This falls to 66% if inguinal nodes are present and 20% if deep pelvic nodes are seen.

## Imaging considerations

Although in other settings (most notably cervical cancer), FDG-PET/CT has been shown to have advantages over CT or MR in staging pelvic and para-aortic lymph nodes, there have been no large-scale studies to show its utility in the initial treatment strategy of vulvar cancer. Diagnosis is made by biopsy of superficially visualizable lesions, and staging is surgical. The most promising niches for PET/CT may lie in the evaluation and re-staging of suspected disease recurrence, and in planning radiation therapy.

The differential FDG avidity of vulvar cancer subtypes has yet to be systematically explored. In our own experience, squamous cell carcinoma and malignant melanoma of the vulva show the same intense uptake seen in histologically similar tumors elsewhere. Individual case reports have described high uptake in an undifferentiated Bartholin's gland carcinoma (1), and in a labial metastasis of a sarcoma of the pelvic floor (2).

## Take-home message

- Literature is scanty, but FDG-PET/CT is likely to have utility for the detection and staging of recurrent vulvar carcinoma, and for guiding radiation therapy.

- Urinary contamination of the vulva is common, and can be easily mistaken for superficial disease. This can be minimized by instructing the patient to utilize strict hygiene when voiding the bladder prior to the study, by rinsing or douching the labia or lower vagina, or by catheterizing the bladder. When present, it can usually be identified by the lack of skin thickening on CT.

## References

1. Imperiale A, Heymann S, Clariá M et al. F-18 FDG PET-CT in a rare case of Bartholin's gland undifferentiated carcinoma managed with chemoradiation and interstitial brachytherapy. *Clin Nucl Med* 2007;**32** (6):498–500.

2. Freudenberg LS, Antoch G, Beyer T et al. Diagnosis of labia metastasis by F-18 FDG PET and CT fusion imaging in sarcoma follow-up. *Clin Nucl Med* 2003;**28**(8):636–7.

A 70-year-old female, who had never had a Pap smear, presented with weight loss, malaise, and intermittent vaginal spot bleeding. Manual pelvic exam detected an irregular, non-tender cervical mass and irregular firmness of the anterior vaginal wall. Ultrasound showed a bulky, nodular, hypoechoic cervical mass and left hydronephrosis. Physical examination under anesthesia found necrotic, malodorous cervical tissue, and a 7 cm mass extending to the pelvic sidewall on the right. A FDG-PET/CT was performed.

## Findings and differential diagnosis

## Diagnosis and clinical follow-up

**Diagnosis of** quamous cell carcinoma of the cervix. The patient was treated with cisplatin chemotherapy, which was discontinued after two cycles due to treatment-induced hearing loss. She then underwent external beam irradiation to the pelvis and para-aortic and left supraclavicular nodes. A follow-up FDG-PET/CT 5 months later showed no residual tumor. Five months after this, she returned to the clinic with acute renal failure and a rectovaginal fistula. A third PET/CT showed no evidence of recurrence; however, there

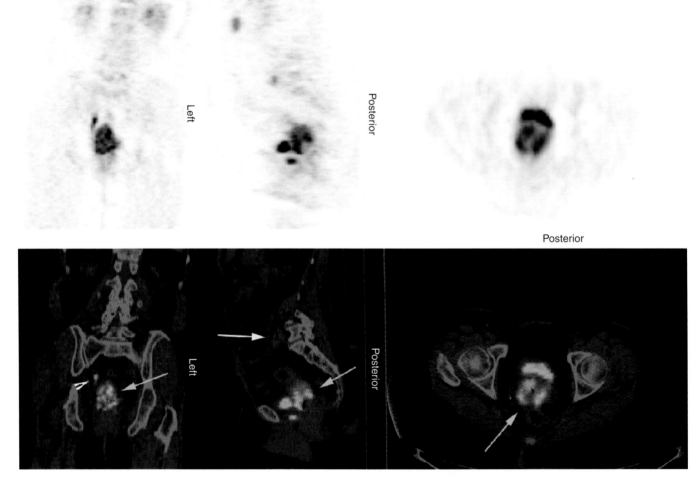

**Figure 12.9** (A) An intensely FDG-avid soft tissue mass is seen in the region of the cervix (blue arrow). Focal uptake anterior to the left side of the sacrum (white arrowhead) and anterior to the spine at the level of L1 (white arrow) reflects physiologic ureteral activity. (B) A small metastatic paraaortic lymph node (blue arrow) is seen medial to the left kidney. (c) Whole-body MIP image shows a second, larger 9-mm metastatic node (long blue arrow) at the level of the renal hila, as well as a left thoracic inlet/supraclavicular lymph node (short blue arrow).

B

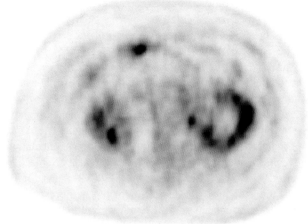

Posterior

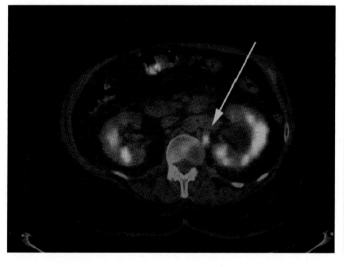

C

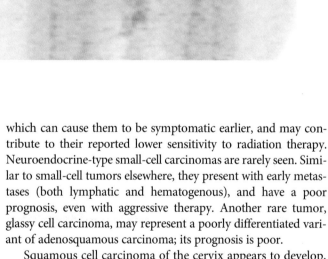

**Figure 12.9** (cont.)

was bilateral hydronephrosis, which appeared to be related to radiation-induced fibrosis in the pelvis. She was treated unsuccessfully with percutaneous nephrostomies and ureteral stents, and died 2 months later of uremia.

## Discussion and teaching points

### Clinical background

Cervical cancer is the eighth most common malignancy in women in the USA, with an annual incidence approaching 13,000 – one-third of whom will die. Both incidence and mortality are declining, however, due largely to preventive measures and early screening via the Papanicolaou exam. As many as 85–90% of cases are of the squamous cell type. Most of the remainder are adenocarcinomas, which are similar to squamous cell tumors in their pattern of spread and survival statistics at a given stage. Some adenocarcinomas have a bulky, "barrel-shaped" appearance,

which can cause them to be symptomatic earlier, and may contribute to their reported lower sensitivity to radiation therapy. Neuroendocrine-type small-cell carcinomas are rarely seen. Similar to small-cell tumors elsewhere, they present with early metastases (both lymphatic and hematogenous), and have a poor prognosis, even with aggressive therapy. Another rare tumor, glassy cell carcinoma, may represent a poorly differentiated variant of adenosquamous carcinoma; its prognosis is poor.

Squamous cell carcinoma of the cervix appears to develop, in many or perhaps most cases, through a sequence of increasing genetic and cytologic derangement (cervical intraepithelial neoplasia, or CIN), chiefly involving metaplastic epithelium at the junction of the squamous exocervix and glandular endocervix. Risk factors include smoking and low socioeconomic status. However, cervical cancer has long been recognized to be a sexually transmitted disease, and recent evidence has fairly conclusively identified infection by high-risk genotypes of human papillomavirus (particularly types 16 and 18) as a causative factor.

Abnormal vaginal bleeding (painless metrorrhagia or post-menopausal bleeding) is an early sign. Other symptoms, such as flank or leg pain, lymphedema, dysuria, obstipation, or rectal or urinary bleeding, are ominous tokens of advanced disease. Spread can occur by lymphatics, or by direct extension into the vagina, lower uterine segment, abutting viscera (chiefly bladder and rectum) or pelvic fascia. Primary lymphatic drainage is through paracervical (ureteral) and parametrial nodes, into obturator, hypogastric, and internal iliac stations. With more advanced disease, common iliac, inguinal, and paraaortic nodes may be involved.

Negative prognostic factors include large tumors, lymphovascular invasion, extracervical extension, deep stromal invasion, and extension to the serosa. Death, when it occurs, is most often due to uremia caused by local extension of tumor, with consequent ureteral obstruction.

Staging is mainly clinical, augmented by PET, CT, MR, or limited surgical exploration. For this purpose, a definitive pelvic physical examination may need to be performed under total anesthesia.

Treatment is highly dependent upon clinical stage. CIN itself may be treated locally, by electrocautery, cryosurgery, laser surgery, LEEP (loop electrosurgical excision procedure), or conization. Low-grade (stage I or IIa) invasive cancer typically requires radical hysterectomy with pelvic lymphadenectomy; post-operative chemotherapy and radiation therapy may be added if positive lymph nodes are found. For higher stage disease, surgery is rarely curative, and the mainstay of treatment is combination radiotherapy (often combining brachytherapy with external-beam radiation) and chemotherapy (usually with cisplatin). Paraaortic nodes are problematical; where these are involved, advanced disease is usually present, and neither radiation therapy nor surgery can offer sufficient benefit to outweigh the very considerable morbidity and mortality of treatment. It has been suggested that extended-field paraaortic irradiation be limited to patients with extensive pelvic nodal disease, but no overt evidence of paraaortic nodal involvement, on the rationale that this subgroup alone may be curable (1).

Pelvic exenteration is regarded by some authorities as the treatment of choice for locally advanced or recurrent disease. Any evidence of extrapelvic spread, or even of pelvic sidewall nodes, is an absolute contraindication for this complex and demanding procedure, as no survivals have been noted in the literature, except in the case of microscopic foci. Thus, accurate pre-operative staging is essential. The 5-year survival after surgery varies from 20% to 62% – considerably higher than for conventional palliative chemotherapy.

As many as 35% of patients with invasive cervical carcinoma will have recurrent or persistent disease, heralded by such symptoms as weight loss, pelvic or thigh pain, leg edema, hemoptysis, or a palpable left supraclavicular lymph node. The most common sites of recurrence include the parametrium and pelvic sidewall, upper vagina, and, more distantly, the liver, lung, and spine. It is extremely important to differentiate true recurrence from benign conditions such as cachexia due to radiation bowel injury, or radiation-induced horseshoe fibrosis of the parametria.

Surgery has little use in the setting of recurrence, although anecdotal cures have been reported after resection of a solitary lung or vaginal metastasis. Re-irradiation is also largely futile, with a salvage rate of no more than 10%, except for patients whose initial radiation therapy was suboptimal. The standard approach is palliative chemotherapy, usually with cisplatin and one or more ancillary agents. Results at present are bleak, with reported 1-year survival rates of 10–15%. Reasons for treatment failure include the development of chemoresistant subclones, poor vascularity of the previously irradiated tumor bed, and nephropathy from ureteral obstruction, which limits the dose for chemotherapy.

## Imaging considerations

For more than a decade, there has been clear and consistent evidence that both primary and metastatic cervical cancer is FDG avid. In recognition of this, cervical cancer was the first gynecologic pelvic malignancy to be approved for PET reimbursement by the Centers for Medicare and Medicaid Services. The high SUV of cervical tumors has been shown to correlate with increased levels of GLUT-1 expression. Intense uptake is seen in all histologic variants, with the highest SUVmax in squamous cell carcinoma, and slightly lower values in adenocarcinoma and adenosquamous tumors. As is the case for many tumors, the intensity of uptake is inversely related to the degree of cellular differentiation.

PET, of course, has no role to play in the diagnosis or treatment of cervical intraepithelial neoplasia (CIN), carcinoma in situ, or minimally invasive cancer (stage Ia). These lesions are all superficially accessible, and metastasis is vanishingly rare. However, several studies have looked at the utility of PET in detecting nodal involvement in patients with early-stage invasive cervical cancer (stages Ib to IIa) (2–5). These have generally shown mediocre sensitivity, particularly for nodes smaller than 5 mm, but high specificity (of 97% or more). Unfortunately, negative predictive values of 87–94% are too low to replace surgical lymphadenectomy for staging of these patients. The maximum SUV of the cervical lesion itself may have some prognostic value, with high values (> 13.4) predicting deep stromal invasion, lymphovascular involvement, and a poorer disease-free survival rate (6).

PET is on firmer ground for more advanced disease. At initial staging, the essential clinical task is the detection of involved lymph nodes and distant metastases, since the nature of the primary lesion is rarely in doubt, and MR and surgical staging are definitive for assessment of local extension of tumor. The advantage of PET over other imaging modalities increases with greater distance from the primary tumor site. PET has been shown to improve detection of paraaortic lymph node metastases (7), and to detect more metastatic sites than CT or MRI (8). However, quite variable sensitivities have been reported for dedicated PET, ranging from a disappointing 38% (9) to a stellar 91% (10); this most likely reflects weakness in detecting small nodes and micrometastases. For example, Roh *et al.* (9) showed that sensitivity increased from 52% to 65% as lymph nodes increased from 5 mm to 10 mm. Hybrid PET/CT performs a little better (11, 12), as does dual-phase PET performed at 40 min and 3 hours post-injection (13, 14). As lackluster as these values are, in head-to-head comparisons, PET still performs better than MRI (10), CT, or lymphangiography (8). PET has also been shown to identify many involved nodes in patients who are node-negative on MRI (15) or CT (16).

The undisputed advantage of PET in initial staging is its very high specificity, which has been reported to lie in the range 94–100% in virtually all studies (10, 12, 15–17).

For patients destined to receive irradiation, including brachytherapy and intensity modulated radiation therapy, PET provides a reliable estimate of tumor volume (18, 19), and improves dose coverage of the tumor, without increasing dose to adjacent organs, such as bladder and rectum (20). These refinements to the treatment protocol have been shown to improve patient survival (21).

As a metabolic indicator, FDG-PET is well-suited for the assessment of treatment response after chemotherapy (22) or irradiation (23). Complete metabolic responders have better survival statistics at both 6 months and 3 years (23, 24) after treatment. Even a mid-treatment PET can be useful for determining whether an alternative therapy should be considered (25). In general, any abnormal post-therapeutic uptake is predictive of recurrent metastasis and death (26). Grigsby *et al.*, for example, reported a 2-year progression-free survival of 86% in patients with negative PET after treatment, but only 40% if uptake persisted. If new sites of abnormal uptake appeared, all patients died (27). As with other tumors, changes in SUV correlate better with histological response than do anatomic findings on MRI (28).

In the pre-treatment setting, PET is a valuable prognostic tool. A large metabolic tumor volume correlates independently with higher FIGO stage and increased likelihood of lymph node metastases and parametrial involvement (29). A high SUVmax of the primary tumor similarly predicts lymph node involvement (30) and a higher rate of recurrence (31). In a study of 287 patients, Kidd *et al.* found a 5-year survival of 95% for patients with tumoral SUVmax less than 5.2, but only 44% with SUVmax greater than 13.3 (32). Thus, a high tumoral SUV may identify patients requiring more aggressive therapy (33). Higher uptake in metastatic nodes is also associated with increased risk of recurrence, post-therapeutic persistence of disease and death (34, 35).

The lymph node uptake pattern is also prognostically significant. Patients with PET-positive pelvic or paraaortic lymph nodes have poorer survival at 20 months (36), 2 years (37), and 3 years (38). In a study of 560 patients, Kidd *et al.* reported a hazard ratio for recurrence in patients with PET-positive pelvic nodes of 2.4, versus 5.88 for paraaortic and 30.27 for supraclavicular nodes (39). In particular, the positive predictive value of abnormal FDG uptake in a left supraclavicular lymph node (Virchow's node), has been reported to be 100% (40). This is an ominous finding, with nearly all patients dying within 2 or 3 years of detection (38–40).

Almost all studies to date have shown uniformly high PET sensitivity (range 80–100%) and specificity (range 76–100%) for disease recurrence, both locally and in the form of distant metastases (41–48). Both positive predictive value and negative predictive value are also high. These numbers hold true, not only for cases with high clinical suspicion, but also for asymptomatic patients undergoing routine surveillance (43, 48–51). As for many other tumors, PET/CT is more accurate than dedicated PET (11). The pick-up rate for metastases to lung and bone appears to be slightly lower than for lymph nodes, particularly for subcentimeter lesions (45, 52). Nonetheless, in general PET performs decidedly better than CT or MRI in direct match-ups (53–55). PET imaging has a significant impact on patient management in 23.1–55% of cases (42, 47, 53, 56).

## Take-home message

- FDG-PET should be considered as a first-line imaging modality for evaluating both symptomatic and asymptomatic patients for disease recurrence.
- FDG-PET or PET/CT is a useful adjunct for initial work-up of patients with invasive cervical cancer (stages IIb and above), providing lesion detection capability and prognostic information that is complementary to MRI.
- FDG-PET promises to be a superior tool for guiding radiation therapy and for assessing the results of neoadjuvant chemotherapy/radiation therapy prior to surgery.
- Any amount of residual uptake after therapy for cervical cancer is a poor prognostic sign. The appearance of new sites of uptake after therapy is particularly ominous.
- FDG-PET should be performed in every patient for whom pelvic exenteration is contemplated, as it can significantly reduce the number of futile procedures.

# References

1. Crawford JS, Harisiadis L, McGowan L, Rogers CC. Paraaortic lymph node irradiation in cervical carcinoma without prior lymphadenectomy. *Radiology* 1987;**164**(1):255–7.

2. Yu L, Jia C, Wang X *et al.* Evaluation of 18 F-FDG PET/CT in early-stage cervical carcinoma. *Am J Med Sci.* 2011;**341**(2):96–100.

3. Bentivegna E, Uzan C, Gouy S *et al.* Correlation between

[18f]fluorodeoxyglucose positron-emission tomography scan and histology of pelvic nodes in early-stage cervical cancer. *Anticancer Res* 2010;**30**(3):1029–32.

4. Boughanim M, Leboulleux S, Rey A *et al.* Histologic results of para-aortic lymphadenectomy in patients treated for stage IB2/II cervical cancer with negative [18F]fluorodeoxyglucose positron emission tomography scans in the para-aortic area. *J Clin Oncol* 2008 20;**26**(15):2558–61.

5. Sironi S, Buda A, Picchio M *et al.* Lymph node metastasis in patients with clinical early-stage cervical cancer: detection with integrated FDG PET/CT. *Radiology* 2006;**238**(1):272–9.

6. Lee YY, Choi CH, Kim CJ *et al.* The prognostic significance of the SUVmax (maximum standardized uptake value for F-18 fluorodeoxyglucose) of the cervical tumor in PET imaging for early cervical cancer: preliminary results. *Gynecol Oncol* 2009;**115**(1):65–8.

7. Tsai CS, Lai CH, Chang TC *et al.* A prospective randomized trial to study the impact of pretreatment FDG-PET for cervical cancer patients with MRI-detected positive pelvic but negative para-aortic lymphadenopathy. *Int J Radiat Oncol Biol Phys* 2010 1;**76**(2):477–84.

8. Grigsby PW, Dehdashti F, Siegel BA. FDG-PET evaluation of carcinoma of the cervix. *Can Positron Imaging* 1999;**2**(2):105–9.

9. Roh JW, Seo SS, Lee S *et al.* Role of positron emission tomography in pretreatment lymph node staging of uterine cervical cancer: a prospective surgicopathologic correlation study. *Eur J Cancer* 2005;**41**(14):2086–92.

10. Reinhardt MJ, Ehritt-Braun C, Vogelgesang D *et al.* Metastatic lymph nodes in patients with cervical cancer: detection with MR imaging and FDG PET. *Radiology* 2001;**218**(3):776–82.

11. Tatsumi M, Cohade C, Bristow RE, Wahl RL. Imaging uterine cervical cancer with FDG-PET/CT: direct comparison with PET. *Mol Imaging Biol* 2009;**11**(4):229–35.

12. Loft A, Berthelsen AK, Roed H *et al.* The diagnostic value of PET/CT scanning in patients with cervical cancer: a prospective study. *Gynecol Oncol* 2007;**106**(1):29–34.

13. Ma SY, See LC, Lai CH *et al.* Delayed (18)F-FDG PET for detection of paraaortic lymph node metastases in cervical cancer patients. *J Nucl Med* 2003;**44**(11):1775–83.

14. Yen TC, Ng KK, Ma SY *et al.* Value of dual-phase 2-fluoro-2-deoxy-d-glucose positron emission tomography in cervical cancer. *J Clin Oncol* 2003;**21**(19):3651–8.

15. Yeh LS, Hung YC, Shen YY *et al.* Detecting para-aortic lymph nodal metastasis by positron emission tomography of 18F-fluorodeoxyglucose in advanced cervical cancer with negative magnetic resonance imaging findings. *Oncol Rep* 2002;**9**(6):1289–92.

16. Lin WC, Hung YC, Yeh LS *et al.* Usefulness of (18)F-fluorodeoxyglucose positron emission tomography to detect para-aortic lymph nodal metastasis in advanced cervical cancer with negative computed tomography findings. *Gynecol Oncol* 2003;**89**(1):73–6.

17. Chung HH, Park NH, Kim JW *et al.* Role of integrated PET-CT in pelvic lymph node staging of cervical cancer before radical hysterectomy. *Gynecol Obstet Invest* 2009;**67**(1):61–6.

18. Malyapa RS, Mutic S, Low DA *et al.* Physiologic FDG-PET three-dimensional brachytherapy treatment planning for cervical cancer. *Int J Radiat Oncol Biol Phys* 2002;**54**(4):1140–6.

19. Dolezelova H, Slampa P, Ondrova B *et al.* The impact of PET with 18FDG in radiotherapy treatment planning and in the prediction in patients with cervix carcinoma: results of pilot study. *Neoplasma* 2008;**55**(5):437–41.

20. Lin LL, Mutic S, Low DA *et al.* Adaptive brachytherapy treatment planning for cervical cancer using FDG-PET. *Int J Radiat Oncol Biol Phys* 2007;**67**(1):91–6.

21. Kidd EA, Siegel BA, Dehdashti F *et al.* Clinical outcomes of definitive intensity-modulated radiation therapy with fluorodeoxyglucose-positron emission tomography simulation in patients with locally advanced cervical cancer. *Int J Radiat Oncol Biol Phys* 2010;**77**(4):1085–91.

22. Siva S, Herschtal A, Thomas JM *et al.* Impact of post-therapy positron emission tomography on prognostic stratification and surveillance after chemoradiotherapy for cervical cancer. *Cancer* 2011;**117**(17):3981–8.

23. Lin LL, Yang Z, Mutic S *et al.* FDG-PET imaging for the assessment of physiologic volume response during radiotherapy in cervix cancer. *Int J Radiat Oncol Biol Phys* 2006;**65**(1):177–81.

24. Schwarz JK, Siegel BA, Dehdashti F, Grigsby PW. Association of posttherapy positron emission tomography with tumor response and survival in cervical carcinoma. *J Am Med Assoc* 2007;**298**(19):2289–95.

25. Schwarz JK, Lin LL, Siegel BA *et al.* 18-F-fluorodeoxyglucose-positron emission tomography evaluation of early metabolic response during radiation therapy for cervical cancer. *Int J Radiat Oncol Biol Phys* 2008;**72**(5):1502–7.

26. Grigsby PW, Siegel BA, Dehdashti F *et al.* Posttherapy [18F] fluorodeoxyglucose positron emission tomography in carcinoma of the cervix: response and outcome. *J Clin Oncol* 2004;**22**(11):2167–71.

27. Grigsby PW, Siegel BA, Dehdashti F, Mutch DG. Posttherapy surveillance monitoring of cervical cancer by FDG-PET. *Int J Radiat Oncol Biol Phys* 2003;**55**(4):907–13.

28. Yoshida Y, Kurokawa T, Kawahara K *et al.* Metabolic monitoring of advanced uterine cervical cancer neoadjuvant chemotherapy by using [F-18]-Fluorodeoxyglucose positron emission tomography: preliminary results in three patients. *Gynecol Oncol* 2004;**95**(3):597–602.

29. Chung HH, Kim JW, Han KH *et al.* Prognostic value of metabolic tumor volume measured by FDG-PET/CT in patients with cervical cancer. *Gynecol Oncol* 2011;**120**(2):270–4.

30. Yilmaz M, Adli M, Celen Z *et al.* FDG PET-CT in cervical cancer: relationship between primary tumor FDG uptake and metastatic potential. *Nucl Med Commun* 2010;**31**(6):526–31.

31. Chung HH, Nam BH, Kim JW *et al.* Preoperative [18F]FDG PET/CT maximum standardized uptake value predicts recurrence of uterine cervical cancer. *Eur J Nucl Med Mol Imaging* 2010;**37**(8):1467–73.

32. Kidd EA, Siegel BA, Dehdashti F, Grigsby PW. The standardized uptake value for F-18 fluorodeoxyglucose is a

sensitive predictive biomarker for cervical cancer treatment response and survival. *Cancer* 2007;**110**(8):1738–44.

33. Yen TC, Lai CH, Ma SY *et al.* Comparative benefits and limitations of 18F-FDG PET and CT-MRI in documented or suspected recurrent cervical cancer. *Eur J Nucl Med Mol Imaging* 2006;**33**(12):1399–407.

34. Yen TC, See LC, Lai CH *et al.* Standardized uptake value in para-aortic lymph nodes is a significant prognostic factor in patients with primary advanced squamous cervical cancer. *Eur J Nucl Med Mol Imaging* 2008;**35**(3):493–501.

35. Kidd EA, Siegel BA, Dehdashti F, Grigsby PW. Pelvic lymph node F-18 fluorodeoxyglucose uptake as a prognostic biomarker in newly diagnosed patients with locally advanced cervical cancer. *Cancer* 2010;**116**(6):1469–75.

36. Unger JB, Lilien DL, Caldito G *et al.* The prognostic value of pretreatment 2-[18F]-fluoro-2-deoxy-D-glucose positron emission tomography scan in women with cervical cancer. *Int J Gynecol Cancer* 2007;**17**(5):1062–7.

37. Grigsby PW, Siegel BA, Dehdashti F. Lymph node staging by positron emission tomography in patients with carcinoma of the cervix. *J Clin Oncol* 2001;**19**(17):3745–9.

38. Singh AK, Grigsby PW, Dehdashti F *et al.* FDG-PET lymph node staging and survival of patients with FIGO stage IIIb cervical carcinoma. *Int J Radiat Oncol Biol Phys* 2003;**56**(2):489–93.

39. Kidd EA, Siegel BA, Dehdashti F *et al.* Lymph node staging by positron emission tomography in cervical cancer: relationship to prognosis. *J Clin Oncol* 2010;**28**(12):2108–13.

40. Tran BN, Grigsby PW, Dehdashti F *et al.* Occult supraclavicular lymph node metastasis identified by FDG-PET in patients with carcinoma of the uterine cervix. *Gynecol Oncol* 2003;**90** (3):572–6.

41. Unger JB, Ivy JJ, Connor P *et al.* Detection of recurrent cervical cancer by whole-body FDG PET scan in asymptomatic and symptomatic women. *Gynecol Oncol* 2004;**94**(1):212–16.

42. Chung HH, Jo H, Kang WJ *et al.* Clinical impact of integrated PET/CT on the management of suspected cervical cancer recurrence. *Gynecol Oncol* 2007;**104**(3):529–34.

43. Kitajima K, Murakami K, Yamasaki E *et al.* Performance of FDG-PET/CT for diagnosis of recurrent uterine cervical cancer. *Eur Radiol* 2008;**18**(10):2040–7.

44. Havrilesky LJ, Wong TZ, Secord AA *et al.* The role of PET scanning in the detection of recurrent cervical cancer. *Gynecol Oncol* 2003;**90**(1):186–90.

45. Ryu SY, Kim MH, Choi SC *et al.* Detection of early recurrence with 18F-FDG PET in patients with cervical cancer. *J Nucl Med* 2003;**44**(3):347–52.

46. Sun SS, Chen TC, Yen RF *et al.* Value of whole body 18F-fluoro-2-deoxyglucose positron emission tomography in the evaluation of recurrent cervical cancer. *Anticancer Res* 2001;**21**(4B):2957–61.

47. van der Veldt AA, Buist MR, van Baal MW *et al.* Clarifying the diagnosis of clinically suspected recurrence of cervical cancer: impact of 18F-FDG PET. *J Nucl Med* 2008;**49**(12):1936–43.

48. Mittra E, El-Maghraby T, Rodriguez CA *et al.* Efficacy of 18F-FDG PET/CT in the evaluation of patients with recurrent cervical carcinoma. *Eur J Nucl Med Mol Imaging* 2009;**36**(12):1952–9.

49. Chang WC, Hung YC, Lin CC *et al.* Usefulness of FDG-PET to detect recurrent cervical cancer based on asymptomatically elevated tumor marker serum levels – a preliminary report. *Cancer Invest* 2004;**22**(2):180–4.

50. Chung HH, Kim SK, Kim TH *et al.* Clinical impact of FDG-PET imaging in post-therapy surveillance of uterine cervical cancer: from diagnosis to prognosis. *Gynecol Oncol* 2006;**103** (1):165–70.

51. Brooks RA, Rader JS, Dehdashti F *et al.* Surveillance FDG-PET detection of asymptomatic recurrences in patients with cervical cancer. *Gynecol Oncol* 2009;**112**(1):104–9.

52. Sakurai H, Suzuki Y, Nonaka T *et al.* FDG-PET in the detection of recurrence of uterine cervical carcinoma following radiation therapy – tumor volume and FDG uptake value. *Gynecol Oncol* 2006;**100**(3):601–7.

53. Lai CH, Huang KG, See LC *et al.* Restaging of recurrent cervical carcinoma with dual-phase [18F]fluoro-2-deoxy-D-glucose positron emission tomography. *Cancer* 2004;**100**(3):544–52.

54. Yen TC, Lai CH, Ma SY *et al.* Comparative benefits and limitations of 18F-FDG PET and CT-MRI in documented or suspected recurrent cervical cancer. *Eur J Nucl Med Mol Imaging* 2006;**33**(12):1399–407.

55. Liu FY, Yen TC, Chen MY *et al.* Detection of hematogenous bone metastasis in cervical cancer: 18F-fluorodeoxyglucose-positron emission tomography versus computed tomography and magnetic resonance imaging. *Cancer* 2009;**115**(23):5470–80.

56. Pallardy A, Bodet-Milin C, Oudoux A *et al.* Clinical and survival impact of FDG PET in patients with suspicion of recurrent cervical carcinoma. *Eur J Nucl Med Mol Imaging* 2010;**37**(7):1270–8.

# Endometrial adenocarcinoma

A 56-year-old female underwent FDG-PET/CT for evaluation of a suspicious lung nodule (later shown to be adenocarcinoma with features of bronchioloalveolar carcinoma). She had previously had a right salpingo-oophorectomy at age 19 for a benign condition.

## Findings and differential diagnosis

but not the cervix. The tumor was grade I based on architectural features, but had focal areas of cytologic atypia which indicated a cytologic grade of II. The tumor invaded 25% of the thickness of the uterine wall.

Although risk of recurrence in the vaginal vault was relatively low (about 9%), the patient elected to have vaginal cylinder brachytherapy 5 weeks after surgery. She has been disease-free since that time.

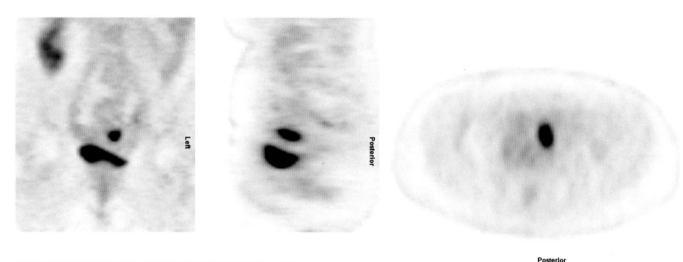

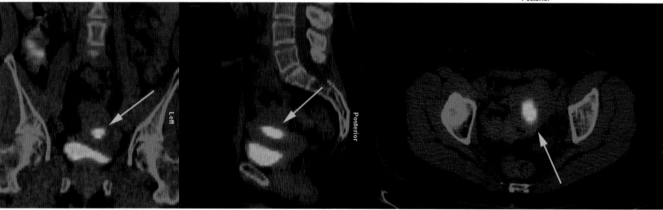

**Figure 12.10** There is uptake in the uterine cavity (blue arrow) which is too intense to be attributable to menstrual endometrial uptake. A 1-cm ground-glass opacity (not shown) was also seen in the upper lobe of the right lung; this later proved to be a well-differentiated pulmonary adenocarcinoma, unrelated to the uterine tumor.

## Diagnosis and clinical follow-up

A biopsy performed the day after PET/CT showed a grade I endometrial adenocarcinoma. A week later, a total abdominal hysterectomy with left sided salpingo-oophorectomy was performed. Post-operative pathologic examination showed endometrial adenocarcinoma involving the lower uterine segment,

## Discussion and teaching points
### Clinical background

This lesion was found incidentally on a FDG-PET/CT study performed for a lung nodule. It underscores the importance of scrutinizing all parts of the exam. Abnormal incidental findings that cannot be explained by the patient's history should be communicated promptly to the referring physician (preferably in person or by telephone), along with the differential diagnosis and any recommendations for follow-up. Simply describing areas of abnormal uptake is not adequate, if their significance is not made clear. Busy referring physicians may overlook such findings if they are not alerted to the possibility that cancer may be present.

Endometrial adenocarcinoma is the most common pelvic malignancy among women in the USA. Most patients are in the sixth decade, although a significant number (5–30%) are premenopausal. Risk factors include obesity, nulliparity, late menopause, unopposed estrogenism, and diabetes. Tamoxifen therapy reportedly carries a slight risk. Endometrial adenocarcinoma has also been associated with hereditary non-polyposis colon cancer syndrome (HNPCC).

Histologically, 84% of these tumors are of an endometrioid type. One-quarter have focal squamous differentiation, which must be distinguished from pure squamous cell carcinoma of the uterus, a rare tumor (0.04% of cases) with a much poorer prognosis. Papillary serous adenocarcinoma (4.5% of cases) is a highly aggressive tumor that tends to show widespread extrauterine involvement (including peritoneal carcinomatosis – otherwise rare for uterine tumors), even for lesions that appear minimally invasive at the primary site. Clear cell adenocarcinoma (2.5% of cases) is seen in older women in the seventh decade. Like similar tumors of the ovary, vagina, and cervix, it has a strong association with exposure *in utero* to diethylstilbestrol (DES), a synthetic non-steroidal estrogen that was formerly prescribed to prevent miscarriages. Mucinous adenocarcinoma (0.9% of cases) is similar to endometrioid adenocarcinoma, in terms of biological behavior, treatment, and prognosis. Metastases to the uterus are occasionally seen. These are most commonly from ovarian and cervical primaries, although tumors of the breast (especially lobular carcinoma), colon, stomach, and pancreas may also turn up.

As many as one-quarter of patients who are initially classified as having locally limited disease (stage I) will show extrauterine involvement on closer examination. Spread is most commonly by direct extension (to the cervix, bladder, rectum, broad ligament, or adnexae), or by lymphatics. Tumors in the upper uterine segment tend to follow ovarian vessels to para-aortic nodes in the upper abdomen. Tumors in the mid- and lower uterus follow the broad ligament toward pelvic nodes, or, less commonly, may pass via the round ligament to superficial inguinal nodes. Peritoneal spread may occur through the fallopian tubes, or from tumors that have broken through the uterine serosa. Hematogenous spread is uncommon, but can occasionally be seen to lung, liver, bone, and brain. Occult metastases to the ovary are seen in 10–15% of cases, particularly from tumors in the lower uterine segment; these should be sought for on every PET/CT scan performed for preoperative staging.

Most endometrioid adenocarcinomas are estrogen-related (probably derived from a precursor lesion, atypical endometrial hyperplasia), and these tend to be better differentiated and show a better prognosis than non-estrogen-related tumors, which typically develop from atrophic endometrium in older patients. Unfavorable prognostic features include a high proportion of squamous component, invasion through more than half the thickness of the myometrial wall, lymphovascular invasion, and extension to the cervix, positive peritoneal cytology, lymph node involvement, or adnexal spread.

Treatment is primarily surgical. The standard protocol for stage I disease consists of extrafascial hysterectomy, with or without salpingo-oophorectomy. If the cervix is involved, a radical hysterectomy is customary. Lymphadenectomy may improve survival, both for stage I and higher-risk disease, and is often elected if there is deep myometrial invasion or involvement of the cervix. The role of radiation therapy is under debate: evidence suggests that it may inhibit local recurrence but offers little improvement in long-term survival (1). Preoperative intracavitary irradiation is commonly performed to prevent vaginal recurrence, particularly if the cervix is involved. For disease that is more advanced, but still confined to the pelvis, post-operative pelvic irradiation may be given. Given the aggressiveness of papillary serous and clear-cell tumors, whole-abdominal irradiation is indicated. If peritoneal carcinomatosis is suggested by cytology, intraperitoneal $^{32}$P may be considered. Chemotherapy with doxorubicin/cisplatin is under investigation; it may have some utility in cases of advanced disease.

Five-year survival is 81–91% for stage I; 71–79% for stage II; 30–60% for stage III; and 15–17% for stage IV (2). Recurrence to the vaginal vault can be treated with surgery and/or radiation therapy. More distant sites of recurrence are problematical; hormonal or chemotherapy is generally performed, although efficacy is limited. Solitary recurrences in some cases may be amenable to external beam irradiation.

## Imaging considerations

To date, only a handful of relatively small-scale studies have evaluated FDG-PET for the initial assessment of endometrial adenocarcinoma. While sensitivity for the primary tumor appears to be high (on the order of 84–96.7%) (3, 4), most tumors will have been diagnosed by direct biopsy. The real task for imaging is to determine the extent of extrauterine disease, and here the results for PET have been mixed. For nodal involvement, both patient-based and lesion-based sensitivities are disappointingly low (ranging from 50% to 77.8%) (3–8), largely reflecting the difficulty of detecting small nodes (6). Specificities, however, are uniformly high (94–100%). Thus, while there is no question of PET replacing surgical lymphadenectomy for staging purposes, PET may help to select patients who may benefit from lymphadenectomy, and rule out this highly invasive procedure in those who already have distant metastases or rampant nodal disease (5).

PET does much better in detecting distant metastases, with a sensitivity of 83.3–100% – better than CT or MRI (3, 8). PET may also have prognostic value, inasmuch as high SUVmax of the primary tumor appears to correlate with increased aggressiveness, as reflected in higher FIGO grade (9).

For detection and staging of recurrence, FDG-PET has performed well on all reports to date. Sensitivity and specificity for dedicated PET, for example, were reported to be 96% and 78%, respectively, with a positive predictive value of 89% and negative predictive value of 91% (10). Several studies have shown that PET statistics improve when combined with CT or MRI (11–13). In the most recent studies with hybrid PET/CT, sensitivity (range 90.9 to 100%) and specificity (range 93.5 to 100%) have both been high (13–15). These are superior to reported values for MRI or CT (sensitivity 68.2–84.6% and specificity 85.7–87%) (12, 13). FDG-PET or PET/CT imaging had a significant impact on patient management in 22.6–48.3% of cases. Given these consistently good results, FDG-PET/CT should be considered as a first-line imaging modality for surveillance of recurrence in patients with a history of endometrial adenocarcinoma.

## Take-home message

- Any amount of endometrial FDG uptake in a postmenopausal woman who is not taking hormone supplements should be regarded as abnormal. The differential diagnosis, which includes endometrial hyperplasia (typical or atypical) versus adenocarcinoma, cannot be resolved by PET/CT imaging, but requires a full gynecologic work-up, including endometrial biopsy if indicated.
- 25% of patients with apparently limited-stage endometrial adenocarcinoma will turn out to have extrauterine spread after complete staging. While FDG-PET/CT cannot replace MRI for evaluation of the parametria and other local structures, it is a useful adjunct for detecting nodal involvement and distant metastases.
- FDG-PET/CT should be considered the imaging modality of choice for detecting and staging recurrence.
- FDG-PET/CT is a useful preliminary to surgical lymphadenectomy, obviating unnecessary procedures in patients with advanced disease. However, it has too little sensitivity for small nodes to replace lymphadenectomy altogether.

## References

1. Onsrud M, Kolstad P, Normann T. Postoperative external pelvic irradiation in carcinoma of the corpus stage I: a controlled clinical trial. *Gynecol Oncol* 1976;**4**(2):222–31.

2. Creasman WT, Odicino F, Maisonneuve P et al. Carcinoma of the corpus uteri. *Int J Gynaecol Obstet* 2003; **83**(Suppl 1):79–118.

3. Picchio M, Mangili G, Samanes Gajate AM et al. High-grade endometrial cancer: value of [18F]FDG PET/CT in preoperative staging. *Nucl Med Commun* 2010;**31**(6):506–12.

4. Horowitz NS, Dehdashti F, Herzog TJ et al. Prospective evaluation of FDG-PET for detecting pelvic and para-aortic lymph node metastasis in uterine corpus cancer. *Gynecol Oncol* 2004; **95**(3):546–51.

5. Signorelli M, Guerra L, Buda A et al. Role of the integrated FDG PET/CT in the surgical management of patients with high risk clinical early stage endometrial cancer: detection of pelvic nodal metastases. *Gynecol Oncol* 2009; **115**(2):231–5.

6. Kitajima K, Murakami K, Yamasaki E et al. Accuracy of integrated FDG-PET/contrast-enhanced CT in detecting pelvic and paraaortic lymph node metastasis in patients with uterine cancer. *Eur Radiol* 2009;**19**(6):1529–36.

7. Nayot D, Kwon JS, Carey MS, Driedger A. Does preoperative positron emission tomography with computed tomography predict nodal status in endometrial cancer? A pilot study. *Curr Oncol* 2008;**15**(3):123–5.

8. Suzuki R, Miyagi E, Takahashi N et al. Validity of positron emission tomography using fluoro-2-deoxyglucose for the preoperative evaluation of endometrial cancer. *Int J Gynecol Cancer* 2007;**17**(4):890–6.

9. Nakamura K, Kodama J, Okumura Y et al. The SUVmax of 18F-FDG PET correlates with histological grade in endometrial cancer. *Int J Gynecol Cancer* 2010;**20**(1):110–15.

10. Belhocine T, De Barsy C, Hustinx R, Willems-Foidart J. Usefulness of (18)F-FDG PET in the post-therapy surveillance of endometrial carcinoma. *Eur J Nucl Med Mol Imaging* 2002; **29**(9):1132–9.

11. Chao A, Chang TC, Ng KK et al. 18F-FDG PET in the management of endometrial cancer. *Eur J Nucl Med Mol Imaging* 2006;**33**(1):36–44.

12. Saga T, Higashi T, Ishimori T et al. Clinical value of FDG-PET in the follow up of post-operative patients with endometrial cancer. *Ann Nucl Med* 2003;**17**(3):197–203.

13. Kitajima K, Murakami K, Yamasaki E et al. Performance of integrated FDG-PET/contrast-enhanced CT in the diagnosis of recurrent uterine cancer: comparison with PET and enhanced CT. *Eur J Nucl Med Mol Imaging* 2009;**36**(3):362–72.

14. Chung HH, Kang WJ, Kim JW et al. The clinical impact of [(18)F]FDG PET/CT for the management of recurrent endometrial cancer: correlation with clinical and histological findings. *Eur J Nucl Med Mol Imaging* 2008; **35**(6):1081–8.

15. Sironi S, Picchio M, Landoni C et al. Post-therapy surveillance of patients with uterine cancers: value of integrated FDG PET/CT in the detection of recurrence. *Eur J Nucl Med Mol Imaging* 2007;**34**(4):472–9.

# Uterine carcinosarcoma

A 19-year-old female presented with weight loss, intensifying pelvic and flank pain, and an 8-month history of vaginal bleeding. Her hematocrit on admission was 22.0, requiring transfusion. Abdominal CT disclosed a 16.7 × 10.2 cm pelvic mass. The patient underwent total abdominal hysterectomy, left salpingo-oophorectomy, omentectomy, and pelvic lymph node dissection; however, a large paraaortic mass was deemed unresectable. Pathologic examination reported a large, fleshy, friable, hemorrhagic, and necrotic mass arising from the uterus, composed of both a poorly differentiated carcinomatous element (30%), and a high-grade, undifferentiated sarcomatous element (70%), with focal myxoid features. One month later, a follow-up FDG-PET/CT was performed.

## Findings and differential diagnosis

## Diagnosis and clinical follow-up

Diagnosis of residual carcinosarcoma of the uterus, with peritoneal carcinomatosis and a metastatic left supraclavicular node. The patient received palliative chemotherapy with gemcitabine and taxotere. She died after resumption of hemorrhage, 2 weeks after her PET/CT scan.

## Discussion and teaching points
### Clinical background

Sarcomas represent up to 8% of uterine malignancies. About half of these tumors are carcinosarcomas, with the remainder composed of leiomyosarcomas, endometrial stromal sarcomas, and adenosarcomas.

Carcinosarcomas, also known as malignant mixed Müllerian tumors, contain both epithelial and stromal elements, both

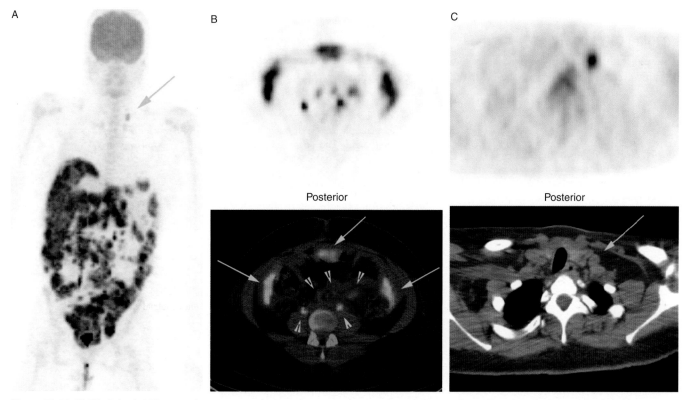

A      B      C

Posterior      Posterior

**Figure 12.11** (A) Whole-body MIP image shows extensive peritoneal carcinomatosis, encasing the liver and extending down both paracolic gutters to envelop the ascending colon and adjacent bowel loops. A metastatic left supraclavicular lymph node is also visible (blue arrow). (B) Peritoneal carcinomatosis (blue arrows) is demonstrated, partly encasing bowel. Numerous metastatic lymph nodes are also present (blue arrowheads). (C) The metastatic left supraclavicular lymph node is clearly visible on both FDG-PET and CT.

of which are malignant. The epithelial component is usually endometrioid in appearance. The stromal component may be of a uterine type, or it may contain heterologous elements, such as bone or cartilage. Pelvic irradiation appears to be a risk factor. Most patients are post-menopausal, and more than 60% of them will have extrauterine spread at the time of diagnosis. Lung metastases, in particular, are common, and often will consist of only the epithelial component of the tumor. The prognosis is correspondingly poor. Treatment is surgical, consisting of total hysterectomy with bilateral salpingo-oophorectomy and thorough pelvic and paraaortic lymph node dissection. Adjuvant therapies are of limited use. Radiation therapy decreases the incidence of local recurrences, but has no effect upon distant metastases or survival. Chemotherapy has not been proven effective, although trials with ifosfamide and cisplatin are ongoing.

Endometrial stromal sarcomas are monophasic tumors, without an epithelial component. Histological grade is significant. A low-grade type is compatible with prolonged survival, although recurrences are common. High-grade tumors have a poor prognosis, similar to that of carcinosarcoma. Treatment is surgical, consisting of total hysterectomy with bilateral salpingo-oophorectomy. The role of lymph node dissection is under debate.

Adenosarcomas are biphasic, combining a malignant stromal component with benign-appearing epithelial elements. They have a relatively low malignant potential.

## Imaging considerations

Although only a handful of studies of FDG-PET imaging of uterine sarcomas have been published, they have uniformly reported high uptake, with detection rates equivalent to or slightly better than CT or MR, both for primary (1, 2) and recurrent tumors (3, 4). In the largest series of 36 patients, who received either FDG-PET or PET/CT scans for sarcoma recurrence, Park *et al.* reported a positive predictive value of 100% for patients with clinical suspicion of recurrence and a negative predictive value of 95.5% for asymptomatic patients (4). Sensitivity, specificity, and accuracy were all uniformly high, ranging from 87.5% to 100%. Sung *et al.* (3) also reported that FDG-PET was particularly good at detecting extrapelvic metastases, which are found in 80% of cases of sarcoma recurrences. This evidence, limited as it is, is unambiguously in favor of a key role for FDG-PET/CT, both for pre-operative staging and detection of recurrence in women with known or suspected uterine sarcoma.

## Take-home message

- Although many uterine sarcomas have a bleak prognosis, there is an important subset of these tumors (chiefly low-grade stromal sarcomas and adenosarcomas) that is eminently treatable.
- Although literature is scanty, FDG-PET/CT appears to have an excellent potential for the detection of tumor recurrence. It may also be useful for primary staging.
- FDG-PET/CT is especially valuable for the detection of distant metastases, which are particularly common for this group of tumors.

## References

1. Nagamatsu A, Umesaki N, Li L, Tanaka T. Use of 18F-fluorodeoxyglucose positron emission tomography for diagnosis of uterine sarcomas. *Oncol Rep* 2010;**23**(4):1069–76.

2. Umesaki N, Tanaka T, Miyama M *et al.* Positron emission tomography with (18)F-fluorodeoxyglucose of uterine sarcoma: a comparison with magnetic resonance imaging and power Doppler imaging. *Gynecol Oncol* 2001; **80**(3):372–7.

3. Sung PL, Chen YJ, Liu RS *et al.* Whole-body positron emission tomography with 18F-fluorodeoxyglucose is an effective method to detect extra-pelvic recurrence in uterine sarcomas. *Eur J Gynaecol Oncol* 2008;**29**(3):246–51.

4. Park JY, Kim EN, Kim DY *et al.* Role of PET or PET/CT in the post-therapy surveillance of uterine sarcoma. *Gynecol Oncol* 2008;**109**(2):255–62.

# Uterine leiomyosarcoma

A 54-year-old menopausal female who had been receiving Coumadin for atrial fibrillation presented with vaginal bleeding, which was treated with dilation and curettage. Two months later she experienced renewed vaginal bleeding, intermittent at first, then massive and requiring blood transfusion and intrauterine tamponade with a Foley catheter. Abdominal CT showed a bulky uterus with multiple leiomyomata, the largest of which measured 11 cm. However, a concurrent chest CT also showed multiple bilateral pulmonary nodules, ranging in size from 3 mm to 2.1 cm. A FDG-PET/CT was performed.

## Findings and differential diagnosis

## Diagnosis and clinical follow-up

Diagnosis of uterine leiomyosarcoma, with metastases to lung. The patient was not considered a surgical candidate. External-beam radiation therapy was planned, but not started. A month later, she complained of diplopia. A head CT showed no evidence of brain metastasis or infarct, and cerebrospinal fluid yielded no malignant cells. A week later, she went into septic shock and died.

## Discussion and teaching points
### Clinical background

Leiomyosarcomas are pure sarcomatous tumors, derived from uterine myometrium. They tend to occur in a younger age

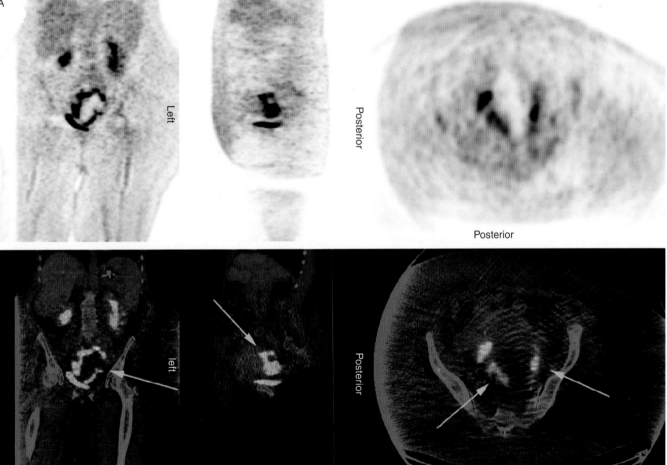

**Figure 12.12.** (A) A 12 × 11 cm soft-tissue mass in the uterus (blue arrows) shows heterogeneous uptake, with a rim of intense FDG avidity, and a large central area of photopenia, representing tumor necrosis. (B) and (C) FDG-avid nodules (blue arrows) are seen in the left lung, consistent with metastases.

317

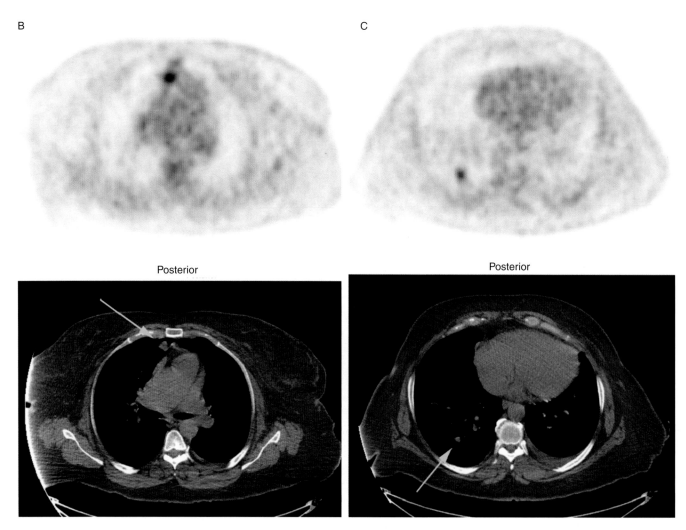

B

C

Posterior

Posterior

**Figure 12.12** (cont.)

group, often heralded by pain or menorrhagia. Many are found incidentally, after resection of a presumed leiomyoma. By conventional anatomic imaging, or even by histology, they can be difficult to distinguish from benign leiomyomas, although necrosis is a tell-tale sign. (This is made even more difficult by the existence of so-called benign metastasizing leiomyomas, which can spread to lungs, lymph nodes, or other organs in the form of non-invasive, benign-appearing nodules.) Spread is mainly hematogenous, typically resulting in metastases to lung (seen in 10% of patients at initial diagnosis), kidney, and liver. Prognosis is poor, even worse than for carcinosarcoma. Premenopausal women fare better, with a 5-year survival of 63.6%; however, for post-menopausal women the outlook is indeed grim, with a 5-year survival of only 5.5%. Treatment is by total hysterectomy. Given the hematogenous predilections of this tumor, the utility of nodal dissection is debatable; for those tumors found incidentally, re-operation for nodal staging is generally avoided. No adjuvant therapy has been shown to prolong survival.

## Imaging considerations

As for other types of uterine sarcomas, published efficacy data for FDG-PET or PET/CT are scanty, but studies consistently report high uptake. Nagamatsu *et al.* (1) showed that PET may be instrumental for making the key distinction between leiomyosarcoma and benign leiomyoma in a primary uterine mass. Although the accuracy of PET alone was only 73%, this rose to 100% when interpreted in conjunction with serum levels of lactate dehydrogenase isoenzyme-3, which are selectively elevated in leiomyosarcomas. Other studies (2, 3) have reported high accuracy for PET or PET/CT in detecting tumor recurrences, particularly distant metastases.

### Take-home message

- Although literature is scanty, FDG-PET/CT appears to be accurate for detecting recurrent leiomyosarcoma.
- Given the consistently high FDG uptake of these tumors, PET/CT may have some utility for differentiating

leiomyosarcomas from benign fibroids, particularly in combination with serum LDH levels.

- The presence of necrosis is a fairly specific sign of leiomyosarcoma.
- In both primary work-up and restaging for suspected recurrence, FDG-PET/CT can be valuable for detecting

distant metastases, which are particularly common among these patients. The lung, kidney, and liver should be scrutinized in every case of leiomyosarcoma.

# References

1. Nagamatsu A, Umesaki N, Li L, Tanaka T. Use of 18F-fluorodeoxyglucose positron emission tomography for diagnosis of uterine sarcomas. *Oncol Rep* 2010;**23**(4):1069–76.

2. Sung PL, Chen YJ, Liu RS *et al.* Whole-body positron emission tomography with 18F-fluorodeoxyglucose is an effective method to detect extra-pelvic recurrence in uterine sarcomas. *Eur J Gynaecol Oncol* 2008;**29**(3):246–51.

3. Park JY, Kim EN, Kim DY *et al.* Role of PET or PET/CT in the post-therapy surveillance of uterine sarcoma. *Gynecol Oncol* 2008;**109**(2):255–62.

A 44-year-old female presented with increasing abdominal girth, bloating, and shortness of breath. Abdominal CT showed extensive ascites, an ovarian mass, and numerous peritoneal implants. The CA125 level was 70. The patient underwent a percutaneous needle biopsy of the ovarian mass, which showed a malignant spindle cell neoplasm, poorly differentiated, with focal areas of necrosis. A FDG-PET/CT was performed.

## Findings and differential diagnosis

## Diagnosis and clinical follow-up

Diagnosis of poorly differentiated ovarian carcinoma, with peritoneal carcinomatosis. The patient was scheduled for neoadjuvant chemotherapy with carboplatin and taxol, to be followed by debulking surgery.

## Discussion and teaching points
### Clinical background

Ovarian cancer is the most common fatal cancer of the female genital tract (53% of deaths), and the fourth most common

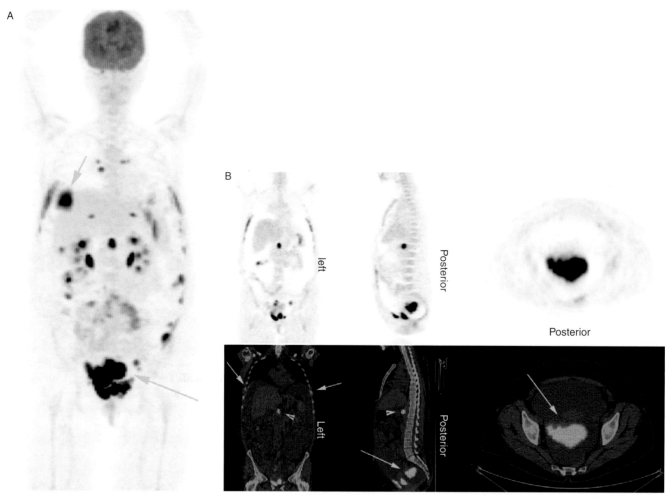

**Figure 12.13** (A) Whole-body MIP image shows an intensely-FDG-avid 8.8 × 5.5 cm right adnexal soft tissue mass (long blue arrow), along with a hepatic metastasis (short blue arrow), and extensive peritoneal carcinomatosis and abdominal and mediastinal lymph nodal spread. (B) The primary adnexal tumor is again identified (long blue arrow), along with sites of peritoneal carcinomatosis (short blue arrows), and a 1.7 cm metastatic lymph node adjacent to the origin of the superior mesenteric artery (blue arrowhead). Extensive ascites is present throughout the abdomen and pelvis.

fatal cancer in women overall. Despite improvements in chemotherapeutic regimens and surgical technique, mortality has changed little over decades. Risk factors are still poorly understood: incidence is higher in industrialized countries; infertility increases risk; and modern combination oral contraceptives and daily acetaminophen appear to be protective. Perhaps 10% of cases are hereditary, with associations to mutations in BRCA1 (or to a lesser extent BRCA2), and to other disorders such as Type II Lynch syndrome.

Due to the overall low incidence, there is no economically viable screening method, which is unfortunate, since most ovarian tumors are asymptomatic until late, when pain may incidentally arise due to torsion, rupture, or infection. Most tumors are detected by manual pelvic exam or by transvaginal ultrasound.

*Epithelial carcinomas.* 85–90% of ovarian malignancies are of epithelial origin: 42% are serous cystadenocarcinomas; 17% undifferentiated; 15% endometrioid; 12% mucinous; and 6% of clear cell type. Most tumors in this group behave similarly; while stage and histological grade are prognostically significant, the specific histological type is not.

For epithelial cancers, spread is predominantly intraperitoneal. This is conventionally assumed to occur through breach of the mesovarium; however, it has been proposed that peritoneal involvement may also result from multifocal disease originating from coelomic epithelium (indeed, peritoneal carcinomatosis of an ovarian serous papillary type has been described in the absence of any identifiable ovarian tumors) (1). Local spread to the uterus, fallopian tubes, and bowel is common. Involvement of pelvic and retroperitoneal nodes may arise through channels in the infundibulopelvic ligament. However, metastasis to distant vital organs is relatively rare, even in advanced stage disease. Death is usually related to obstruction of the gastrointestinal tract (malnutrition and electrolyte imbalance) or to protein loss from repeated paracenteses.

A much better prognosis is seen in the case of tumors of so-called borderline malignant potential. Seen most often in younger patients, these tumors have a 95% 10-year survival, with even cases of advanced-stage disease tending to do well. A quarter of these patients, however, will eventually die from recurrences (typically peritoneal), which can appear decades after initial treatment. Hence, long-term – even life-long – follow-up is mandatory. Standard treatment is by total hysterectomy with bilateral salpingo-oophorectomy; however, a more conservative approach has been advocated for patients of childbearing age who wish to preserve fertility.

For invasive tumors, staging is critical for determining a plan of treatment. For stage I disease, the preferred course is total hysterectomy/bilateral salpingo-oophorectomy, usually with omentectomy and pelvic and periaortic lymphadenectomy; however, for younger stage Ia patients who want to preserve fertility, unilateral salpingo-oophorectomy may be considered. For stage II disease, adjuvant chemotherapy is often added (typically with platinum-based agents). Stage III and IV disease, by definition, is not to be cured with the knife; treatment usually consists of surgical debulking, followed by chemotherapy (usually with multiple agents such as carboplatin and paclitaxel), and often by a second-look laparotomy if the response to chemotherapy is good. For high-risk patients, neoadjuvant chemotherapy may sometimes be used to shrink tumors prior to debulking.

Radiation therapy is of limited usefulness, since once disease begins to spread, the entire pelvis and abdomen must be targeted. Intraperitoneal administration of radioisotopic therapy agents (phosphorus-32-chromic phosphate, gold-198) has little effect upon bulky disease, or upon retroperitoneal lymph nodes (metastatic lymph nodes are non-functional and do not take up the radioisotopes). Some studies have shown potentiation of chemotherapy by co-injection of immunogenic organisms such as *Corynebacterium parvum*, or **Bacillus Calmette–Guérin** (BCG), however this technique is still under investigation.

*Sex cord-stromal tumors.* Five percent of ovarian tumors are of sex cord-stromal derivation. Many of these are hormonally active. **Granulosa-cell tumors** can be highly estrogenic, to the extent that up to 10% of patients may develop a secondary estrogen-dependent endometrial carcinoma, which should always be sought for during pre-operative staging. Inhibin is a specific tumor marker used for following post-menopausal patients. **Juvenile granulosa-cell tumors** can cause sexual precocity in children. 98% of these are stage I at diagnosis; however, advanced stage disease, when present, can be very aggressive. **Thecomas** are also estrogenic; they typically have a benign course. **Fibromas** are hormonally inactive. They, too, are benign, but are often associated with ascites or hydrothorax (Meigs' syndrome), due to increased capillary permeability due to secretion of vascular endothelial growth factor (VEGF). **Sertoli–Leydig cell tumors** (androblastomas) are typically virilizing due to secretion of testosterone or other androgens. They are of low malignant potential, unless poorly differentiated or heterologous elements are present.

Treatment of sex cord-stromal tumors reflects their relatively indolent behavior, and consists of salpingo-oophorectomy (unilateral in younger patients, bilateral after menopause) ± hysterectomy. Chemotherapy is reserved for those uncommon tumors with advanced stage or high-risk features on histology.

*Germ cell tumors.* These are derived from primitive germ cells of the embryonic gonad. They include numerous histologic subtypes, such as dysgerminoma, gonadoblastoma, endodermal sinus tumor, embryonal carcinoma, polyembroma and mature and immature teratoma. Many of these have strikingly similar male counterparts. Ninety-seven percent of them are benign. They are typically found in younger women (often during pregnancy), presenting as a palpable abdominal mass or pain. Most are highly chemosensitive and radiosensitive, and even aggressive, advanced-stage tumors are curable in a large majority of cases. The standard approach consists of surgical resection or debulking, followed by combination chemotherapy (the standard regimen consisting of bleomycin,

**Table 12.1** Primary ovarian carcinoma. Imaging statistics

| Study Ref. | # Patients | Sensitivity | Specificity | Accuracy | PPV | NPV |
|---|---|---|---|---|---|---|
| **PET/CT** | | | | | | |
| 2 | 108 | 82.4 | 76.9 | 81.1 | – | – |
| 3 | 133 | – | – | 92.1 | – | – |
| 4 | 30 | 71.4 | 81.3 | – | – | – |
| 5 | 40 | 69.4 | 97.5 | 94 | – | – |
| 6 | 59 | 87 | 100 | 92 | 81 | 100 |
| Weighted average | 370 | 80.0 | 86.7 | 88.8 | – | – |
| **Dedicated PET** | | | | | | |
| 7 | 49 | 78 | 87 | 82 | – | – |
| 8 | 99 | 58 | 76 | – | – | – |
| 9 | 103 | 58 | 78 | 76 | – | – |
| 10 | 101 | – | 80 | – | – | – |
| 11 | 51 | – | – | – | 86 | 76 |
| 12 | 19 | 100 | 67 | 86 | – | – |
| Weighted average | 422 | 64.6 | 78.6 | 78.8 | – | – |
| **CT/MRI** | | | | | | |
| 3 | 133 | – | – | 74.9 | – | – |
| 7 | 49 | 91 | 87 | 92 | – | – |
| 8 | 141 | 83 | 84 | – | – | – |
| 9 | 103 | 83 | 84 | 83 | – | – |
| 10 | 101 | – | 84 | – | – | – |
| 12 | 19 | 86 | 100 | 89 | – | – |
| Weighted average | 546 | 84.4 | 85.1 | 81.3 | – | – |
| **Ultrasound** | | | | | | |
| 3 | 133 | – | – | 83 | – | – |
| 6 | 50 | 90 | 61 | 80 | 78 | 80 |
| 8 | 99 | 92 | 60 | – | – | – |
| 9 | 103 | 92 | 59 | 63 | – | – |
| 10 | 101 | 92 | 60 | – | – | – |
| Weighted average | 486 | 91.7 | 59.8 | 75.3 | – | – |

etoposide, and cisplatin). Fertility-sparing surgery is frequently adopted. To date, there have been no studies specifically examining the role of PET in managing this group of tumors.

## Imaging considerations

FDG-PET is a relative newcomer to ovarian cancer imaging, and its role is still to be defined. From the foregoing discussion, the potential applications would be expected to include: (1) diagnosis of the primary adnexal mass; (2) pre-operative staging and surgical planning; (3) evaluation of response to

chemotherapy in non-surgical cases or after debulking; and (4) detection of recurrence (see Case 7).

**Diagnosis of the primary adnexal mass.** At present, no imaging approach is completely satisfactory. Transvaginal ultrasound is widely employed for screening, due to its low cost and high sensitivity. However, its specificity is poor, and an abnormal ultrasound may still need to be confirmed by follow-up imaging. At present, MRI is most commonly used for that purpose, however, PET/CT is emerging as a viable competitor. A tabulation of all published studies of FDG-PET/CT performance on a per-patient basis (2–12; see Table 12.1) shows closely comparable sensitivities and specificities for FDG-PET/CT compared with MRI.

The reported sensitivity of FDG-PET/CT would be even higher, except for the contribution of false negatives due to borderline ovarian tumors, which have low uptake (SUV typically < 3), similar to benign lesions (1, 13). When borderline tumors are excluded (typically about 15% of all tumors in the ovarian carcinoma spectrum), FDG-PET performance improves; Yamamoto et al., for example, showed an increase in sensitivity from 71.4% to 100% (4). The bottom line is that, using current interpretative criteria, a negative PET/CT scan does not exclude a borderline tumor. However, this drawback can be turned to advantage. Combining PET with MRI can provide a three-way classification of lesions: (1) PET(–)/MRI (–): likely benign; (2) PET(–) /MR(+): suspicious for borderline tumor; and (3) PET(+)/MR(+): suspicious for invasive malignancy (13). Since the optimal surgical approach can differ for borderline and invasive tumors, particularly in younger women who may want to preserve fertility, such a dual-imaging protocol would allow for informed pre-surgical planning (fine-needle biopsy has suboptimal specificity in this setting (14)). It remains to be shown whether the pairing of FDG-PET/CT with transvaginal ultrasound can provide the same differentiation.

***Pre-operative staging and surgical planning.*** The great advantage of FDG-PET/CT is that it is a sensitive, whole-body imaging modality that can simultaneously evaluate local disease, pelvic and retroperitoneal lymph nodes, far-flung peritoneal recesses and distant metastases. Thus, it is particularly well suited for pre-operative staging. For example, in a series by Nam et al. (3), 95 of 133 patients had spread of disease to extra-abdominal nodes which were not clinically predicted and were detected solely by PET/CT. These authors recommended the use of FDG-PET/CT for routine pre-operative evaluation.

The intraperitoneal route is a major route of spread for ovarian carcinoma, and it is here that the record of PET/CT is mixed, given that many peritoneal implants are microscopic. PET has poor sensitivity for lesions smaller than 0.5 cm. Contrast CT has been reported to be superior to dedicated

PET for this application (15); however, as yet there have been no studies specifically comparing CT and hybrid PET/CT with contrast. It should be noted that nothing perfectly detects microscopic disease. Surgical staging, the gold standard, also has less than 100% sensitivity, due to sampling errors, and the occasional inaccessibility of some sectors and pockets due to adhesions or other obstructions. When positive, or at least equivocal, FDG-PET/CT may be useful for directing attention to optimal sites for surgical exploration and biopsy.

***Therapy planning/evaluation of response to therapy.*** Most studies to date have dealt with neoadjuvant chemotherapy. A post-treatment SUV of less than 3.8 (16) or less than 2 after three cycles (17) reportedly predicts a good response. Patients with more than a 55% decrease in SUV after three cycles had a mean survival of 38.9 months, compared with 19.7 months for those with less than a 55% decrease (18). In this setting, PET was a better predictor than histopathology or clinical criteria.

FDG-PET/CT has the potential to provide tumor volumes for external-beam radiation therapy, although radiation therapy has a limited role in the treatment of ovarian carcinoma. Two authors (19, 20) have reported the use of a hand-held intraoperative gamma probe to identify involved lymph nodes during second-look surgery.

## Take-home message

- Many patients will have advanced-stage disease at the time of presentation.
- Spread is predominantly intraperitoneal, with nodal and distant metastases appearing only rarely or late in the disease (although both are present in the case history above).
- FDG-PET/CT may be useful for distinguishing borderline tumors from invasive adenocarcinoma; however, it fails to distinguish borderline tumors from normal tissue.
- Endometrial adenocarcinoma is seen in 10% of patients with granulosa-cell tumors, and uterine FDG uptake should be scrutinized in every case.

## References

1. Tobacman JK, Greene MH, Tucker MA et al. Intra-abdominal carcinomatosis after prophylactic oophorectomy in ovarian-cancer-prone families. *Lancet* 1982;2(8302):795–7.

2. Kitajima K, Suzuki K, Senda M et al. FDG-PET/CT for diagnosis of primary ovarian cancer. *Nucl Med Commun* 2011;32:549–53.

3. Nam EJ, Yun MJ, Oh YT et al. Diagnosis and staging of primary ovarian cancer: correlation between PET/CT, Doppler US, and CT or MRI. *Gynecol Oncol* 2010;116(3):389–94.

4. Yamamoto Y, Oguri H, Yamada R et al. Preoperative evaluation of pelvic masses with combined 18F-fluorodeoxyglucose positron emission tomography and computed tomography. *Int J Gynaecol Obstet* 2008;102(2):124–7.

5. Kitajima K, Murakami K, Yamasaki E et al. Diagnostic accuracy of integrated FDG-PET/contrast-enhanced CT in staging ovarian cancer: comparison with enhanced CT. *Eur J Nucl Med Mol Imaging* 2008;35(10):1912–20.

6. Castellucci P, Perrone AM, Picchio M et al. Diagnostic accuracy of 18F-FDG PET/CT in characterizing ovarian lesions and staging ovarian cancer: correlation with transvaginal ultrasonography, computed tomography, and histology. *Nucl Med Commun* 2007;28(8):589–95.

7. Kawahara K, Yoshida Y, Kurokawa T et al. Evaluation of positron emission tomography with tracer 18-fluorodeoxyglucose in addition to magnetic resonance imaging in the diagnosis of ovarian cancer in selected women after ultrasonography. *J Comput Assist Tomogr* 2004; 28(4):505–16.

8. Fenchel S, Grab D, Nuessle K et al. Asymptomatic adnexal masses:

correlation of FDG PET and histopathologic findings. *Radiology* 2002;**223**(3):780–8.

9. Rieber A, Nüssle K, Stöhr I *et al.* Preoperative diagnosis of ovarian tumors with MR imaging: comparison with transvaginal sonography, positron emission tomography, and histologic findings. *Am J Roentgenol* 2001;**177**(1):123–9.

10. Grab D, Flock F, Stöhr I *et al.* Classification of asymptomatic adnexal masses by ultrasound, magnetic resonance imaging, and positron emission tomography. *Gynecol Oncol* 2000;**77**(3):454–9.

11. Hubner KF, McDonald TW, Niethammer JG *et al.* Assessment of primary and metastatic ovarian cancer by positron emission tomography (PET) using 2-[18F]deoxyglucose (2-[18F]FDG). *Gynecol Oncol* 1993;**51**(2):197–204.

12. Kubik-Huch RA, Dörffler W, von Schulthess GK *et al.* Value of (18F)-FDG positron emission tomography, computed tomography, and magnetic resonance imaging in diagnosing primary and recurrent ovarian carcinoma. *Eur Radiol* 2000;**10**(5):761–7.

13. Jung DC, Choi HJ, Ju W *et al.* Discordant MRI/FDG-PET imaging for the diagnosis of borderline ovarian tumors. *Int J Gynecol Cancer* 2008;**18**(4):637–41.

14. Athanassiadou P, Grapsa D. Fine needle aspiration of borderline ovarian lesions. Is it useful? *Acta Cytol* 2005;**49**:278–85.

15. Pfannenberg C, Königsrainer I, Aschoff P *et al.* (18)F-FDG-PET/CT to select patients with peritoneal carcinomatosis for cytoreductive surgery and hyperthermic intraperitoneal chemotherapy. *Ann Surg Oncol* 2009;**16**(5):1295–303.

16. Nishiyama Y, Yamamoto Y, Kanenishi K *et al.* Monitoring the neoadjuvant therapy response in gynecological cancer patients using FDG PET. *Eur J Nucl Med Mol Imaging* 2008;**35**(2):287–95.

17. Martoni AA, Fanti S, Zamagni C *et al.* [18F]FDG-PET/CT monitoring early identifies advanced ovarian cancer patients who will benefit from prolonged neo-adjuvant chemotherapy. *Q J Nucl Med Mol Imaging* 2011;**55**(1):81–90.

18. Avril N, Sassen S, Schmalfeldt B *et al.* Prediction of response to neoadjuvant chemotherapy by sequential F-18-fluorodeoxyglucose positron emission tomography in patients with advanced-stage ovarian cancer. *J Clin Oncol* 2005;**23**(30):7445–53.

19. Barranger E, Kerrou K, Petegnief Y *et al.* Laparoscopic resection of occult metastasis using the combination of FDG-positron emission tomography/computed tomography image fusion with intraoperative probe guidance in a woman with recurrent ovarian cancer. *Gynecol Oncol.* 2005;**96**(1):241–4.

20. Cohn DE, Hall NC, Povoski SP *et al.* Novel perioperative imaging with 18F-FDG PET/CT and intraoperative 18F-FDG detection using a handheld gamma probe in recurrent ovarian cancer. *Gynecol Oncol* 2008;**110**(2):152–7.

A 54-year-old female with a BRCA1 mutation underwent prophylactic bilateral salpingo-oophorectomy. Despite this, she presented 2 years later with ascites, and was found to have a CA125 level of 1,387. Abdominal CT showed extensive peritoneal carcinomatosis, which was biopsied and was shown to be due to a papillary serous adenocarcinoma of ovarian type. A debulking procedure was performed, including omentectomy, upper vaginectomy, large bowel resection, and splenectomy. She was then treated with carboplatin and taxol chemotherapy. A second-look laparotomy 8 months later was positive for residual disease, and she was re-treated with gemzar and cisplatin chemotherapy. Another second-look laparotomy 5 months later was negative. However, her CA125 levels continued to rise, and for the next 6 years she underwent multiple rounds of chemotherapy with different regimens. A FDG-PET/CT scan was then performed.

## Findings and differential diagnosis

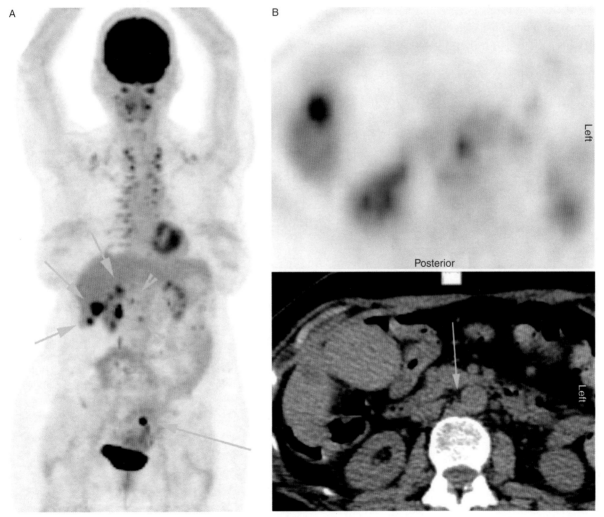

**Figure 12.14** (A) Whole-body MIP image shows a 1.8-cm intensely FDG-avid mesenteric/serosal implant (long blue arrow), along with multiple hepatic metastases (short blue arrows) and paraaortic lymph nodes (blue arrowheads). Bilateral supraclavicular and paraspinal uptake is due to hypermetabolic brown fat, and is not metastatic. (B) A small paraaortic lymph node metastasis is visible (blue arrow).

## Diagnosis and clinical follow-up

Diagnosis of recurrent ovarian adenocarcinoma, with peritoneal carcinomatosis and metastases to liver and lymph nodes. The patient continues to receive palliative chemotherapy.

## Discussion and teaching points

### Clinical background

The optimal strategy for follow-up of ovarian carcinoma is still undetermined, which is regrettable, since many, if not most, of these patients will relapse. As Copeland states (1): "there is no current evidence that intensive investigative monitoring has any significant positive impact on survival or quality of life." Serum levels of CA-125, a mucin-like glycoprotein found in many coelomic derivatives, but not in normal ovaries, are elevated in more than 80% of non-mucinous ovarian carcinomas. A rise in this marker can precede symptomatic relapse by about 5 months. However, it is not specific, and can also be elevated in a number of conditions, including chronic liver disease, congestive heart failure, pancreatitis, colitis, and arthritis. Second-look laparotomies were formerly used rather frequently for restaging, but less often now: stage I or II disease is usually negative; and half of stage III or IV patients with negative laparotomies will still go on to recurrence, due to missed microscopic disease. The technique still has some use in research protocols, or to assess response to chemotherapy or obtain a prognostic staging "snapshot" – niches, however, that are potentially also available to FDG-PET/CT.

Chemotherapy is the mainstay of second-line therapy, although re-treatment response rates are only in the range of 14–38%. Surgical intervention is useful mainly for palliative treatment of bowel and urinary tract obstruction.

## Imaging considerations

Perhaps the best documented role for FDG-PET/CT in the context of ovarian carcinoma is as a follow-up for rising CA-125 serum titers in women with a history of clinical remission after first-line treatment with surgery and/or chemotherapy. Table 12.2 (2–22) summarizes the studies published so far. The weighted mean sensitivity and specificity of FDG-PET/CT is

**Table 12.2** Recurrent ovarian carcinoma. Imaging statistics.

| Study Ref. | # Patients | Sensitivity | Specificity | Accuracy | PPV | NPV |
|---|---|---|---|---|---|---|
| **PET/CT** | | | | | | |
| 2 | 60 | 95.5 | 93.3 | 95 | 97.7 | 87.7 |
| 3 | 37 | 100 | 85 | 94 | 91 | 100 |
| 4 | 60 | 97 | 90 | – | – | – |
| 5 | 43 | 88.4 | 88.2 | – | – | – |
| 6 | 70 | 93 | 55.6 | 78.6 | 76.9 | 83.3 |
| 7 | 132 | 74.3 | 90 | 82.6 | – | – |
| 8 | 36 | 73 | – | 81 | – | – |
| 9 | 51 | – | – | 92 | – | – |
| 10 | 77 | 93.3 | 96.9 | 94.8 | 97.7 | 91.2 |
| 11 | 41 | 88.2 | 71.4 | 85.4 | – | – |
| 12 | 22 | 83.3 | – | 81.8 | 93.8 | – |
| Weighted average | 629 | 87.6 | 84.8 | 86.5 | 91.0 | 89.4 |
| **Dedicated PET** | | | | | | |
| 13 | 86 | 86.9 | 78.8 | 84.8 | 91.9 | 68.4 |
| 14 | 29 | 84.6 | 100 | 86.2 | 100 | 42.9 |
| 15 | 28 | 95 | 87.5 | 92.9 | – | – |
| 16 | 25 | 80 | 100 | 84 | – | – |
| 17 | 24 | 90.9 | 92.3 | 91.7 | – | – |
| 18 | 106 | 83 | 83 | – | – | – |
| 19 | 20 | – | – | 93 | – | – |
| 20 | 19 | 100 | 50 | 90 | – | – |
| Weighted average | 337 | 86.6 | 83.9 | 87.7 | 93.9 | 62.0 |

**Table 12.2** (*cont.*)

| Study Ref. | # Patients | Sensitivity | Specificity | Accuracy | PPV | NPV |
|---|---|---|---|---|---|---|
| **CT/MRI** | | | | | | |
| 2 | 60 | 55.5 | 66.6 | 58.3 | 83.3 | 33.3 |
| 3 | 60 | 81 | 90 | – | – | – |
| 8 | 36 | 91 | 89 | – | – | – |
| 9 | 51 | – | – | 83 | – | – |
| 13 | 86 | 53.3 | 81.8 | 60.8 | 89 | 38.6 |
| 16 | 25 | 55 | 100 | 64 | – | – |
| 17 | 24 | 90.9 | 46.2 | 66.7 | – | – |
| 20 | 19 | 86 | 100 | 89 | – | – |
| 21 | 25 | 69.6 | 83.3 | 74.3 | – | – |
| 22 | 24 | 72.7 | 75 | 73.3 | – | – |
| Weighted average | 410 | 68.9 | 80.0 | 68.4 | – | – |
| **Serum CA125 Level** | | | | | | |
| 13 | 86 | 57.6 | 93.9 | 67.2 | – | – |
| 16 | 25 | 75 | 100 | 80 | – | – |
| 17 | 24 | 90.9 | 76.9 | 66.7 | – | – |
| Weighted average. | 135 | 66.7 | 92.0 | 69.5 | – | – |
| Ultrasound | | | | | | |
| 4 | 60 | 66 | 90 | – | – | – |
| Laparoscopy | | | | | | |
| 6 | 70 | 95 | 64 | 83.1 | 80.8 | 88.9 |

superior to ultrasound, CT, or MRI. Similar values have been reported for CA-125 levels as low as 30 U/mL (23), or even 18 U/mL, where the detection rate was 85.6% (24). FDG-PET/CT has even detected recurrences in patients with normal CA-125 levels (25). Results were good for all recurrence patterns, including intraperitoneal and retroperitoneal disease. The use of PET/CT resulted in a significant change in management in 24.7–62% of patients (7, 10, 26–30).

As might be expected, the weakest point of PET/CT imaging is in the detection of very small foci of early recurrence, particularly microscopic peritoneal carcinomatosis. As noted above, even surgical staging does poorly in this context, given that half of all patients with negative second-look laparatomies go on to relapse. Since recurrence is inevitable for many of these patients, the most useful role of imaging surveillance is perhaps not to document curative extirpation of disease (which is quite possibly a mirage), but to identify the proper time-point for initiating second-line therapy. From this point of view, FDG-PET/CT may be ideal, as it can identify disease well ahead of clinical symptoms of recurrence, when CA-125 levels are only slightly elevated. It can also assess the total tumor burden, and offer guidance as to the form of therapy to be attempted (i.e., re-excision, palliative surgery, or chemotherapy).

## Take-home message

- Ovarian carcinoma (in the form of peritoneal implants) may occur years after bilateral oophorectomies.
- Recurrent disease may be present (and may be detectable by FDG-PET/CT) even when the serum CA125 levels are low.
- FDG-PET/CT is superior to ultrasound, CT, or MRI for detecting recurrent ovarian carcinoma.
- FDG-PET/CT may be able to fulfill the role of second-look laparatomy in reassessing patients after treatment. At the very least, it is capable of minimizing futile laparotomies if performed in advance of surgery.

# References

1. Copeland LJ. Epithelial ovarian cancer. In PJ DiSaia, WT Creasman (Eds.), *Clinical Gynecologic Oncology*, 7th edn. Philadelphia, PA: Mosby-Elsevier, 2007, pp. 313–67.

2. Bilici A, Ustaalioglu BB, Seker M *et al.* Clinical value of FDG PET/CT in the diagnosis of suspected recurrent ovarian cancer: is there an impact of FDG PET/CT on patient management? *Eur J Nucl Med Mol Imaging* 2010; 37(7):1259–69.

3. Pan HS, Lee SL, Huang LW, Chen YK. Combined positron emission tomography-computed tomography and tumor markers for detecting recurrent ovarian cancer. *Arch Gynecol Obstet* 2011;283(2):335–41.

4. Risum S, Høgdall C, Markova E *et al.* Influence of 2-(18F) fluoro-2-deoxy-D-glucose positron emission tomography/computed tomography on recurrent ovarian cancer diagnosis and on selection of patients for secondary cytoreductive surgery. *Int J Gynecol Cancer* 2009; 19(4):600–4.

5. Iagaru AH, Mittra ES, McDougall IR *et al.* 18F-FDG PET/CT evaluation of patients with ovarian carcinoma. *Nucl Med Commun* 2008;29(12):1046–51.

6. Fagotti A, Fanfani F, Rossitto C *et al.* A treatment selection protocol for recurrent ovarian cancer patients: the role of FDG-PET/CT and staging laparoscopy. *Oncology* 2008;75(3–4):152–8.

7. Kitajima K, Murakami K, Yamasaki E *et al.* Performance of integrated FDG-PET/contrast-enhanced CT in the diagnosis of recurrent ovarian cancer: comparison with integrated FDG-PET/non-contrast-enhanced CT and enhanced CT. *Eur J Nucl Med Mol Imaging* 2008;35(8):1439–48.

8. Kim CK, Park BK, Choi JY *et al.* Detection of recurrent ovarian cancer at MRI: comparison with integrated PET/CT. *J Comput Assist Tomogr* 2007;31(6):868–75.

9. Sebastian S, Lee SI, Horowitz NS *et al.* PET-CT vs. CT alone in ovarian cancer recurrence. *Abdom Imaging* 2008;33(1):112–8.

10. Chung HH, Kang WJ, Kim JW *et al.* Role of [18F]FDG PET/CT in the assessment of suspected recurrent ovarian cancer: correlation with clinical or histological findings. *Eur J Nucl Med Mol Imaging* 2007;34(4):480–6.

11. Nanni C, Rubello D, Farsad M *et al.* (18)F-FDG PET/CT in the evaluation of recurrent ovarian cancer: a prospective study on forty-one patients. *Eur J Surg Oncol* 2005;31(7):792–7.

12. Bristow RE, del Carmen MG, Pannu HK *et al.* Clinically occult recurrent ovarian cancer: patient selection for secondary cytoreductive surgery using combined PET/CT. *Gynecol Oncol*;90(3):519–28.

13. García-Velloso MJ, Jurado M *et al.* Diagnostic accuracy of FDG PET in the follow-up of platinum-sensitive epithelial ovarian carcinoma. *Eur J Nucl Med Mol Imaging* 2007;34(9):1396–405.

14. Takekuma M, Maeda M, Ozawa T *et al.* Positron emission tomography with 18F-fluoro-2-deoxyglucose for the detection of recurrent ovarian cancer. *Int J Clin Oncol* 2005;10(3):177–81.

15. Chang WC, Hung YC, Kao CH *et al.* Usefulness of whole body positron emission tomography (PET) with 18F-fluoro-2-deoxyglucose (FDG) to detect recurrent ovarian cancer based on asymptomatically elevated serum levels of tumor marker. *Neoplasma* 2002;49(5):329–33.

16. Torizuka T, Nobezawa S, Kanno T *et al.* Ovarian cancer recurrence: role of whole-body positron emission tomography using 2-[fluorine-18]-fluoro-2-deoxy-D-glucose. *Eur J Nucl Med Mol Imaging* 2002;29(6):797–803.

17. Yen RF, Sun SS, Shen YY *et al.* Whole body positron emission tomography with 18F-fluoro-2-deoxyglucose for the detection of recurrent ovarian cancer. *Anticancer Res* 2001;21(5):3691–4.

18. Zimny M, Siggelkow W, Schröder W *et al.* 2-[Fluorine-18]-fluoro-2-deoxy-d-glucose positron emission tomography in the diagnosis of recurrent ovarian cancer. *Gynecol Oncol* 2001;83(2):310–15.

19. Jiménez-Bonilla J, Maldonado A, Morales S *et al.* Clinical impact of 18F-FDG-PET in the suspicion of recurrent ovarian carcinoma based on elevated tumor marker serum levels. *Clin Positron Imaging* 2000;3(6):231–6.

20. Kubik-Huch RA, Dörffler W *et al.* Value of (18F)-FDG positron emission tomography, computed tomography, and magnetic resonance imaging in diagnosing primary and recurrent ovarian carcinoma. *Eur Radiol* 2000;10(5):761–7.

21. Picchio M, Sironi S, Messa C *et al.* Advanced ovarian carcinoma: usefulness of [(18)F]FDG-PET in combination with CT for lesion detection after primary treatment. *Q J Nucl Med* 2003;47(2):77–84.

22. Nakamoto Y, Saga T, Ishimori T *et al.* Clinical value of positron emission tomography with FDG for recurrent ovarian cancer. *Am J Roentgenol* 2001;176(6):1449–54.

23. Menzel C, Döbert N, Hamscho N *et al.* The influence of CA 125 and CEA levels on the results of (18)F-deoxyglucose positron emission tomography in suspected recurrence of epithelial ovarian cancer. *Strahlenther Onkol* 2004;180(8):497–501.

24. Palomar A, Nanni C, Castellucci P *et al.* Value of FDG PET/CT in patients with treated ovarian cancer and raised CA125 serum levels. *Mol Imaging Biol.* 2011;14:123–9.

25. Murakami M, Miyamoto T, Iida T *et al.* Whole-body positron emission tomography and tumor marker CA125 for detection of recurrence in epithelial ovarian cancer. *Int J Gynecol Cancer* 2006;16(Suppl 1):99–107.

26. Simcock B, Neesham D, Quinn M *et al.* The impact of PET/CT in the management of recurrent ovarian cancer. *Gynecol Oncol* 2006;103(1):271–6.

27. Mangili G, Picchio M, Sironi S *et al.* Integrated PET/CT as a first-line re-staging modality in patients with suspected recurrence of ovarian cancer. *Eur J Nucl Med Mol Imaging* 2007;34(5):658–66.

28. Soussan M, Wartski M, Cherel P *et al.* Impact of FDG PET-CT imaging on the decision making in the biologic suspicion of ovarian carcinoma recurrence. *Gynecol Oncol* 2008;108(1):160–5.

29. Fulham MJ, Carter J, Baldey A *et al.* The impact of PET-CT in suspected recurrent ovarian cancer: A prospective multi-centre study as part of the Australian PET Data Collection Project. *Gynecol Oncol.* 2009;112(3):462–8.

30. Gadducci A, Cosio S. Surveillance of patients after initial treatment of ovarian cancer. *Crit Rev Oncol Hematol* 2009;71(1):43–52.

# Lymphoma

Lale Kostakoglu

## Introduction

Hodgkin's (HL) and aggressive non-Hodgkin's lymphomas (NHL) are potentially curable neoplasms owing to their marked chemo- and radiosensitivity as well as to recent introduction of more effective treatment strategies (1, 2). In these patients individualized therapy schemes based on well-defined risk categories can be devised with the prerequisite of an accurate staging system for evaluation of disease extent. Accurate risk profiling based on staging and established predictors of outcome as well as effective response evaluation during or following therapy and restaging are essential to determine the optimal treatment strategies. Anatomic imaging modalities, including both computed tomography (CT) and magnetic resonance imaging (MRI) cannot differentiate between active lymphoma and a benign process or inflammation-induced reactive changes in relatively small lymph node groups.

The increasing availability of positron emission tomography using $^{18}$F-fluorodeoxyglucose, particularly fused with computed tomography (FDG-PET/CT) has lead to the integration of this modality into the routine staging and restaging algorithms for lymphoma, providing comprehensive information about tumor glucose metabolism combined with anatomic data. The metabolic information can potentially impact patient management and survival, if decisions about additional therapy or to make a change in treatment regimen could be reliably based on FDG-PET imaging. There is now convincing evidence that FDG-PET is a more accurate imaging modality in the staging and evaluation of treatment response of lymphomas compared with conventional imaging techniques, including CT. Furthermore, persistent FDG uptake during and after chemotherapy has high sensitivity and specificity to differentiate residual viable disease from inflammatory post-therapy changes.

This chapter summarizes the data on the proven and potential utility of FDG-PET imaging in combination with CT for staging, restaging, and predicting therapy response using multiple case studies. In addition, current limitations of this imaging modality will also be presented with examples.

## Histopathologic classification and FDG-PET/CT imaging

The subtypes of lymphoma largely vary in morphologic and biologic characteristics. The Revised European and American Lymphoma classification was the first system to incorporate morphology, phenotype, genetic analysis, and clinical features for lymphoproliferative disorders. The World Health Organization (WHO) has refined this system elucidating the origin of these neoplasms. More recently, the updated WHO classification has defined several new distinct and provisional categories based on the biological overlap between classical HL and diffuse large B-cell lymphomas (DLBCL) (3). Among the peripheral T-cell lymphomas (PTCL), more precise definitions were introduced for several entities, including anaplastic large cell lymphoma, and angioimmunoblastic lymphoma. Because of the complexity and diversity of this integrated system, a simplified approach subdividing lymphomas into two broad categories is adopted based on management implications; HL and NHL.

The common lymphoma histologies including HL, DLBCL (most common subtype of aggressive NHLs), and follicular lymphoma (FL) (most common subtype of indolent NHL) are FDG avid in the majority of cases with a sensitivity at 80–90% (4–6). FDG-PET usually upstages patients with additional sites of disease that are not detected on the accompanying high-dose CT, particularly in lymph nodes that fall in the normal category based on CT criteria or in solid organs with diffuse involvement. Although FDG-PET is an invaluable staging tool, pre-therapy contrast enhanced CT maintains its significance due to better delineation of tumor from adjacent organs or anatomic planes with respect to disease extent (7, 8).

Hodgkin's lymphoma is rare and accounts for 10–15% of lymphomas. It is essential to distinguish two distinct entities of HL; nodular lymphocyte predominant HL (NLPHL, 3–7% of HL cases) and the classical HL (cHL) which encompasses the mixed cellularity, lymphocyte rich and lymphocyte depleted, and nodular sclerosing (65–80% of HL cases) subtypes (2). These two major variants, NLPHL and cHL, have distinct disease biologies and clinical presentation patterns. Patients with NLPHL usually present with isolated peripheral lymph node involvement and has a less aggressive disease course. With combination chemotherapy, the cure rate for HL is greater than 80% with first-line therapy. FDG-PET's sensitivity is quite high (~100%) in both subtypes.

Non-Hodgkin's lymphomas account for more than 85% of the lymphomas and the vast majority of NHL is of B-cell origin (~90% of NHL cases) (1). NHL can be broadly classified into **aggressive** and **indolent lymphomas**; the most common histology consists of DLBCL and FL, respectively. One important issue to remember is that the treatment strategy for aggressive NHL is determined based upon not only the anatomic extent but also immunophenotype of the tumor. Thus, aggressive NHLs are treated exclusively with chemotherapy except in some cases in which local radiotherapy may be added. DLBCL comprises almost 40% of all lymphomas (1). Although more than 60% of DLBCL patients are cured with combination chemotherapy and rituximab, relapses frequently occur. In addition to DLBCL, specific variants of large B-cell lymphomas (BCL) include primary mediastinal LBCL (MLBCL) and T-cell/histiocyte-rich BCL (T/HRBCL) (1). One important feature of B-cell lymphomas is that there has been a greater appreciation of morphologic and immunophenotypic overlap between classical HL and some large B-cell lymphomas, mainly primary MLBCL and mediastinal nodular sclerosis HL (9). Early-stage DLBCL is curable in more than three-quarters of patients, however, advanced stage is curable in only half (1, 9). DLBCL sometimes occurs concurrently or subsequently in patients with NLPHL with a cumulative risk of about 10% at 10 years (10). The sensitivity of FDG-PET is considerably high at 95–100% in DLBCL.

AIDS-related lymphomas, both NHL and HL, are clinically characterized by advanced stage associated with constitutional symptoms, extra-nodal involvement, and clinical aggressiveness with poor therapeutic outcomes (10, 11). Recently a primary effusion lymphoma (PEL) has been described involving exclusively serous body cavities (i.e., peritoneum, pleura, or pericardium) (12).

Low-grade NHL (LGL) is a group of indolent B-cell lymphomas that accounts for more than 50% of all lymphomas (1). There are 10 distinct entities described according to the most recent WHO classification (3). FL is the most common subtype that makes up for 70% of LGLs. The other subtypes include marginal zone lymphoma (MZL) and chronic lymphocytic leukemia/small lymphocytic lymphoma (CLL/SLL). LGLs are associated with a good response to initial therapy but followed by frequent relapses, and duration of responses shortens after each additional therapy. The treatment options range from "watch and wait" to hematopoietic stem cell transplantation (13). The management in indolent lymphomas is defined by clinical symptoms rather than disease extent; therefore, the majority of clinicians do not believe that management would be significantly influenced by staging evaluation.

However, new approaches combining dose-intense chemotherapy with "tumor-specific" anti-CD20 monoclonal antibody targeting, unconjugated or with a radiolabel (radioimmunotherapy) have shown promise for a survival benefit (14). Thus, response evaluation would be clinically relevant to timely modify therapy when necessary. Among the three grades (grade 1–3) of FL, grade 1–2 FL are characterized by an indolent clinical course, while grade 3 FL harbors more aggressive characteristics (refer to further discussions in the "transformation to a more aggressive subtype" section). The sensitivity of FDG-PET is high at 90–95% for detection of FL involvement for all grades. Similar results were observed with nodal MZL (6, 15, 16), however, the FDG-PET sensitivity does not exceed 50% in CLL/SLL and 60% in extranodal MZL including the splenic MZL and mucosa-associated lymphoid tissue (MALT) with SUVs in the very low (SUVmax 1.0–2.0) to low range (SUVmax 3.0–5.0) (17, 18).

Mantle cell lymphoma (MCL) is a distinct entity of B-cell lymphomas representing 3–10% of NHLs, and occurs primarily among elderly individuals (3). Although some patients may follow an indolent clinical evolution, the prognosis is usually poor due to an aggressive and progressive clinical course with no currently available effective therapy strategies. The MCL has two major histologic variants that demonstrate different biological and clinical characteristics; the classic variant (80–90% of cases) and the blastoid variant. Although MCL proliferation activity may vary individually in each case, it is generally low in the former subtype and high in the latter (Ki-67 index > 40%). The blastoid variant is associated with more aggressive clinical evolution. The diagnostic sensitivity of FDG-PET for MCL was reported to be 90–100% (18–20); however, the sensitivity for bone marrow and gastrointestinal involvement is low. There are limited data showing that when SUVs are significantly high (> 15) there may be a tendency for more aggressive disease behavior as evidenced by histopathologic features demonstrating a blastoid variant with high Ki-67 index (18), while others found a relationship between high SUVs and more advanced disease and unfavorable outcome when SUVs exceeded 6.0 (20). Additionally, combining PET and international workshop criteria (IWC) identified high-risk patients for early relapse. Positive and negative predictive values of IWC+PET for relapse at 1 year were 62.5 and 100%. These results warrant further prospective investigation towards designing risk-adapted strategies (20).

FDG avidity is reportedly insignificant in more than 50% of patients with some rare lymphomas subtypes including peripheral T-cell (6) and anaplastic large T-cell lymphomas (17, 21).

The International Harmonization Project (IHP) (22) recommends FDG-PET imaging before treatment for HL and DLBCL on the basis of biologic characteristics of consistent FDG-avidity and potential curability. For other subtypes, FDG-PET imaging is recommended to be used in clinical trials, particularly when response rate is the primary objective. The National Comprehensive Cancer Network guidelines

(NCCN) currently recommend FDG-PET imaging as an essential test in HL, DLBCL, AIDS-related B-cell lymphomas and as a useful test in selected cases in FL, MZL, MCL, Burkitt's lymphoma, lymphoblastic lymphoma, peripheral T-cell lymphoma, primary cutaneous B-cell lymphoma, and mycosis fungoides, but does not recommend FDG-PET in CLL/SLL (23, 24).

## Pre-treatment evaluation

The staging work-up includes medical history, physical examination and laboratory procedures (complete blood cell count with differential, peripheral blood smear, lactate dehydrogenase, β2 microglobulin, serum chemistry and protein electrophoresis, sedimentation rate, and blood chemistries (1, 2). A bone marrow aspirate with a biopsy is necessary, particularly for NHL. The patient should also be assessed for human immunodeficiency virus (HIV) status, and other infection-associated lymphomas. Advanced technologies, including molecular and cytogenetic studies, such as bcl-2 or bcl-6, and DNA microarray analysis may improve diagnostic accuracy and refine prognostically divergent histologic subsets.

The most commonly obtained imaging studies include chest, abdomen and pelvis CT, MRI, and lately FDG-PET/CT scans. The size of all lesions should be recorded by 2-D measurements as a baseline against which to compare subsequent post-therapy determinations.

## Staging of lymphomas

Pre-treatment staging is the mainstay for guiding therapy decisions by means of determining the extent of disease. The Ann Arbor staging system, the most widely used staging system for HL and NHL, has evolved over the past 40 years with modifications (25, 26). The gradual evolution of this system was driven by changes in the management and by advances in imaging technology. There are four main stages of lymphomas as demonstrated in Table 13.1. Subscript suffixes are affixed to any stage for more detailed information. The presence of constitutional symptoms: fevers less than 38 °C, night sweats, or weight loss of greater than 10% of body weight during 6 months and bulky disease (tumor > 10 cm) portend worse prognosis. Stages I and IIA are considered early-stage disease, however up to 35% of patients with early stage HL can have occult abdominal nodal or splenic involvement. Stages IIB (particularly bulky), III, and IV are considered advanced-stage disease. The Ann Arbor system has long used physical examination, bone marrow (BM) evaluation, and CT scans to determine the stage of disease. FDG-PET is a sensitive imaging tool to detect nodal and extranodal lymphoma and provides complementary information to conventional staging (further discussed later in this chapter). FDG-PET is now incorporated into the staging algorithm of most histologic subtypes although not firmly in several subtypes like indolent lymphomas and mantle cell lymphoma (23, 24).

**Table 13.1** Ann Arbor staging system of lymphomas.

**Stage I**

Involvement of a single lymph node region **or** involvement of a single extralymphatic organ

**Stage II**

Involvement of two **or** more lymph node regions on the same side of the diaphragm or localized involvement of an extralymphatic organ or site plus an involved lymph node region on the same side of the diaphragm

**Stage III**

Involvement of lymph nodes on **both sides of the diaphragm**; can be accompanied by extralymphatic organ involvement including the spleen

**Stage IV**

Diffuse or disseminated involvement of one or more extralymphatic organs with or without associated lymph node involvement

The presence or absence of the following symptoms should be noted with each stage designation.
A = asymptomatic.
B = fever, sweats, or weight loss greater than 10% of body weight.
X = a mediastinal mass exceeding one-third of the intrathoracic diameter or greater than 10 cm in diameter.
E = extranodal disease.

## FDG-PET/CT imaging patterns of lymphomas

Appreciation of the patterns of distribution and relapse of various lymphoma subtypes equips the imager and the clinician alike with the necessary knowledge for accurate interpretation of imaging findings for selection of better management plans.

**cHL vs. DLBCL.** Classical HL usually spreads contiguously in neighboring nodal stations, while NHL usually skips into disparate nodal stations and typically presents with a widespread distribution. Extrinsic infiltration of bones and muscles by neighboring lymph node masses is seen in both HL and DLBCL (27), however, intrinsic bone marrow (BM) involvement is more common in DLBCL. Intrathoracic presentations are common with involvement of mediastinal nodes, particularly those in the superior mediastinal location. In general, extranodal involvement of the lung parenchyma, pleura and pericardium is more common with NHL than with HL, because of the frequent vascular invasion and hematogeneous spread associated with the former (28). Imaging plays a significant role for recognizing bulky mediastinal HL as these patients have a worse prognosis due to higher risk of disease recurrence compared with those with non-bulky disease. **Bulky disease** is defined as a mediastinal mass exceeding one-third of the chest diameter or greater than 10 cm in diameter.

**Nodular lymphocyte predominant HL** is a rare subtype and seen in 5–10% of HL cases. More than 80% of cases present with supradiaphragmatic early stage, or less commonly with non-bulky IIIA disease. Extranodal involvement, bulky splenic or subdiaphragmatic disease, or B symptoms are unusual in nodular lymphocyte predominant HL but can be a sign of coincident NHL, particularly DLBCL or T-cell rich B-cell lymphoma (29). **HIV-associated HL**, although rare, has a more aggressive pattern with frequent involvement of extra-nodal organs (75–90%) (10–12). The highly active antiretro-viral therapy used to treat these patients has resulted in substantial improvement in their survival, due to allowance of more aggressive chemotherapy.

**MCL** often presents with disseminated disease, generalized lymphadenopathy and BM involvement, although bulky dis-ease and B symptoms are less common (30). Extranodal involvement is almost invariable involving mostly the Wal-deyer's ring and gastrointestinal tract. Central nervous system involvement and an extranodal presentation without nodal involvement are rare (31). The diagnosis of BM involvement relies on immunohistochemistry as imaging studies can be false negative in many cases (30). Imaging for staging purposes does not have a major influence on management due to the invariably disseminated nature of the disease, however, evalu-ation of therapy response is important for potential thera-peutic changes.

**LGL** is similar to MCL in its initial presentation, character-ized by advanced stage disease with generalized nodal and BM or other extranodal organ involvement (1). Of note, CLL/SLL is considered as the tissue infiltrate of CLL, and upon presen-tation most patients have disseminated disease affecting per-ipheral lymph nodes and/or bone marrow, while only about 30% have limited stage disease. A characteristic of LGLs is the phenomenon of spontaneous regression but this is usually partial and short-lived. Imaging can help determine the disease status which may prompt therapy during the active course of the disease. Other characteristics of indolent lymphomas include synchronous discordant lymphomas (20–30% of newly diagnosed patients) and transformation to an aggressive sub-type with a rate of 3–5% per year during the first 10 years following diagnosis (32). In these situations, imaging may help determine a better management strategy.

**LGL transformation to a more aggressive subtype.** There are three grades (grade 1–3) of FL corresponding to an increas-ing number of centroblasts per high power field as recognized in the recent WHO-classification of lymphomas (33). Trans-formation of low grade lymphoma (grades I–III) to an aggres-sive phenotype, mostly to DLBCL histology, occurs during the course of disease in as many as 60% of patients (32, 34, 35). Transformation should be suspected in patients with indolent lymphoma with high SUVs in any group of lymph nodes on FDG-PET (36). In a prior study, the SUV of the biopsy-proven site of transformation ranged from 3 to 38, with a mean of 14 and median of 12 (37). Approximately 50% of patients had an SUV > 13. This finding is in line with a prior study which showed that an SUV > 10 predicted an aggressive lymphoma with >80% certainty and an SUV > 13 with >90% certainty

(38). Consequently, biopsies should be directed to those sites showing the highest FDG avidity to diagnose transformation and timely institute proper treatment.

# FDG-PET/CT imaging for staging of lymphoma

FDG-PET imaging is more sensitive and specific than CT imaging which yields more false negative results in normal-size lymph nodes that harbor lymphoma. A meta-analysis revealed a pooled sensitivity and a false-positive rate of 91% and 10% on patient-based data (39). On a lesion basis analysis, the maximum joint sensitivity and specificity was close to 96% and exceeded corresponding values for contrast-enhanced CT and bone marrow biopsy (5, 39–41).

Discordance of PET and CT findings occurs in approxi-mately 30% of patients at initial staging (7, 39, 41, 42, 43). FDG-PET results typically lead to upstaging because of the identification of additional sites of disease. Schaefer et al. reported that the sensitivity of PET/CT and contrast-enhanced CT for nodal disease in HL and aggressive NHL was 94% and 88% respectively, while the specificity was 100% vs. 86% (44). For organ involvement, the sensitivity of PET/CT was almost twice as much as contrast-enhanced CT (88% vs. 50%) while the specificities were similar (100% vs. 90%).

Contrast-enhanced CT has more diagnostic value in the abdomen than in the chest for delineating lymph nodes from the vessels and bowel loops. The CT portion of the PET/CT examination for initial staging may permit a more accurate assessment of the liver and spleen when combined with a dual- or triple-phase contrast enhanced CT. In a recent prospective study of 103 HL patients, 30% of the patients staged with FDG-PET/contrast-enhanced CT were found to have splenic involvement and 10% liver involvement, whereas with separate procedures only one-third of these patients could be identified (42). More than 50% of relapses in the historical cohort were localized in the spleen and/or liver. FDG-PET/contrast-enhanced CT-guided treatment resulted in a 95% event-free survival (EFS), whereas separate FDG-PET and diagnostic CT-guided treatment resulted in an 81% EFS ($P = 0.002$) (45). Hence using intravenous contrast administration should be considered for PET/CT protocols when necessary, particularly in advanced stage and abdominal lymphomas. In a recent systematic review, Kwee et al. reported that the sensitivity and specificity of CT and FDG-PET were 87.5% and 85.6% vs. 87.5% and 100%, respectively for initial staging of lymph-omas (46), although the sensitivity of PET was somewhat lower in NHL at 83% with no change in specificity. While PET/CT was found to be superior to either modality alone, the investigators felt that further studies are warranted to deter-mine the most accurate and cost-effective method for lymph-oma staging.

**FDG-PET in extranodal lymphoma.** Extranodal NHL consists of heterogeneous group of disease presentations. The most common extranodal sites include BM, spleen, liver, cen-tral nervous system (CNS), gastrointestinal tract (GIT), and the Waldeyer's ring (1). The therapeutic strategy in patients with primary extranodal lymphomas is, in general, analogous to that of nodal lymphomas.

Accurate assessment of bone BM is of great importance in staging lymphoma as it indicates stage IV and changes disease management with therapeutic and prognostic implications (1, 2). Lymphoma involvement of the BM or the cortical bone is common in NHL and detected in 20–60% of patients, especially in LGL, CLL/SLL, and MCL (1). BM biopsy is the mainstay of BM evaluation despite its high rate of mislocalizations of focal marrow infiltration distal to the biopsy site. Notwithstanding the superior sensitivity of MRI in detecting BM infiltration, it is not practical to routinely assess the entire marrow given the time and the cost associated with the technique. The normal BM localization of FDG is a function of physiologic marrow turnover, which may be quite prominent in many cases. However, focal and irregular FDG uptake is usually considered pathological. Diffusely increased BM uptake, however, is non-specific and can be observed in cases with reactive BM hyperplasia induced by erythropoietin or colony stimulating growth factors (47, 48). FDG-PET alone is unreliable for detecting BM involvement with a reported agreement of 78% with the biopsy data (40), hence cannot substitute BM biopsy, although in patients with focal or disseminated BM involvement it usually yields positive results (45, 47, 48). Consequently, in cases with PET-positive BM marrow findings either biopsy or MRI should be considered for confirmation if the therapy decision is likely to be influenced. In a systematic review of 32 studies, PET/CT was found to have a high pooled sensitivity at 92% and specificity at 90% compared to corresponding values of 90% and 76% for MRI (49). However, the sensitivity of the PET/CT studies was highly heterogeneous. Nonetheless, PET/CT data should be compared with that of whole-body MRI rather than a segmental MRI which offers an advantageous stance to PET/CT imaging.

Lymphoma involvement of the spleen is more common than of the liver. Approximately one-third of patients with lymphoma have splenic involvement regardless of its size while only up to 10% HL patients and 15% NHL patients have hepatic involvement (50). Nodular disease is usually associated with aggressive NHL and diffuse disease with LGL. The sensitivity and specificity of FDG-PET for the detection of splenic involvement by lymphoma exceeds that of CT at above 90%. In a recent prospective study, when FDG-PET was fused with contrast-enhanced CT, three times more patients were found to have hepatic and splenic involvement compared with staging with each test alone (42). As alluded to before, FDG-PET/contrast-enhanced CT can be used as an accurate front-line single imaging tool enabling effective management.

The most common gastrointestinal (GIT) site is the stomach, accounting for 50% of the GIT lymphomas (1). In the Western world the most frequent lymphomas in adults are B-cell lymphomas: the mucosa-associated lymphoid tissue-lymphomas (MALT lymphoma) and DLBCL in the stomach

and DLBCL in the small bowel (1, 3). In marginal zone lymphomas, the lesions are often FDG-PET-negative, thus PET imaging has not become a routine staging procedure in this group of patients (51). MALT-type gastric lymphoma can transform into a DLBCL. FDG-PET can help in grading/subtyping of gastric MALT lymphoma and DLBCL, however, its role should be established with sufficient clinical data.

Primary CNS lymphoma is invariably of the NHL subtype (> 80% B-cell) (3). Chemoradiotherapy is the standard of care for CNS lymphoma, however, approximately half of the patients in complete remission will relapse, and 15% patients have primary refractory CNS lymphoma (52). These tumors are more frequently seen in immunocompromised patients including those with prior organ transplantation or AIDS. Although CT and MRI generally provide characteristic findings that are suggestive of CNS lymphoma, imaging characteristics can be similar in CNS lymphoma and toxoplasmosis (53–55). Essentially, a lesion with an FDG uptake higher than the adjacent gray matter indicates a malignant process which prompts a confirmatory biopsy rather than empirical treatment (54). Challenges arise, however, when the CNS mass undergoes necrosis or is below the resolution limits of PET systems (< 7.0 mm). Single or multiple periventricular lesions with gadolinium enhancement on MRI are typical findings in immunocompetent patients, whereas ring-enhancing lesions are only observed in immunocompromised patients (52). FDG-PET has a high sensitivity for detecting brain (~90%) and spinal lesions (80%), but small lesions diagnosed by MRI can go undetected in FDG-PET due to resolution limits (55). FDG-PET is also capable of detecting occult systemic lymphoma in close to 10% of cases whose disease is not detected by conventional work-up (55). Despite the considerable advances in diagnostic imaging procedures, none of these techniques supplant a diagnostic biopsy but they can be used to guide the site of biopsy (see Chapter 20). FDG-PET may suit better in the follow-up of patients with CNS lymphoma rather than at diagnosis.

## FDG-PET impact on patient management

Although PET identifies more lesions than CT, it is not universally accepted that PET can replace CT for staging, mostly due to expense concerns and a low benefit yield from detection of additional disease sites. Stage migration occurs in up to 30% of patients, and this change alters management in only 10–15% of the cases (56, 57). Essentially, the broad use of chemotherapy mitigates the need for the exact definition of anatomic disease extent. However, the recent trend to abbreviate treatment and limit radiotherapy to involved lymph nodes requires more accurate information on anatomic disease extent. PET/CT may be of particular value before therapy for those patients who apparently have stage I–II disease and for whom field radiation therapy is being considered. Advanced-stage HL or NHL may be curable with combination chemotherapy. Hence one should realize that additional information derived from an imaging modality can upstage or downstage disease but may not lead to management changes. As emphasized before, accurate staging is more clinically relevant in aggressive NHL and HL than in indolent and mantle cell lymphoma as the latter pair is associated with advanced stage disease in a vast majority of patients.

## Special considerations

**Thymic uptake**. Thymic hyperplasia is a common phenomenon that occurs after completion of treatment (58). It has been proposed that this finding is due to an immunologic rebound characterized by thymic aplasia followed by hyperplasia. FDG uptake in the hyperplastic thymus may lead to false positive readings, particularly in those with a mediastinal lymphoma (59, 60).

**BM uptake after administration of colony stimulators**. In patients treated with chemotherapy followed by bone marrow stimulants such as granulocyte colony-stimulating factor and granulocyte-macrophage colony-stimulating factor, the BM will have diffuse, increased FDG accumulation (61). Therefore, diffuse BM FDG uptake is commonly attributable to the effect of hematopoietic cytokines. However, diffuse bone marrow FDG uptake can also be caused by bone marrow involvement by lymphoma which may be indistinguishable from hematopoietic cytokine-mediated FDG bone marrow uptake.

**Post-transplant lymphoproliferative disorder**. Post-transplant lymphoproliferative disorder (PTLD) is a complication of both solid organ and allogeneic bone marrow transplantations. In most cases, PTLD is associated with Epstein–Barr virus (EBV) infection of B cells. The niche for FDG-PET/CT appears to be in assessing response to therapy, rather than aiding in diagnosis of PTLD. In a limited study there was no difference between anatomical and PET imaging at staging of disease although PET showed promise in detecting extranodal disease in the BM.

## FDG-PET/CT for evaluation of therapy response and at restaging during follow-up

Assessment of residual disease during or after therapy and evaluation for recurrence during follow-up is an integral part of patient management schemes. Overall close to 50% of patients with NHL or HL will have a persistent mass after treatment while only 20% of these patients will relapse (62, 63). FDG-PET is an effective imaging modality and superior to CT in the differentiation of post-therapy fibrotic masses from residual or recurrent disease. Further treatment solely based on morphologic characteristics in those with post-therapy fibrotic masses only increases morbidity, the risk of developing solid tumors, and cardiovascular disease in the years following therapy even if a cure is achieved.

**Post-therapy prediction of therapy outcome**. The existing prognostic risk factors, International Prognostic Score (IPS) and International Prognostic Index (IPI), for HL and NHL,

respectively, were developed to stratify the risk of recurrence and survival in an attempt to determine the most proper management strategy (64). More recently, several studies have demonstrated that post-therapy FDG-PET imaging has a role in the prediction of tumor recurrence (65–67). In a mixed group of 44 patients with abdominal HL and aggressive NHL, Zinzani et al. reported a 2-year actuarial relapse-free survival rate of 95% for a negative PET result compared with 0% for a positive result regardless of a residual mass on CT (68). Similarly, in a prospective study, Spaepen et al. reported a negative and a positive predictive value of 80% and 100% for FDG-PET after completion of first-line chemotherapy in patients with aggressive NHL (67). Exclusively in HL patients, similar results were reproduced with significantly short disease-free survivals at 0–4% for the PET-positive group while those patients in the PET-negative group had longer survivals at 85–95% (69–70).

**Integrated International Workshop Criteria (IWC) and FDG-PET**. Post-therapy FDG-PET has recently been integrated into IWC response criteria for lymphoma based on encouraging results (22). The term "complete remission/unconfirmed (CRu)" was originally coined to describe persistence of a post-therapy mass, which had decreased in size by at least 75% on CT scan with complete resolution of all clinical symptoms. However, in the majority of cases CRu resulted in overtreatment when the residual mass in fact represented fibrosis rather than active tumor (62, 63). In one study, it was observed that CRu patients mostly had negative FDG-PET findings and also had a longer than 32-month progression-free survival (PFS) leading to the reclassification of these patients into CR category (71). Consequently, in the revised IWC-PET criteria, the challenge associated with CRu has been eliminated by FDG-PET (22, 71). Currently, those patients without metabolic evidence of residual disease are classified as CR regardless of CT response, while those with positive PET findings are classified as PR, SD, or PD based on CT measurements. Although several retrospective studies reported results employing IHP criteria, prospective trials are ongoing using IHP criteria; hence, further data will be obtained to validate these results.

**Stem cell transplantation**. For relapsed lymphoma, high-dose chemotherapy with autologous stem cell transplantation (HDT/SCT) can yield a 5-year event-free survival (EFS) of up to 50% (1, 2). However, the success of this highly toxic treatment relies on tumor chemosensitivity, which requires a dynamic biologic marker (72). Those patients with a positive pre-transplant PET are considered at risk, and should have close follow-up after transplantation. In earlier studies, the relapse-free survival was reported to be five times higher in the PET-negative group compared to the PET-positive group when PET was performed after HDT and immediately prior to SCT (73–75). In a meta-analysis of 12 pre-SCT PET studies including 630 patients, the joint sensitivity and specificity were 69% and 81%. PET was found to have superior accuracy in the prediction of treatment outcome (76). Nonetheless, there are limited FDG-PET data showing that chemosensitive patients have a better prognosis than those with chemoresistant disease based on persistent FDG uptake after induction therapy. A retrospective analysis in 42 DLBCL reported that during a median follow-up of 34.5 months, the median EFS was significantly lower for both pre-SCT and post-SCT PET positive groups (27.4 months) and after transplantation there was no difference in the EFS between the pre-transplant negative and positive groups if the PET result was negative after transplantation (77).

A meta-analysis demonstrated a strong correlation between pre-SCT PET results and the outcome of autologous SCT. A negative pre-SCT PET not only indicates a longer PFS, but also a significant gain in overall survival (OS) (78). A negative PET after salvage chemotherapy confers complete remission and high chemosensitivity. In the case of a positive PET finding after salvage chemotherapy, one should consider intensifying treatment or altering treatment before autologous SCT. If this is not an option, other strategies, such as tandem autologous SCT, allogeneic SCT or treatment with antibodies, can be implemented (79). In summary, more prospective data are warranted for a definitive conclusion with regards to the role of PET in the setting of HDT/SCT.

**Incurable lymphomas**. In low-grade lymphomas and other rare lymphoma subtypes, although limited, data exist supporting the utility of PET/CT imaging in FL and MCL. In other rare subtypes, due to lack of a systematic evaluation, FDG-PET results should be individually analyzed and interpreted based on the particular histologic subtype. Despite its often indolent clinical course, FL is a heterogeneous disease entity. Current criteria for early identification of patients with a poor prognosis are suboptimal using the Follicular Lymphoma International Prognostic Index (FLIPI) (80) for individual patients. Similarly in MCL, the limitations of the prognostic criteria MIPI have been acknowledged (81). Unlike HL and DLBCL, there is paucity of data about the role of PET/CT for response assessment of these lymphoma subtypes.

In MCL, Bodet-Milin *et al.* reported a positive and negative predictive value of 62.5 and 100% respectively, for identifying MCL relapse at 1 year with the use of revised IWG response criteria incorporating PET results (82). With a median follow-up of 21 months, only the revised IWC criteria were accurate to identify patients with high risk for early relapse among other established prognostic parameters. In a study of 49 patients with relapsed or refractory FL or MCL patients who received a similar therapy regimen, after completion of therapy, the percent reduction in SUVmax (70% vs. 29%) and in maximum perpendicular diameter (78% vs. 48%) were significantly greater in patients with a CR than in those with non-CR (83). The positive and negative predictive value of SUVmax at a threshold of 61% was similar at 77% and 78%, respectively. These are encouraging results towards designing risk-adapted strategies although validation with larger series is warranted to establish the value of PET in FL and MCL. Early during therapy as a predictor of response measuring chemosensitivity,

82 advanced-stage MCL patients undergoing HDT/SCT, post two or three cycles, FDG-PET status was not found to be associated with PFS or OS after a median follow-up of 23 months (84). In corroboration with prior studies, however, end-therapy PET status was statistically significantly associated with PFS and trended towards significance for OS. Although, these data do not support the prognostic utility of an interim PET in MCL, a prospective multicenter trial using a uniform PET protocol and set of interpretation criteria is still warranted to prove or refute its role in this setting.

In FL, Le Dortz *et al.* reported that in 45 untreated patients, the specificity and positive predictive value of PET/CT performed after 4 or 6 cycles of chemoimmunotherapy induction treatment was higher than that of CT (97% vs. 51% and 92% vs. 43%, respectively), in the determination of response (85). The median progression-free survival was 48 months in the PET/CT-negative group, compared with 17.2 months for the group with residual uptake (85). In a retrospective review of 31 treated FL patients (only grades I and II), FDG-PET had a high sensitivity of 95% and a specificity of 88% for lesion detection (86). Post-induction PET positive patients had shorter mean PFS compared with PET negative patients; post-salvage PET positive patients trended toward shorter mean response duration compared with negative patients. These results indicate that PET is accurate in the diagnostic assessment of treated FL-1 and FL-2, and post-treatment PET positive patients are likely to relapse faster than PET negative patients.

**Evaluation of response to radioimmunotherapy**. Despite its established utility in lymphoma, data on the value of FDG-PET to assess response to radioimmunotherapy are scarce. In a retrospective analysis of 59 relapsed or refractory FL patients treated with radioimmunotherapy, the post-radioimmunotherapy PET documented a 46% CR, 25% PR, and 29% no response, with an overall survival of 71%. With a median follow-up period of 23 months, the multivariate analysis confirmed that the post-radioimmunotherapy PET was the sole independent predictor of PFS (87). In a recent study of 23 relapsed or refractory FL patients, PET/CT performed at 2 months revealed complete or partial metabolic response in 69.5% of patients while indicating refractory disease in the remaining patients (all confirmed at 6-month scanning). Better overall survival was observed for patients when SUVs decreased by at least 49% both at 2 and 6 months after radioimmunotherapy ($P < .05$). Despite a rather small sample size, these data suggest that early assessment of radioimmunotherapy response using PET/CT may be beneficial in the identification of patients who would require additional therapy (88).

**Early response evaluation during therapy in curable lymphomas**. Chemotherapy for both DLBCL and HL is planned with a curative intent, with the first-line therapy having the greatest chance for achieving this goal (1, 2). Rapidity of chemotherapy response is reported to be a good measure of chemosensitivity; consequently, the patients who do not achieve a CR with several cycles of chemotherapy have shorter PFS compared with those who had a rapid response.

Regardless of subsequent achievement of a remission, the slowly responding patients may benefit from early administration of dose-intense salvage therapy (89). Interim FDG-PET results could help de-escalate therapy by abbreviation of treatment cycles or avoid RT in patients who achieve an early CR. In a meta-analysis of 13 studies involving 360 advanced-stage HL patients and 311 DLBCL patients, interim FDG-PET had an overall sensitivity of 81% and a specificity of 97% for advanced-stage HL, and a sensitivity of 78% and a specificity of 87% for DLBCL (89).

For DLBCL, while FDG-PET has a clear role in the evaluation of the post-therapy response, its predictive value at an interim time-point in this setting is controversial due to heterogeneity of disease biology and treatment strategies (89). Although several studies reported that FDG-PET performed after two to four cycles of chemotherapy has demonstrated prognostic value, these results varied significantly among patient groups (90–92). The 2-year PFS for the PET-negative groups was comparable at 82–93%, while the PFS for the PET-positive group varied from 0 to 43%. In another study, using three response groups, the estimated 5-year PFS was 89% for the PET-negative group, 59% for the minimal residual uptake (MRU) group, and 16% for the PET-positive group (91). After one cycle of therapy, in 24 patients the 2-year progression-free survival for those who had a negative FDG-PET result was 100%, compared with only 12.5% in those with a positive result (93). PET after two cycles was independent of B symptoms, age, stage, the presence of extranodal disease and bulky disease and emerged as the strongest single prognostic factor of all (90–92). The above-mentioned differences in PET results may be due to varying follow-up periods, patient population trends, and different types of treatments employed (i.e., the use of standard chemotherapy alone versus the use of chemotherapy plus Rituximab). It is also possible that the different interpretation guidelines used for interim PET studies might have contributed to the variability of results.

More recently, in newly diagnosed aggressive NHL, a positive interim FDG-PET often carried an adverse prognosis, with reported 2-year PFS rates of 0 to 50% after standard first-line therapy. However, some patients treated with immunochemotherapy (R-CHOP) experienced a favorable long-term outcome despite a positive interim FDG-PET scan (94). To further clarify the clinical relevance of interim FDG-PET scans in a risk-adapted sequential immunochemotherapy program in 97 patients, overall 61% had a negative PET scan, 86.4% of whom remained progression free at a median follow-up of 44 months. In patients with a positive PET result (39%) repeat biopsy revealed no disease in 87%, and 51% of these patients remained progression free after consolidation therapy during the follow-up period. Progression-free survival of interim FDG-PET-positive/biopsy-negative patients was identical to that in patients with a negative interim FDG-PET scan. Consequently, interim or post-treatment FDG-PET did not predict outcome in this dose-dense, sequential immunochemotherapy program.

Hence, these heterogeneous data do not provide grounds to use PET-based response-stratification strategies without a predefined prognosis determined for PET negative and positive groups in homogeneous patient populations receiving standard regimens and using similar response criteria. Nonetheless, there is also evidence that early treatment intensification based on midtreatment PET-positive disease, improves patient outcome. In a phase II trial of risk-adapted therapy of 59 B-cell lymphoma patients, on intention-to-treat analysis, the 2-year EFS was 67% in PET-positive patients and 89% in PET-negative patients (95). No association was found between the IPI categories and the midtreatment PET results. The favorable outcome achieved here in historically poor-risk patients warrants further, more definitive investigation of treatment modification based on early PET scanning.

In HL, unlike DLBCL, early interim PET imaging is strongly predictive of advanced-stage disease (96). Persistent FDG uptake after a few cycles of chemotherapy is associated with relapse rates ranging from 50–100% while the relapse rate in patients with complete resolution of FDG uptake during therapy is usually lower than 10% (97–99). Interestingly, HL harbors only scattered tumor cells, and Hodgkin and Reed–Sternberg (HRS) cells, accounting for approximately 1% of the total cell count in biopsy specimens, while the predominant fraction is composed of non-neoplastic mononuclear bystander cells (100). Chemokines selectively attract inflammatory cells including eosinophils, histiocytes, macrophages, plasma cells, and T lymphocytes. Although the majority of HL patients show normalization of the FDG uptake after a few courses of standard ABVD (adriamycin, bleomycin, vinblastine, and dacarbazine) therapy, the relationship between these inflammatory cells and FDG uptake becomes crucial in the post-therapy setting as they may lead to false-positive readings in as much as 40% of patients. In this regard, FDG-PET when used early during therapy as a response surrogate has shown to be an independent predictor of outcome. Individualizing therapy using FDG-PET as a prognostic indicator may give rise to a paradigm shift from the use of full-course chemotherapy to abbreviated cycles of therapy or the avoidance of adjuvant radiation therapy in the right subgroup of patients.

Studies utilizing FDG-PET for assessment of response have reported that at least 85% of early-stage HL patients achieve a metabolic CR after two or three cycles of chemotherapy (97–99). In patients with early stage HL, after two or three cycles of chemotherapy, with a positive interim PET (15%) the relapse rate was only 30%, while all advanced-stage patients relapsed within 2 years. When minimal residual uptake (MRU = slightly above the background) was regarded as negative for residual disease, 94% were progression free after a median follow-up of 3.3 years compared with only 39% of patients with a definitively positive PET finding (97). Similar findings were reported after two cycles of chemotherapy in another study of HL patients (98). In another study that evaluated the prognostic value of PET after one cycle (PET1) in a mixed cohort of HL and DLBCL, 26% of patients had a PET1-positive result in the HL group and

83% relapsed (93). The 2-year PFS rate for PET-negative patients after one cycle of therapy was 100%, compared with only 12.5% in those with a PET1-positive result.

In advanced stage HL, after two cycles in 40 patients, all patients with positive PET results either had refractory disease or relapsed (101). All PET2-negative patients remained in CR while in the group with MRU, 75% achieved a CR with a median follow-up of 18 months. In a larger group of HL patients (n = 260) with either advanced-stage (n = 190) or stage IIA disease with adverse prognostic factors, after two cycles, 86% of the PET2-positive patients had treatment failure during a median follow-up of 2.2 years. In PET2–negative patients, 95% were in CR. The positive and negative predictive value of PET-2 for predicting 2-year PFS were 93% and 92%, respectively. Early interim FDG-PET results have also been shown to have a stronger prognostic value for prediction of PFS than any of the other pretreatment prognostic factors such as IPS (98, 99). Recently, Cerci et al. reported that treatment failure was seen in 53% of PET2-positive patients and in only 8% of PET2-negative patients regardless of disease stage. EFS was 53.4% for PET2-positive patients and 90.5% for PET2-negative ones (P < 0.001). When patients were categorized according to low or high IPS risk and according to early or advanced stage of disease, PET2 was also significantly associated with treatment outcome (102).

There are also conflicting results, however, in which early response did not prove to be a good prognostic factor. In 96 patients with non-bulky limited-stage HL, interim PET did not predict outcome, with a PFS of 87% vs. 91% (P = 0.6) in the positive and negative PET groups, respectively. End-of-treatment PET results were predictive of outcome however, with PFS of 94% in PET-negative patients versus 54% in PET-positive patients. In conclusion, interim PET scans were not predictive of outcome, compared with completion of therapy scans which were highly predictive of PFS. Of note, in this low-risk patient population, even patients with interim positive PET scans show a favorable prognosis (103).

In a pre-therapy risk- and interim PET- or Ga67-adapted therapy of 108 HL patients with adverse prognostic factors, the CR, 5-year EFS, and overall survival rates were 97%, 85%, and 90%, respectively. Similar EFS and OS rates were observed for patients in both risk groups. Relapse or progression occurred in 27% of patients with interim positive PET/CT versus 2.3% of those with negative scans (P < 0.02) justifying a role for early interim PET/CT as a useful tool for adjustment of chemotherapy (104). In another study of 45 advanced-stage, high risk (IPS > 3) HL patients, PET2 was used to de-escalate therapy. At the end of all therapy, 40 (89%) patients were in CR (disappearance of all clinical evidence of disease and PET negativity). After a median follow-up of 48 months, PFS and overall survival at 4 years were 78% and 95%, respectively. The 4-year PFS for early PET-negative patients (n = 31) and early PET-positive patients (n = 13) were 87% and 53%, respectively (P = 0.01). These data indicate that combined escalated BEACOPP therapy (bleomycin, etoposide, adriamycin, cyclophosphamide, vincristine, procarbazine and prednisone) and standard therapy (ABVD) may improve the outcome of patients with high-risk advanced HL (105).

**Recurrent lymphoma after first-line therapy and surveillance.** Despite improvements in survival rates relapses can occur in approximately 30–50% of lymphoma patients following first-line therapy (106). In a meta-analysis, the sensitivity and specificity of FDG-PET to predict disease relapse were reported to be 50–100% and 67–100%, respectively, for HL and 33–77% and 82–100%, respectively, for NHL, irrespective of whether there was a residual mass on CT (96). Surveillance strategies aim to detect early relapse for a potentially more effective second-line therapy. However, the effectiveness of therapy is also limited by tumor chemoresistance and the eligibility of patients for more toxic therapy protocols (1, 2). PET/CT is a more sensitive tool than other existing imaging modalities in the detection of residual disease; however, it is yet to be proven that subclinical detection of relapse leads to survival benefit.

Frequent follow-up with 3–4 monthly FDG-PET studies may be necessary for patients with advanced stage or unfavorable risks or, alternatively, for those who have a slow response to therapy as determined by interim PET studies. On the other hand, a large fraction of false-positive findings may be obtained in the limited-stage or favorable-risk group or in those who have a rapid response to therapy. Current practice guidelines include clinical visits every 3–6 months for 3–5 years and annually thereafter (23, 24, 107). Imaging studies are ordered at the discretion of the referring physician and this practice is heterogeneous across various centers.

In a recent study of 125 HL and aggressive NHL patients, more than 60% of relapses were diagnosed clinically, especially in aggressive NHL and in cases with extranodal involvement; however, HL relapses were more commonly detected by FDG-PET imaging (108). Overall, 2.6 times more HL relapses were diagnosed by routine imaging compared with those with aggressive NHL. While clinical examination remains the most common mode of detecting relapse, these results suggest a potential role for routine PET/CT surveillance in HL patients; however, survival did not appear to be affected by the mode of detection. In another study of 421 patients with mixed histologies including HL, aggressive NHL and FL, all of whom achieved the first complete remission, serial 6-month FDG-PET scans enabled detection of lymphoma relapse within 18 months of therapy (109). There are also conflicting results reporting detection rates of recurrence as low as 8% for FDG-PET during a median follow-up of 31 months in classical HL patients. The positive predictive value of surveillance PET/CT and CT was found to be lower than 30%. Factors that were found to improve the PPV in detecting recurrent HL included concordant findings on PET and CT, recurrence at a prior disease site, or the occurrence of a radiographic abnormality within 12 months (110).

Despite its high negative predictive value, one should realize that false-negative findings will be inevitable in cases with residual microscopic disease, particularly in those that fall into the pre-therapy high-risk category. Nevertheless, patients with relapsing lymphoma can still be salvaged with second-line therapy in as many as 80% of HL and 60% of DLBCL patients (111). In this regard, the low positive predictive value of FDG-PET raises more important questions for its clinical value in identifying patients who would need immediate additional treatment. While a negative test provides reassurance regarding continued remission, there may be false-positive results that may result in unnecessary tests, biopsies, economic burden, and anxiety. Particularly, in patients with early-stage non-bulky, low-risk HL, unnecessary imaging should be avoided given the rather low recurrence rates of less than 15% (112, 113). In this patient population, annual PET/CT may be performed without a high-dose CT, especially in those with supradiaphragmatic disease. It is also important to recognize that the radiation dose received from whole-body PET/CT (8 mSv) is much lower than that from high-dose dedicated CT of the chest, abdomen, and pelvis (16 mSv) (114).

One caution to be exercised should be that necrotic areas within tumors may have a poor exchange between blood and tissue, therefore, a lower volume of distribution of radiotracer that may lead to false negative findings during monitoring of therapy. These patients should be followed more frequently than others with no appreciable necrotic components in their tumors.

In summary, further multicenter large-scale studies are warranted to determine the role of FDG-PET in the follow-up setting as well as to determine whether or not it leads to a survival advantage.

**Timing of FDG-PET imaging.** Interim PET should be scheduled at least 2 weeks, preferably 3 weeks after the initiation of therapy (71, 115), or within 4–5 days of the start of the subsequent therapy cycle. This approach should be adopted to improve the positive predictive value by minimizing false-positive findings introduced by the inflammatory response that usually peaks between 10 and 15 days of therapy administration (115). The timing of FDG-PET studies after completion of therapy is more flexible, however, a 3-week window after end of therapy should be observed to allow time for inflammation to subside. Needless to say is that the time interval between radiation therapy and FDG-PET imaging should not be less than 6 weeks.

**Standardization of the interpretation criteria.** In practice, interim FDG-PET scans can be evaluated qualitatively (visually) or semiquantitatively using SUVs. Defining the positive and negative PET reading and categorizing minimal residual uptake (MRU) by visual assessment alone can be challenging. In an attempt to avoid the wide variability among readers, the imaging subcommittee of the International Harmonization Project (IHP) in Lymphoma provided a definition for a negative FDG-PET scan after completion of therapy, recommending that the mediastinal blood pool (MBP) be used as an internal reference for lesions of 2.0 cm or larger (22, 71) to discriminate a positive finding from a negative one. However,

for lesions measuring less than 2 cm, background uptake remains the reference irrespective of the lesion location. For interim PET readings, a higher cut-off may be used given that these scans measure chemosensitivity rather than response and it has been proven that the prognosis of the MRU group is similar to that of PET-negative patients at interim PET evaluation (97, 98). More recently, the London criteria were adopted at a consensus meeting in Deauville to allow for a continuous reading scheme using a 5-point scoring system and also to minimize false-positive results by employing a higher threshold using liver uptake as the reference (116, 117). The advantages of the 5-point scoring system include flexibility, reproducibility, and provision of a relatively continuous response scheme based on the degree of residual positivity. The 5-point scoring system lends itself as a flexible reading scale depending on whether the study question involves escalation or de-escalation of treatment. In a de-escalation treatment a higher threshold can be used (liver) to ensure highest likelihood of true-negative PET, while in the setting of treatment escalation the threshold can be lowered to select patients with the highest likelihood of resistant disease. A recently published result series of a multicenter study confirmed a high level of agreement (Kappa = 0.85 (95% CI 0.74–0.96)) amongst different reviewers using this 5-point scoring system (117).

**Semi-quantitative evaluation.** Visual evaluation of response on FDG-PET imaging has been shown to be reliable although quantitative analysis is desirable in certain situations, particularly in DLBCL and in other rare and incurable forms of lymphoma. Metabolic changes measured by standard uptake values are continuous, rather than binary variables; consequently, may parallel an in vivo therapy response scale, which presents a range of metabolic changes with potentially different prognostic outcomes. However, SUV measurements heavily depend on several factors related to PET protocols, e.g., wait time after injection, blood glucose concentration, body weight, partial volume effect, and individual scanner-dependent features. Thus, strict adherence to protocols is necessary for all imaging periods. For an optimized response assessment, the minimum requirement would be that the same protocol and scanner be utilized, and that the wait time after FDG injection is maintained with a 10–15 min window allowance (118). The SUV cut-off as a prognostic indicator may be different for defining response early during therapy compared with that after completion of therapy. In HL, a SUVmax cut-off of 4.0 provided the best joint sensitivity and specificity for the prediction of progression after two cycles of chemotherapy (98). In DLBCL after two cycles of chemotherapy, the optimum threshold SUVmax for prediction of EFS was 5.0 and the 2-year estimate for EFS was 21% in patients with a SUVmax reduction of < 66% compared with 79% in those with reduction > 66% (119). In light of these studies, the cut-off values of 4.0 or 5.0 exceed that of the SUVmax of the mediastinal blood pool or of the liver (usually around 2.0–3.0). Further studies are needed to define a widely accepted semiquantitative approach for lymphoma, probably with slightly different values for each subtype.

In summary, FDG-PET is useful when performed after completion of therapy in lymphoma, in both HL and DLBCL. Although FDG-PET reliably detects disease resistance early in the course of therapy, its effectiveness as a surrogate for chemoresistance or chemosensitivity has been proven at interim evaluation only in advanced stage HL.

Furthermore, there is no evidence to suggest that an early change of therapy in poorly responding patients will translate into a survival benefit. Prospective, randomized, multicenter trials are underway to further define the benefit of individualized therapies using FDG-PET as a surrogate for tumor response.

# References

1. Friedberg JW, Mauch PM, Rimsza LM, Fisher RI. Non-Hodgkin's lymphomas. In VT DeVita, TS Lawrence, SA Rosenberg (Eds.), *DeVita, Hellman, and Rosenberg's Cancer: Principles and Practice of Oncology*, 8th edn. Philadelphia, PA: Lippincott Williams & Wilkins, 2008, pp. 2098–166.

2. Diehl V, Re D, Harris NL, Mauch PM. Hodgkin lymphoma. In VT DeVita, TS Lawrence, SA Rosenberg (Eds.), *DeVita, Hellman, and Rosenberg's Cancer: Principles and Practice of Oncology*, 8th edn. Philadelphia, PA: Lippincott Williams & Wilkins, 2008, pp. 2167–213.

3. Swerdlow SH, Campo E, Harris NL et al. *WHO Classification of Tumours of Haematopoietic and Lymphoid Tissues*, 4th edn. Lyon: International Agency for Research on Cancer, 2008.

4. Thill R, Neuerburg J, Fabry U et al. Comparison of findings with 18-FDG PET and CT in pretherapeutic staging of malignant lymphoma. *Nuklearmedizin* 1997;36:234–9.

5. Buchmann I, Reinhardt M, Elsner K et al. 2-(fluorine-18)fluoro-2-deoxy-D-glucose positron emission tomography in the detection and staging of malignant lymphoma. A bicenter trial.*Cancer* 2001;91:889–99.

6. Elstrom R, Guan L, Baker G et al. Utility of FDG-PET scanning in lymphoma by WHO classification. *Blood* 2003;101:3875–6.

7. Bangerter M, Moog F, Buchmann I et al. Whole-body 2-[18F]-fluoro-2-deoxy-D-glucose positron emission tomography (FDG-PET) for accurate staging of Hodgkin's disease. *Ann Oncol* 1998;9:1117–22.

8. Jerusalem G, Beguin Y, Fassotte MF et al. Whole-body positron emission tomography using 18F-fluorodeoxyglucose compared to standard procedures for staging patients with Hodgkin's disease. *Haematologica* 2001; 86:266–73.

9. Jaffe ES, Wilson WH. Gray zone, synchronous, and metachronous lymphomas: diseases at the interface of non-Hodgkin's lymphomas and Hodgkin's lymphoma. In PM Mauch, JO Armitage, B Coiffier et al. (Eds.), *Non-Hodgkin's Lymphoma*. Philadelphia, PA: Lippincott, Williams, and Wilkins, 2004, pp. 69–80.

10. Mounier N, Spina M, Gabarre J et al. AIDS-related non-Hodgkin lymphoma. *Blood* 2006;107:3832–40.

11. Mounier N, Spina M, Spano JP. Hodgkin lymphoma in HIV positive patients. *Curr HIV Res* 2010;8:141–6.

12. Tirelli U, Spina M, Gaidano G et al. Epidemiological, biological and clinical features of HIV-related lymphomas in the era of highly active antiretroviral therapy. *AIDS* 2000;14:1675–88.

13. Hiddemann W, Buske C, Dreyling M et al. Treatment strategies in follicular lymphomas: current status and future perspectives. *J Clin Oncol* 2005;23:6394–9.

14. Illidge T, Chan C. How have outcomes for patients with follicular lymphoma changed with the addition of monoclonal antibodies? *Leuk Lymphoma* 2008;49(7):1263–73.

15. Le Dortz L, De Guibert S, Bayat S et al. Diagnostic and prognostic impact of (18)F-FDG PET/CT in follicular lymphoma. *Eur J Nucl Med Mol Imaging* 2010;37:2307–14.

16. Wöhrer S, Jaeger U, Kletter K et al. 18F-fluorodeoxy-glucose positron emission tomography (18F-FDG-PET) visualizes follicular lymphoma irrespective of grading. *Ann Oncol* 2006;17:780–4.

17. Weiler-Sagie M. 18F-FDG avidity in lymphoma readdressed: a study of 766 patients. *J Nucl Med* 2010;51:25–30.

18. Shrikanthan S, Zhuang HM, Schuster S, Alavi A. FDG-PET imaging in diagnosis of mantle cell lymphoma. *J Nucl Med* 2004;45:93P.

19. Brepoels L, Stroobants S, De Wever W et al. Positron emission tomography in mantle cell lymphoma. *Leuk Lymphoma* 2008;49:1693–701.

20. Bodet-Milin C, Touzeau C, Leux C et al. Prognostic impact of 18F-fluorodeoxyglucose positron emission tomography in untreated mantle cell lymphoma: a retrospective study from the GOELAMS group. *Eur J Nucl Med Mol Imaging* 2010;37(9):1633–42.

21. Kako S, Izutsu K, Ota Y et al. FDG-PET in T-cell and NK-cell neoplasms. *Ann Oncol* 2007;18:1685–90.

22. Cheson BD, Pfistner B, Juweid ME et al. Revised response criteria for malignant lymphoma. *J Clin Oncol* 2007;25:579–86.

23. National Comprehensive Cancer Network, Hodgkin Lymphoma. *NCCN* **v1** 2011 http://www.nccn.org/professionals/physician_gls/pdf/hodgkins.pdf

24. National Comprehensive Cancer Network, non-Hodgkin Lymphoma. *NCCN* **v2** 2011 http://www.nccn.org/professionals/physician_gls/pdf/nhl.pdf

25. Lister TA, Crowther D, Sutcliffe SB et al. Report of a committee convened to discuss the evaluation and staging of patients with Hodgkin's disease: Cotswald meeting. *J Clin Oncol* 1989;7:1630–6.

26. Rosenberg S. Validity of the Ann Arbor staging system classification for the non-Hodgkin's lymphomas. *Cancer Treat Rep* 1977;61:1023–7.

27. Chew FS, Schellingerhout D, Kee SB. Primary lymphoma of skeletal muscle. *Am J Roentgenol* 1999;172:1370.

28. Cazals-Hatem D, Lepage E, Brice P et al. Primary mediastinal large B-cell lymphoma: a clinicopathologic study of 141 cases compared with 916 nonmediastinal large B-cell lymphomas – a GELA ("Groupe d'Etude des Lymphomas de l'Adulte") study. *Am J Surg Pathol* 1996;20: 877–88.

29. Greiner TC, Gascoyne RD, Anderson ME et al. Nodular lymphocyte-predominant Hodgkin's disease associated with large-cell lymphoma:

analysis of Ig gene rearrangements by V-J polymerase chain reaction. *Blood* 1996;**88**:657–66.

30. Jares P, Campo E. Advances in the understanding of mantle cell lymphoma. *Br J Haematol* 2008;**142**:149–65.

31. Ferrer A, Bosch F, Villamor N et al. Central nervous system involvement in mantle cell lymphoma. *Ann Oncol* 2008;**19**:135–41.

32. Tan D, Horning SJ. Follicular lymphoma: clinical features and treatment. *Hematol Oncol Clin North Am* 2008;**22**:863–82, viii.

33. Ott G, Katzenberger T, Lohr A et al. Cytomorphologic, immunohistochemical, and cytogenetic profiles of follicular lymphoma: 2 types of follicular lymphoma grade 3. *Blood* 2002;**99**:3806–12.

34. Montoto S, Davies AJ, Matthews J et al. Risk and clinical implications of transformation of follicular lymphoma to diffuse large B-cell lymphoma. *J Clin Oncol* 2007;**25**:2426–33.

35. Yuen AR, Kamel OW, Halpern J et al. Long-term survival after histologic transformation of low-grade follicular lymphoma. *J Clin Oncol* 1995;**13**:1726–33.

36. Noy A, Schöder H, Gönen M et al. The majority of transformed lymphomas have high standardized uptake values (SUVs) on positron emission tomography (PET) scanning similar to diffuse large B-cell lymphoma (DLBCL). *Ann Oncol* 2009; **20**:508–12.

37. Partridge S, Timothy A, O'Doherty MJ et al. 2-Fluorine-18-fluoro-2-deoxy-D glucose positron emission tomography in the pretreatment staging of Hodgkin disease: influence on patient management in a single institution. *Ann Oncol* 2000;**11**:1273–9.

38. Schoder H, Noy A, Gonen M et al. Intensity of 18fluorodeoxyglucose uptake in positron emission tomography distinguishes between indolent and aggressive non-Hodgkin's lymphoma. *J Clin Oncol* 2005;**23**(21):4643–51.

39. Isasi CR, Lu P, Blaufox MD A metaanalysis of 18F-2-deoxy-2-fluoro-D-glucose positron emission tomography in the staging and restaging of patients with lymphoma. *Cancer* 2005;**104**:1066–74.

40. Moog F, Bangerter M, Diederichs CG et al. Extranodal malignant lymphoma: detection with FDG PET versus CT. *Radiology* 1998:**206**:475–81.

41. Hutchings M, Loft A, Hansen M et al. Position emission tomography with or without computed tomography in the primary staging of Hodgkin's lymphoma. *Haematologica* 2006;**91**:482–9.

42. Picardi M, Soricelli A, Grimaldi F et al. Fused FDG-PET/contrast-enhanced CT detects occult subdiaphragmatic involvement of Hodgkin's lymphoma thereby identifying patients requiring six cycles of anthracycline-containing chemotherapy and consolidation radiation of spleen. *Ann Oncol* 2011;**22** (3):671–80.

43. Tatsumi M, Cohade C, Nakamoto Y et al. Direct comparison of FDG PET and CT findings in patients with lymphoma: initial experience. *Radiology* 2005;**237**:1038–45.

44. Schaefer NG, Hany TF, Taverna C et al. Non-Hodgkin lymphoma and Hodgkin disease: coregistered FDG PET and CT at staging and restaging – do we need contrast-enhanced CT? *Radiology* 2004;**232**:823–9.

45. Rodriguez-Vigil B, Gomez-Leon N, Pinilla I et al. PET/CT in lymphoma: prospective study of enhanced full-dose PET/CT versus unenhanced low-dose PET/CT. *J Nucl Med* 2006;**47**:1643–8.

46. Kwee TC, Kwee RM, Nievelstein RA. Imaging instagin of malignant lymphoma: a systematic review. *Blood* 2008;**111**:504–16.

47. Carr R, Barrington SF, Madan B et al. Detection of lymphoma in bone marrow by whole-body positron emission tomography. *Blood* 1998;**91**:3340–6.

48. Pakos EE, Fotopoulos AD, Ioannidis JP. 18F-FDG PET for evaluation of bone marrow infiltration in staging of lymphoma: a meta-analysis. *J Nucl Med* 2005;**46**:958–63.

49. Wu LM, Chen FY, Jiang XX et al. (18)F-FDG PET, combined FDG-PET/CT and MRI for evaluation of bone marrow infiltration in staging of lymphoma: A systematic review and meta-analysis. *Eur J Radiol* 2012;**81**:303–11.

50. Gospodarowicz MK, Ferry JA, Cavalli F. Unique aspects of primary extranodal lymphomas. In PM Mauch, JO Armitage, B Coiffier et al. (Eds.), *Non-Hodgkin's Lymphoma*. Philadelphia, PA: Lippincott, Williams, and Wilkins, 2004, pp. 685–707.

51. Enomoto K, Hamada K, Inohara H et al. Mucosa-associated lymphoid tissue lymphoma studied with FDG-PET: a comparison with CT and endoscopic findings, *Ann Nucl Med* 2008;**22**:261–7.

52. Morris PG, Zacharia TT, Law M, Naidich TP, Leeds NE. Central nervous system lymphoma characterization by diffusion-weighted imaging and MR spectroscopy. *J Neuroimaging* 2008;**18**:411–17.

53. Herrlinger U, Schabet M, Clemens M et al. Clinical presentation and therapeutic outcome in 26 patients with primary CNS lymphoma. *Acta Neurol Scand* 1998;**97**:257–64.

54. Heald AE, Hoffman JM, Bartlett JA, Waskin HA. Differentiation of central nervous system lesions in AIDS patients using positron emission tomography (PET). *Int J STD AIDS* 1996;**7**:337–46.

55. Mohile NA, Deangelis LM, Abrey LE. Utility of brain FDG-PET in primary CNS lymphoma. *Clin Adv Hematol Oncol* 2008; **6**: 818–820, 840.

56. Blum RH, Seymour JF, Wirth A et al. Frequent impact of [18F] Fluorodeoxyglucose positron emission tomography on the staging and management of patients with indolent non-Hodgkin lymphoma. *Clin Lymphoma* 2004;**4**:43–9.

57. Freudenberg LS, Antoch G, Schütt P et al. FDG PET/CT in restaging of patients with lymphoma. *Eur J Nucl Med Mol Imaging* 2004;**31**:325–9.

58. Kissin CM, Husband JE, Nicholas D, Eversman W. Benign thymic enlargement in adults after chemotherapy: CT demonstration. *Radiology* 1987;**163**:67–70.

59. Nasseri F, Eftekhari F. Clinical and radiologic review of the normal and abnormal thymus: pearls and pitfalls. *Radiographics* 2010;**30**:413–28.

60. Ferdinand B, Gupta P, Kramer EL. Spectrum of thymic uptake at 18F-FDG PET. *Radiographics* 2004;**24**:1611–16.

61. Abdel-Dayem HM, Rosen G, El-Zeftawy H et al. Fluorine-18 fluorodeoxyglucose splenic uptake from extramedullary hematopoiesis after granulocyte colony-stimulating factor

stimulation. *Clin Nucl Med* 1999;**24**:319–22.

62. Surbone A, Longo DL, DeVita VT *et al.* Residual abdominal masses in aggressive non-Hodgkin lymphoma after combination chemotherapy: significance and management. *J Clin Oncol* 1988;**6**:1832–7.

63. Radford JA, Cowan RA, Flanagan M *et al.* The significance of residual mediastinal abnormality on the chest radiograph following treatment for Hodgkin disease. *J Clin Oncol* 1988;**6**:940–6.

64. Hasenclever D, Diehl V, for the International Prognostic Factors Project on Advanced Hodgkin's Disease. A prognostic score for advanced Hodgkin's disease. *New Engl J Med* 1998;**339**:1506–14.

65. Cremerius U, Fabry U, Neuerburg J *et al.* Positron emission tomography with 18F-FDG to detect residual disease after therapy for malignant lymphoma. *Nucl Med Commun* 1998;**19**:1055–63.

66. Dittmann H, Sokler M, Kollmannsberger C *et al.* Comparison of 18FDG-PET with CT scans in the evaluation of patients with residual and recurrent Hodgkin's lymphoma. *Oncol Rep* 2001;**8**:1393–9.

67. Spaepen K, Stroobants S, Dupont P *et al.* Prognostic value of positron emission tomography (PET) with fluorine-18 fluorodeoxyglucose ([$^{18}$F]FDG after first line chemotherapy in non-Hodgkins lymphoma: Is ([$^{18}$F]FDG PET a valid alternative to conventional diagnostic methods? *J Clin Oncol* 2001;**19**:414–19.

68. Zinzani PL, Magagnoli M, Chierichetti F *et al.* The role of positron emission tomography (PET) in the management of lymphoma patients. *Ann Oncol* 1999;**10**:1181–4.

69. Mikhaeel NG, Mainwaring P, Nunan T, Timothy AR. Prognostic value of interim and post treatment FDG-PET scanning in Hodgkin lymphoma [abstract]. *Ann Oncol* 2002; **13**(Suppl 2):21.

70. Wiedmann E, Baican B, Hertel A *et al.* Positron emission tomography (PET) for staging and evaluation of response to treatment in patients with Hodgkin's disease. *Leuk Lymphoma* 1999;**34**:545–51.

71. Juweid ME, Stroobants S, Hoekstra OS *et al.* Use of positron emission tomography for response assessment of lymphoma: consensus of the Imaging Subcommittee of International Harmonization Project in Lymphoma. *J Clin Oncol* 2007;**25**:571–8.

72. Robinson SP, Goldstone AH, Mackinnon S *et al.* Chemoresistant or aggressive lymphoma predicts for a poor outcome following reduced-intensity allogeneic progenitor cell transplantation: an analysis from the Lymphoma Working Party of the European Group for Blood and Bone Marrow Transplantation. *Blood* 2002;**100**:4310–16.

73. Spaepen K, Stroobants S, Dupont P *et al.* Prognostic value of pretransplantation positron emission tomography using fluorine 18-fluorodeoxyglucose in patients with aggressive lymphoma treated with high-dose chemotherapy and stem cell transplantation. *Blood* 2003;**102**:53–9.

74. Cremerius U, Fabry U, Wildberger JE *et al.* Pre-transplant positron emission tomography using fluorine-18-fluoro-deoxyglucose predicts outcome in patients treated with high-dose chemotherapy and autologous stem cell transplantation for non-Hodgkin's lymphoma. *Bone Marrow Transpl* 2002;**30**:103–11.

75. Becherer A, Mitterbauer M, Jaeger U *et al.* Positron emission tomography with [18F]2-fluoro-D-2-deoxyglucose (FDG-PET) predicts relapse of malignant lymphoma after high-dose therapy with stem cell transplantation. *Leukemia* 2002;**16**:260–7.

76. Terasawa T, Dahabreh IJ, Nihashi T. Fluorine-18-fluorodeoxyglucose positron emission tomography in response assessment before high-dose chemotherapy for lymphoma: a systematic review and meta-analysis. *Oncologist* 2010;**15**(7):750–9.

77. Roland V, Bodet-Milin C, Moreau A *et al.* Impact of high-dose chemotherapy followed by auto-SCT for positive interim [(18)F] FDG-PET diffuse large B-cell lymphoma patients. *Bone Marrow Transpl* 2011;**46**:393–9.

78. Poulou LS, Thanos L, Ziakas PD. Unifying the predictive value of pretransplant FDG PET in patients with lymphoma: a review and meta-analysis of published trials. *Eur J Nucl Med Mol Imaging* 2010;**37**:156–62.

79. Gisselbrecht C, Vose J, Nademanee A, Gianni AM, Nagler A. Radioimmunotherapy for stem cell transplantation in non-Hodgkin's lymphoma: in pursuit of a complete response. *Oncologist* 2009;**14**(Suppl 2):41–51.

80. Buske C, Gisselbrecht C, Gribben J *et al.* Refining the treatment of follicular lymphoma. *Leuk Lymphoma* 2008;**49** (Suppl 1):18–26.

81. Schaffel R, Hedvat CV, Teruya-Feldstein J *et al.* Prognostic impact of proliferative index determined by quantitative image analysis and the International Prognostic Index in patients with mantle cell lymphoma. *Ann Oncol* 2010;**21**(1):133–9.

82. Bodet-Milin C, Touzeau C, Leux C *et al.* Prognostic impact of 18F-fluoro-deoxyglucose positron emission tomography in untreated mantle cell lymphoma: a retrospective study from the GOELAMS group. *Eur J Nucl Med Mol Imaging* 2010;**37**:1633–42.

83. Tateishi U, Tatsumi M, Terauchi T *et al.* Relevance of monitoring metabolic reduction in patients with relapsed or refractory follicular and mantle cell lymphoma receiving bendamustine: a multicenter study. *Cancer Sci* 2011;**102**:414–18.

84. Mato AR, Svoboda J, Feldman T *et al.* Post-treatment (not interim) PET-CT scan status is highly predictive of outcome in mantle cell T lymphoma treated with R-HyperCVAD. *Cancer* 2011;Abstract online:DOI:10.1002/ cncr.26731.

85. Le Dortz L, De Guibert S, Bayat S *et al.* Diagnostic and prognostic impact of 18F-FDG PET/CT in follicular lymphoma. *Eur J Nucl Med Mol Imaging* 2010;**37**:2307.

86. Bishu S, Quigley JM, Bishu SR *et al.* Predictive value and diagnostic accuracy of F-18-fluoro-deoxy-glucose positron emission tomography treated grade 1 and 2 follicular lymphoma. *Leuk Lymphoma* 2007;**48**:1548–55.

87. Lopci E, Santi I, Derenzini E *et al.* FDG-PET in the assessment of patients with follicular lymphoma treated by ibritumomab tiuxetan Y 90: multicentric study. *Ann Oncol* 2010;**21**(9):1877–83.

88. Storto G, De Renzo A, Pellegrino T *et al*. Assessment of metabolic response to radioimmunotherapy with 90Y-ibritumomab tiuxetan in patients with relapsed or refractory B-cell non-Hodgkin lymphoma. *Radiology* 2010;**254**:245–52.

89. Terasawa T, Lau J, Bardet S *et al*. Fluorine-18-fluorodeoxyglucose positron emission tomography for interim response assessment of advanced-stage Hodgkin's lymphoma and diffuse large B-cell lymphoma: a systematic review. *J Clin Oncol* 2009;**27**(11):1906–14.

90. Haioun C, Itti E, Rahmouni A *et al*. [18F]Fluoro-2-deoxy-D-glucose positron emission tomography (FDG-PET) in aggressive lymphoma: an early prognostic tool for predicting patient outcome. *Blood* 2005;**106**:1376–81.

91. Mikhaeel NG, Hutchings M, Fields PA, O'Doherty MJ, Timothy AR. FDG-PET after two to three cycles of chemotherapy predicts progression-free and overall survival in high-grade non-Hodgkin lymphoma. *Ann Oncol* 2005;**16**:1514–23.

92. Spaepen K, Stroobants S, Dupont P *et al*. Early restaging positron emission tomography with (18)F-fluorodeoxyglucose predicts outcome in patients with aggressive non-Hodgkin's lymphoma. *Ann Oncol* 2002;**13**:1356–63.

93. Kostakoglu L, Goldsmith SJ, Leonard JP *et al*. FDG-PET after 1 cycle of therapy predicts outcome in diffuse large cell lymphoma and classic Hodgkin disease. *Cancer* 2006;**107**:2678–87.

94. Moskowitz CH, Schöder H, Teruya-Feldstein J *et al*. Risk-adapted dose-dense immunochemotherapy determined by interim FDG-PET in advanced-stage diffuse large B-Cell lymphoma. *J Clin Oncol* 2010;**28**(11):1896–903.

95. Kasamon YL, Wahl RL, Ziessman HA *et al*. Phase II study of risk-adapted therapy of newly diagnosed, aggressive non-Hodgkin lymphoma based on midtreatment FDG-PET scanning. *Biol Blood Marrow Transplant* 2009;**15**(2):242–8.

96. Terasawa T, Nihashi T, Hotta T *et al*. 18F-FDG PET for posttherapy assessment of Hodgkin's disease and aggressive non-Hodgkin's lymphoma: a systematic review. *J Nucl Med* 2008;**49**:13–21.

97. Hutchings M, Mikhaeel NG, Fields PA *et al*. Prognostic value of interim FDG-PET after two or three cycles of chemotherapy in Hodgkin lymphoma. *Ann Oncol* 2005;**16**:1160–8.

98. Hutchings M, Loft A, Hansen M *et al*. FDG-PET after two cycles of chemotherapy predicts treatment failure and progression-free survival in Hodgkin lymphoma. *Blood* 2006;**107**:52–9.

99. Gallamini A, Hutchings M, Rigacci L *et al*. Early interim 2-[18F]fluoro-2-deoxy-D-glucose positron emission tomography is prognostically superior to international prognostic score in advanced-stage Hodgkin's lymphoma: a report from a joint Italian–Danish study. *J Clin Oncol* 2007;**25**:3746–52.

100. Steidl C, Lee T, Shah SP, Farinha P *et al*. Tumor-associated macrophages and survival in classic Hodgkin's lymphoma. *New Engl J Med* 2010;**362**:875–85.

101. Zinzani PL, Tani M, Fanti S *et al*. Early positron emission tomography (PET) restaging: a predictive final response in Hodgkin's disease patients. *Ann Oncol* 2006;**17**:1296–1300.

102. Cerci JJ, Pracchia LF, Linardi CC *et al*. 18F-FDG PET after 2 cycles of ABVD predicts event-free survival in early and advanced Hodgkin lymphoma. *J Nucl Med* 2010;**51**(9):1337–43. Erratum in *J Nucl Med* 2010;**51**(10):1658.

103. Barnes JA, Lacasce AS, Zukotynski K **et al**. End-of-treatment but not interim PET scan predicts outcome in nonbulky limited-stage Hodgkin's lymphoma. *Ann Oncol* 2011;**22**(4):910–15.

104. Dann EJ, Bar-Shalom R, Tamir A *et al*. Risk-adapted BEACOPP regimen can reduce the cumulative dose of chemotherapy for standard and high-risk Hodgkin lymphoma with no impairment of outcome. *Blood* 2007;**109**(3):905–9.

105. Avigdor A, Bulvik S, Levi I *et al*. Two cycles of escalated BEACOPP followed by four cycles of ABVD utilizing early-interim PET/CT scan is an effective regimen for advanced high-risk Hodgkin's lymphoma. *Ann Oncol* 2010;**21**(1):126–32.

106. Quddus F, Armitage JO. Salvage therapy for Hodgkin's lymphoma. *Cancer J* 2009;**15**:161–3.

107. Engert A, Eichenauer DA, Dreyling M. Hodgkin's lymphoma: ESMO clinical recommendations for diagnosis, treatment and follow-up. *Ann Oncol* 2009;**20**(Suppl 4):108–9.

108. Goldschmidt N, Or O, Klein M, Savitsky B, Paltiel O. The role of routine imaging procedures in the detection of relapse of patients with Hodgkin lymphoma and aggressive non-Hodgkin lymphoma. *Ann Hematol* 2011;**90**(2):165–71.

109. Zinzani PL, Stefoni V, Tani M *et al*. Role of [18F]fluorodeoxyglucose positron emission tomography scan in the follow-up of lymphoma. *J Clin Oncol* 2009;**27**:1781–7.

110. Lee AI, Zuckerman DS, Van den Abbeele AD *et al*. Surveillance imaging of Hodgkin lymphoma patients in first remission: a clinical and economic analysis. *Cancer* 2010;**116**:3835–42.

111. Josting A, Diehl V. Current treatment strategies in early stage Hodgkin's disease. *Curr Treat Options Oncol* 2003;**4**:297–305.

112. Cheson B. The case against heavy PETing. *J Clin Oncol* 2009;**11**:1742–3.

113. Meyer RM, Gospodarowicz MK, Connors JM *et al*. Randomized comparison of ABVD chemotherapy with a strategy that includes radiation therapy in patients with limited stage Hodgkin's lymphoma: National Cancer Institute of Canada Clinical Trials Group and the Eastern Cooperative Oncology Group. *J Clin Oncol* 2005;**23**:4634–42.

114. Brix G, Lechel U, Glatting G *et al*. Radiation exposure of patients undergoing whole-body dual-modality 18F-FDG PET/CT examinations. *J Nucl Med* 2005;**46**:608–13.

115. Spaepen K, Stroobants S, Dupont P *et al*. [(18)F]FDG PET monitoring of tumour response to chemotherapy: does [(18)F]FDG uptake correlate with the viable tumour cell fraction? *Eur J Nucl Med Mol Imaging* 2003;**30**:682–8.

116. Meignan M, Gallamini A, Haioun C. Report on the First International Workshop on Interim-PET-Scan in

Lymphoma. *Leuk Lymphoma* 2009;**50**:1257–60.

117. Barrington SF, Qian W, Somer E *et al.* Concordance between four European centres of PET reporting criteria designed for use in multicentre trials in Hodgkin lymphoma. *Eur J Nucl Med Mol Imaging* 2010;**37**:1824–33.

118. Thie JA, Hubner KF, Smith GT. Optimizing imaging time for improved performance in oncology PET studies. *Mol Imaging Biol* 2002;**4**:238–44.

119. Lin C, Itti E, Haioun C *et al.* Early 18F-FDG PET for prediction of prognosis in patients with diffuse large B-cell lymphoma: SUV-based assessment versus visual analysis. *J Nucl Med* 2007;**48**:1626–32.

**Case 1**: A 35-year-old female recently diagnosed with classical Hodgkin's lymphoma (cHL).

**Case 2**: A 46-year-old male recently diagnosed with nodular lymphocyte predominant HL (NLPHL).

Both patients underwent a FDG-PET/CT scan to evaluate the extent of disease prior to therapy initiation.

## Acquisition and processing parameters

Following a fasting period of 6 hours, the patients (similar protocols for both patients) were intravenously injected with approximately 20 mCi of FDG, and an uptake phase of 90 min was allowed prior to PET/CT imaging. Plasma glucose levels were less than 100 mg/dL at the time of FDG injection. The patients voided before the start of imaging acquisition, and images were obtained from the orbits to the proximal thighs using a combined PET/CT scanner. Imaging was performed in the supine position, with arms placed above their heads, in an attempt to reduce beam-hardening artifacts in the torso. The low-dose CT protocol acquisition parameters were as follows; 140 kVp, 80 mA, 0.8 s per CT rotation, pitch of 1.35 : 1, and a reconstructed slice thickness of 5.0 mm. The CT data were reconstructed using a filtered back-projection algorithm and a $512 \times 512$ matrix, with a transaxial field of view of 50 cm. The CT images were used to generate the transmission maps for attenuation correction of the PET acquisitions and anatomic localization. Immediately after the

CT scan, and without changing the patient's position, the tabletop moved automatically to the PET position. The emission scans were acquired starting at the mid-thighs toward the head, in six 4 minutes/bed positions (14.5 cm longitudinal field of view). PET data were reconstructed using an ordered-subset expectation maximization iterative algorithm (28 subsets, 2 iterations).

## Findings and differential diagnosis

**Case 1**: Coronal CT, PET, PET/CT fused slices and the volumetric/maximum intensity projection image (MIP) (Figure 13.1A, B, C, D, respectively) demonstrate multiple foci of increased FDG uptake in the left neck and left chest corresponding to the lower cervical, supraclavicular, paratracheal and multiple anterior superior mediastinal lymph node stations. The majority of these lymph nodes are coalescing in a contiguous pattern which is characteristic for cHL. There is no evidence of splenic and other site of extranodal involvement.

**Case 2**: Coronal CT, PET, PET/CT fused slices and the volumetric/maximum intensity projection image (MIP) (Figure 13.2A, B, C, D, respectively) demonstrate increased FDG uptake in the neck and chest corresponding to right lower cervical, bilateral supraclavicular, right paratracheal and right superior mediastinal lymph node stations. There is no evidence of splenic or extranodal involvement. There is apparently lesser degree of FDG accumulation within the

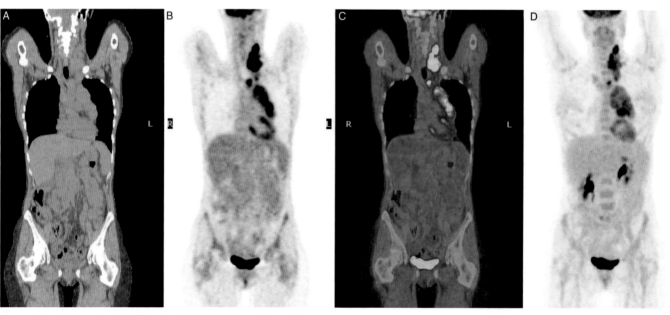

**Figure 13.1** (A) Coronal CT; (B) FDG-PET; (C) FDG-PET/CT fused slices; (D) maximum intensity projection (MIP) image.

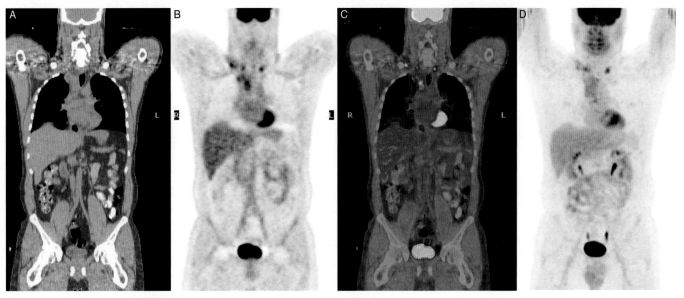

**Figure 13.2** (A) Coronal CT; (B) FDG-PET; (C) FDG-PET/CT fused slices; (D) maximum intensity projection (MIP) image.

involved lymph nodes compared with Case 1 which suggests a different histologic subtype of HL.

Differential diagnosis: Case 1: Stage II cHL; Case 2: Stage II NLPHL.

## Diagnosis and clinical follow-up

**Case 1**: Excisional biopsy of a left cervical lymph node was positive for classical HL.

**Case 2**: Excisional biopsy of a right cervical lymph node was positive for nodular lymphocyte predominant HL (NLPHL).

## Discussion and teaching points

Pretreatment staging determines the extent of disease and helps direct therapy. The TNM (tumor, node, metastasis) staging system is not applicable in lymphomas because usually the specific origin of tumor is not clearly identified. The Ann Arbor staging system has been adopted for staging of both HL and NHL (1, 2). There are four main stages of lymphomas (Table 13.1). The presence of constitutional symptoms: fevers less than 38 °C, night sweats, or weight loss of greater than 10% of body weight during the 6 months (B) and bulky disease (X) portend worse prognosis. Stages I and IIA are considered early-stage disease and stages IIB (particularly bulky), III, and IV are considered advanced-stage disease. PET/CT has proven to be more sensitive and specific than contrast-enhanced high-dose CT for evaluation of lymphoma involvement (3–8) (further discussed later in this chapter). Thus, more recently, FDG-PET has been incorporated into the staging algorithm of most histologic subtypes, particularly in HL and DLBCL (9, 10). In a meta-analysis of FDG-PET staging of patients who had lymphoma, the pooled sensitivity for 14 studies with patient-based data was 91% with a false-positive rate of only

10%, with an apparently higher sensitivity and false-positive rate in HL patients compared with NHL (7). The maximum sensitivity and specificity were 95.6%. In Case 1, contiguous involvement of the neck and chest lymph nodes is characteristic to cHL. Initial disease is located in the chest in more than 80% of cases and superior mediastinal lymph nodes are more frequently involved (≥ 85%) compared to non-Hodgkin's lymphoma (NHL). Mediastinal HL is characterized by the presence of a discrete anterior superior mediastinal mass with surface lobulation due to conglomeration of multiple involved lymph nodes (11). In general, involvement of extranodal organs is not common in HL. FDG-PET usually upstages disease because it finds additional sites of nodal and extranodal disease. Concordance of PET and CT occurs in approximately 80% of HL patients (3–5). Nonetheless, it may be preferable that both FDG-PET and high-resolution CT are obtained for pretreatment staging for better definition of disease extent and size measurements that may prove useful for assessment of response (3–5). PET detects additional disease sites in 10–20% of patients that modify clinical stage, and even fewer patients for whom this modification alters management or outcome (3, 12).

As noted in Case 2, the nodular lymphocyte predominant HL (NLPHL) differs in histological and clinical presentation from cHL with a more indolent course, favorable therapy response, and even at times spontaneous remission. The NLPHL cells are positive for CD45, CD19, CD20, CD22, but lack expression of CD15 and CD30, the typical markers for cHL (13, 14). NLPHL more often presents in early stages (~60%) and only 6% present with stage IV disease. B symptoms are observed only in 10% of NLPHL which contrasts with cHL (13). The prognostically significant factors of bulky disease and mediastinal involvement are rare in NLPHL. NLPHL seems to be confined more often to peripheral sites, such as upper neck, epitrochlear, and inguinal nodes (14). In NLPHL skip areas are more common compared with the contiguous pattern seen with classical H, and involvement of mediastinum and hilar regions is not as common as in classical HL. Curable relapses are frequent and the disease may progress to NHL (13, 14). Similar to cHL, FDG-PET sensitivity is close to 100% in patients with NLPHL (15).

## Take-home message

- The Ann Arbor staging system has been adopted for staging of both HL and NHL. There are four main stages of lymphomas.
- The sensitivity of FDG-PET for staging of HL is high at above 90% with a low false-positive rate, hence FDG-PET

imaging may provide complementary information to CT and bone-marrow biopsy.

- Involvement of intrathoracic lymph nodes are common in HL, moreover, the distribution pattern is usually contiguous rather than widespread in the body.
- The disease distribution pattern is different between cHL and NLPHL which can be easily recognized by observing the characteristics of FDG-PET imaging with respect to disease distribution patterns and FDG uptake. Differentiation between the two subtypes may have management consequences as NLPHL has a more indolent course, favorable therapy response, and even at times spontaneous remission.

## References

1. Lister TA, Crowther D, Sutcliffe SB *et al.* Report of a committee convened to discuss the evaluation and staging of patients with Hodgkin's disease: Cotswald meeting. *J Clin Oncol* 1989;7:1630–6.

2. Rosenberg S. Validity of the Ann Arbor staging system classification for the non-Hodgkin's lymphomas. *Cancer Treat Rep* 1977;61:1023–7.

3. Jerusalem G, Beguin Y, Najjar F *et al.* Positron emission tomography (PET) with 18F-fluorodeoxyglucose (18F-FDG) for the staging of low-grade non-Hodgkin lymphoma (NHL). *Ann Oncol* 2001;12:825–30.

4. Naumann R, Beuthien-Baumann B, Reiss A *et al.* Substantial impact of FDG PET imaging on the therapy decision in patients with early-stage Hodgkin lymphoma. *Br J Cancer* 2004;90:620–5.

5. Hutchings M, Loft A, Hansen M *et al.* Positron emission tomography with or without computed tomography in the primary staging of Hodgkin lymphoma. *Haematologica* 2006;91:482–9.

6. Buchmann I, Reinhardt M, Elsner K *et al.* 2-(fluorine-18)fluoro-2-deoxy-D-glucose positron emission tomography in the detection and staging of malignant lymphoma. A bicenter trial. *Cancer* 2001;91:889–99.

7. Isasi CR, Lu P, Blaufox MD. A metaanalysis of 18F-2-deoxy-2-fluoro-D-glucose positron emission tomography in the staging and restaging of patients with lymphoma. *Cancer* 2005;104:1066–74.

8. Schaefer NG, Hany TF, Taverna C *et al.* Non-Hodgkin lymphoma and Hodgkin disease: coregistered FDG PET and CT at staging and restaging – do we need contrast-enhanced CT? *Radiology* 2004;232:823–9.

9. National Comprehensive Cancer Network, Hodgkin Lymphoma, *NCCN* v1 2011. http://www.nccn.org/professionals/physician_gls/pdf/hodgkins.pdf

10. National Comprehensive Cancer Network, non-Hodgkin Lymphoma, *NCCN* v2 2011. http://www.nccn.org/professionals/physician_gls/pdf/nhl.pdf

11. Tateishi U, Muller NL, Johkoh T *et al.* Primary mediastinal lymphoma: characteristic features of the various histological subtypes on CT. *J Comput Assist Tomogr* 2004;28:782–9.

12. Rodriguez-Vigil B, Gomez-Leon N, Pinilla I *et al.* PET/CT in lymphoma: prospective study of enhanced full-dose PET/CT versus unenhanced low-dose PET/CT. *J Nucl Med* 2006;47:1643–8.

13. Nogova L, Reineke T, Josting A *et al.* Lymphocyte-predominant and classical Hodgkin's lymphoma – comparison of outcomes. *Eur J Haematol* 2005;75 (Suppl 66):106–110.

14. Diehl V, Sextro M, Franklin J *et al.* Clinical presentation, course, and prognostic factors in lymphocyte-predominant Hodgkin's disease and lymphocyte-rich classical Hodgkin's disease: report from the European Task Force on Lymphoma Project on Lymphocyte-Predominant Hodgkin's Disease. *J Clin Oncol* 1999;17:776–83.

15. Elstrom R, Guan L, Baker G *et al.* Utility of FDG-PET scanning in lymphoma by WHO classification. *Blood* 2003;101:3875–6.

**Case 3**: A 50-year-old female recently diagnosed with diffuse large B-cell lymphoma (DLBCL).

**Case 4**: A 42-year-old male with a history of HIV positive serology and AIDS (CD4+ T cells < 200 per cubic millimeter of blood) for the past 5 years, recently diagnosed with DLBCL.

**Case 5**: A 52-year-old male with a history of HIV positive serology with no diagnosis of AIDS or lymphoma (CD4+ T cells: 400 per cubic millimeter of blood).

Cases 3 and 4 underwent FDG-PET/CT imaging to evaluate the extent of disease prior to initiation of therapy. Case 5 underwent FDG-PET/CT imaging to evaluate for lymphadenopathy and to determine the site for biopsy.

## Acquisition and processing parameters

Following a fasting period of 6 hours, the patients (similar protocols for all three patients) were intravenously injected with approximately 18–20 mCi of FDG, and an uptake phase of 60 min was allowed prior to PET/CT imaging. Plasma glucose levels were less than 100 mg/dL at the time of FDG injection. The patients voided before the start of imaging acquisition, and images were obtained from the orbits to the proximal thighs using a combined PET/CT scanner. Imaging was performed in the supine position, with arms placed above their heads, in an attempt to reduce beam-hardening artifacts in the torso. The low-dose CT protocol acquisition parameters

were as follows; 140 kVp, 80 mA, 0.8 s per CT rotation, pitch of 1.35 : 1, and a reconstructed slice thickness of 5.0 mm. The CT data were reconstructed using a filtered back-projection algorithm and a 512 × 512 matrix, with a transaxial field of view of 50 cm. The CT images were used to generate the transmission maps for attenuation correction of the PET acquisitions and anatomic localization. Immediately after the CT scan, and without changing the patient's position, the tabletop moved automatically to the PET position. The emission scans were acquired starting at the mid-thighs toward the head, in six 4 minutes/bed positions (14.5 cm longitudinal field of view). PET data were reconstructed using an ordered-subset expectation maximization iterative algorithm (28 subsets, 2 iterations).

## Findings and differential diagnosis

**Case 3**: Coronal CT, PET, PET/CT fused slices and the maximum intensity projection image (MIP) (Figure 13.3A, B, C, D, respectively) demonstrate multiple foci of increased FDG uptake in the chest, abdomen, and pelvis, corresponding to the mediastinal (subcarinal), retroperitoneal, pelvic, and left inguinal lymph node stations following a non-contiguous widespread pattern. Also noted is the heterogeneous focal uptake within an enlarged spleen, consistent with splenic involvement. Focal sites of increased uptake within the axial skeleton (multiple ribs, left iliac crest, left greater trochanter) as well as in a linear pattern in the proximal appendicular

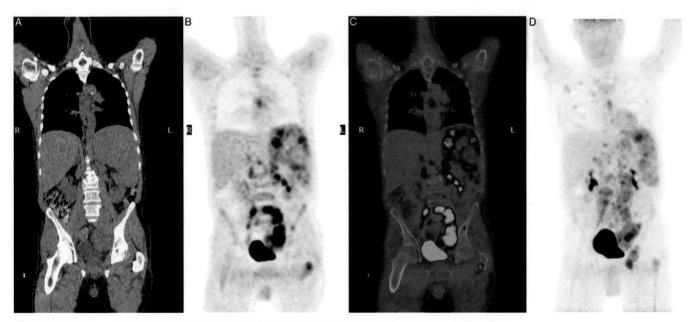

**Figure 13.3** (A) Coronal CT; (B) FDG-PET; (C) FDG-PET/CT fused slices; (D) maximum intensity projection (MIP) image.

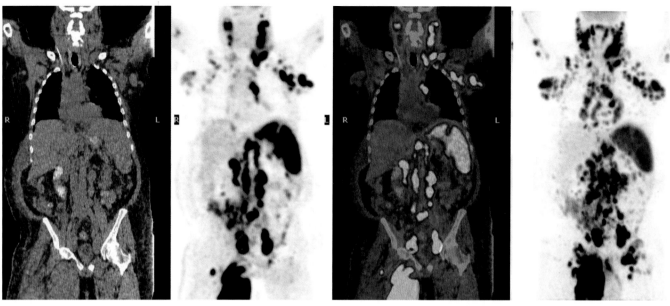

**Figure 13.4** (A) Coronal CT; (B) FDG-PET; (C) FDG-PET/CT fused slices; (D) maximum intensity projection (MIP) image.

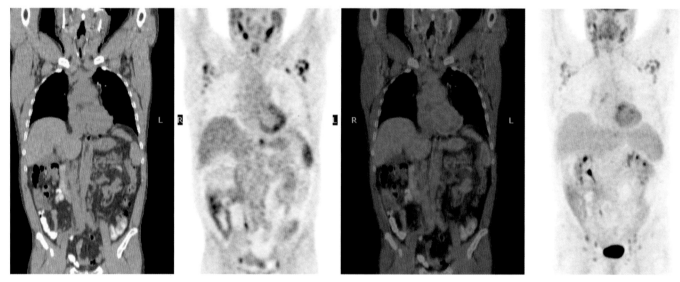

**Figure 13.5** (A) Coronal CT; (B) FDG-PET; (C) FDG-PET/CT fused slices; (D) maximum intensity projection (MIP) image.

skeleton, particularly in the right humerus and left femur, compatible with bone and bone marrow involvement. Differential diagnosis: Stage IV DLBCL.

**Case 4**: Coronal CT, PET, PET/CT fused slices and maximum intensity projection image (MIP) (Figure 13.4A, B, C, D, respectively) demonstrate multiple foci of significantly increased FDG uptake corresponding to markedly enlarged bilateral cervical, axillary, mediastinal, hilar, diaphragmatic, retroperitoneal, mesenteric, pelvic, and inguinal lymph node stations compatible with widespread involvement of disease in the lymph nodes. Additionally, there is intense uptake within the spleen as well as in a mass situated in the right upper medial thigh. Note the uptake within the right proximal humerus and more vaguely and focally in multiple ribs, consistent with bone marrow involvement.

Although both patients in Case 3 and 4 have stage IV DLBCL, note the more aggressive disease distribution pattern and the intensity of FDG uptake in Case 4, suggestive of a highly aggressive clinical behavior. The histology in Case 4 demonstrated high Ki67 staining reflecting high proliferative index, thus, more aggressive disease biology.

Differential diagnosis: Stage IV, HIV-associated lymphoma, probably DLBCL in etiology. However, HL, Burkitt's lymphoma, and plasmablastic lymphoma (PBL) should be considered in the differential diagnosis as these are also associated with HIV-positive serology.

**Case 5**: Coronal CT, PET, PET/CT fused slices and maximum intensity projection image (MIP) (Figure 13.5A, B, C, D, respectively) demonstrate multiple foci of mild-to-moderately increased FDG uptake in mildly enlarged bilateral cervical, axillary, and inguinal lymph node stations.

Differential diagnosis: HIV-related lymphadenopathy with no definite evidence of high-grade lymphoma. HIV-associated lymphoma can be considered in the differential diagnosis although the peripheral distribution, absence of marked lymph node enlargement and low-grade FDG uptake are not in line with a high-grade lymphoma that is expected in the setting of HIV disease.

## Diagnosis and clinical follow-up

**Case 3**: Excisional biopsy of a left inguinal lymph node was positive for DLBCL.

**Case 4**: Core biopsy of the right thigh mass was positive for DLBCL.

**Case 5**: No biopsy. During a clinical follow-up of 12 months the patient has been stable with no clinical suspicion of lymphoma.

## Discussion and teaching points

In general, the nodal involvement is usually widespread and non-contiguous, extranodal involvement of the lung parenchyma, pleura, and pericardium is more common with NHL than with HL because of the frequent vascular invasion and hematogenous spread associated with the former (1). Extrinsic infiltration of bones and muscles by neighboring lymph node masses is seen in both HL and DLBCL (2, 3). Intrathoracic involvement is less common in DLBCL compared with HL and usually is an extension of widespread disease process. The sensitivity of FDG-PET is highest in DLBCL (> 95%) among other NHL subtypes (4). Bone marrow (BM) involvement is more common in DLBCL compared with HL. FDG-PET can detect BM involvement even if the BM biopsy is negative (5–7). However, FDG-PET alone is unreliable in detecting low disease volume in the BM and degenerative changes (7) and reactive BM hyperplasia can lead to false-positive findings, thus, PET cannot substitute BM biopsy in lymphoma staging.

DLBCL is the most common type of HIV-associated lymphoma, accounting for 80–90% of cases; however, primary CNS lymphoma, Burkitt's lymphoma, HL, plasmablastic lymphoma (PCNSL), and primary effusion lymphoma (PEL) can occur in HIV-positive patients (8). These lymphomas are characterized clinically by aggressiveness as evidenced by advanced stage, extra-nodal involvement and poor therapeutic outcomes, however, outcomes have been improved after the introduction of highly active antiretroviral therapy (HAART) (9, 10). The most common sites of extranodal involvement include the bone marrow, gastrointestinal tract, spleen, and the central nervous system. FDG-PET imaging demonstrates extensive disease with significantly high SUV values. However, one has to realize that the spectrum of HIV infection ranges from an asymptomatic seropositive stage to a syndrome characterized by persistent generalized lymphadenopathy which eventually evolves to the final stage of severe immune dysfunction. HIV mediates its impact on the immune system primarily through an interaction with the CD4 membrane antigen that is expressed on the surface of the T-helper cells. In HIV-related lymphadenopathy, the morphologic feature is dominated by florid hyperplasia of lymphoid cells with secondary follicles and expanded germinal centers in the lymph nodes (11). The increased FDG uptake is, therefore, manifested in multiple lymph node groups, usually distributed in the peripheral and superficial stations such as cervical, axillary, and inguinal regions (12). A progressive pattern of lymphoid tissue activation was reported starting from the head and neck during acute disease, a generalized pattern of peripheral lymph node activation during mid-stages, and involvement of abdominal lymph nodes during late disease, suggesting that lymphoid tissues are engaged in a predictable sequence depending on the viral load and HAART therapy response (13–16). Moreover, AIDS-related opportunistic infections including cytomegalovirus, *Cryptococcus neoformans*, and classic or atypical tuberculosis (17) are common when CD4+ T-cell numbers decline below a critical level, and impair cell-mediated immunity. If the patient does not have a prior diagnosis of lymphoma the differentiation between malignancy, reactive hyperplasia, and infectious causes can be challenging. Nonetheless, a good clinical history, patient's viral load, CD4 levels and the response to HAART status may help the image interpreter avoid false-positive readings.

## Take-home message

- PET-positive bone marrow findings should be confirmed by biopsy or MR imaging particularly if a stage migration and thereby a change in treatment strategy will be based on these findings.
- In DLBCL, the nodal involvement is usually widespread and non-contiguous; extranodal involvement and BM involvement are more common than with HL. On the other hand, intrathoracic involvement is less common compared with HL.
- AIDS-associated lymphomas are clinically characterized by advanced stage, extra-nodal involvement and clinical aggressiveness with poor therapeutic outcomes. FDG-PET demonstrates extensive disease involvement with significantly higher SUV values due to the aggressive nature of these lymphomas.
- In the HIV (+) population without the presence of malignant disease, a progressive pattern of lymphoid tissue activation is noted, characterized by a generalized pattern of lymph node involvement starting from the head and neck and evolving to the abdominal and inguinal lymph nodes depending on the viral load and response to HAART therapy, suggesting that lymphoid tissues are affected in a predictable sequence.
- The PET reader should be cognizant of the susceptibility of HIV-positive individuals to infectious processes including cytomegalovirus, *Cryptococcus neoformans*, and tuberculosis, to avoid false-positive reading of FDG images.

# References

1. Cazals-Hatem D, Lepage E, Brice P *et al.* Primary mediastinal large B-cell lymphoma: a clinic-pathologic study of 141 cases compared with 916 nonmediastinal large B-cell lymphomas – a GELA ("Groupe d'Etude des Lymphomas de l'Adulte") study. *Am J Surg Pathol* 1996;**20**:877–8.

2. Chew FS, Schellingerhout D, Kee SB. Primary lymphoma of skeletal muscle. *Am J Roentgenol* 1999;**172**:1370.

3. Malloy PC, Fishman EK, Magid D. Lymphoma of bone, muscle, and skin: CT findings. *Am J Roentgenol* 1992;**159**(4):805–9.

4. Elstrom R, Guan L, Baker G *et al.* Utility of FDG-PET scanning in lymphoma by WHO classification. *Blood* 2003;**101**:3875–6.

5. Moog F, Bangerter M, Kotzerke J *et al.* 18F-fluorodeoxyglucose-positron emission tomography as a new approach to detect lymphomatous bone marrow. *Blood* 1998;**16**:603–9.

6. Carr R, Barrington SF, Madan B *et al.* Detection of lymphoma in bone marrow by whole-body positron emission tomography. *Blood* 1998;**91**:3340–6.

7. Pakos EE, Fotopoulos AD, Ioannidis JP. 18F-FDG PET for evaluation of bone marrow infiltration in staging of lymphoma: a meta-analysis. *J Nucl Med* 2005;**46**:958–63.

8. Mounier N, Spina M, Gabarre J *et al.* AIDS-related non-Hodgkin lymphoma. *Blood* 2006;**107**:3832–40.

9. Mounier N, Spina M, Spano JP. Hodgkin lymphoma in HIV positive patients. *Curr HIV Res* 2010;**8**:141–6.

10. Tirelli U, Errante D, Dolcetti R *et al.* Hodgkin's disease and human immunodeficiency virus infection: clinicopathologic and virologic features of 114 patients from the Italian Cooperative Group on AIDS and Tumors. *J Clin Oncol* 1995;**13**:1758–67.

11. Biberfeld P, Chayt KJ, Marselle LM *et al.* HTVL-III expression in infected lymph nodes and relevance to pathogenesis of lymphadenopathy. *Am J Pathol* 1986;**125**:436.

12. Goshen E, Davidson T, Avigdor A, Zwas T, Levy I. PET/CT in the evaluation of lymphoma in patients with HIV-1 with suppressed viral loads. *Clin Nucl Med* 2008;**33**:610–14.

13. Scharko A, Perlman S, Pyzalski R *et al.* Whole-body positron emission tomography in patients with HIV-1 infection. *Lancet* 2003;**20**:959–61.

14. Iyengar S, Chin B, Margolick J, Beulah P, Schwartz D. Anatomical loci of HIV-associated immune activation and association with viraemia. *Lancet* 2003;**20**:945–50.

15. Brust D, Polis M, Davey R *et al.* Fluorodeoxyglucose imaging in healthy subjects with HIV infection: impact of disease stage and therapy on pattern of nodal activation. *AIDS* 2006;**20**:495–503.

16. Lucignani G, Orunesu E, Cesari M *et al.* FDG-PET imaging in HIV-infected subjects: relation with therapy and immunovirological variables. *Eur J Nucl Med Mol Imaging* 2009;**36**:640–7.

17. Samuel R, Bettiker R, Suh B. AIDS related opportunistic infections, going but not gone. *Arch Pharm Res* 2002;**25**:215–28.

**Case 6**: A 67-year-old male recently diagnosed with small lymphocytic lymphoma/chronic lymphocytic leukemia (CLL/SLL). The patient underwent a pre-therapy PET/CT study to evaluate the extent of disease.

**Case 7**: A 62-year-old male diagnosed with grade-II FL, 8 years prior, treated with Rituximab and recurred twice and now presenting with B symptoms (night sweats and weight loss) and elevated LDH, suspicious for histologic transformation to DLBCL. The patient underwent a PET/CT study to evaluate for transformation to a higher-grade lymphoma to determine the biopsy site if any suspicion arises on imaging.

## Acquisition and processing parameters

Following a fasting period of 6 hours, the patients (similar protocols for both patients) were intravenously injected with approximately 20 mCi of FDG, and an uptake phase of 90 min was allowed prior to PET/CT imaging. Plasma glucose levels were less than 100 mg/dL at the time of FDG injection. The patients voided before the start of imaging acquisition, and images were obtained from the orbits to the proximal thighs using a combined PET/CT scanner. Imaging was performed in the supine position, with arms placed above their heads, in an attempt to reduce beam-hardening artifacts in the torso. The low-dose CT protocol acquisition parameters were as follows; 140 kVp, 80 mA, 0.8 s per CT rotation, pitch of 1.35 : 1, and a reconstructed slice thickness of 5.0 mm. The CT data were reconstructed using a filtered back-projection algorithm and a $512 \times 512$ matrix, with a transaxial field of view of 50 cm. The CT images were used to generate the transmission maps for attenuation correction of the PET acquisitions and anatomic localization. Immediately after the CT scan, and without changing the patient's position, the tabletop moved automatically to the PET position. The emission scans were acquired starting at the mid-thighs toward the head, in six 4 minutes/bed positions (14.5 cm longitudinal field of view). PET data were reconstructed using an ordered-subset expectation maximization iterative algorithm (28 subsets, 2 iterations).

## Findings and differential diagnosis

**Case 6**: Axial CT, PET, and PET/CT fused slices (Figure 13.6, left to right, respectively) demonstrate multiple foci of mildly increased

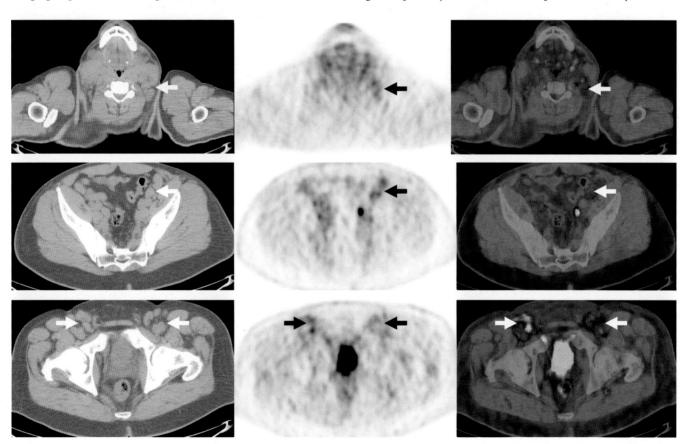

**Figure 13.6** From left to right: axial CT, FDG-PET, and FDG-PET/CT fused slices.

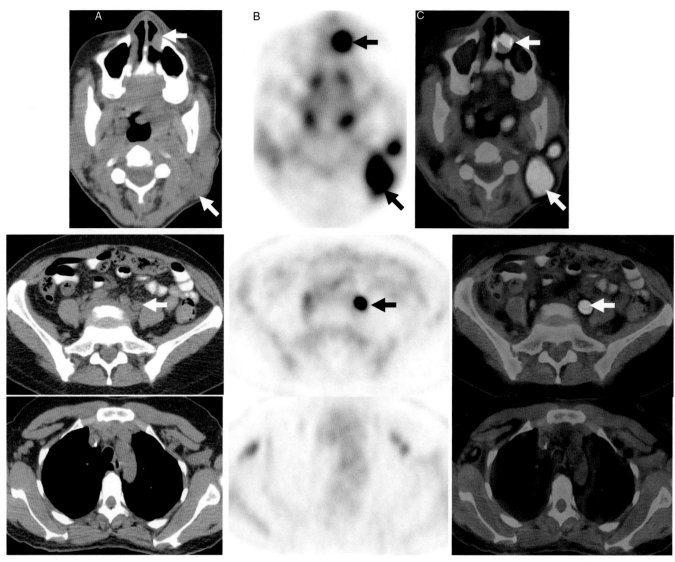

**Figure 13.7** From left to right: axial CT, FDG-PET, and FDG-PET/CT fused slices.

FDG uptake (SUVmax 2.0–3.0) in the neck and pelvis corresponding to bilateral enlarged cervical, external iliac, and inguinal lymph nodes. Note that these lymph nodes can be overlooked if an accompanying CT does not exist as a morphologic reference.

Differential diagnoses: Broad differential diagnosis encompasses a spectrum of entities including all low-grade lymphomas – CLL/SLL, nodal marginal zone lymphoma, FL, prolymphocytic leukemia (PLL), monoclonal, and benign polyclonal B-cell lymphocytosis.

**Case 7**: Axial CT, PET, and PET/CT fused slices (Figure 13.7, left to right, respectively) demonstrate multiple foci of significantly increased FDG uptake corresponding to enlarged left cervical lymph nodes (SUVmax 12.5) and a non-enlarged left retroperitoneal lymph node (left common iliac) (SUVmax 11.4), consistent with high-grade lymphoma. There is also significant uptake in a mass in the left nasal cavity that may represent an additional site of lymphoma or an unrelated neoplasm. Note the

small axillary lymph nodes with mild uptake (SUVmax 3.2) which probably represent low-grade lymphoma in line with the patient's original diagnosis of grade II FL.

Differential diagnoses: Transformed low-grade lymphoma, particularly based on the discrepancy between the high-grade uptake seen in the neck as well as in the retroperitoneal lymph node and the low-grade uptake in the axillary lymph nodes. Other differential diagnoses include high-grade lymphoma such as *de novo* DLBCL, Burkitt's lymphoma, and other high-grade lymphomas such as lymphoblastic lymphoma and anaplastic large-cell lymphoma.

## Diagnosis and clinical follow-up

**Case 6**: Core biopsy of a left cervical lymph node was positive for CLL/SLL.

**Case 7**: Core biopsy of a left cervical lymph node was positive for transformation to DLBCL.

## Discussion and teaching points

CLL/SLL is a clonal lymphoproliferative disorder characterized by proliferation of mature lymphocytes. Of note, in the WHO classification, SLL is considered as the tissue infiltrate of CLL (1, 2). CLL/SLL is primarily a disease of older adults of > 50 years age (2). The onset of CLL is insidious, most often localized to the lymph nodes but some cases eventually progress to involve the peripheral blood, and it is then that the disease is referred to as CLL/SLL. After the bone marrow and lymph nodes, the spleen is the most common site of involvement by CLL. In this entity, the most consistent clinical finding is diffuse lymphadenopathy demonstrating varying degrees of FDG uptake (usually low to undetectable). In various series, when subsets of indolent lymphoma were evaluated, FDG-PET detected only up to 60% of nodal disease sites in the CLL/SLL present on CT images (3–6). For this disease subtype a high-resolution CT study would be helpful to complement FDG-PET to better define the extent of disease.

FL is the most common subtype and makes up for 70% of LGLs. Clinically, patients present with peripheral lymphadenopathy involving the cervical, axillary, inguinal, or femoral regions. Upon complete staging, however, stage III or IV disease is observed in more than 80% of cases. Intrathoracic adenopathy, if present, is rarely bulky. Extranodal disease other than in the bone marrow is uncommon (7). BM involvement occurs in close to 70% of cases. Clinical heterogeneity in advanced disease led to development of The Follicular Lymphoma International Prognostic Index (FLIPI: age > 60 years, more than four nodal sites, hemoglobin < 12 gm/dL, advanced stage, and elevated lactate dehydrogenase level), which separates patients into three distinct risk categories based on overall survival (8). The sensitivity of FDG-PET exceeds 90% in all grades of FL and it detects far more lesions than does CT scan, especially extranodal lesions (> 89%) (3–6).

In the natural history of low-grade NHL a prolonged indolent phase of the disease may be followed by clinical progression to intermediate and high-grade disease. The frequency of histologic transformation to an aggressive lymphoma is about 3% per year (9). The median survival from the time of histological transformation is less than 2 years. Recent reports indicate that treatment for transformed lymphoma has improved in the last several years (10). The histologic transformation to a higher grade has also been described for CLL/SLL and is characterized by development of a high-grade NHL, most frequently an immunoblastic variant of DLBCL, referred to as "Richter transformation" (11). Clinically, transformation is suspected when there is rapid enlargement of the lymph nodes or B symptoms. However, the size of a tumor mass is not a reliable predictor of transformation as indolent disease can gradually reach a large size without transformation. In this setting, FDG-PET may be helpful by demonstrating lymph node groups that are significantly more hypermetabolic compared with other lymph nodes (12–15). PET/CT imaging can correctly exclude Richter's transformation with an overall sensitivity, specificity, positive and negative predictive values of 91%, 80%, and 53% and 97%, respectively (12). The SUVmax in transformed lymphoma is similar to that obtained for *de novo* DLBCL, usually with a median value of ≥ 12 (13). A cut-off SUVmax of 10 provided a better balance with specificity of 80% and sensitivity of 70% of detecting transformation (15). Thus, transformation should be suspected in patients with indolent lymphoma with high SUVs in any group of lymph nodes on FDG-PET. Consequently, biopsies should be directed to those sites showing the highest FDG avidity, to diagnose transformation and timely institute proper treatment.

## Take-home message

- In CLL/SLL, the most consistent clinical finding is diffuse lymphadenopathy demonstrating varying degrees of low-grade FDG uptake. In the CLL/SLL, FDG-PET imaging can detect only up to 60% of nodal disease sites that are better observed on a high-resolution CT scan.

- In patients with indolent NHL, transformation to an aggressive phenotype is the harbinger of clinical decline and the impetus for more aggressive therapy.

- Clinically, transformation is suspected when there is rapid enlargement of the lymph nodes or B symptoms. In this setting, FDG-PET may be helpful by demonstrating lymph node groups that are significantly more hypermetabolic compared with other lymph nodes.

- PET/CT has an overall sensitivity and specificity of 90% and 80%, respectively for the detection of transformation to a higher grade, particularly in Richter's syndrome.

- The FDG uptake in transformed low-grade lymphoma is similar to that obtained for *de novo* DLBCL exceeding a SUVmax of 10.0, thus, transformation should be suspected in patients with indolent lymphoma with high SUVs, usually 2.5–3 times higher than those non-transformed lymph nodes of low-grade lymphoma histology.

## References

1. Swerdlow SH, Campo E, Harris NL *et al.* *WHO Classification of Tumours of Haematopoietic and Lymphoid Tissues*, 4th edn. Lyon: International Agency for Research on Cancer, 2008.

2. Wierda WG, Chiorazzi N, Dearden C *et al.* Chronic lymphocytic leukemia: new concepts for future therapy. *Clin Lymphoma Myeloma Leuk* 2010;**10**(5):369–78.

3. Le Dortz L, De Guibert S, Bayat S *et al.* Diagnostic and prognostic impact of (18)F-FDG PET/CT in follicular lymphoma. *Eur J Nucl Med Mol Imaging* 2010;**37**:2307–14.

4. Wohrer S, Jaeger U, Kletter K *et al.* 18F-fluoro-deoxy-glucose positron emission tomography (18F-FDG-PET) visualizes follicular lymphoma irrespective of grading. *Ann Oncol* 2006;**17**:780–784.

5. Elstrom R, Guan L, Baker G *et al.* Utility of FDG-PET scanning in

lymphoma by WHO classification. *Blood* 2003;**101**:3875–6.

6. Jerusalem G, Beguin Y, Najjar F *et al.* Positron emission tomography (PET) with 18F-fluorodeoxyglucose (18F-FDG) for the staging of low-grade non-Hodgkin lymphoma (NHL). *Ann Oncol* 2001;**12**:825–30.

7. Tan D, Horning SJ. Follicular lymphoma: clinical features and treatment. *Hematol Oncol Clin North Am* 2008;**22**:863–82.

8. Solal-Celigny P, Roy P, Colombat P *et al.* Follicular Lymphoma International Prognostic Index. *Blood* 2004;**104**:1258–65.

9. Montoto S, Davies AJ, Matthews J *et al.* Risk and clinical implications of transformation of follicular lymphoma to diffuse large B-cell lymphoma. *J Clin Oncol* 2007;**25**:2426–33.

10. Tan D, Rosenberg SA, Lavori P *et al.* Improved prognosis after histologic transformation of follicular lymphoma: the Stanford experience 1960–2003. Programs and abstracts of the 10th International Conference on Malignant Lymphoma. *Lugano*, 2008, p. 111.

11. Tsimberidou AM, Keating MJ. Richter syndrome: biology, incidence, and therapeutic strategies. *Cancer* 2005;**103**:216–28.

12. Bruzzi JF, Macapinlac H, Tsimberidou AM *et al.* Detection of Richter's transformation of chronic lymphocytic leukemia by PET/CT. *J Nucl Med* 2006;**47**(8):1267–73.

13. Noy A, Schöder H, Gönen M *et al.* The majority of transformed lymphomas have high standardized uptake values (SUVs) on positron emission tomography (PET) scanning similar to diffuse large B-cell lymphoma (DLBCL). *Ann Oncol* 2009;**20**:508–12.

14. Anis M, Irshad A. Imaging of abdominal lymphoma. *Radiol Clin North Am* 2008;**46**:265–85.

15. Schoder H, Noy A, Gonen M *et al.* Intensity of 18fluorodeoxyglucose uptake in positron emission tomography distinguishes between indolent and aggressive non-Hodgkin's lymphoma. *J Clin Oncol* 2005;**23**:4643–51.

A 48-year-old male with a history of abdominal DLBCL, treated with 6 cycles of standard R-CHOP, referred for a FDG-PET/CT study to evaluate disease extent 6 months (Figure 13.8, upper panel) and 12 months (Figure 13.8, lower panel) after completion of therapy. The patient did not experience any constitutional, laboratory, or any other clinical symptoms at the time of the PET imaging.

## Acquisition and processing parameters

Following a fasting period of 6 hours, the patient was intravenously injected with approximately 11.5 mCi of FDG, and an uptake phase of 70 min was allowed prior to PET/CT imaging. Plasma glucose levels were less than 100 mg/dL at the time of FDG injection. The patient voided before the start of imaging acquisition, and images were obtained from the orbits to the proximal thighs using a combined PET/CT scanner. Imaging was performed in the supine position, with arms placed above the head, in an attempt to reduce beam-hardening artifacts in the torso. The low-dose CT protocol acquisition parameters were as follows; 140 kVp, 80 mA, 0.8 s per CT rotation, pitch of 1.35 : 1, and a reconstructed slice thickness of 5.0 mm. The CT data were reconstructed using a filtered back-projection algorithm and a 512 × 512 matrix, with a transaxial field of view of 70 cm. The CT images were used to generate the transmission maps for attenuation correction of the PET acquisitions and anatomic localization. Immediately after the CT scan, and without changing the patient's position, the tabletop moved automatically to the PET position. The emission scans were acquired starting at the mid-thighs toward the head, in six 4 minutes/bed positions (15.1 cm longitudinal field of view). PET data were reconstructed using an ordered-subset expectation maximization iterative algorithm (28 subsets, 4 iterations).

## Findings and differential diagnosis

Figure 13.8, upper panel (6 months after therapy): Axial CT, PET, PET/CT fused slices demonstrate focal FDG uptake in the abdomen that persists at 12 months with additional foci appearing as well, consistent with disease relapse in mesenteric nodules (lower panel).

Differential diagnosis: Recurrence of high-grade lymphoma and sclerosing mesenteritis (panniculitis), granulomatous disease not limited to but including tuberculosis.

## Diagnosis and clinical follow-up

Biopsy was not performed. Clinical and FDG-PET imaging follow-up at 3 months showed progression of disease in the

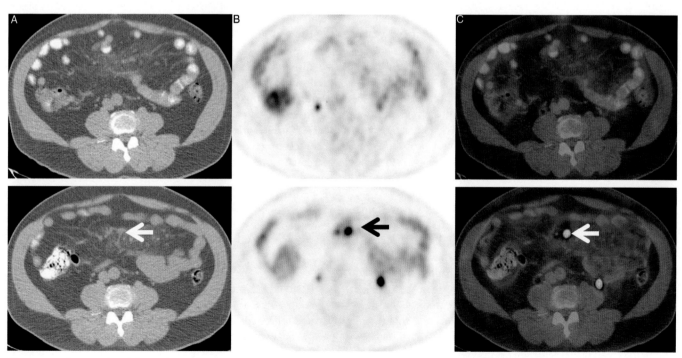

**Figure 13.8** Top row: from left to right: Axial CT, FDG-PET, and FDG-PET/CT fused slices 6 months after six cycles of standard R-CHOP. Bottom row: from left to right: axial CT, FDG-PET, and FDG-PET/CT fused slices 12 months after six cycles of standard R-CHOP.

abdomen with enlargement of the mesenteric nodules, and increase in FDG uptake (not shown here) confirming disease recurrence. The patient subsequently underwent salvage therapy with HDT/SCT.

## Discussion and teaching points

Despite improvements in survival rates, relapses can occur in approximately 30–50% of lymphoma patients following first-line therapy (1). While residual CT masses are associated with a relapse rate of less than 50%, disease recurrence or progression should be anticipated in the majority of patients with positive post-therapy FDG-PET findings (2–5). In a meta-analysis, the sensitivity and specificity of FDG-PET to predict relapse were reported to be 50–100% and 67–100%, respectively, for HL and 33–77% and 82–100%, respectively, for NHL, irrespective of whether there is a residual mass on CT or not (6). Nonetheless, it should also be recognized that, owing to its high spatial resolution, CT scans can delineate organ involvement that is not apparent on the FDG-PET imaging, reinforcing the need for combined PET and CT interpretations, particularly for disease in the neck and abdomen, the sites where physiologic uptake by normal structures may hinder interpretation without well-defined anatomic markers.

There is no current consensus regarding the optimal method for surveillance of HL and DLBCL patients after first remission. The National Comprehensive Cancer Network (NCCN) recently published recommendations for follow-up of patients who have HL and NHL (7, 8): for patients who have NHL in an initial complete remission, follow-up should include an interim history and physical examination every 2–4 months for 1–2 years, then every 3–6 months for the next 3–5 years, with annual monitoring for late effects after 5 years. For follicular or other indolent histology lymphoma patients in complete remission, the recommendation for follow-up is every 3 months for a year, and then every 3–6 months. For diffuse large B-cell NHL, the guidelines proposed every 3 months for 24 months and then every 6 months for 36 months. Imaging studies should be performed when clinically indicated. An individual patient will have a high probability of positive findings with a high pre-test likelihood of recurrence defined by clinical, biochemical, or interim PET imaging results (9). Thus, the testing frequency should be based on the probability of disease recurrence. Overall, a lymphoma relapse is expected in about 65% of those with a positive finding; only one-third of these patients will have a concomitant positive result on CT. Interestingly, when the PET was positive after two cycles, 74% of patients had a PET-proven relapse while only 20% of patients had a relapse in the low-risk group (9). More recently, following a strategy of obtaining a PET every 3–4 months in the first 2 years, every 6 months in the 3 following years, and yearly thereafter, most relapses (62%) were diagnosed clinically, especially in aggressive-NHL patients, however, HL relapses were more commonly detected by PET/CT ($P < 0.05$) (10). These results confirm FDG-PET to

be a valid tool for follow-up of lymphoma patients, however, one should bear in mind that false-positive findings may occur in approximately 30% of cases and the rate of recurrence may not be high enough to justify a frequent PET strategy. Of note, false-positive findings are most commonly obtained in infectious or inflammatory processes, however, the pattern of FDG uptake in these situations is usually recognizable in experienced hands unless a granulomatous disease coexists with lymphoma. Interval development of FDG accumulation in the region of original disease should be recognized as compelling evidence for further therapy. According to the revised IWG response criteria (11) disease relapse is defined as appearance of any new lesion greater than 1.5 cm in any axis during or at the end of therapy, even if others are decreasing in size. Increased FDG uptake in a previously unaffected site only should be considered relapse or progressive disease after confirmation with other modalities. In patients who have no prior history of pulmonary lymphoma, new lung nodules on CT should be considered benign. Thus, a therapeutic decision should not be supported by histologic confirmation. Lesions should be PET-positive in a typical FDG-avid lymphoma or one that was PET positive before therapy unless the lesion is too small to be detected (less than 1.5 cm in its long axis by CT) (11).

In patients with previously treated abdominal lymphoma, the presence of mesenteric accompanied by adjacent fat stranding may be confused with mesenteric panniculitis (MP) or sclerosing mesenteritis. MP is a benign condition that is associated with non-specific inflammation involving the adipose tissue of the mesentery leading to acute inflammatory changes and fat necrosis. Differentiating MP from tumoral involvement of mesenteric lymph nodes is imperative as the CT features of MP are not specific and may be confused with granulomatous disease, primary or secondary abdominal neoplasms and lymphoma (12). Although the evidence is still preliminary, FDG-PET/CT appears to be a highly specific test for differentiating a malignant condition from a benign one in the mesentery. In a limited study of 19 oncology patients, in 33 PET/CTs, a negative study was found to have a high diagnostic accuracy in excluding neoplastic mesenteric processes while increased uptake suggested the co-existing malignant mesenteric deposits, particularly in patients with lymphoma (13). In all patients with CT findings of mesenteritis and a negative PET result, no malignant involvement of the mesentery was diagnosed.

## Take-home message

- Residual CT masses are non-specific and associated with a relapse rate of less than 50%. However, disease recurrence or progression should be anticipated in the majority of patients with positive post-therapy FDG-PET findings as FDG-PET is highly sensitive and specific in predicting disease relapse irrespective of whether there is a residual mass on CT.

- There is no current consensus regarding the optimal method for surveillance of HL and DLBCL patients after completion of first-line therapy. The NCCN guidelines do not include PET/CT as a surveillance tool but rather recommend a follow-up with interim history and physical examination every 2–4 months for 1–2 years, then every 3–6 months for the next 3–5 years, with annual monitoring for late effects after 5 years.

- A patient will have an increased risk of recurrence when the interim PET result is positive; thus, the testing frequency should be based on the probability of disease recurrence and follow-up should be conducted more often in those patients with a PET positive finding after several cycles during therapy.

- Most relapses are diagnosed clinically in aggressive NHL patients, however, HL relapses are more commonly detected by PET/CT.

- FDG-PET may be a valid tool for follow-up of lymphoma patients, however, one should bear in mind that false-positive findings may occur in approximately 30% of cases who are in a surveillance program.

- Interval development of FDG accumulation in the region of original disease should be recognized as compelling evidence for further therapy, while increased FDG uptake in a previously unaffected site should be considered relapse or progressive disease only after confirmation with other modalities or biopsy.

# References

1. Quddus F, Armitage JO. Salvage therapy for Hodgkin's lymphoma. *Cancer J* 2009;**15**:161–3.

2. Mikhaeel NG, Timothy AR, O'Doherty MJ, Hain S, Maisey MN. 18-FDG-PET as a prognostic indicator in the treatment of aggressive Non-Hodgkin's Lymphoma – comparison with CT. *Leuk Lymphoma* 2000;**39**:543–53.

3. Spaepen K, Stroobants S, Dupont P *et al*. Prognostic value of positron emission tomography (PET) with fluorine-18 fluorodeoxyglucose ([18F]FDG) after firstline chemotherapy in non-Hodgkin lymphoma: is [18F]FDG-PET a valid alternative to conventional diagnostic methods? *J Clin Oncol* 2001;**19**:414–19.

4. Barnes JA, Lacasce AS, Zukotynski K *et al*. End-of-treatment but not interim PET scan predicts outcome in nonbulky limited-stage Hodgkin's lymphoma. *Ann Oncol* 2011;**22**(4):910–15.

5. Sher DJ, Mauch PM, Van Den Abbeele A *et al*. Prognostic significance of mid- and post-ABVD PET imaging in Hodgkin's lymphoma: the importance of involved-field radiotherapy. *Ann Oncol* 2009;**20**:1848–53.

6. Terasawa T, Nihashi T, Hotta T *et al*. 18F-FDG PET for posttherapy assessment of Hodgkin's disease and aggressive Non-Hodgkin's lymphoma: a systematic review. *J Nucl Med* 2008;**49**:13–21.

7. National Comprehensive Cancer Network, Hodgkin Lymphoma. *NCCN* **v1** 2011 http://www.nccn.org/professionals/physician_gls/pdf/hodgkins.pdf

8. National Comprehensive Cancer Network, non-Hodgkin Lymphoma. *NCCN* **v2** 2011 http://www.nccn.org/professionals/physician_gls/pdf/nhl.pdf

9. Zinzani PL, Stefoni V, Tani M *et al*. Role of [18F]fluorodeoxyglucose positron emission tomography scan in the follow-up of lymphoma. *Clin Oncol* 2009;**27**:1781–7.

10. Goldschmidt N, Or O, Klein M, Savitsky B, Paltiel O. The role of routine imaging procedures in the detection of relapse of patients with Hodgkin lymphoma and aggressive non-Hodgkin lymphoma. *Ann Hematol* 2011;**90**:165–71.

11. Cheson BD, Pfistner B, Juweid ME *et al*. Revised response criteria for malignant lymphoma. *J Clin Oncol* 2007;**25**:579–86.

12. Horton KM, Lawler LP, Fishman EK. CT findings in sclerosing mesenteritis (panniculitis): spectrum of disease. *Radiographics* 2003;**23**:1561–7.

13. Zissin R, Metser U, Hain D, Even-Sapir E. Mesenteric panniculitis in oncologic patients: PET-CT findings. *Br J Radiol* 2006;**79**:37–43.

**Case 9**: A 26-year-old female with a history of stage II classical Hodgkin's lymphoma (cHL), treated with six cycles of standard ABVD therapy, referred for a PET/CT study for evaluation of response 3 weeks after completion of first-line therapy (Figure 13.9, upper panel). Thereafter patient was followed with a PET/CT 2 months later (middle panel). An additional FDG-PET/CT study was obtained four cycles after initiation of second-line therapy with ICE (bottom panel).

**Case 10**: A 29-year-old female with a history of stage II classical Hodgkin's lymphoma (cHL), treated with six cycles of standard ABVD therapy, referred for PET/CT imaging for evaluation of response 3 weeks after completion of first-line therapy (Figure 13.10, upper panel). Thereafter patient was

followed with a FDG-PET/CT study 3 months later to reevaluate disease status (lower panel). Of note, the patient had a complete response with no evidence of FDG uptake within the mediastinal mass after two cycles (not shown here).

## Acquisition and processing parameters

Following a fasting period of 6 hours, the patients (similar protocols for both patients) were intravenously injected with approximately 18–20 mCi of FDG, and an uptake phase of 60 min was allowed prior to PET/CT imaging. Plasma glucose levels were less than 100 mg/dL at the time of FDG injection. The patients voided before the start of imaging acquisition, and images were obtained from the orbits to the proximal

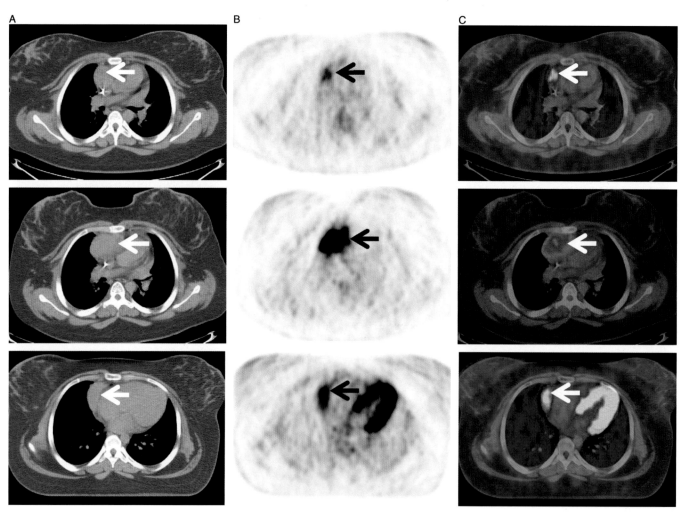

**Figure 13.9** Axial CT, FDG-PET, and FDG-PET/CT fused slices. Upper panel: 3 weeks after completion of six cycles of first-line therapy. Middle panel: 2 months after completion of first-line therapy. Lower panel: after four cycles of second-line therapy.

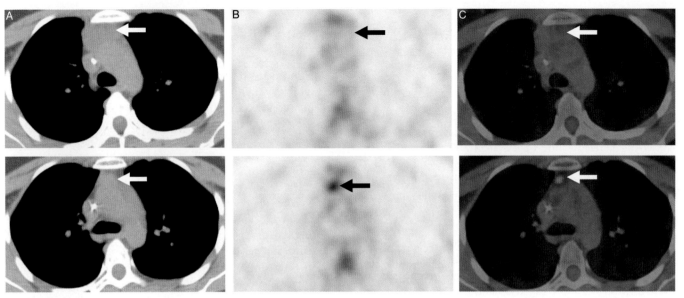

**Figure 13.10** Axial CT, FDG-PET, and FDG-PET/CT fused slices. Upper panel: 3 weeks after completion of first-line therapy. Lower panel: 3 months later to reevaluate disease status.

thighs using a combined PET/CT scanner. Imaging was performed in the supine position, with arms placed above their heads, in an attempt to reduce beam-hardening artifacts in the torso. The low-dose CT protocol acquisition parameters were as follows; 140 kVp, 80 mA, 0.8 s per CT rotation, pitch of 1.35 : 1, and a reconstructed slice thickness of 5.0 mm. The CT data were reconstructed using a filtered back-projection algorithm and a $512 \times 512$ matrix, with a transaxial field of view of 50 cm. The CT images were used to generate the transmission maps for attenuation correction of the PET acquisitions and anatomic localization. Immediately after the CT scan, and without changing the patients' position, the tabletop moved automatically to the PET position. The emission scans were acquired starting at the mid-thighs toward the head, in six 4 minutes/bed positions (14.5 cm longitudinal field of view). PET data were reconstructed using an ordered-subset expectation maximization iterative algorithm (28 subsets, 2 iterations).

## Findings and differential diagnosis

**Case 9**: Axial CT, PET, and PET/CT fused slices (Figure 13.9A, B, C, upper panel) demonstrate increased FDG uptake in the right anterior mediastinum corresponding to a mass measuring > 2.0 cm, that is situated superior and anterior to the right heart (arrows). The uptake within this mass is greater than that seen in the mediastinal blood pool structures (SUVmax: 4.0 vs. 1.9). This finding is consistent with residual lymphoma with non-complete resolution of disease given that the patient completed all six cycles of therapy. After 2 months the mediastinal mass demonstrates interval increase in metabolism (SUVmax 8.7) and size (arrows), consistent with progression of disease (middle panel). After four cycles of second-line (salvage) therapy since the last PET/CT study, the mediastinal mass has decreased in metabolism and size, however, the FDG uptake still persists (arrows), consistent with residual lymphoma (lower panel).

Differential diagnosis: Residual lymphoma, post-therapy inflammatory changes, thymic rebound.

**Case 10**: Axial CT, PET, and PET/CT fused slices demonstrate increased FDG uptake slightly greater than that seen in the mediastinal blood pool structures in the right anterior mediastinum corresponding to a heterogeneous mass measuring > 2.0 cm, situated anterior to the aortic arch (Figure 13.10, arrows, upper panel). This finding is consistent with treated lymphoma given that the patient completed all six cycles of therapy. The subsequent PET/CT study performed 3 months later demonstrates increased FDG uptake within the anterior mediastinum corresponding to a soft tissue density (lower panel). Although this mass coincides with the original disease site, considering the facts that the patient had early-stage HL, with rapid response to therapy (CR at two cycles) and no evidence of disease after completion of therapy, this finding at 3 months post completion of therapy most likely represents thymic rebound.

Differential diagnosis: Residual lymphoma, post-therapy inflammatory changes, thymic rebound.

## Diagnosis and clinical follow-up

**Case 9**: 3-month follow-up FDG-PET/CT followed by biopsy of the mediastinal mass revealed relapsed cHL. Subsequently, the patient was started on a salvage therapy with ICE and another follow-up PET/CT was obtained at four cycles of second-line therapy.

**Case 10**: No biopsy or interim therapy between the two PET/CT studies. A follow-up study at 6 months after the last PET/CT study revealed significant decrease of uptake and regression of the anterior mediastinal mass noted on the second PET/CT study (not shown), confirming the diagnosis of thymic rebound peaking at around 3 months and regressing in the following 3 months.

## Discussion and teaching points

Following therapy, a multitude of studies has shown that FDG-PET is a sensitive and specific diagnostic tool for identification of residual lymphoma in the post-therapy setting (1–8). According to these results, more than 90% of lymphoma patients with a positive post-therapy FDG-PET are expected to succumb to disease progression while residual post-therapy masses identified on CT do not have a strong predictive value conferring a relapse rate of less than 50%. A meta-analysis performed for end-of-treatment evaluation using FDG-PET, revealed a sensitivity, specificity, PPV, and NPV of 76%, 94%, 82%, and 92%, respectively (9). Another systematic review reported considerable differences between the pooled sensitivity and specificity for detection of residual disease in HL and DLBCL; 84% and 90%, vs. 72% and 100%, respectively, at completion of first-line chemotherapy (10). These differences can be attributed to biologic dissimilarities between the two disease entities, a more florid inflammatory tumor response (lower specificity) and the higher cure rates seen in patients with HL compared with those with DLBCL. Alternatively, as DLBCL is a less curable disease entity than HL, FDG-PET cannot definitively exclude minimal residual disease (chemoresistant or chemorefractory clones), which translates into lower sensitivity. Based on the established compelling data, FDG-PET is now an integral part of IWG response criteria for lymphoma as a result of its ability to eliminate the unconfirmed complete remission category "Cru" culminating to better separation of the progression-free survival curves between CR and partial response categories (11, 12). According to these guidelines, visual assessment is considered adequate for a definition of a positive PET result. After completion of chemotherapy, a positive FDG-PET scan is defined as focal or diffuse FDG uptake above background in a location incompatible with normal anatomy. Residual masses of at least 2.0 cm in greatest transverse diameter with FDG activity exceeding that of mediastinal blood pool structures are considered positive, while smaller masses are considered PET-positive only if their activity exceeds surrounding background activity (11, 12). Using these new definitions, in a preliminary study of a mixed group of patients with HL and DLBCL, the 2-year event-free survival in patients who had PET-positive residual masses was 0% compared with 95% in patients who had PET-negative residual masses and 85% in patients without residual masses (13). It is important to emphasize that the minimum recommended interval between chemotherapy administration and FDG PET is 3 weeks for evaluation after completion of therapy, for inflammation to subside to avoid false-positive readings (12).

Thymic hyperplasia or rebound is a common phenomenon after corticosteroid therapy, radiation therapy, and chemotherapy particularly in young adults and pediatric patients (14, 15). The thymic gland volume may reduce by 40% of its original volume, likewise, during the rebound phase it can grow as much as 50% larger and it usually returns to its original size within a year (14, 16). Among patients who undergo chemotherapy, approximately 20% develop thymic rebound and this phenomenon usually starts within 3 months of completion of chemotherapy. The diagnostic challenge remains in the differentiation between thymic rebound and residual or recurrent lymphoma. Thymic rebound typically shows diffuse enlargement, a concave and smooth contour with no mass association on CT (16). Streaks of fat should be identified and the gland should maintain a bilobed appearance. FDG-PET invariably demonstrates uptake with a wide variation of patterns and intensities from focal and high grade to diffuse and low grade (17). Hence SUV measurements are not deemed to be helpful. In a pediatric population with malignant disease, thymic FDG uptake was significantly higher after chemotherapy than during chemotherapy (mean SUVmax 2.7 vs. 1.7) (18). A significant relationship was observed between thymic FDG uptake and interval after completion of chemotherapy. The peak period is between 3–6 months after therapy and thereafter it regresses to normal levels and should return to normal after 12 months. In challenging cases, the individual risk factors may help make the differential diagnosis. These include the patient pre-therapy risk profile, particularly the stage, B symptoms, and the bulk of the tumor, the response profile during interim PET evaluation (if available), and the time window in which the patient is evaluated (thymic rebound most seen 3–6 months after therapy).

## Take-home message

- More than 90% of lymphoma patients with a positive post-therapy FDG-PET result have disease progression, while only less than 50% of patients relapse when there is a residual post-therapy mass on CT.

- The considerable differences in FDG-PET performance between the HL and DLBCL at completion of chemotherapy for detection of residual disease are due to distinct disease biologies between these two entities. As more florid inflammatory response (false positives) and higher cure rates (true negatives) are expected in patients with HL compared with those with DLBCL, the specificity of PET is lower and its NPV is higher for HL and vice versa for DLBCL.

- According to the revised IWG response guidelines, visual assessment is adequate for response assessment in lymphoma. After completion of chemotherapy, those residual masses of ≥ 2 cm with FDG activity exceeding that of mediastinal blood pool structures are considered positive, while smaller masses are considered PET-positive only if their activity exceeds adjacent background activity.

- FDG-PET invariably demonstrates uptake in the thymus due to rebound after therapy, with a wide variation of patterns and intensities ranging from focal and high grade to diffuse and low grade. The FDG uptake within the hyperplastic thymus peaks between 3–6 months after therapy and should return to normal after 12 months.

# References

1. Naumann R, Vaic A, Beuthien-Baumann B et al. Prognostic value of positron emission tomography in the evaluation of post-treatment residual mass in patients with Hodgkin's disease and non-Hodgkin's lymphoma. *Br J Haematol* 2001; **115**:793–800.

2. Spaepen K, Stroobants S, Dupont P et al. Prognostic value of positron emission tomography (PET) with fluorine-18 fluorodeoxyglucose ([18F]FDG) after first-line chemotherapy in non-Hodgkin's lymphoma: is [18F]FDG-PET a valid alternative to conventional diagnostic methods? *J Clin Oncol* 2001;**19**:414–19.

3. Spaepen K, Stroobants S, Dupont P et al. Can positron emission tomography with [(18)F]-fluorodeoxyglucose after first-line treatment distinguish Hodgkin's disease patients who need additional therapy from others in whom additional therapy would mean avoidable toxicity? *Br J Haematol* 2001;**115**: 272–8.

4. Zinzani PL, Fanti S, Battista G et al. Predictive role of positron emission tomography (PET) in the outcome of lymphoma patients. *Br J Cancer* 2004;**91**;850–4.

5. Weihrauch MR, Scheidhauer K, Ansen S, Dietlein M, Bischoff S. Thoracic positron emission tomography using 18F-fluorodeoxyglucose for the evaluation of residual mediastinal Hodgkin disease. *Blood* 2001;**98**:2930–4.

6. Mikhaeel NG, Timothy AR, Hain SF, O'Doherty MJ. 18-FDG-PET for the assessment of residual masses on CT following treatment of lymphomas. *Ann Oncol* 2000;**11**(Suppl 1):147–50.

7. Friedberg JW, Fischman A, Neuberg D et al. FDG-PET is superior to gallium scintigraphy in staging and more sensitive in the follow-up of patients with de novo Hodgkin lymphoma: a blinded comparison. *Leuk Lymphoma* 2004;**45**:85–92.

8. Panizo C, Pérez-Salazar M, Bendandi M et al. Positron emission tomography using 18F-fluorodeoxyglucose for the evaluation of residual Hodgkin's disease mediastinal masses. *Leuk Lymphoma.* 2004;**45**:1829–33.

9. Jerusalem G, Hustinx R, Beguin Y, Fillet G. Evaluation of therapy for lymphoma. *Semin Nucl Med* 2005;**35**:186–96.

10. Zijlstra JM, Lindauer-van der Werf G, Hoekstra OS et al. 18F-fluoro-deoxyglucose positron emission tomography for post-treatment evaluation of malignant lymphoma: a systematic review. *Haematologica* 2006;**91**:522–9.

11. Cheson BD, Pfistner B, Juweid ME et al. Revised response criteria for malignant lymphoma. *J Clin Oncol* 2007;**25**:579–86.

12. Juweid ME, Stroobants S, Hoekstra OS et al. Use of positron emission tomography for response assessment of lymphoma: consensus of the Imaging Subcommittee of International Harmonization Project in Lymphoma. *J Clin Oncol* 2007;**25**:571–8.

13. Olsen K, Sohi J, Abraham T et al. Initial validation of standardized quantitative (visual) criteria for FDG PET assessment of residual masses following lymphoma therapy. *Proc Radiol Soc North Am* 2006;**323** [abstract 355:E323–302].

14. Webb RW. The mediastinum: mediastinal masses. In RW Webb, C Higgins (Eds.), *Thoracic Imaging: Pulmonary and Cardiovascular Radiology.* Philadelphia, PA: Lippincott Williams & Wilkins, 2005, pp. 212–70.

15. Kissin CM, Husband JE, Nicholas D, Eversman W. Benign thymic enlargement in adults after chemotherapy: CT demonstration. *Radiology* 1987;**163**: 67–70.

16. Nasseri F, Eftekhari F. Clinical and radiologic review of the normal and abnormal thymus: pearls and pitfalls. *Radiographics* 2010;**30**:413–28.

17. Ferdinand B, Gupta P, Kramer EL. Spectrum of thymic uptake at 18F-FDG PET. *Radiographics* 2004;**24**:1611–16.

18. Kawano T, Suzuki A, Ishida A et al. The clinical relevance of thymic fluorodeoxyglucose uptake in pediatric patients after chemotherapy. *Eur J Nucl Med Mol Imaging* 2004;**31**:31–6.

**Case 11**: A 38-year-old male with a recent diagnosis of stage IIA classical Hodgkin's lymphoma (cHL), referred for a PET/CT study to evaluate disease extent prior to first-line therapy (Figure 13.11, upper panel). Thereafter patient was followed with an interim PET/CT after two cycles of therapy (lower panel) for evaluation of response/determination of chemosensitivity.

**Case 12**: A 44-year-old female with a recent diagnosis of stage IIB classical Hodgkin's lymphoma (cHL) referred for a PET/CT study for evaluation of disease extent prior to first-line therapy (Figure 13.12, upper panel). Thereafter patient was followed with an interim PET/CT after two cycles of therapy (lower panel) for evaluation of response/determination of chemosensitivity.

## Acquisition and processing parameters

Following a fasting period of 6 hours, the patients (similar protocols for both patients) were intravenously injected with approximately 20 mCi of FDG, and an uptake phase of 60 min was allowed prior to PET/CT imaging. Plasma glucose levels were less than 100 mg/dL at the time of FDG injection. The patients voided before the start of imaging acquisition, and images were obtained from the orbits to the proximal thighs using a combined PET/CT scanner. Imaging was performed in the supine position, with arms placed above the head, in an attempt to reduce beam-hardening artifacts in the torso. The low-dose CT protocol acquisition parameters were as follows: 140 kVp, 80 mA, 0.8 s per CT rotation, pitch of 1.35 : 1, and a reconstructed slice thickness of 5.0 mm. The CT data were reconstructed using a filtered back-projection algorithm and a 512 × 512 matrix, with a transaxial field of view of 50 cm. The CT images were used to generate the transmission maps for attenuation correction of the PET acquisitions and anatomic localization. Immediately after the CT scan, and without changing the patient's position, the tabletop moved automatically to the PET position. The emission scans were acquired starting at the mid-thighs toward the head, in six 4 minutes/bed positions (14.5 cm longitudinal field of view). PET data were reconstructed using an ordered-subset expectation maximization iterative algorithm (28 subsets, 2 iterations).

## Findings and differential diagnosis

**Case 11**: Axial CT, PET, and PET/CT fused slices demonstrate (Figure 13.11, upper panel) increased FDG uptake (SUVmax 8.4) in the left axilla, corresponding to a mass with infiltrative changes in the surrounding fat planes (arrows), these findings are consistent with the diagnosis of cHL. The interim PET/CT study after two cycles of therapy (lower panel) demonstrates significant decrease in size (> 2.0 cm) and FDG uptake within the axillary mass (arrows) that slightly exceeds (SUVmax 2.6)

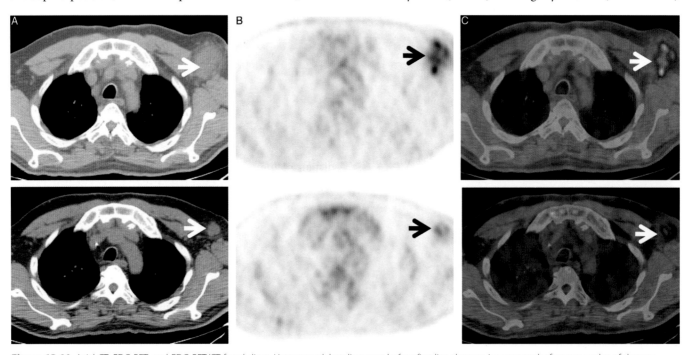

**Figure 13.11** Axial CT, FDG-PET, and FDG-PET/CT fused slices. Upper panel: baseline scan before first-line therapy. Lower panel: after two cycles of therapy.

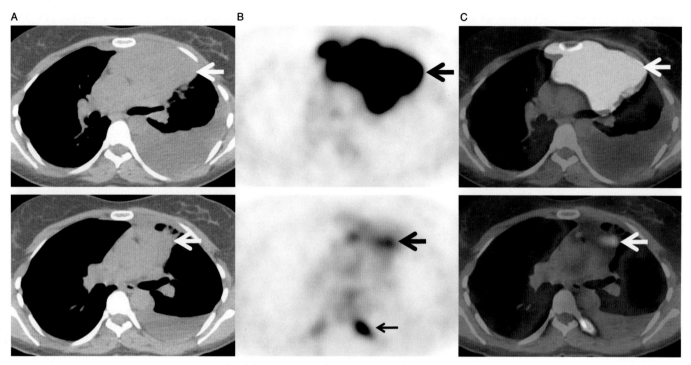

**Figure 13.12** Axial CT, FDG-PET, and FDG-PET/CT fused slices. Upper panel: baseline scan before first-line therapy. Lower panel: after two cycles of therapy.

that seen in mediastinal blood pool structures (SUVmax 1.9), however, lower than that seen in the liver (SUVmax 3.4) (not shown). By London criteria developed for interim PET reading, this finding is consistent with inflammatory changes/chemosensitive disease. Note that if the patient is being evaluated for response after completion of all six cycles with similar findings this level of uptake would qualify for a positive PET reading by IHP criteria.

Differential diagnosis: Residual lymphoma, post-therapy inflammatory changes.

**Case 12**: Axial CT, PET, and PET/CT fused slices demonstrate (Figure 13.12, upper panel) increased FDG uptake (SUVmax: 12.7) in the left anterior mediastinum, corresponding to a large conglomerate mass, consistent with the patient's diagnosis of cHL (arrows). The interim PET/CT study after two cycles of therapy (lower panel) demonstrates significant decrease in size (> 2.0 cm), however, FDG uptake (SUVmax 5.4) within the mass exceeds that seen in both mediastinal blood pool structures (SUVmax 2.0) and the liver uptake (SUVmax 3.5). This finding is consistent with residual lymphoma/chemoresistant disease. The fusiform area of uptake in the left posterior chest adjacent to the pleural effusion, almost overlapping the rib (small arrow) represents brown fat uptake in the paravertebral space.

Differential diagnosis: Residual lymphoma, post-therapy inflammatory changes.

## Diagnosis and clinical follow-up

**Case 11**: Clinical (laboratory tests and physical exam) and imaging (PET/CT) follow-up at completion of therapy (after

six cycles) and for the subsequent 18 months have been negative for residual or recurrent lymphoma (PFS: not reached). No biopsy was performed during the follow-up period.

**Case 12**: The therapy was not changed based on interim PET results. Clinical (laboratory tests and physical exam) and imaging (PET/CT) follow-up at completion of therapy (after six cycles) was negative (not shown). However, the disease relapsed at 5 months of follow-up within the same mediastinal mass. A biopsy was performed prior to the planned HDT/ASCT and confirmed residual/relapsed lymphoma. The patient had a favorable response to HDT/ASCT and has been progression-free for 8 months and currently still under surveillance.

## Discussion and teaching points

Post-therapy FDG-PET imaging has a definite role in the prediction of tumor recurrence. The 2-year relapse-free survival rates are usually high at > 90% for a negative PET result compared with 0–20% for a positive scan regardless of a residual mass on CT (1–5). Post-therapy FDG-PET has recently been integrated into the International Workshop Group (IWG) response criteria for lymphoma (6). In the revised IWC-PET criteria, the challenge associated with complete response, unconfirmed complete remission (Cru) has been eliminated by FDG-PET (6, 7). Currently, those patients without metabolic evidence of residual disease are classified as CR regardless of CT response, while those with positive PET findings are classified as PR, SD, or PD based on CT measurements. In an attempt to standardize interpretation of PET images at completion of therapy, the imaging subcommittee of the International Harmonization Project (IHP) in lymphoma recommended that the mediastinal blood pool (MBP) be set as a background for lesions of 2.0 cm or larger as an internal reference (6, 7) to discriminate a positive finding from a negative. However, in lesions measuring less than 2.0 cm, adjacent background uptake is used as the reference irrespective of the lesion location.

Rapid response to chemotherapy is a determinant of tumor biological homogeneity which translates into a more uniform chemosensitivity across the entire tumor volume. This also connotes a low probability of developing resistant cell variants and ultimately more effective cell kill resulting in an improved DFS. The rapidly responding tumors are more likely to be eradicated by several cycles of chemotherapy, thus, these patients may not need the full-course standard therapy. In a systematic analysis, interim FDG-PET had an overall sensitivity of 81% and a specificity of 97%, while the sensitivity and specificity were 78% and 87%, respectively for DLBCL (8). Consequently, in advanced-stage HL, FDG-PET performed after a few cycles of standard chemotherapy was determined to be a reliable prognostic test to identify poor responders, warranting prospective studies to assess PET-based treatment strategies. For DLBCL, no reliable conclusions can be drawn due to heterogeneity. The number of chemotherapy cycles can be abbreviated to avoid unnecessary therapy-related morbidity. More than 90% of patients with limited stage or favorable risk HL achieve a durable response (9); consequently, the current disease management focuses on the strategies that would reduce the long-term treatment-related risks. The conventional therapy options for this group of patients include combined modality therapy with chemotherapy (ABVD) with or without involved field radiotherapy (IFRT) (9). The treatment with chemotherapy alone is a more attractive alternative as it is expected to be associated with fewer late effects compared with combined modality therapy with IFRT. Ongoing trials using interim FDG-PET results to de-escalate therapy including reduction of radiation dose or radiation field size, and abbreviated chemotherapy, may help in decreasing the number of treatment-related long-term complications.

For interim PET readings, a relatively continuous visual reading scheme may be used given that these scans measure chemosensitivity rather than ultimate response. The minimal residual uptake (MRU) is a frequent phenomenon seen during PET interpretation. It has been proven that the prognosis of the MRU group is similar to that of PET-negative patients at interim PET evaluation (10–12). For interim PET analysis, the London criteria were developed to fill the need for a continuous reading scheme using a 5-point scoring system employing a higher threshold using liver uptake as the reference (13, 14). Any FDG uptake that is equal to or is lower than that of the liver parenchyma is considered negative. A recently published result series of a multicenter study confirmed a high level of agreement among different reviewers using this scoring system (14). One important issue to highlight is that interim PET should be scheduled at least 2 weeks, preferably 3 weeks after the initiation of therapy (7, 15) or within 4–5 days of start of the subsequent therapy cycle. This approach should be adopted to improve the positive predictive value by minimizing false-positive findings introduced by the inflammatory response that usually peaks at between 10 and 15 days of therapy administration (15).

## Take-home message

- The 2-year relapse-free survival rates are usually high at > 90% for a negative PET result compared with 0–20% for a positive result regardless of a residual mass on CT.
- According to International Workshop Group (IWG) response criteria, currently, those patients without metabolic evidence of residual disease on FDG-PET imaging are classified as CR regardless of CT response, while those with positive PET findings are classified as PR, SD, or PD based on CT measurements.
- At end-therapy response evaluation, the mediastinal blood pool (MBP) is set as a background for lesions of 2.0 cm or larger as an internal reference by IHP criteria to discriminate a positive from a negative finding.
- In advanced-stage HL including stage IIB, FDG-PET performed after a few cycles of standard chemotherapy is a reliable prognostic test to identify poor responders. For DLBCL, no reliable conclusions can be drawn due to disease and therapy heterogeneity.
- For interim PET readings, a continuous visual reading scheme is preferred to determine response or rather to measure chemosensitivity.
- For interim PET analysis, the London criteria were developed to fill the need for a continuous reading scheme using a 5-point scoring system employing liver uptake as the reference. Any FDG uptake that is equal to or is lower than that of the liver parenchyma is considered negative.
- Interim FDG-PET scans should be scheduled at least 2 weeks after the initiation of therapy or within 4–5 days of the start of the subsequent therapy cycle to minimize false-positive findings introduced by the inflammatory response that usually peaks at between 10 and 15 days of therapy administration.

## References

1. Zinzani PL, Magagnoli M, Chierichetti F et al. The role of positron emission tomography (PET) in the management of lymphoma patients. *Ann Oncol* 1999:**10**:1181–4.

2. Cremerius U, Fabry U, Neuerburg J et al. Positron emission tomography with 18F-FDG to detect residual disease after therapy for malignant lymphoma. *Nucl Med Commun* 1998;**19**:1055–63.

3. Mikhaeel NG, Timothy AR, O'Doherty MJ, Hain S, Maisey MN. 18-FDG-PET as a prognostic indicator in the treatment of aggressive Non-Hodgkin's Lymphoma – comparison with CT. *Leuk Lymphoma* 2000;**39**:543–53.

4. Dittmann H, Sokler M, Kollmannsberger C *et al*. Comparison of 18FDG-PET with CT scans in the evaluation of patients with residual and recurrent Hodgkin's lymphoma. *Oncol Rep* 2001;**8**:1393–9.

5. Spaepen K, Stroobants S, Dupont P *et al*. Prognostic value of positron emission tomography (PET) with fluorine-18 fluorodeoxyglucose ([$^{18}$F]FDG) after first line chemotherapy in non-Hodgkins lymphoma: is [$^{18}$F]FDG PET a valid alternative to conventional diagnostic methods? *J Clin Oncol* 2001;**19**:414–19.

6. Cheson BD, Pfistner B, Juweid ME *et al*. Revised response criteria for malignant lymphoma. *J Clin Oncol* 2007;**25**:579–86.

7. Juweid ME, Stroobants S, Hoekstra OS *et al*. Use of positron emission tomography for response assessment of lymphoma: consensus of the Imaging Subcommittee of International Harmonization Project in Lymphoma. *J Clin Oncol* 2007;**25**:571–8.

8. Terasawa T, Lau J, Bardet S *et al*. Fluorine-18-fluorodeoxyglucose positron emission tomography for interim response assessment of advanced-stage Hodgkin's lymphoma and diffuse large B-cell lymphoma: a systematic review. *J Clin Oncol* 2009;**27**:1906–14.

9. Diehl V, Re D, Harris NL, Mauch PM. Hodgkin Lymphoma. In VT DeVita, TS Lawrence, SA Rosenberg (Eds.), *DeVita, Hellman, and Rosenberg's Cancer: Principles and Practice of Oncology*, 8th edn. Philadelphia, PA: Lippincott Williams & Wilkins, 2008, 2167–213.

10. Hutchings M, Mikhaeel NG, Fields PA *et al*. Prognostic value of interim FDG-PET after two or three cycles of chemotherapy in Hodgkin lymphoma. *Ann Oncol* 2005;**16**:1160–8.

11. Hutchings M, Loft A, Hansen M **et al**. FDG-PET after two cycles of chemotherapy predicts treatment failure and progression-free survival in Hodgkin lymphoma. *Blood* 2006;**107**:52–9.

12. Gallamini A, Rigacci L, Merli F *et al*. The predictive value of positron emission tomography scanning performed after two courses of standard therapy on treatment outcome in advanced stage Hodgkin's disease. *Haematologica* 2006;**91**:475–81.

13. Meignan M, Gallamini A, Haioun C. Report on the First International Workshop on Interim-PET-Scan in Lymphoma. *Leuk Lymphoma* 2009;**50**:1257–60.

14. Barrington SF, Qian W, Somer E *et al*. Concordance between four European centres of PET reporting criteria designed for use in multicentre trials in Hodgkin lymphoma. *Eur J Nucl Med Mol Imaging* 2010;**37**:1824–33.

15. Spaepen K, Stroobants S, Dupont P *et al*. [(18)F]FDG PET monitoring of tumour response to chemotherapy: does [(18)F]FDG uptake correlate with the viable tumour cell fraction? *Eur J Nucl Med Mol Imaging* 2003;**30**:682–8.

**Chapter**

# 14

# Melanoma

Kent P. Friedman and Stephan Probst

## Introduction

Malignant melanoma, a neoplasm of melanocytes, has a lifetime risk of 1 per 75 people in North America, and accounts for only 5% of skin cancers, but is responsible for three times as many deaths as non-melanoma skin cancers (1). Both the incidence rate and mortality from the disease have increased significantly since the 1970s, though the former may be partly attributed to increased awareness and screening (2, 3). Melanoma is primarily a disease of white people; rates are up to 20 times higher in whites than in African Americans. Major risk factors apart from race include family history of melanoma, atypical or numerous nevi, sun sensitivity, a history of excessive UV exposure, immunosuppressed states, and occupational exposure to carcinogens (1).

## Staging

Melanoma is staged using the widely accepted American Joint Committee on Cancer's (AJCC) TNM staging system, which was most recently updated in 2009 (4). This system defines stage by features of the primary tumor (T), the presence or absence of tumor spread to regional lymph nodes (N) and the presence or absence of metastasis to distant sites (M) (Table 14.1). The TNM classifications are then organized into anatomic stage groupings, which dictate prognosis, treatment options and are predictive of other expected features of the disease in a given patient (Table 14.2).

## Treatment

Surgery is the definitive treatment for early-stage melanoma, and is curative in localized disease. Unfortunately, few therapies exist that have a significant impact on survival in patients with regional or distant tumor spread. Surgical resection of involved regional lymph nodes is important for local disease control and staging, and removal of distant metastases may be beneficial in some individuals with limited sites of disease (5). Melanomas are highly radioresistant and no combination conventional chemotherapy regimen has proven to be significantly better than single-agent dacarbazine, which yields only a

10–15% response rate (6). Biological therapies such as high-dose interferon-alfa-2b, interleukin-2, and most recently immunotherapy with tumor vaccines have shown only modest benefit with few patients responding and even fewer showing a complete response (7, 8). Targeted therapies such as those interfering with BRAF signaling offer much promise, but for the most part are at pre-clinical stages of evaluation (9). The 5-year survival of patients with stage IV disease is about 15%, and currently there are no standard systemic therapeutic regimens that offer significant survival advantage for patients with metastatic melanoma without significant risk of toxicities.

## FDG-PET imaging of melanoma

Positron emission tomography (PET) particularly with fluorodeoxyglucose (FDG) has proven to be a useful non-invasive imaging modality for the initial staging and follow-up of melanoma. In the early 1990s, when it became clear that melanoma cells avidly concentrated radiolabeled glucose analogs, researchers lauded the elegance of the modality and early work seemed to endorse this enthusiasm, with small series in humans reporting perfect sensitivity and specificity (10). More than 15 years later, FDG-PET and PET/CT remain strong tools in the armamentarium of clinicians who manage patients with melanoma, albeit with many since-discovered caveats. FDG-PET has found utility in a number of clinical scenarios, however, due to the nature of cutaneous melanoma, namely its accessibility to biopsy and its distinct visual characteristics on physical exam, it is unlikely that FDG-PET will ever replace or compete with histopathology in the diagnosis of primary melanoma. However, once a diagnosis has been established, FDG-PET has been successfully utilized in initial staging, assessment of local or distant recurrence, and the evaluation of response to therapy (8). Given the sharp differences in survival rates amongst the varied stages of the disease, accurate staging is paramount for appropriate patient management. The following cases will illustrate the potential value and also highlight some of the limitations of FDG-PET/CT in these and other clinical scenarios.

**Table 14.1** Tumor, node, metastasis (TNM) staging categories for cutaneous melanoma. (Adapted with permission from (4).)

| Classification | Thickness (mm) | Ulceration status/ mitoses |
|---|---|---|
| T | | |
| Tis | NA | NA |
| T1 | ≤ 1.00 | a: Without ulceration and mitosis $< 1/mm^2$ b: With ulceration or mitoses $\geq 1/mm^2$ |
| T2 | 1.01–2.00 | a: Without ulceration b: With ulceration |
| T3 | 2.01–4.00 | a: Without ulceration b: With ulceration |
| T4 | > 4.00 | a: Without ulceration b: With ulceration |
| N | No. of metastatic nodes | Nodal metastatic burden |
| N0 | 0 | NA |
| N1 | 1 | a: Micrometastasis* b: Macrometastasis† |
| N2 | 2–3 | a: Micrometastasis* b: Macrometastasis† c: In transit metastases/satellites without metastatic nodes |
| N3 | 4+ metastatic nodes, or matted nodes, or in transit metastases/satellites with metastatic nodes | |
| M | Site | Serum LDH |
| M0 | No distant metastases | NA |
| M1a | Distant skin, subcutaneous, or nodal metastases | Normal |
| M1b | Lung metastases | Normal |
| M1c | All other visceral metastases | Normal |
| | Any distant metastasis | Elevated |

NA, not applicable; LDH, lactate dehydrogenase.
*Micrometastases are diagnosed after sentinel lymph node biopsy.
†Macrometastases are defined as clinically detectable nodal metastases confirmed pathologically.

**Table 14.2** Anatomic stage groupings for cutaneous melanoma. (Adapted with permission from (4).)

| | Clinical staging* | | | | Pathologic staging† | | |
|---|---|---|---|---|---|---|---|
| | T | N | M | | T | N | M |
| 0 | Tis | N0 | M0 | 0 | Tis | N0 | M0 |
| IA | T1a | N0 | M0 | IA | T1a | N0 | M0 |
| IB | T1b | N0 | M0 | IB | T1b | N0 | M0 |
| | T2a | N0 | M0 | | T2a | N0 | M0 |
| IIA | T2b | N0 | M0 | IIA | T2b | N0 | M0 |
| | T3a | N0 | M0 | | T3a | N0 | M0 |
| IIB | T3b | N0 | M0 | IIB | T3b | N0 | M0 |
| | T4a | N0 | M0 | | T4a | N0 | M0 |
| IIC | T4b | N0 | M0 | IIC | T4b | N0 | M0 |
| III | Any T | N>N0 | M0 | IIIA | T1-4a | N1a | M0 |
| | | | | | T1-4a | N2a | M0 |
| | | | | IIIB | T1-4b | N1a | M0 |
| | | | | | T1-4b | N2a | M0 |
| | | | | | T1-4a | N1b | M0 |
| | | | | | T1-4a | N2b | M0 |
| | | | | | T1-4a | N2c | M0 |
| | | | | IIIC | T1-4b | N1b | M0 |
| | | | | | T1-4b | N2b | M0 |
| | | | | | T1-4b | N2c | M0 |
| | | | | | Any T | N3 | M0 |
| IV | Any T | Any N | M1 | IV | Any T | Any N | M1 |

*Clinical staging includes microstaging of the primary melanoma and clinical/ radiologic evaluation for metastases. By convention, it should be used after complete excision of the primary melanoma with clinical assessment for regional and distant metastases.
†Pathologic staging includes microstaging of the primary melanoma and pathologic information about the regional lymph nodes after partial (i.e. sentinel node biopsy) or complete lymphadenectomy. Pathologic stage 0 or stage IA patients are the exception; they do not require pathologic evaluation of their lymph nodes.

## PET/CT acquisition and processing parameters at our institution

We ask patients to fast for at least 6 hours prior to the study and to refrain from strenuous exercise for 24 hours preceding the scan. Pre-test serum glucose should be below 200 mg/dL prior to FDG injection. For adult oncology studies, the standard dose is 15 mCi (555 MBq) of FDG, and we generally let 60 minutes of uptake time elapse prior to scanning.

All scans are performed on a Siemens Biograph 6 integrated PET/CT scanner. Patients do not routinely get IV contrast, but we do use READI-CAT 1.2% barium sulfate as oral contrast. Melanoma imaging is performed from the vertex to the toes (true whole-body imaging) most often with the patient's arms down; this is sometimes done in two separate acquisitions, although both acquisitions are not always shown in the case examples. Our CT parameters are as follows: 6 × 4 mm detector configuration, 5 mm slice reconstruction thickness with B40 kernel, 5 mm slice interval, 95 mA (Siemens Care Dose4D), 130 kVp, and 70 cm scan field of view.

We generally scan patients for 2–4 minutes per bed position, using longer times for larger patients, patients whose injected FDG doses were in the lower range of normal, or where uptake time was inadvertently delayed much beyond 60 minutes. Our PET parameters are as follows: $168 \times 168$ matrix, 4 iterations with 8 subsets of OSEM reconstruction utilizing a Gaussian prefilter. Both attenuation corrected and non-attenuation corrected images are generated. Our clinical reports and those in this text always reference maximum lesion SUV corrected for actual body weight (SUVmax-bw).

# References

1. American Cancer Society. Cancer Facts & Figures 2009. Available at http://www.cancer.org/downloads/STT/500809web.pdf.

2. Hall HI, Miller DR, Rogers JD et al. Update on the incidence and mortality from melanoma in the United States. *J Am Acad Dermatol* 1999;**40**(1):35–42.

3. Welch HG, Woloshin S, Schwartz LM. Skin biopsy rates and incidence of melanoma: population based ecological study. *Br Med J* 2005;**331**(7515):481.

4. Balch CM, Gershenwald JE, Soong SJ et al. Final version of 2009 AJCC melanoma staging and classification. *J Clin Oncol* 2009;**27**(36):6199–206.

5. Essner R. Surgical treatment of malignant melanoma. *Surg Clin North Am* 2003;**83**:109–156.

6. Fecher LA, Flaherty KT. Where are we with adjuvant therapy of stage III and IV melanoma in 2009? *J Natl Compr Canc Netw* 2009;**7**(3): 295–304.

7. Atkins MB, Lotze MT, Dutcher JP et al. High-dose recombinant interleukin 2 therapy for patients with metastatic melanoma: analysis of 270 patients treated between 1985 and 1993. *J Clin Oncol* 1999;**17**(7):2105–16.

8. Kirkwood JM, Strawderman MH, Ernstoff MS et al. Interferon alfa-2b adjuvant therapy of high-risk resected cutaneous melanoma: the Eastern Cooperative Oncology Group Trial EST 1684. *J Clin Oncol* 1996; **14**(1):7–17.

9. Dhomen N, Marais R. BRAF signaling and targeted therapies in melanoma. *Hematol Oncol Clin North Am* 2009;**23**(3):529–45, ix.

10. Gritters LS, Francis IR, Zasadny KR et al. Initial assessment of positron emission tomography using 2-fluorine-18-fluoro-2-deoxy-D-glucose in the imaging of malignant melanoma. *J Nucl Med* 1993;**34**:1420–7.

11. Friedman KP, Wahl RL. Clinical use of positron emission tomography in the management of cutaneous melanoma. *Semin Nucl Med* 2004;**34**(4):242–53.

# Initial nodal staging

A 66-year-old female with melanoma of the right heel, status post sentinel node biopsy.

## Acquisition and processing parameters

Approximately 60 minutes following the intravenous administration of 14.9 mCi of FDG in the left antecubital fossa, PET/CT images from the vertex to toes were obtained. Serum glucose level was 105 mg/dL at the time of injection.

## Findings and differential diagnosis

There is intense FDG uptake within multiple intrapelvic nodes, including right iliac (Figure 14.1) and right pelvic sidewall masses (up to 3 cm with SUV of 14). There is an intensely FDG-avid mass within the left inguinal region that measures 2.3 cm with an SUV of 12.2 (Figure 14.2). There are surgical clips and post-operative change within the right inguinal region associated with no significant FDG uptake (Figure 14.3).

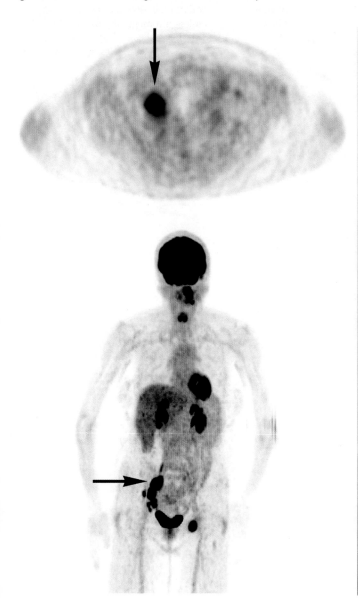

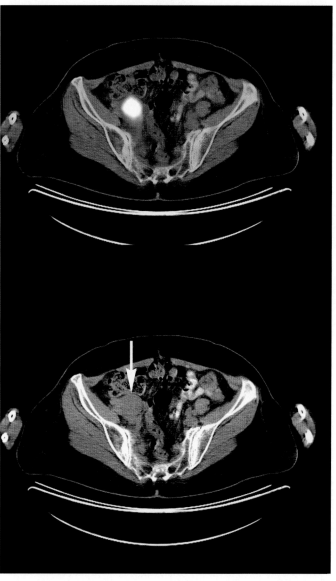

**Figure 14.1** Selected axial FDG-PET, fused, and CT image with maximum intensity projection (MIP) localizer: very intense FDG accumulation can be seen in an enlarged right iliac node indicated by the arrow.

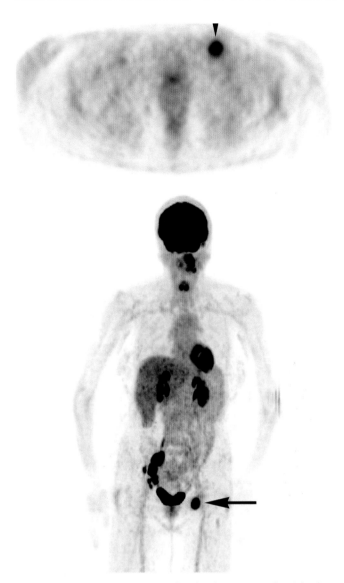

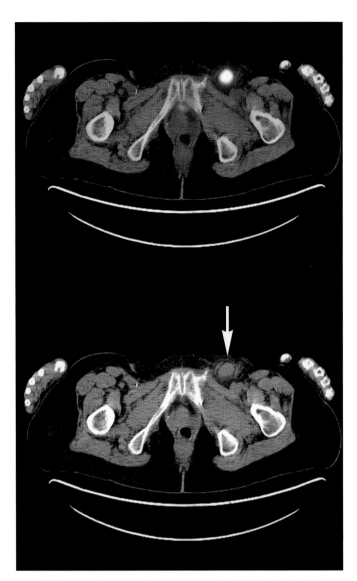

**Figure 14.2** Selected axial FDG-PET, fused, and CT image with MIP localizer: very intense FDG accumulation can be seen in an enlarged left inguinal node indicated by the arrow.

Incidentally noted on the maximum intensity projection image is physiologic vocal cord and oropharyngeal uptake.

## Diagnosis and clinical follow-up

Multiple FDG avid melanoma metastases to the right pelvic sidewall, right iliac and left inguinal nodal stations. Normal post-operative appearance of the distal right inguinal region (Figure 14.3). These lesions were biopsy proven shortly thereafter.

## Discussion and teaching points

Following the initial diagnosis of cutaneous melanoma, prognosis weighs heavily on three parameters, namely the depth of invasion of the primary tumors, presence or absence of ulceration, and nodal or distant metastatic status. Wide local

excision to ensure complete removal of the primary tumor is standard of care in almost all instances, and for lesions less than 1 mm in thickness, no further treatment is required. For any greater depth of primary tumor, sentinel node biopsy is typically recommended to assess the histologic status of locally draining lymph nodes (1). Interested in a non-invasive staging tool, investigators examined the possible role for FDG-PET in nodal staging. Early reports of regional lymph node status assessment with FDG-PET in primary diagnosis were very favorable with sensitivities of 85–100% and specificities of 92–100%, however, these were heavily selected patients in which clinically palpable disease was present in many cases (2, 3). Once the selection bias was removed and patients with clinically N0 disease were enrolled in further trials, sensitivities plummeted into an unacceptably low range of 0–8% (4, 5). Of note, specificity remained high in all of the published series

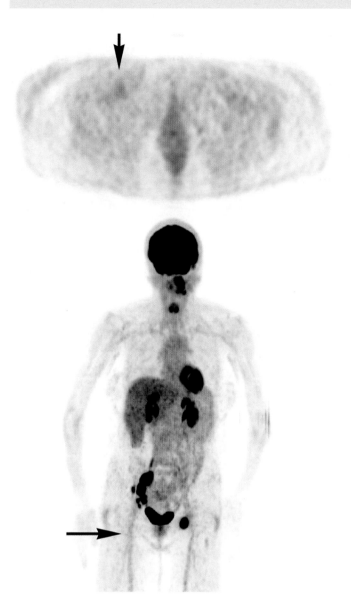
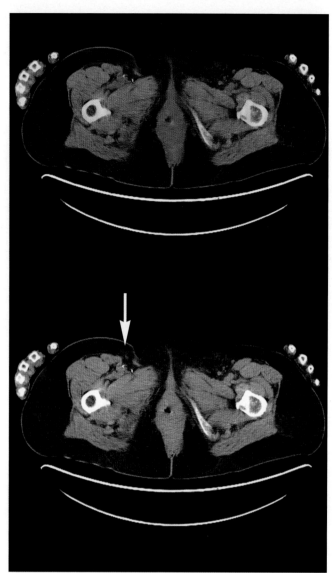

**Figure 14.3** Selected axial FDG-PET, fused, and CT image with MIP localizer: right inguinal prior nodal sampling site is identified with mild, benign FDG uptake and surgical clips.

(5, 6). The earlier bias towards patients with large-volume macroscopic nodal disease unfairly increased the sensitivity of FDG-PET, and as nodal metastasis begin microscopically, the physical limitations of PET in small volume lesions became readily apparent in this group of patients. It is now clear that FDG-PET cannot replace sentinel lymph node biopsy in the initial nodal staging of clinically localized melanoma.

## Take-home message

1. FDG-PET/CT cannot replace sentinel lymph node biopsy in the initial staging of clinically localized (N0 M0) melanoma, because of very poor sensitivity for small volume and microscopic disease.
2. Specificity of FDG-PET for evaluation of sentinel lymph nodes is high (90–100%).

## References

1. Morton DL, Cochran AJ, Thompson JF *et al*. Sentinel node biopsy for early-stage melanoma: accuracy and morbidity in MSLT-I, an international multicenter trial. *Ann Surg* 2005;**242**(3):302–11.

2. Wagner JD, Schauwecker D, Hutchins G *et al*. Initial assessment of positron emission tomography for detection of nonpalpable regional lymphatic metastases in melanoma. *J Surg Oncol* 1997; **64**(3):181–9.

3. Macfarlane DJ, Sondak V, Johnson T *et al*. Prospective evaluation of 2-[18F]-2-deoxy-D-glucose positron emission tomography in staging of regional lymph nodes in patients with cutaneous malignant melanoma. *J Clin Oncol* 1998;**16**(5):1770–6.

4. Acland KM, Healy C, Calonje E *et al.* Comparison of positron emission tomography scanning and sentinel node biopsy in the detection of micrometastases of primary cutaneous malignant melanoma. *J Clin Oncol* 2001;**19**(10): 2674–8.

5. Hafner J, Schmid MH, Kempf W *et al.* Baseline staging in cutaneous malignant melanoma. *Br J Dermatol* 2004;**150**(4):677–86.

6. Belhocine T, Pierard G, De Labrassinne M *et al.* Staging of regional nodes in AJCC stage I and II melanoma: 18FDG PET imaging versus sentinel node detection. *Oncologist* 2002;7(4):271–8.

## Initial distant staging

A 50-year-old male with melanoma of the right posterior scalp and recent right neck wide excision.

## Acquisition and processing parameters

Approximately 60 min following the intravenous administration of 12.9 mCi of FDG in the left antecubital fossa, tomographic studies from the vertex to toes were obtained. Serum glucose level was 109 mg/dL at the time of injection.

## Findings and differential diagnosis

There is extensive diffuse reticulonodular infiltration of both lungs associated with moderate FDG uptake, most prominent at the bases and involving the pleural surfaces extensively (Figure 14.4).

The unenhanced liver demonstrates a small right lobe hypodensity with intense hypermetabolism, SUV 9.3 (Figure 14.6). Multiple other hypermetabolic lesions are apparent in the liver, without corresponding CT abnormality. There are

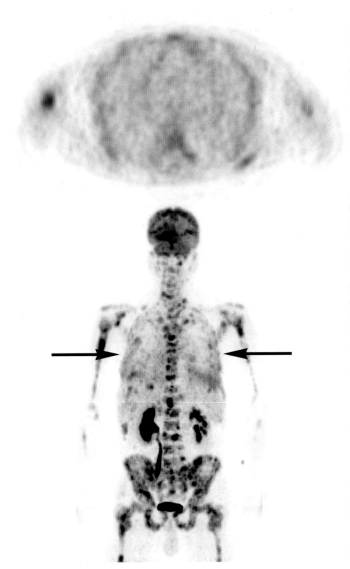
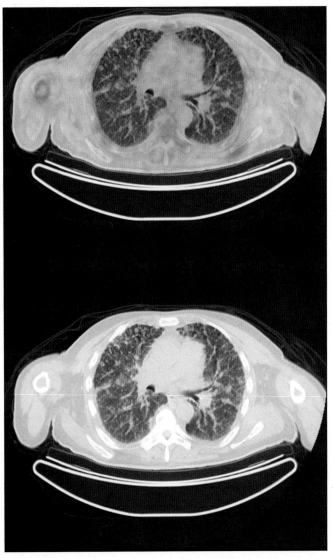

**Figure 14.4** Selected axial FDG-PET, fused, and CT images with MIP localizer: moderately intense FDG uptake is identified diffusely throughout extensive bilateral micro-nodular lung disease, in keeping with diffuse melanoma metastases.

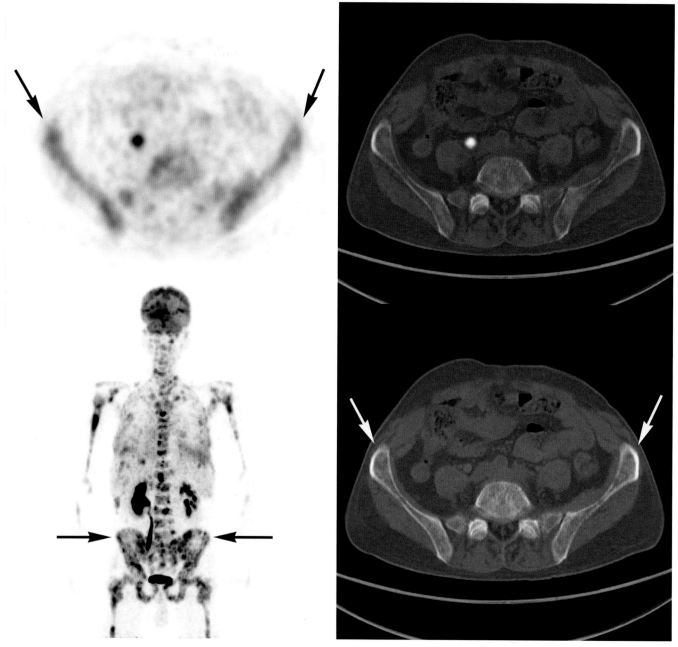

**Figure 14.5** Selected axial FDG-PET, fused, and CT images with MIP localizer: moderately intense FDG uptake is identified diffusely throughout both iliac bones with associated sclerosis, in keeping with melanoma metastases.

innumerable coalescing intensely FDG-avid foci throughout the axial and appendicular skeleton associated with focal areas of trabecular and cortical bone lysis. This is especially apparent in the pelvis (Figure 14.5) and the proximal humeri (Figure 14.7). Also noted on the maximum intensity projection image is moderate right hydroureteronephrosis with tracer stasis.

## Diagnosis and clinical follow-up

Innumerable FDG-avid bone metastases to the axial and appendicular skeleton. Metastatic pulmonary carcinomatosis. Multiple liver metastases. The patient's clinical course

deteriorated rapidly, and no attempt was made to correlate the findings histopathologically.

## Discussion and teaching points

Following the identification of an intermediate to high-risk primary melanoma lesion ($\geq 1.0$ mm Breslow thickness), sentinel node staging is indicated, but as seen in the previous case's discussion, it cannot be performed by FDG-PET/CT. In the case of negative sentinel lymph nodes, the risk of distant metastasis is low and the yield of imaging seems to be poor. For example in a series of 49 clinically N0 patients with up to

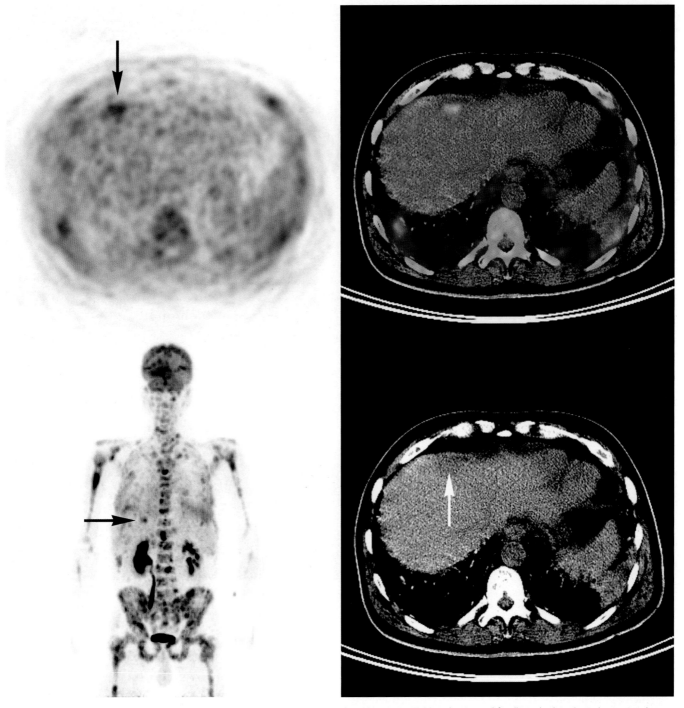

**Figure 14.6** Selected axial FDG-PET, fused and CT image with MIP localizer: moderately intense FDG uptake is noted focally in the liver (arrow), associated with CT hypodensity, in keeping with melanoma metastasis.

T3b lesion who underwent PET/CT, only one patient (2%) had a confirmed unsuspected metastasis and three out of five suspicious lesions on PET/CT ended up being false-positives (1). In the instance of node positive disease, it is of interest to look at pathologically positive, clinically negative (microscopic) nodal disease and pathologically positive, clinically positive (macroscopic) nodal disease separately, as differing tumor extent should impact the prevalence of M1 disease in these different patient populations. Macroscopic nodal metastases are recognized as carrying a worse prognosis compared with microscopic lymph node involvement. Horn and colleagues studied 33 patients with subclinical pathology-proven microscopic sentinel node metastases and found a not-insignificant 12% true-positive fraction, with a further 6% of patients in which positive FDG-PET findings could not be confirmed (2). More recently a larger series of 251 patients

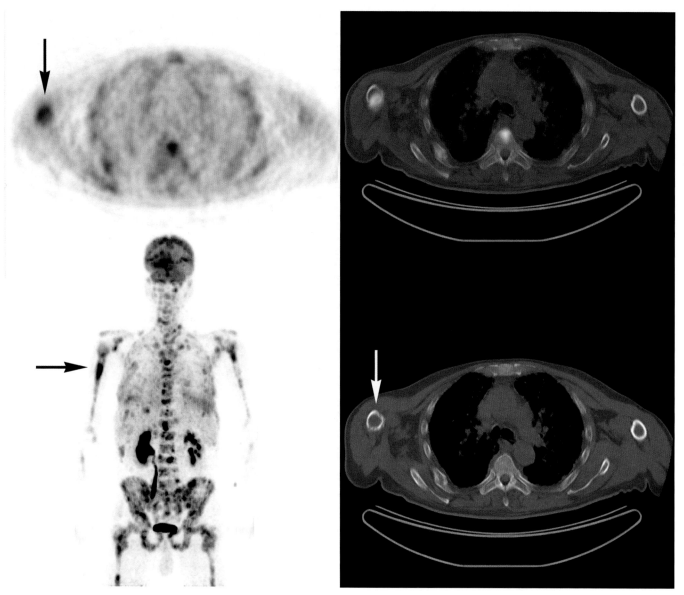

**Figure 14.7** Selected axial FDG-PET, fused and CT images with MIP localizer: intense FDG uptake is seen in the proximal right humeral diaphysis, with notable cortical disruption on CT (arrow), consistent with melanoma metastasis.

with clinically evident macroscopic nodal disease, 27% were correctly upstaged to stage IV by FDG-PET, and the planned treatment was changed in 15% (3). Slightly more than half (60%) of the upstaged patients had solitary sites of metastatic disease whereas the remainder had multiple sites of involvement. An earlier series by Tyler *et al.* in 95 stage III melanoma patients also suggested clinical value of FDG-PET with a 20% true-positive fraction and a 15% rate of management alteration (4). Another small series by Wagner *et al.*, suggested that FDG-PET can up-stage a significant number of patients (3 of 11, or 27%) who would otherwise have been considered to harbor only local lymph node metastases (5). As an aside, FDG-PET seems superior to CT in terms of sensitivity and specificity for the detection of stage IV disease in this setting (3, 6, 7).

A recent pooled analysis of 28 studies involving 2,095 patients suggested a sensitivity of 83%, a specificity of 85%, and a diagnostic odds ratio of 19.8 for the detection of metastases at initial staging of high-risk melanoma (8).

## Take-home message

1. FDG-PET/CT is indicated in clinical and subclinical node-positive disease (stage III) as up to one-quarter of patients can be upstaged and up to one-fifth will have their treatment changed.
2. FDG-PET/CT is probably not useful in histopathologically node-negative disease as a low prevalence of metastatic lesions dictates that many findings reported as suspicious will in fact be false-positives.

# References

1. Yancovitz M, Finelt N, Warycha MA *et al.* Role of radiologic imaging at the time of initial diagnosis of stage T1b-T3b melanoma. *Cancer* 2007;**110**(5):1107–14.

2. Horn J, Lock-Andersen J, Sjostrand H *et al.* Routine use of FDG-PET scans in melanoma patients with positive sentinel node biopsy. *Eur J Nucl Med Mol Imaging* 2006;**33**(8):887–92.

3. Bastiaannet E, Wobbes T, Hoekstra OS *et al.* Prospective comparison of [18F] fluorodeoxyglucose positron emission tomography and computed tomography in patients with melanoma with palpable lymph node metastases: diagnostic accuracy and impact on treatment. *J Clin Oncol* 2009;**27** (28):4774–80.

4. Tyler DS, Onaitis M, Kherani A *et al.* Positron emission tomography scanning in malignant melanoma. *Cancer* 2000;**89**:1019–25.

5. Wagner JD, Schauwecker D, Hutchins G *et al.* Initial assessment of positron emission tomography for detection of nonpalpable regional lymphatic metastases in melanoma. *J Surg Oncol* 1997;**64**:181–9.

6. Holder WD Jr, White RL Jr, Zuger JH *et al.* Effectiveness of positron emission tomography for the detection of melanoma metastases. *Ann Surg* 1998;**227**:764–9.

7. Swetter SM, Carroll LA, Johnson DL *et al.* Positron emission tomography is superior to computed tomography for metastatic detection in melanoma patients. *Ann Surg Oncol* 2002;**9**:646–53.

8. Krug B, Crott R, Lonneux M *et al.* Role of PET in the initial staging of cutaneous malignant melanoma: systematic review. *Radiology* 2008;**249**(3):836–44.

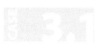 

A 34-year-old female with a history of melanoma involving the distal left arm posteriorly, status post primary resection and radiotherapy to the left axilla.

## Acquisition and processing parameters

Approximately 60 min following the intravenous administration of 14.7 mCi of FDG in the left antecubital fossa, tomographic studies from the vertex to toes were obtained.

Serum glucose level was 93 mg/dL at the time of injection.

## Findings and differential diagnosis

Intense metabolic activity is visualized fusing to a lobulated, serpiginous-appearing soft tissue lesion in the subcutaneous fat of the left arm extensor compartment extending from the mid to distal humerus, measuring up to 1.9 × 2.4 cm (transaxial plane) with SUV 6.9 (Figures 14.8, 14.9, 14.10). This soft tissue lesion courses in the subcutaneous adipose tissue without involving the adjacent triceps muscles. Also noted on the maximum intensity projection image, are several soft tissue nodules in the left upper arm adjacent to the lesion described above. Post-radiation inflammatory uptake is noted on the musculature of the left upper chest and shoulder.

## Diagnosis and clinical follow-up

Tumor growing within and extending from the lymphatics in the left upper arm. This diagnosis was confirmed via clinical follow-up.

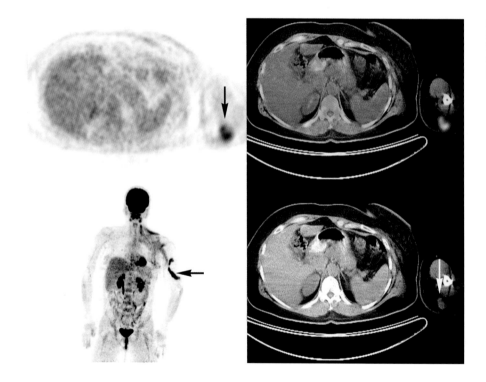

**Figure 14.8** Selected axial FDG-PET, fused and CT images with MIP localizer: Intense FDG uptake in dilated lymphatic channel in the left upper arm, consitent with in-transit melanoma metastasis (arrow).

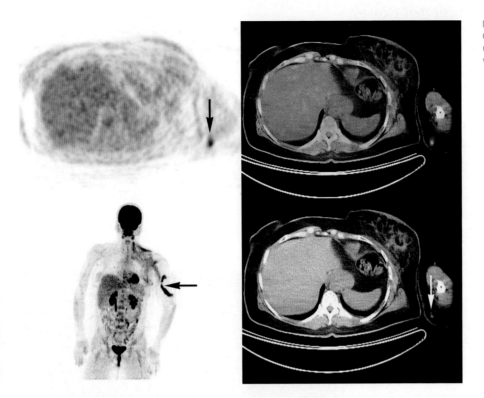

**Figure 14.9** Selected axial FDG-PET, fused and CT images with MIP localizer: again, intense FDG uptake in dilated lymphatic channel, in keeping with in-transit melanoma metastasis (arrow).

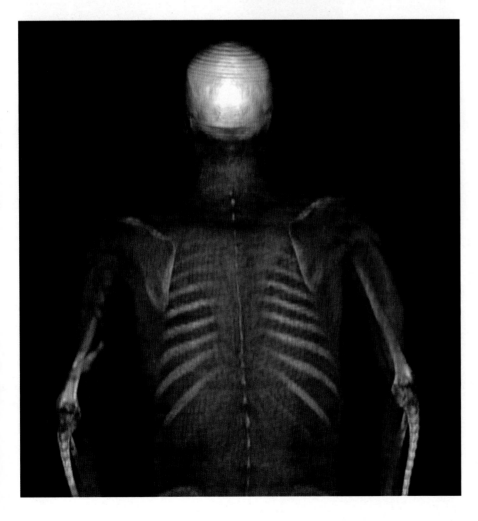

**Figure 14.10** Posterior view of CT volumetric reconstruction, with FDG-PET in red overlay, depicting uptake in dilated lymphatic channel of the left upper arm.

A 70-year-old female with a history of melanoma on the left ankle with positive inguinal nodal metastases, status post left inguinal dissection and radiotherapy.

### Acquisition and processing parameters

Approximately 60 min following the intravenous administration of 15.4 mCi of FDG in the left antecubital fossa, tomographic studies from the vertex to toes were obtained. Serum glucose level was 117 mg/dL at the time of injection.

### Findings and differential diagnosis

There are several small subcutaneous and cutaneous soft tissue nodules with intense FDG activity involving the left leg, most prominently at the left ankle (Figures 14.11, 14.12). An intensely

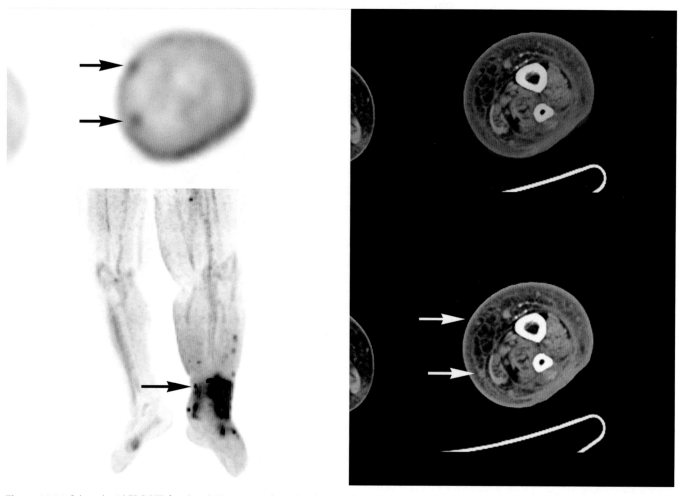

**Figure 14.11** Selected axial FDG-PET, fused, and CT images with MIP localizer: moderately intense FDG uptake is identified focally in small cutaneous and subcutaneous soft-tissue satellite metastases in the left lower leg. There is incidentally noted subcutaneous edema from prior left inguinal lymphatic dissection.

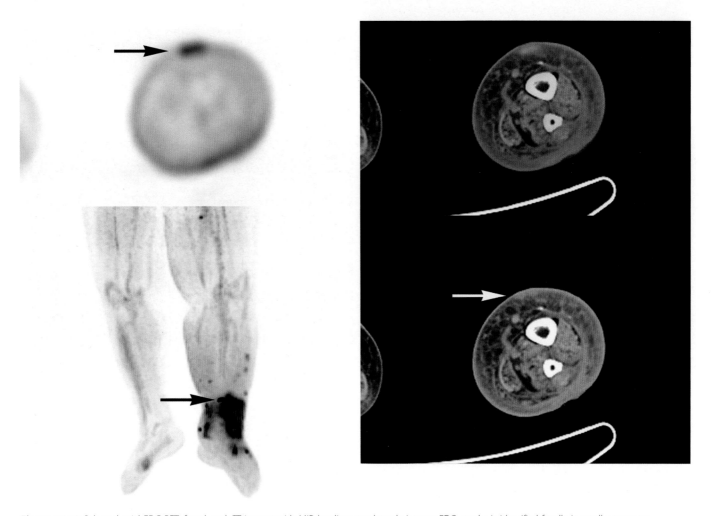

**Figure 14.12** Selected axial FDG-PET, fused, and CT images with MIP localizer: moderately intense FDG uptake is identified focally in small cutaneous and subcutaneous soft-tissue satellite metastases in the left lower leg. There is incidentally noted subcutaneous edema from prior left inguinal lymphatic dissection.

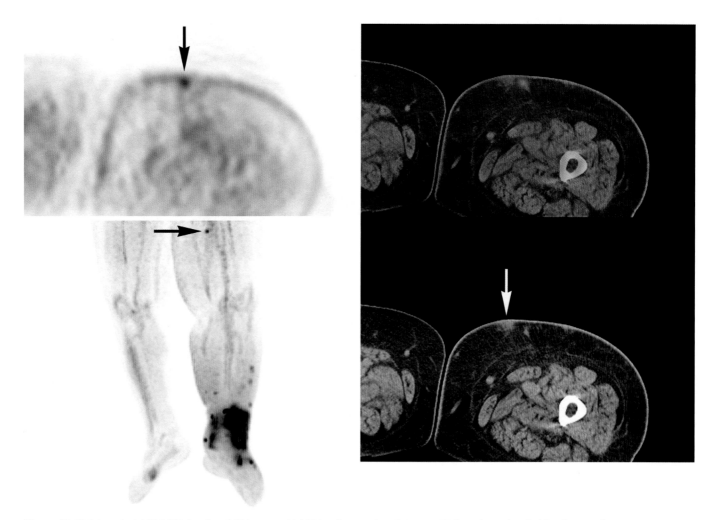

**Figure 14.13** Selected axial FDG-PET, fused, and CT images with MIP localizer: moderately intense FDG uptake is identified focally in small cutaneous and subcutaneous soft-tissue satellite metastases in the left lower leg. There is incidentally noted subcutaneous edema from prior left inguinal lymphatic dissection.

FDG-avid tiny cutaneous lesion is noted at the left anterior thigh (Figure 14.13). Also noted on the maximum intensity projection image, are multiple other very small lesions in the left foot and ankle. There is also marked edema of the left leg and intense uptake diffusely throughout the soft tissues of the right ankle in keeping with post-radiotherapy inflammation.

## Diagnosis and clinical follow-up

Numerous cutaneous and subcutaneous foci of punctuate intense activity involving the left leg, ankle, and foot consistent with extensive local recurrence of melanoma. Post-radiation changes and marked edema of the left leg.

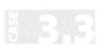
An 80-year-old female with melanoma involving the left great toe.

## Acquisition and processing parameters

Approximately 60 min following the intravenous administration of 16.0 mCi of FDG in the left antecubital fossa, tomographic studies from the vertex to toes were obtained. Serum glucose level was 98 mg/dL at the time of injection.

## Findings and differential diagnosis

Intense FDG uptake is identified in at least six soft tissue nodules in the left leg measuring up to 2.2 × 1.9 cm with SUV 25.9 (Figures 14.14–14.17). Also noted on the maximum intensity projection image, multiple other small hypermetabolic lesions are seen in the left leg and left inguinal region. A solitary focal lesion is noted in the medial right calf. Bilateral pulmonary metastases are present, right more intense than left.

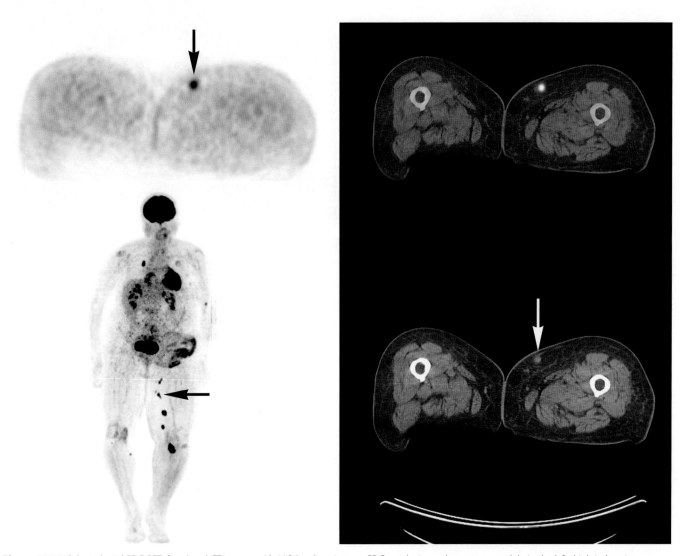

**Figure 14.14** Selected axial FDG-PET, fused and CT images with MIP localizer: intense FDG uptake in a subcutaneous nodule in the left thigh in keeping with melanoma metastasis.

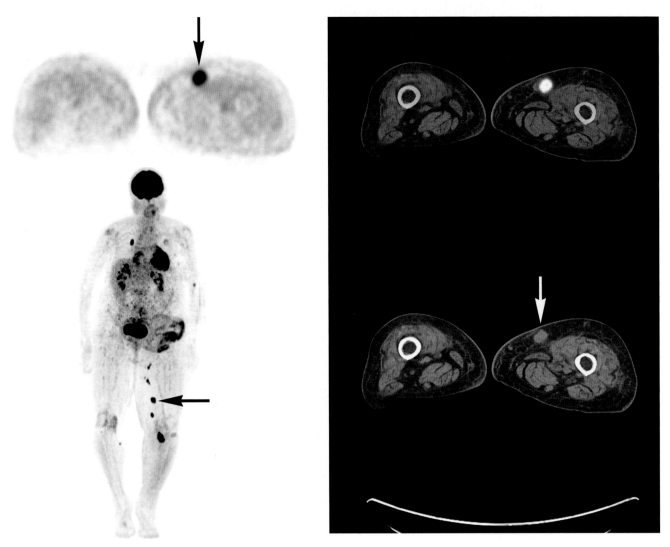

**Figure 14.15** Selected axial FDG-PET, fused and CT images with MIP localizer: intense FDG uptake in a subcutaneous nodule in the left thigh consistent with melanoma metastasis.

## Diagnosis and clinical follow-up

Up to six tumor nodules growing within the lymphatics in the left leg, consistent with in-transit melanoma metastases. Follow-up imaging was consistent with this diagnosis.

## Discussion and teaching points

As well as nodal and distant spread, the presence or absence of local satellite (2 cm or less from the primary lesion) or in-transit (> 2 cm from the primary lesion) metastases can be strong prognostic indicators (1). Although the data are limited, scattered reports suggest that given the higher risk, FDG-PET imaging may be warranted as it uncovers unsuspected stage IV disease. In a small subset of nine patients with local satellite lesions, one (11%) was confirmed to have true-positive distant disease (2). In another limited set of 18 patients with recurrent disease and satellite or in-transit metastases, FDG-PET led to a change in management in three (17%) (3).

## Take-home message

1. Patients with local satellite or in-transit metastasis from melanoma are at higher risk and may benefit from FDG-PET imaging to detect additional locoregional tumor foci as well as unsuspected distant disease, but further study is warranted.

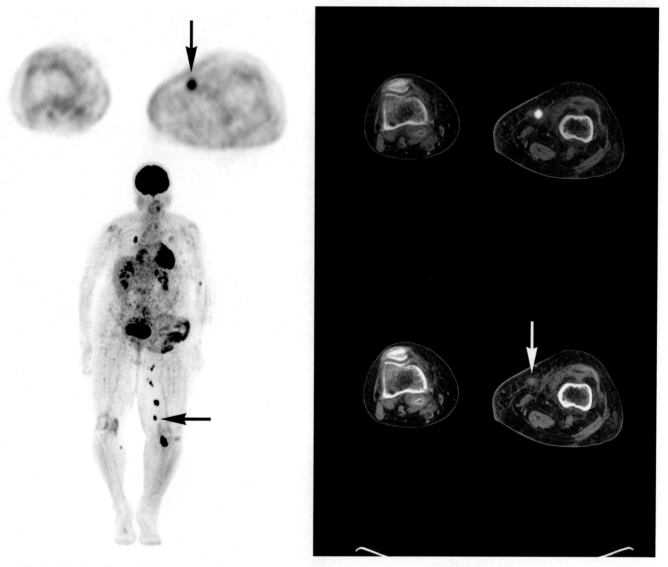

**Figure 14.16** Selected axial FDG-PET, fused and CT images with MIP localizer: intense FDG uptake in a subcutaneous nodule in the left thigh in keeping with melanoma metastasis.

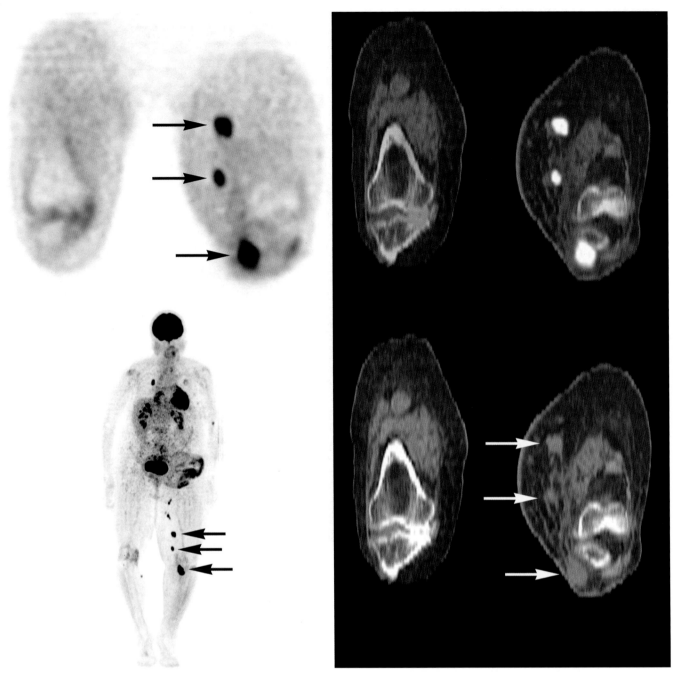

**Figure 14.17** Selected coronal FDG-PET, fused and CT images with MIP localizer: intense FDG uptake is identified in multiple subcutaneous nodules in the left leg in keeping with in-transit melanoma metastases.

# References

1. Payette MJ, Katz M 3rd, Grant-Kels JM. Melanoma prognostic factors found in the dermatopathology report. *Clin Dermatol* 2009;**27**(1):53–74.

2. Acland KM, O'Doherty MJ, Russell-Jones R. The value of positron emission tomography scanning in the detection of subclinical metastatic melanoma. *J Am Acad Dermatol* 2000;**42**(4):606–11.

3. Stas M, Stroobants S, Dupont P *et al.* 18-FDG PET scan in the staging of recurrent melanoma: additional value and therapeutic impact. *Melanoma Res* 2002;**12**(5): 479–90.

A 53-year-old male with melanoma of the scalp, with known metastatic lesions to the neck, lung, and brain, status post brain radiotherapy.

## Acquisition and processing parameters

Approximately 60 min following the intravenous administration of 14.2 mCi of FDG in the left antecubital fossa, tomographic studies from the vertex to toes were obtained. Serum glucose level was 113 mg/dL at the time of injection.

## Findings and differential diagnosis

Multiple foci of intramuscular intense hypermetabolism are noted, including in the left gluteal muscle (Figure 14.18), in the extensor muscles of the left thigh (Figure 14.19), and in the right posterior chest wall muscles (Figure 14.20). These lesions are difficult to appreciate on non-contrast CT. Moderate hypermetabolism, SUV 6.4, is identified in a 2.2-cm lesion intimately associated with the pancreas (Figure 14.21). Also noted on the MIP are multiple chest nodal metastases including subcarinal, AP window, right hilar, and paratracheal

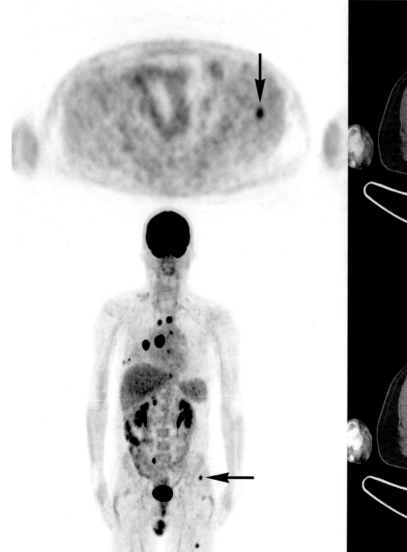

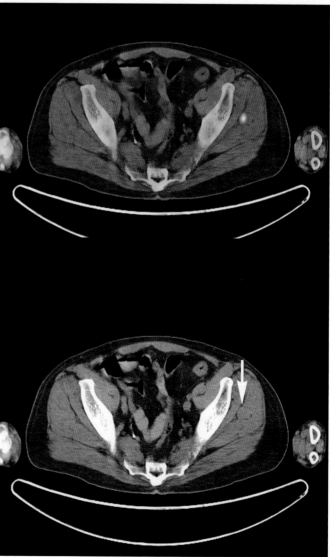

**Figure 14.18** Selected axial FDG-PET, fused, and CT images with MIP localizer: intensely FDG avid metastasis is seen focally in the left gluteus musculature.

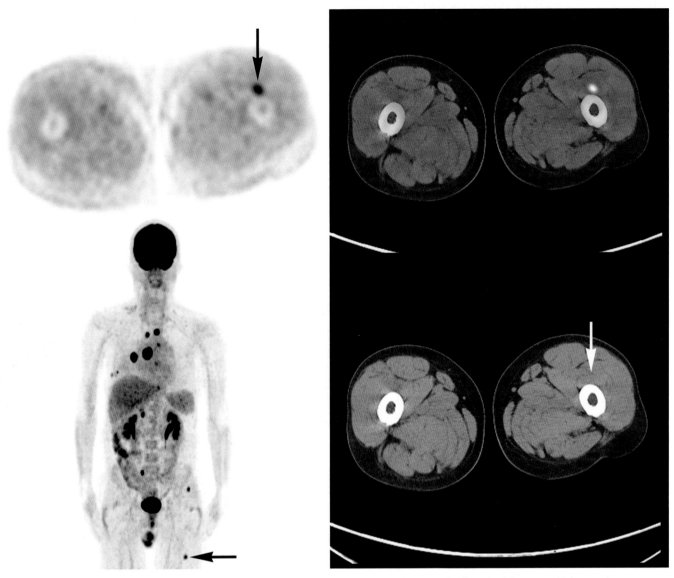

**Figure 14.19** Selected axial FDG-PET, fused, and CT images with MIP localizer: intense FDG uptake is seen focally in the left anterior thigh musculature, in keeping with melanoma metastasis.

nodes. Also, a second right chest wall metastasis is noted lateral to the one described above. The intense focus in the right pelvis corresponds to the ureter, and likely represents focal urine stasis.

## Diagnosis and clinical follow-up

Multifocal metastatic melanoma with subcarinal, paratracheal, AP window, right hilar, right chest wall, pancreatic/peripancreatic, and intramuscular lower extremity metastases. The clinical course confirmed this diagnosis.

## Discussion and teaching points

Despite certain limitations, FDG-PET remains more accurate than computed tomography (CT) in the distant staging of high-risk melanoma. Rinne *et al.* reported on 100 consecutive high-risk patients, both at follow-up and at initial presentation, and found the sensitivity, specificity, and accuracy of PET to be 92%, 94%, and 92%, respectively on a per-lesion basis. This compared very favorably to CT where the sensitivity, specificity, and accuracy were 58%, 45%, and 56%, respectively, again on a per-lesion basis. Even on a per-patient basis, CT failed to identify many patients with disease progression. PET was superior in detecting cervical metastases (100% vs. 67%) and abdominal metastases (100% vs. 27%), however it did come up short for small lung lesions (70% vs. 87%) (1). Lower sensitivity for small lung nodules has been previously noted in other series where only four of 27 small (< 1 cm) lung nodules were detected by PET (2). Holder *et al.* confirmed the superiority of FDG-PET with an overall sensitivity and specificity of 94% and 83%, respectively, compared with 55% and 84% for CT (3). Several other studies as well attest to the increased

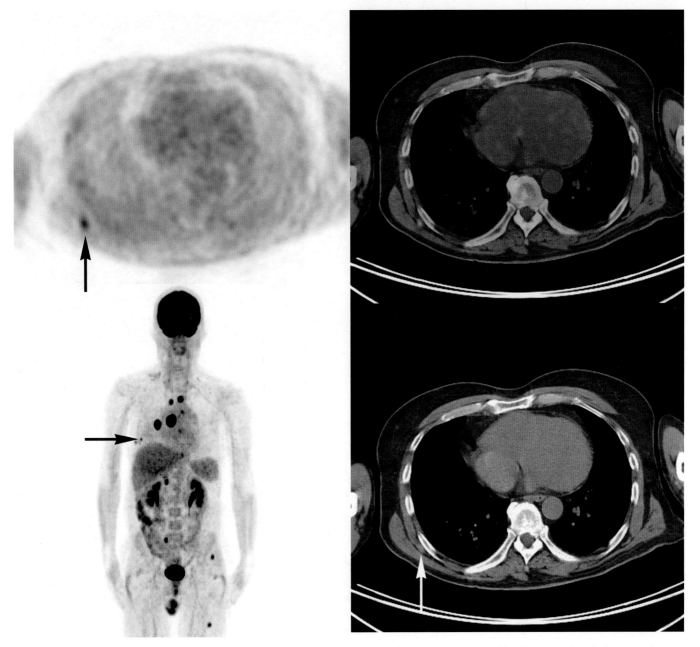

**Figure 14.20** Selected axial FDG-PET, fused, and CT images with MIP localizer: intense FDG avid metastasis is noted focally deep to the right latissimus dorsi.

accuracy of FDG-PET compared with conventional imaging for M-staging of melanoma (4, 5). However, confirming previously suspected limitations, Dietlein *et al.* reported on a lower sensitivity for small pulmonary nodules and intracerebral lesions (6).

Clinical PET-only scanners are no longer being manufactured, and increasingly PET/CT is the norm, particularly in modern medical centers, as reflected in more recent research. Reinhardt *et al.* reported that the accuracy of FDG-PET/CT was significantly higher than that of either FDG-PET or CT alone for M-staging (98% vs. 93% and 84%, respectively) and

significantly higher than that of CT for N-staging (98% vs. 86%) in a retrospective study of 250 patients (7). In a high-risk series by Strobel *et al.*, FDG-PET/CT was shown to be superior to either modality alone, where the sensitivity, specificity, and accuracy of PET-only for the detection of melanoma metastases were 85%, 96%, and 91%, respectively, jumping to 98%, 94%, and 96%, when low-dose CT was added. In 13% of their patients, metastases were detected only on CT, and a high proportion of these were small lung lesions (8).

Evaluation of the brain for metastatic disease remains problematic on FDG-PET/CT due to high physiologic uptake

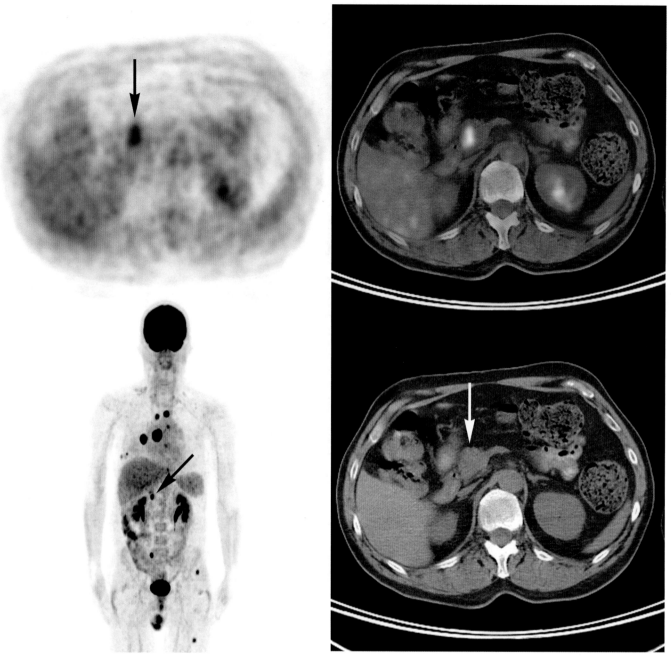

**Figure 14.21** Selected axial FDG-PET, fused, and CT images with MIP localizer: intense FDG uptake is noted focally in the region of the head of the pancreas, consistent with melanoma metastasis.

of FDG, and the inability of non-enhanced low-dose CT to detect small intra-axial lesions. MRI is routinely recommended in stage IV and often performed in stage III disease even in the setting of negative FDG-PET/CT neuroimaging (6, 9, 10).

## Take-home message

1. FDG-PET is superior in overall accuracy to CT alone for distant staging of high-risk melanoma, but may miss small pulmonary nodules that fall below the limit of resolution of PET. FDG-PET/CT is superior in overall accuracy to either modality alone for distant staging of high-risk melanoma and is standard of care where available.

2. Complete staging of stage IV, and probably stage III cutaneous melanoma, requires MRI of the brain even if this region is normal on FDG-PET/CT as physiologic FDG uptake can mask lesions.

# References

1. Rinne D, Baum RP, Hor G *et al.* Primary staging and follow-up of high risk melanoma patients with whole-body 18F-fluorodeoxyglucose positron emission tomography: results of a prospective study of 100 patients. *Cancer* 1998;**82**:1664–71.

2. Gritters LS, Francis IR, Zasadny KR *et al.* Initial assessment of positron emission tomography using 2-fluorine-18-fluoro-2-deoxy-D-glucose in the imaging of malignant melanoma. *J Nucl Med* 1993;**34**:1420–7.

3. Holder WD Jr, White RL Jr, Zuger JH *et al.* Effectiveness of positron emission tomography for the detection of melanoma metastases. *Ann Surg* 1998;**227**:764–9; discussion 769–71.

4. Eigtved A, Andersson AP, Dahlstrom K *et al.* Use of fluorine-18 fluorodeoxyglucose positron emission tomography in the detection of silent metastases from malignant melanoma. *Eur J Nucl Med* 2000;**27**:70–5.

5. Swetter SM, Carroll LA, Johnson DL *et al.* Positron emission tomography is superior to computed tomography for metastatic detection in melanoma patients. *Ann Surg Oncol* 2002;**9**:646–53.

6. Dietlein M, Krug B, Groth W *et al.* Positron emission tomography using 18F-fluorodeoxyglucose in advanced stages of malignant melanoma: a comparison of ultrasonographic and radiological methods of diagnosis. *Nucl Med Commun* 1999;**20**:255–61.

7. Reinhardt MJ, Joe AY, Jaeger U *et al.* Diagnostic performance of whole body dual modality 18F-FDG PET/CT imaging for N- and M-staging of malignant melanoma: experience with 250 consecutive patients. *J Clin Oncol* 2006;**24**(7):1178–87.

8. Strobel K, Dummer R, Husarik DB *et al.* High-risk melanoma: accuracy of FDG PET/CT with added CT morphologic information for detection of metastases. *Radiology* 2007; **244**(2):566–74.

9. Mohr P, Eggermont AM, Hauschild A, Buzaid A. Staging of cutaneous melanoma. *Ann Oncol* 2009; **20**(Suppl 6):vi14–21.

10. Strobel K, Dummer R, Steinert HC *et al.* Chemotherapy response assessment in stage IV melanoma patients – comparison of 18F-FDG-PET/CT, CT, brain MRI, and tumor marker S-100B. *Eur J Nucl Med Mol Imaging* 2008;**35**(10):1786–95.

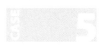

# FDG-PET/CT's prognostic value

A 77-year-old male with melanoma of the left foot diagnosed in 2003, now presents with new left groin adenopathy.

## Acquisition and processing parameters

Approximately 60 min following the intravenous administration of 11.3 mCi of FDG in the right antecubital fossa, tomographic studies from the vertex to toes were obtained. Serum glucose level was 117 mg/dL at the time of injection.

## Findings and differential diagnosis

Innumerable intensely hypermetabolic (SUV 10) small hepatic metastases are noted (Figure 14.22). Multiple small metastases are identified throughout virtually all bones of the axial and appendicular skeleton. There is involvement of both humeri, the sternum, the spine diffusely, the pelvis (Figure 14.23), and the femora (Figure 14.24). No significant blastic or lytic change is identified on CT at the majority of these sites.

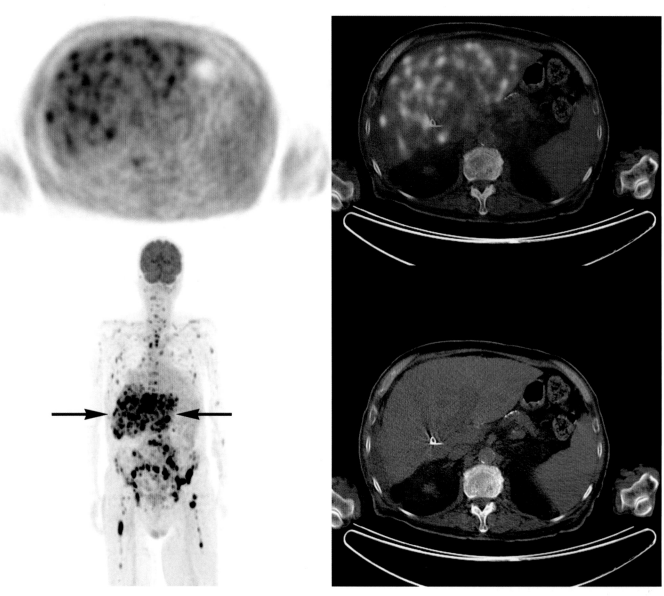

**Figure 14.22** Selected axial FDG-PET, fused, and CT images with MIP localizer: the liver is riddled with innumerable small metastases with intense hypermetabolism (SUV up to 10).

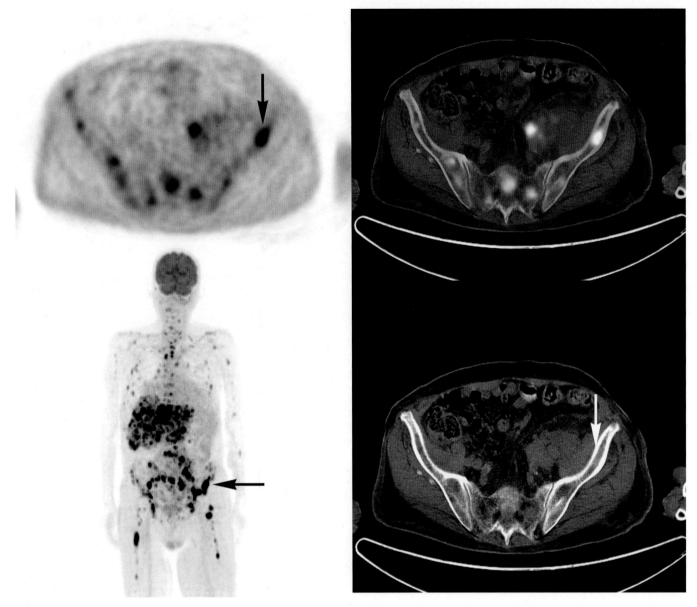

**Figure 14.23** Selected axial FDG-PET, fused and CT images with MIP localizer: intense FDG uptake is identified in multiple lesions throughout both iliac bones, in keeping with melanoma metastases.

Pathologic enlarged intensely hypermetabolic nodes are identified in the paraaortic retroperitoneal (Figure 14.25), left common, and left external iliac stations. Also noted on the maximum intensity projection are bilateral hilar and chest nodal metastases and bilateral small lung metastases.

## Diagnosis and clinical follow-up

Widespread metastatic melanoma with extensive bone and liver metastatic disease as well as lung and nodal retroperitoneal lesions. Histopathology was obtained from the left groin prior to the scan and the clinical course was consistent with this diagnosis.

## Discussion and teaching points

The burden of disease paradigm in oncologic imaging is that patients with extensive metastatic disease have a worse prognosis than those with limited number of lesions, despite being identically staged. A related paradigm has evolved within FDG-PET imaging whereas the standard uptake values (SUV) of tumors also portend prognosis, with worse outcomes attached to higher SUVs (1). This is biologically plausible, as FDG uptake has been correlated with proliferation rate, and thus, the degree of malignancy of a given tumor (2).

Some early work has been done in melanoma by Bastiaan-net *et al.* who determined that a high local nodal SUVmean

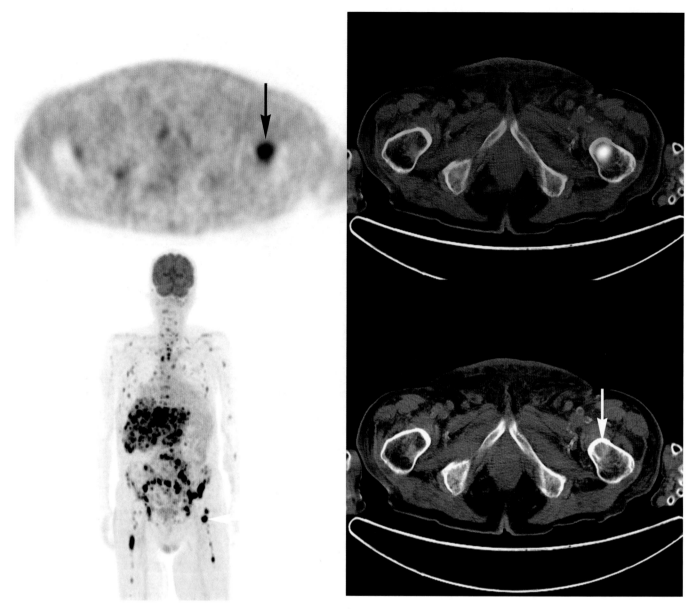

**Figure 14.24** Selected axial FDG-PET, fused and CT images with MIP localizer: intense FDG uptake is identified in the proximal left femur, consistent with melanoma metastases.

($> 5.2$) was associated with a shorter duration of disease-free survival compared with a low SUVmean, although overall survival was similar in both groups (3). Pleiss *et al.* graded FDG uptake on a qualitative 4-point scale where grade III was defined as above liver uptake but lower than cerebellum and grade IV was equal or above cerebellar uptake. The 5-year survival was 71% for patients with grade III lesions vs. 38% for those with grade IV lesions, although the authors did admit that some of the grade III lesions could have been false-positives, as not all were histopathologically confirmed. Of course

staging as seen on FDG-PET was a strong predictor of overall survival at 5 years (2). In a small series of 14 patients with choroidal melanoma, SUVs also correlated positively with surrogate features linked to metastatic potential (4).

## Take-home message

1. Although preliminary, early work suggests that FDG-PET, via SUV and disease burden quantification, has prognostic value beyond traditional staging in patients with advanced melanoma.

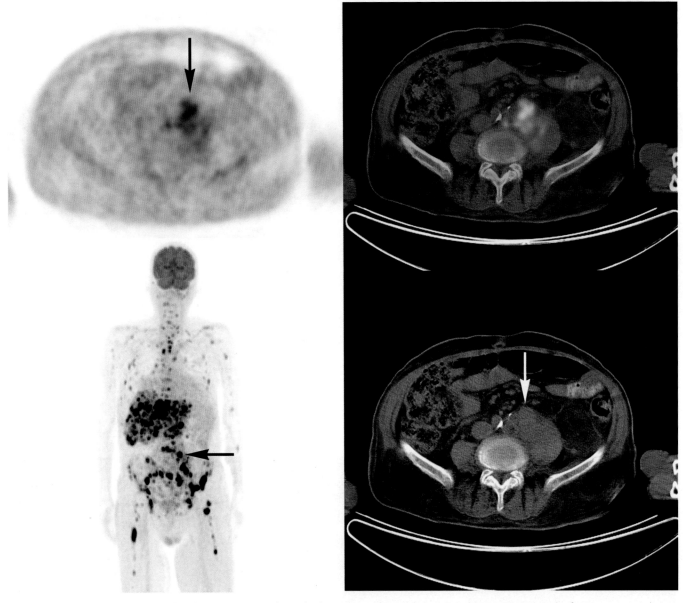

**Figure 14.25** Selected axial FDG-PET, fused and CT images with MIP localizer: intense FDG uptake is seen in a large retroperitoneal soft tissue metastatic lesion.

# References

1. Pastorino U, Landoni C, Marchianò A *et al*. Fluorodeoxyglucose uptake measured by positron emission tomography and standardized uptake value predicts long-term survival of CT screening detected lung cancer in heavy smokers. *J Thorac Oncol* 2009; **4**(11):1305–6.

2. Pleiss C, Risse JH, Biersack HJ, Bender H. Role of FDG-PET in the assessment of survival prognosis in melanoma. *Cancer Biother Radiopharm* 2007;**22**(6):740–7.

3. Bastiaannet E, Hoekstra OS, Oyen WJ *et al*. Level of fluorodeoxyglucose uptake predicts risk for recurrence in melanoma patients presenting with lymph node metastases. *Ann Surg Oncol* 2006;**13**(7):919–26.

4. Finger PT, Chin K, Iacob CE. 18-Fluorine-labelled 2-deoxy-2-fluoro-D-glucose positron emission tomography/computed tomography standardised uptake values: a non-invasive biomarker for the risk of metastasis from choroidal melanoma. *Br J Ophthalmol* 2006;**90**(10):1263–6.

An 80-year-old female with melanoma, with known metastases to the lung and brain. Two scans of the same patient are separated by 4 months and 18 days with interval systemic chemotherapy, last administered 2 weeks prior to the later study.

## Acquisition and processing parameters

Approximately 60 min following the intravenous administration of 14.1 mCi of FDG in the left antecubital fossa, tomographic studies from the vertex to toes were obtained. Serum glucose level was 100 mg/dL at the time of injection.

## Findings and differential diagnosis

There has been excellent interval response to therapy in the pulmonary metastatic disease. To illustrate, the left upper lobe mass, previously 6.3 × 5.0 cm with SUV 11.9, currently measures 1.4 × 1.2 cm with SUV 1.9, an excellent anatomic and metabolic response (Figure 14.26). There has been excellent metabolic

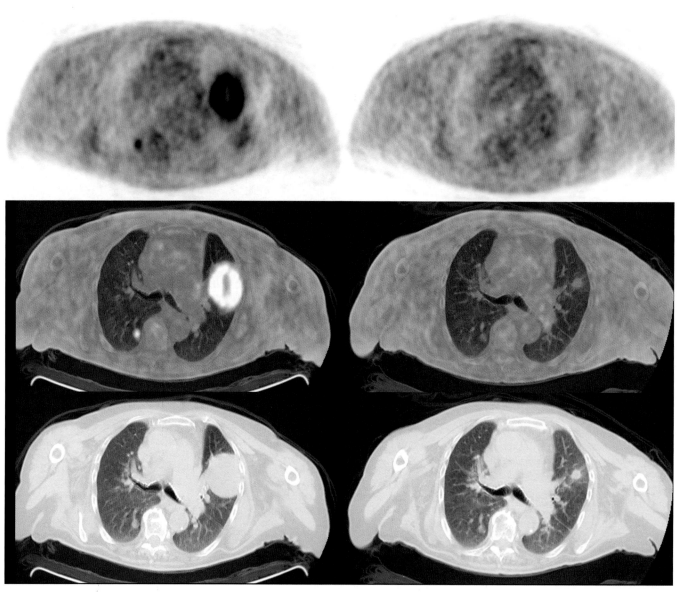

**Figure 14.26** Two scans of the same patient separated by 4 months and 18 days; the three left panels are prior to therapy, the three right panels are post-treatment. Very intense FDG uptake is identified in two melanoma lung metastases, before and after chemotherapy. There is excellent interval anatomic and metabolic response to treatment.

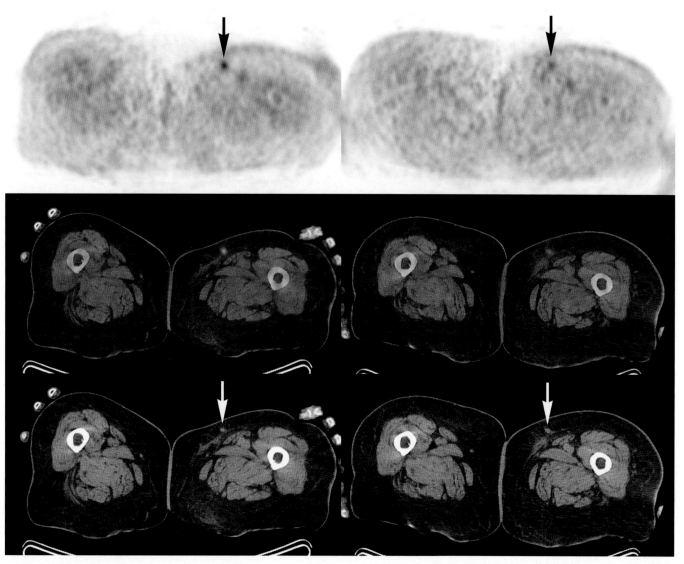

**Figure 14.27** Two scans of the same patient separated by 4 months and 18 days; the three left panels are prior to therapy, the three right panels are post-treatment. Moderately intense FDG uptake is identified in small left thigh subcutaneous lesion, before and after chemotherapy. There is good metabolic response to treatment, but there is little anatomic change.

response in the previously identified 1.2 cm right lower lobe nodule, with SUV decrease from 5.0 to 2.0, although this lesion is stable anatomically (Figure 14.26).

Good metabolic response is noted in the left upper thigh nodular soft tissue metastasis (Figure 14.27).

Also noted on the maximum intensity projection image is some metabolic response in the five other left medial thigh and knee soft tissue nodules, with others gaining in intensity (Figure 14.28). Post-radiotherapy change and edema of the left leg is also noted. Physiologic bowel uptake is seen on both studies.

## Diagnosis and clinical follow-up

Near-complete metabolic response with marked partial anatomic response in multiple metastatic lung nodules. Mixed metabolic response in multiple subcutaneous lesions of the left

leg. The lung lesions continued to demonstrate good response on a follow-up FDG-PET/CT scan.

## Discussion and teaching points

FDG-PET and PET/CT are increasingly being used to monitor response to therapy in patients with malignancy. Rates of glycolysis – and therefore FDG uptake – are strongly linked to mitotic rate, cellular density and viability, all of which can be non-invasively measured with PET to assess a tumor's response to therapy well before anatomic change is apparent.

Mercier *et al.* investigated a small number of patients before and after isolated limb perfusion surgery and found a reduction in the number of visualized lesions in all patients studied, corresponding to a therapeutic response – others have also replicated these findings (1, 2). In a pilot trial of FDG-PET

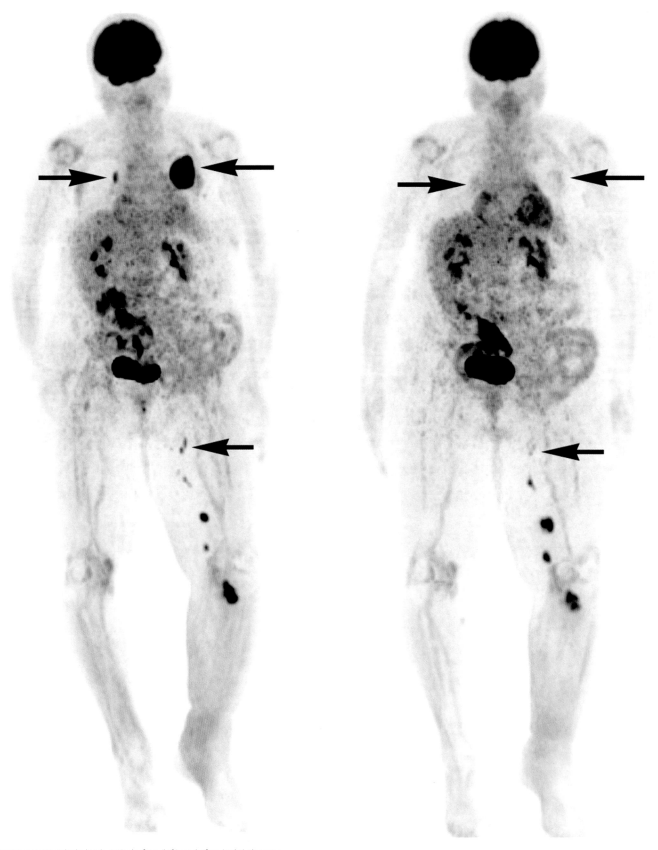

**Figure 14.28** Whole-body MIPs before (left) and after (right) therapy.

to assess response to systemic chemotherapy in stage IV melanoma, the single patient with a complete metabolic response survived 679 days compared with a median of 206 days in those with a partial metabolic response and 129 days in those with progressive diseases on FDG-PET, suggesting a strong predictive role for the modality (3). Pre-clinical work with investigational therapies also points to reduction of FDG uptake post-treatment as an indicator of success, and early data have been promising for response assessment to radiotherapy in neurotropic desmoplastic melanoma (4, 5).

Strobel *et al.* investigated 25 stage IV cutaneous melanoma patients with FDG-PET/CT before and after three cycles of chemotherapy and found a 1-year overall survival of 40% in PET non-responders (n = 15) as compared with 80% in PET responders (n = 10). The group concluded that FDG-PET/CT was an excellent tool for chemotherapy response assessment but cautioned that MRI was required to detect brain recurrences, although these conclusions applied only to cutaneous melanoma and did not hold true in uveal melanoma (6–8).

## Take-home message

1. FDG-PET offers a meaningful way to assess response to a multitude of different therapies in the setting of advanced melanoma, and is predictive of overall survival.
2. MRI is probably required as an adjunct to FDG-PET to assess response to therapy in the brain and to detect intra-axial recurrences.

## References

1. Mercier GA, Alavi A, Fraker DL. FDG positron emission tomography in isolated limb perfusion therapy in patients with locally advanced melanoma: preliminary results. *Clin Nucl Med* 2001;**26**:832–6.

2. Ryan ER, Hill AD, Skehan SJ. FDG PET/CT demonstrates the effectiveness of isolated limb infusion for malignant melanoma. *Clin Nucl Med* 2006;**31**(11):707–8.

3. Hofman MS, Constantinidou A, Acland K *et al.* Assessing response to chemotherapy in metastatic melanoma with FDG PET: early experience. *Nucl Med Commun* 2007;**28**(12):902–6.

4. Yip D, Le MN, Chan JL *et al.* A phase 0 trial of riluzole in patients with resectable stage III and IV melanoma. *Clin Cancer Res* 2009;**15**(11):3896–902.

5. Hannah A, Feigen M, Quong G *et al.* Use of [F]-fluorodeoxyglucose positron emission tomography in monitoring response of recurrent neurotropic desmoplastic melanoma to radiotherapy. *Otolaryngol Head Neck Surg* 2000;**122**(2):304–6.

6. Strobel K, Dummer R, Steinert HC *et al.* Chemotherapy response assessment in stage IV melanoma patients-comparison of 18F-FDG-PET/CT, CT, brain MRI, and tumormarker S-100B. *Eur J Nucl Med Mol Imaging* 2008;**35**(10):1786–95.

7. Strobel K, Skalsky J, Steinert HC *et al.* S-100B and FDG-PET/CT in therapy response assessment of melanoma patients. *Dermatology* 2007;**215**(3): 192–201.

8. Strobel K, Bode B, Dummer R *et al.* Limited value of 18F-FDG PET/CT and S-100B tumour marker in the detection of liver metastases from uveal melanoma compared to liver metastases from cutaneous melanoma. *Eur J Nucl Med Mol Imaging* 2009;**36**(11):1774–82.

A 73-year-old male with melanoma of the right third finger.

## Acquisition and processing parameters

Approximately 60 min following the intravenous administration of 13.9 mCi of FDG in the left antecubital fossa,

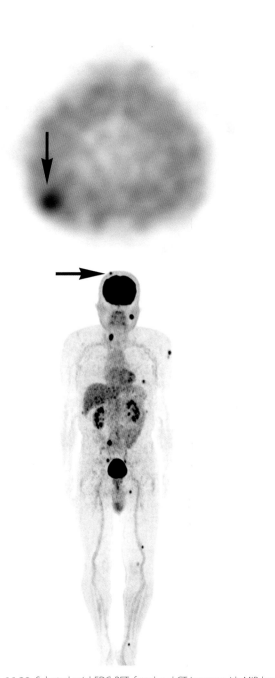
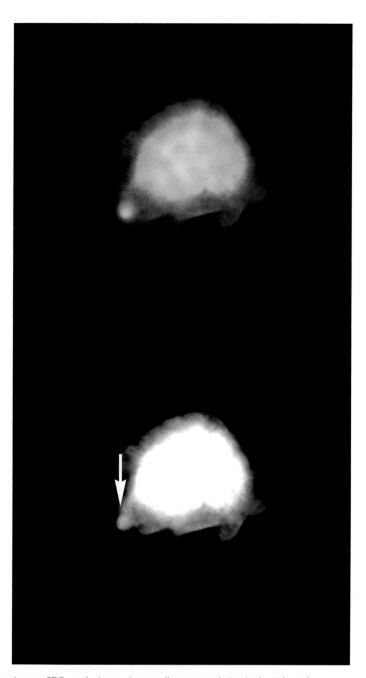

**Figure 14.29** Selected axial FDG-PET, fused and CT images with MIP localizer: intense FDG uptake is seen in a small cutaneous lesion in the right scalp, consistent with melanoma metastasis.

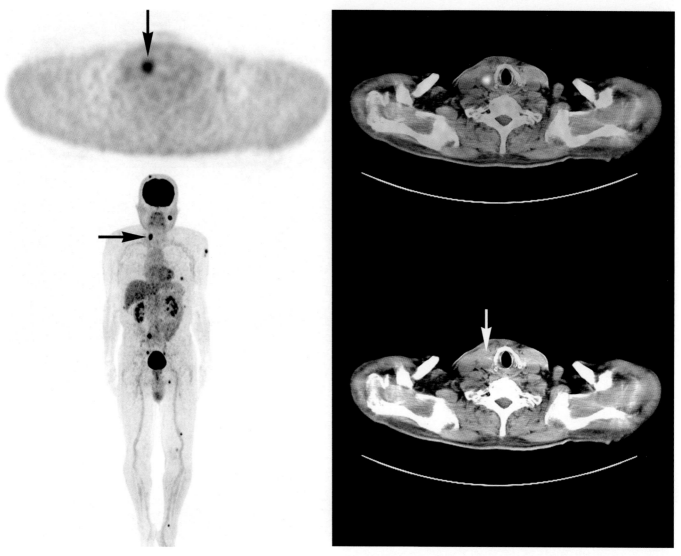

**Figure 14.30** Selected axial FDG-PET, fused and CT images with MIP localizer: intense FDG uptake is seen in a small right thyroid metastatic lesion.

tomographic studies from the vertex to toes were obtained. Serum glucose level was 89 mg/dL at the time of injection.

## Findings and differential diagnosis

Intense FDG activity is noted in an 8 mm subcutaneous nodule in the right scalp, SUV 5.2 (Figure 14.29). Intense uptake is seen in a 1.1 cm left internal jugular node with SUV 9.4 (Figure 14.30).

There is a focus of intense increased uptake fusing to a blastic lesion in the marrow space of the right sacral body with SUV 8.6, (Figure 14.32), and another similar lesion is noted in the marrow space of the left distal femur with SUV 5.7 (Figure 14.31). A 1.8 × 0.7 cm subcutaneous nodule is seen in the left shoulder with SUV 5.8 (Figure 14.33). A 1.4 cm nodule is noted at the left lung base SUV 5.0 (Figure 14.34). Multiple other findings are noted on the MIP image including a small bone lesion in the distal left tibia and a tiny subcutaneous

nodule in the right upper quadrant. Right retroperitoneal nodes and a left inguinal lymph node metastasis are appreciated. A small muscular metastasis is seen in the left knee just posterior to the medial femoral condyle.

## Diagnosis and clinical follow-up

Metastatic soft tissue nodules in right scalp, right neck, left shoulder, lungs, right abdominal wall, retroperitoneum, left inguinal region, and left knee. Osseous metastases of the right sacrum, left femur, and left tibia. Clinical follow-up confirmed these diagnoses.

## Discussion and teaching points

The imaging follow-up of patients with cutaneous melanoma is controversial. Meyers *et al.* followed 118 patients with stage II and III melanoma for at least 2 years, and found that during that time only three asymptomatic patients had unsuspected

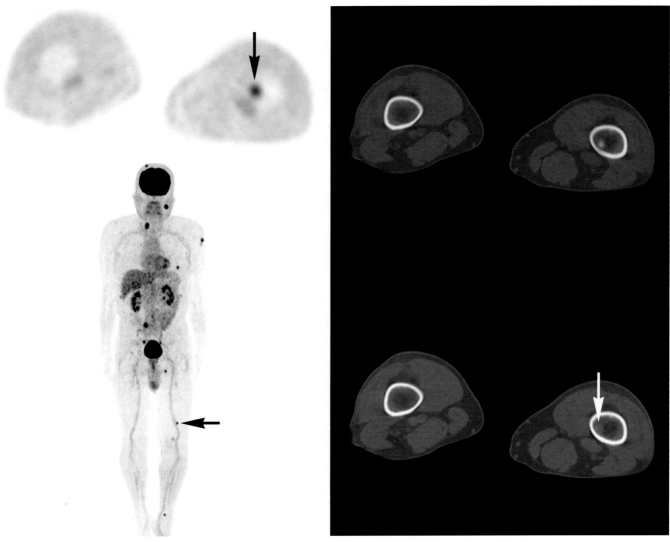

**Figure 14.31** Selected axial FDG-PET, fused and CT images with MIP localizer: intense FDG uptake is seen in a small left femoral diaphysis metastasis from melanoma.

recurrences discovered by conventional imaging, and they concluded that imaging follow-up in stage II/III was of little value, although it must be noted that none of their patients underwent FDG-PET (1). A different group – again in a series lacking FDG-PET – found that the method of detecting a relapse of initially stage I to III melanoma, whether by conventional imaging or clinical follow-up, did not impact patient outcome and only served to add to costs (2).

In the only series to specifically look at FDG-PET in this setting, Koskivuo *et al.* scanned 30 asymptomatic stage IIB–IIIC melanoma patients between 7 and 48 months after initial surgery and found 6 (20%) recurrences by PET, with most of the recurrences occurring in the 7th to 14th month post-operatively. In all patients with a PET-proven recurrence, treatment strategy was altered, either in the form of additional surgery or chemotherapy. Although the study was not designed to show a survival benefit of routine PET scanning,

the authors commented that solitary distant metastases excision confers survival benefit (3).

As an aside, most centers routinely perform true whole-body PET/CT – vertex to toes – as opposed to a limited whole-body scan (base of the skull to the mid-thighs), as is common in other malignancies, because melanoma has a higher rate of non-visceral soft-tissue metastases (4).

## Take-home message

1. There is little evidence in favor of conventional imaging for the routine follow-up of high-risk melanoma patients.
2. FDG-PET can detect subclinical recurrence in intermediate and high-risk melanoma in up to 20% of patients, and will often dictate changes in treatment, however it remains to be seen if this early detection confers a survival advantage.

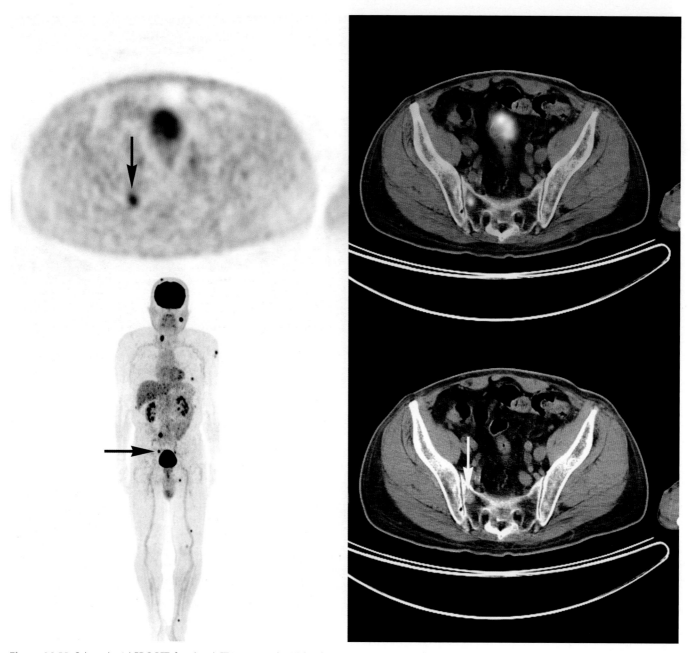

Figure 14.32 Selected axial FDG-PET, fused and CT images with MIP localizer: intense FDG uptake is seen in a small right sacral lesion, in keeping with melanoma bone metastasis. Note subtle sclerosis on CT.

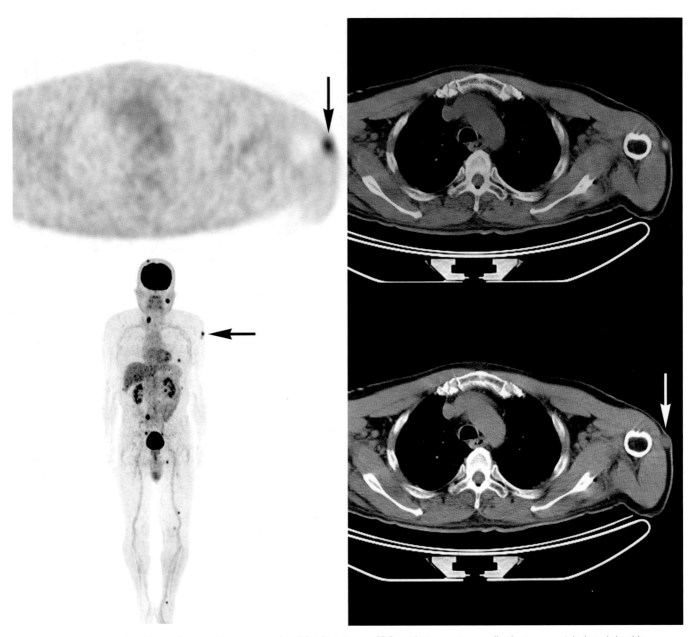

**Figure 14.33** Selected axial FDG-PET, fused and CT images with MIP localizer: intense FDG uptake is seen in a small subcutaneous right lateral shoulder metastasis from melanoma.

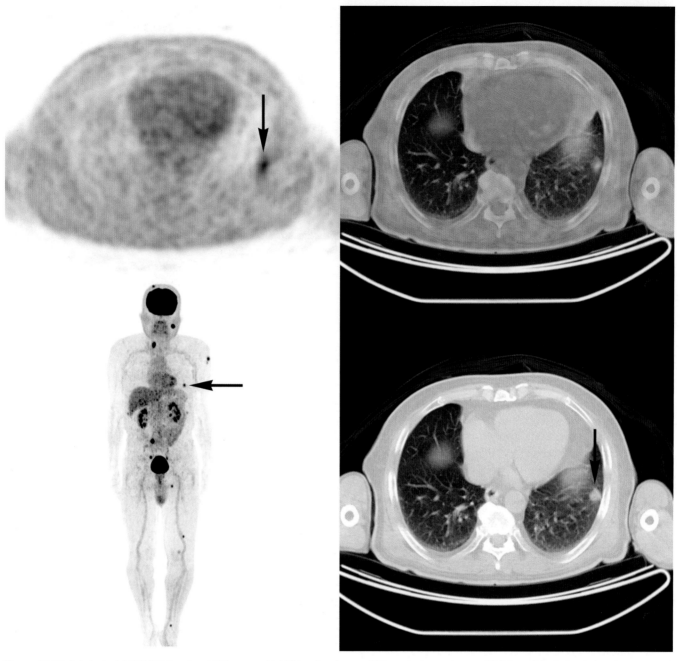

**Figure 14.34** Selected axial FDG-PET, fused and CT images with MIP localizer: intense FDG uptake is seen in a small left lower lobe lesion, in keeping with melanoma lung metastasis.

# References

1. Meyers MO, Yeh JJ, Frank J et al. Method of detection of initial recurrence of stage II/III cutaneous melanoma: analysis of the utility of follow-up staging. *Ann Surg Oncol* 2009;**16**(4): 941–7.

2. Hofmann U, Szedlak M, Rittgen W, Jung EG, Schadendorf D. Primary staging and follow-up in melanoma patients – monocenter evaluation of methods, costs and patient survival. *Br J Cancer* 2002;**87**(2):151–7.

3. Koskivuo IO, Seppänen MP, Suominen EA, Minn HR. Whole body positron emission tomography in follow-up of high risk melanoma. *Acta Oncol* 2007;**46**(5):685–90.

4. Nguyen NC, Chaar BT, Osman MM. Prevalence and patterns of soft tissue metastasis: detection with true whole-body F-18 FDG PET/CT. *BMC Med Imaging* 2007;7:8.

**Chapter**

# 15

# Bone

Einat Even-Sapir and Ora Israel

## Introduction

The vast majority of malignant bone lesions initiate as bone marrow deposits of malignant cells. As the lesion enlarges, the surrounding bone undergoes osteoclastic (resorptive) and osteoblastic (depositional) activity. Based on the balance between these two processes, lesions may appear radiographically, as lytic, sclerotic (blastic), or mixed (1–3).

Osteosarcoma is the most frequent primary bone malignancy in children and second in adults following multiple myeloma. The Ewing sarcoma family of tumors is the second most frequent primary bone malignancy in children and young adults (4). Bone metastases are the most common malignant bone tumor, with breast cancer being the leading primary tumor in women and prostate cancer in men, followed by lung cancer. The type of metastases and the incidence of metastatic skeletal spread depend on the type of malignancy and the disease stage, respectively (5).

The purpose of imaging is to identify malignant skeletal involvement as early as possible, to determine the extent of the disease, to evaluate the presence of clinically relevant complications (such as fractures or lesions which harbor risk for neurologic deficit), to monitor response to therapy, and at times, to guide biopsy (5, 6).

Scintigraphy plays a major role in the assessment of malignant bone involvement. There are various radiopharmaceuticals, which may be used for this goal, both single photon-emitting tracers detected by gamma cameras and positron-emitting tracers detected by positron emission tomography (PET) technology. Detection of malignant involvement of the skeleton is based on either direct accumulation of tracer in the tumor cells or indirectly reflecting bone changes that occur secondary to the presence of malignant cells. For instance, $^{67}$Ga-citrate, $^{131}$I, $^{123}$I, and $^{111}$I-Somatostatin are SPECT tracers and $^{18}$F-fluorodeoxyglucose ($^{18}$F-FDG or FDG), $^{11}$C-choline or acetate and $^{68}$Ga-somatostatin are PET tracers which accumulate in the tumor tissue itself. Uptake of $^{99m}$Tc-methylene diphosphonate ($^{99m}$Tc-MDP), the tracer routinely used for bone scintigraphy (BS) and of $^{18}$F-fluoride, a PET bone-seeking agent, in malignant bone lesions reflect mostly

secondary reactive osteoblastic changes. Tracers, which directly accumulate in the tumor cells, may therefore identify malignant involvement at earlier stages before cortical bone reaction has occurred (7–9).

Integrated systems composed of SPECT or PET with CT (SPECT/CT and PET/CT), have been recently introduced in the routine imaging practice. Morphological characterization of scintigraphic lesions in the skeleton can potentially improve the specificity of the functional study, separating between benign and malignant lesions (10). Another major contribution of the CT images from the integrated study, is their ability to better localize the lesion, especially when using radiotracers, which accumulate in both bone and in soft tissue. For example, accurate localization of the scintigraphic finding on CT allows diagnosis of invasion of the epidural space and neural foramen found in approximately 10% of vertebral lesions (11). These findings are clinically significant as they may cause spinal cord compression. Early identification followed by appropriate treatment in this clinical scenario is essential to avoid permanent neurological deficit (12).

FDG-PET/CT has become a routine modality for the imaging algorithm of oncologic patients. The normal red marrow demonstrates low FDG uptake, and increased activity suggests early malignant involvement of the marrow, which may precede the bone reaction that needs to occur in order to be detected by BS and CT (7). The advantages of FDG-PET/CT over BS in detecting malignant bone involvement has been reported in various types of cancers, obviating in many patients with FDG-avid tumors the need to perform an additional BS (13–15). In addition to its ability to detect metastases confined to the marrow component, FDG-PET/CT is highly sensitive for detection of lytic type cortical bone metastases characterized by their high rate of glycolysis and hypoxia. In contrast, BS is relatively insensitive for detection of this type of lesion. Although FDG-PET/CT has been reported as appropriate for detecting all types of bone metastases, it is somewhat less sensitive for detection of sclerotic metastases that are generally less aggressive (16–18). Detection of the latter can be achieved by reviewing the CT data of PET/CT, or by performing complementary BS or $^{18}$F-fluoride-PET, which are highly sensitive for detection of blastic lesions.

New therapeutic strategies for metastatic skeletal spread are being developed. Treatment of bone metastases has improved over the last decade with the introduction of bisphosphonates. These are pyrophosphate analogs that potently inhibit osteoclast-induced bone resorption and have proved to be highly effective in reducing the incidence of skeletal-related complications (6). After successful therapy, imaging aims at accurately differentiating between an active metastasis and bone repair, a task that often cannot be achieved by BS using $^{99m}$Tc-MDP or by CT, since the process of bone repair similarly to active metastasis is associated with increased bone turnover and cortical changes. Post-therapeutic bone morphology is altered and associated with the appearance of sclerotic changes, which may persist even when metastases are no longer active. In contrast, as the mechanism of detection of bone malignancy by FDG-PET is based on direct accumulation of the tracer in viable tumor cells, successful treatment is reflected on FDG-PET as decrease or disappearance of radiotracer uptake (19, 20).

Follow-up FDG-PET/CT should be performed with attention to the time elapsed from last therapy, since anti-cancer treatment,

either chemo- or radiotherapy, or more recently hormonal and biologic drugs, have an effect on the uptake of FDG by tumor cells. Performing FDG-PET/CT too soon after therapy may result in metabolic shutdown of the tumor cells and a false-negative study. Treatment with granulocyte colony stimulating factors (GCSF) may induce diffusely increased FDG uptake in the marrow, thus masking malignant infiltration (21–23).

The use of FDG-PET/CT for assessment of malignant skeletal involvement is however, valuable only in tracer-avid tumors. As will be discussed below, FDG is not always the tracer of choice for imaging patients with prostate cancer or with neuroendocrine tumors. Other PET tracers can be used to image the latter. The cases that follow will illustrate the benefit of FDG-PET/CT for the detection of early metastatic spread; the detection of clinical significant complications of skeletal spread by fused PET and CT data; the role of FDG-PET/CT in monitoring response of metastatic bone disease to therapy, and its role in hematologic and primary bone malignancies. In two additional cases, the detection of malignant bone involvement by PET/CT using radiotracers other than FDG will be illustrated, including $^{68}$Ga-somatostatin in a patient with carcinoid, and $^{11}$C-choline in a patient with prostate cancer.

# References

1. Roodman GD. Mechanisms of bone metastasis. *New Engl J Med* 2004;**350**:1655–64.

2. Blake GM, Park-Holohan SJ, Cook GJ, Fogelman I. Quantitative studies of bone with the use of 18F-fluoride and 99mTc-methylene diphosphonate. *Semin Nucl Med* 2001;**31**:28–49.

3. Galasko CS. Mechanisms of lytic and blastic metastatic disease of bone. *Clin Orthop* 1982;**169**:20–7.

4. Hawkins DS, Schuetze SM, Butrynski JE et al. [18F]Fluorodeoxyglucose positron emission tomography predicts outcome for Ewing sarcoma family of tumors. *J Clin Oncol* 2005;**23**:8828–34.

5. Padhani A, Husband J. Bone metastases. In JES Husband, RH Reznek (Eds.), *Imaging in Oncology*. Oxford: Isis Medical Media, 1998, pp. 765–87.

6. Clamp A, Danson S, Nguyen H, Cole D, Clemons M. Assessment of therapeutic response in patients with metastatic bone disease. *Lancet Oncol* 2004;**5**(10):607–16.

7. Cook GJ, Fogelman I. The role of positron emission tomography in the management of bone metastases. *Cancer* 2000;**88**:2927–33.

8. Hamaoka T, Madewell JE, Podoloff DA, Hortobagyi GN, Ueno NT. Bone imaging

in metastatic breast cancer. *J Clin Oncol* 2004;**22**(14):2942–53.

9. Even-Sapir E. Imaging of malignant bone involvement by morphologic, scintigraphic, and hybrid modalities. *J Nucl Med* 2005;**46**:1356–67.

10. Nakamoto Y, Cohade C, Tatsumi M, Hammoud D, Wahl RL. CT appearance of bone metastases detected with FDG PET as part of the same PET/CT examination. *Radiology* 2005;**237**(2):627–34.

11. Metser U, Lerman H, Blank A et al. Malignant involvement of the spine: assessment by 18F-Fluorodeoxyglucose PET/CT. *J Nucl Med* 2004;**45**:279–84.

12. Van Goethem JW, van den Hauwe L, Ozsarlak O, De Schepper AM, Parizel PM. Spinal tumors. *Eur J Radiol* 2004;**50**:159–76.

13. Franzius F, Sciuk J, Daldrup-Link HE, Jurgens H, Schober O. FDG-PET for detection of osseous metastases from malignant primary bone tumors: comparison with bone scintigraphy. *Eur J Nucl Med* 2000;**27**:1305–11.

14. Liu FY, Chang JT, Wang HM et al. [18F]fluorodeoxyglucose positron emission tomography is more sensitive than skeletal scintigraphy for detecting bone metastasis in endemic nasopharyngeal carcinoma

at initial staging. *J Clin Oncol* 2006; **24**(4):599–604.

15. Krüger S, Buck AK, Mottaghy FM et al. Detection of bone metastases in patients with lung cancer: 99mTc-MDP planar bone scintigraphy, 18F-fluoride PET or 18F-FDG PET/CT. *Eur J Nucl Med Mol Imaging* 2009; **36**(11):1807–12.

16. Cook GJ, Houston S, Rubens R, Maisey MN, Fogelman I. Detection of bone metastases in breast cancer by 18FDG PET: differing metabolic activity in osteoblastic and osteolytic lesions. *J Clin Oncol* 1998;**16**:3375–9.

17. Burgman P, Odonoghue JA, Humm JL, Ling CC. Hypoxia-induced increase in FDG uptake in MCF7 cells. *J Nucl Med* 2001;**42**:170–5.

18. Nakai T, Okuyama C, Kubota T et al. Pitfalls of FDG-PET for the diagnosis of osteoblastic bone metastases in patients with breast cancer. *Eur J Nucl Med Mol Imaging* 2005;**32**(11):1253–8.

19. Gallowitsch HJ, Kresnik E, Gasser J et al. F-18 fluorodeoxyglucose positron-emission tomography in the diagnosis of tumor recurrence and metastases in the follow-up of patients with breast carcinoma: a comparison to conventional imaging. *Invest Radiol* 2003;**38**:250–6.

20. Du Y, Cullum I, Illidge TM, Ell PJ. Fusion of metabolic function

and morphology: sequential [18F]fluorodeoxyglucose positron-emission tomography/ computed tomography studies yield new insights into the natural history of bone metastases in breast cancer. *J Clin Oncol* 2007;**25**(23):3440–7.

21. Sugawara Y, Fisher SJ, Zasadny KR *et al.* Preclinical and clinical studies of bone marrow uptake of fluorine-18-fluorodeoxyglucose with or without granulocyte colony-stimulating factor during chemotherapy. *J Clin Oncol* 1998;**16**:173–80.

22. Clamp A, Danson S, Nguyen H, Cole D, Clemons M. Assessment of therapeutic response in patients with metastatic bone disease. *Lancet Oncol* 2004;**5**:607–16.

23. Kazama T, Swanston N, Podoloff DA, Macapinlac HA. Effect of colony-stimulating factor and conventional- or high-dose chemotherapy on FDG uptake in bone marrow. *Eur J Nucl Med Mol Imaging* 2005; **32**:1406–11.

A 61-year-old male was evaluated for staging of a newly diagnosed non-small cell lung carcinoma. $^{99m}$Tc-MDP planar bone scan (BS) and FDG-PET/CT were performed, 6 days apart. The patient underwent fusion surgery of the two lower lumbar vertebrae 7 years prior to the current imaging tests.

## Acquisition and processing parameters

$^{99m}$Tc-MDP-bone scan: Planar images of the entire skeleton were obtained using a dual-headed gamma camera with high-resolution collimators 2 hours after the intravenous injection of 740 MBq (20 mCi) $^{99m}$Tc-MDP. A total of 1.5 million counts were collected.

FDG-PET/CT scan: After a fasting period of 4 hours, blood sugar levels were 105 mg/dL. A dose of 555 MBq (15 mCi) of FDG was injected intravenously, and oral contrast was given. After 95 min distribution time, reduced-dose CT acquisition performed with the patient in the supine position with his arms up was followed by the PET acquisition. The unenhanced CT acquisition protocol was the following: 140 kVp, 80 mA, 0.8 s per CT rotation, pitch of 6 and a table speed of 22.5 mm/s. The PET acquisition protocol included six bed positions of 4 min each over the head and neck, chest, abdomen, pelvis, and proximal femurs. Transaxial images (35 per field of view) were reconstructed as 128 × 128 pixel images with a pixel size of 4 × 4 mm and a slice thickness of 4.25 mm. The axial field of view (FOV) was 14.5 cm. An ordered subsets expectation maximization (OSEM) algorithm using 2 iterations and 28 subsets was used for reconstructing the 2-D whole-body data from the PET projections (1).

## Findings

Figure 15.1: Anterior (left panel) and posterior (right panel) whole body bone scan demonstrates increased tracer uptake along the lateral aspect of the lower lumbar spine representing the fusion mass. There are no lesions suggestive of metastatic skeletal spread.

Figures 15.2 and 15.3: FDG-PET/CT images, each composed of four panels: unenhanced transaxial CT (top left), PET (top right), PET/CT (bottom-left) and maximal intensity projection (MIP). The MIP image illustrates uptake in extensive disease in the lung, lymph nodes above and below the diaphragm, the right adrenal gland and the liver. PET/CT image at the level of the lumbar spine (Figure 15.2) illustrates the presence of a lytic metastasis in the left lamina of L2. At the level of the lower pelvis (Figure 15.3) PET/CT shows a tiny lytic metastasis in the posterior aspect of the right acetabulum. Bone metastases are noted by red markers.

## Diagnosis and clinical follow-up

Lung carcinoma metastatic to lung, lymph nodes, liver, and bone. The patient was referred for chemotherapy.

## Discussion and teaching points

Prognosis of patients with non-small cell lung carcinoma (NSCLC) depends on the stage and resectability status of the tumor. Skeletal morbidity is an important concern in patients with NSCLC. The incidence of skeletal-related events is expected to increase as survival improves with the introduction of novel therapies. Delay in detection of metastatic spread and incorrect staging can potentially result in suboptimal treatment decisions including the implementation of major surgery or aggressive chemoradiation therapy in patients with metastatic spread (2, 3). It should be kept in mind that about 40% of patients with proven bone metastases are asymptomatic (4–6). For decades, the staging algorithm of patients with NSCLC included the use of bone scintigraphy (BS). However, nowadays FDG-PET/CT is performed in newly diagnosed NSCLC for staging purposes. As illustrated in the current case FDG-PET/CT is more sensitive than BS for detection of early metastatic spread in bone. Comparing the sensitivity of FDG-PET and BS for detection of metastatic skeletal disease, the former has been reported by various authors to be superior, thus obviating the need to perform a separate BS (5, 6). Bury et al. investigated 110 consecutive patients with NSCLC, and reported a higher positive predictive value (PPV) and lower false-positive rate for FDG-PET when compared with BS (4). In a recent study by Krüger et al., FDG-PET/CT and BS were performed within 7 days in 126 patients with NSCLC. FDG-PET/CT was superior, primarily for detection of lytic type metastases (7). In another recent study by Ak et al., detection of bone metastases by FDG-PET/CT and BS was retrospectively compared in 95 lung cancer patients. In 19 patients (20%), FDG-PET/CT identified metastatic skeletal spread while BS was false negative (8). These findings reflect the high sensitivity of FDG imaging to detect early metastases confined to the bone marrow, or lytic metastases (the common type of metastases in NSCLC), whereas BS is relatively insensitive for detection of these types of lesion.

## Take-home message

- FDG-PET/CT is more sensitive than $^{99m}$Tc-MDP bone scintigraphy for the assessment of malignant skeletal spread in patients with NSCLC, accurately identifying marrow-based and lytic metastases for which bone scintigraphy is insensitive.

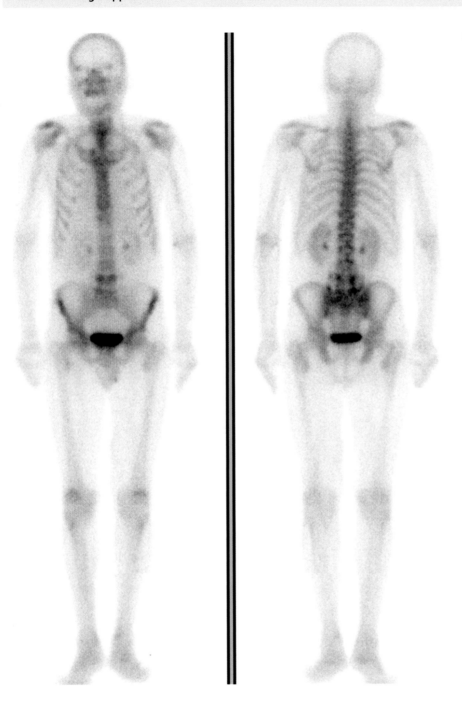

Figure 15.1 Bone scintigraphy.

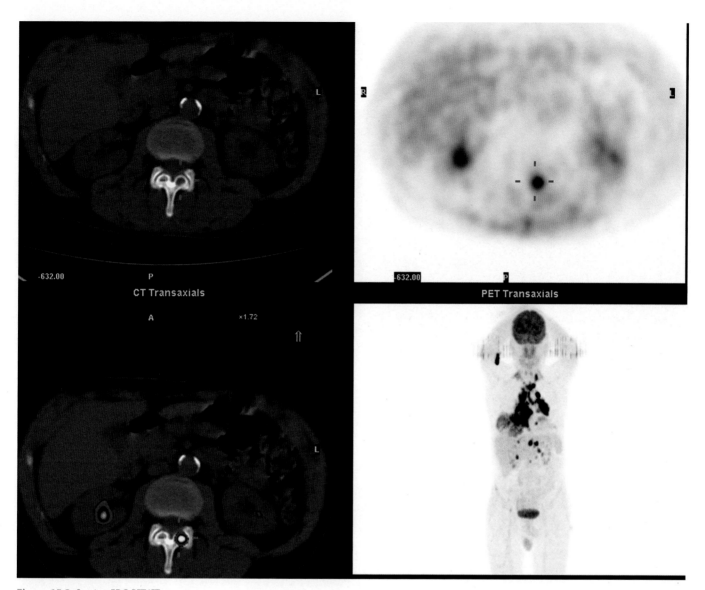

CT Transaxials

PET Transaxials

**Figure 15.2** Staging FDG-PET/CT.

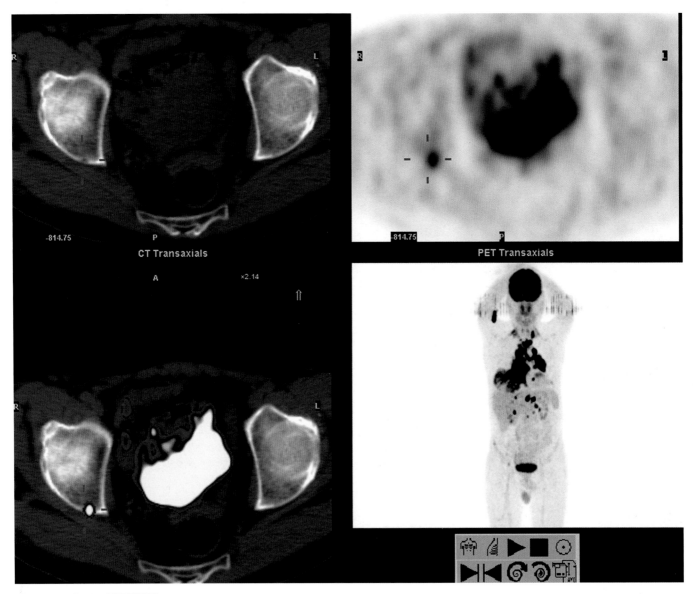

**Figure 15.3** Staging FDG-PET/CT.

# References

1. Kennedy JA, Israel O, Frenkel A, Bar-Shalom R, Azhari H. Improved image fusion in PET/CT using hybrid image reconstruction and Super-Resolution. *Int J Biomed Imaging* **2007**;2007:46846.

2. Langer C, Hirsh V. Skeletal morbidity in lung cancer patients with bone metastases: demonstrating the need for early diagnosis and treatment with bisphosphonates. *Lung Cancer* 2010; **67**(1):4–11.

3. Hirsh V. Skeletal disease contributes substantially to morbidity and mortality in patients with lung cancer. *Clin Lung Cancer* 2009;**10**(4):223–9.

4. Bury T, Barreto A, Daenen F *et al.* Fluorine-18 deoxyglucose positron emission tomography for the detection of bone metastases in patients with non-small cell lung cancer. *Eur J Nucl Med* 1998; **25**:1244–7.

5. Lardinois D, Weder W, Hany TF *et al.* Staging of non-small-cell lung cancer with integrated positron-emission tomography and computed tomography. *New Engl J Med* 2003; **348**:2500–7.

6. Cheran SK, Herndon JE, Patz EF. Comparison of whole-body FDG-PET to bone scan for detection of bone metastases in patients with a new diagnosis of lung cancer. *Lung Cancer* 2004;**44**:317–25.

7. Krüger S, Buck AK, Mottaghy FM *et al.* Detection of bone metastases in patients with lung cancer: 99mTc-MDP planar bone scintigraphy, 18F-fluoride PET or 18F-FDG PET/CT? *Eur J Nucl Med Mol Imaging* 2009; **36**(11):1807–12.

8. Ak I, Sivrikoz MC, Entok E, Vardareli E. Discordant findings in patients with non-small-cell lung cancer: absolutely normal bone scans versus disseminated bone metastases on positron-emission tomography/computed tomography. *Eur J Cardiothorac Surg* 2010;**37**(4): 792–6.

A 72-year-old male, after thyroidectomy and [131]I ablation due to papillary thyroid carcinoma, was referred for FDG-PET/CT due to elevated thyroglobulin serum levels and upper back pain.

## Acquisition and processing parameters

After fasting for a period of 12 hours, blood sugar levels were 110 mg/dL. A dose of 499.5 MBq (13.5 mCi) of FDG was administered intravenously, and oral contrast was used. After 90 min distribution time, reduced-dose CT acquisition was performed with the patient in the supine position with his arms up followed by PET acquisition. The unenhanced CT and PET acquisition protocols and reconstruction parameters were as described in Case 1 (1).

## Findings

Figure 15.4 is composed of four panels: unenhanced transaxial CT (top left), PET (top right), PET/CT (bottom-left) and MIP. Increased uptake is detected on a soft tissue mass that replaces normal bone in the posterior left elements of the T3 vertebra. In addition to lysis of bone this tumoral mass appears to invade the epidural space (red marker).

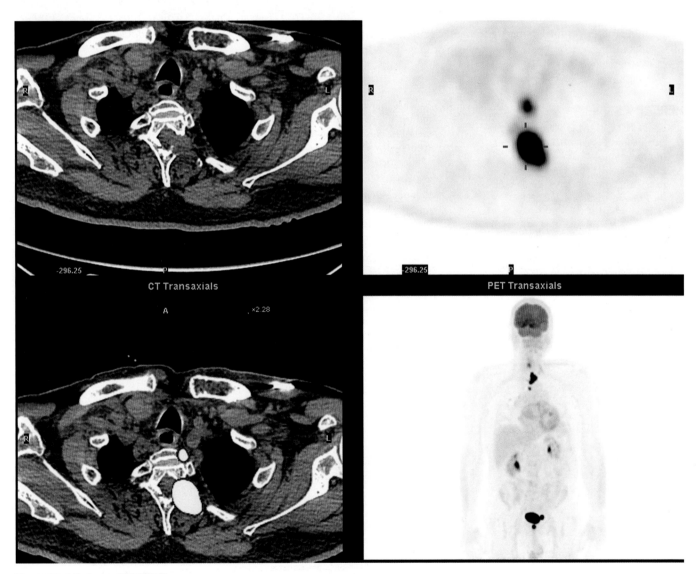

**Figure 15.4** Restaging FDG-PET/CT.

## Diagnosis and clinical follow-up

Metastatic involvement of T3 vertebra and the corresponding epidural space in a patient with thyroid carcinoma. The patient was further referred for radiotherapy of this region.

## Discussion and teaching points

Patients with metastatic bone disease are at increased risk for skeletal-related events (SREs) including pathologic fractures, hypercalcemia, and neural compression, mainly in the spine, the most common site of skeletal metastases (2, 3). Spinal metastases can be classified according to their anatomic location as intra- or extradural. The latter account for up to 95% of spinal lesions; they originate from the vertebra and subsequently impinge on the thecal sac. There have been several reports on the prognosis of patients with skeletal metastases with special attention to the presence of vertebral metastases. Tokuhashi *et al.* proposed a prognostic scoring system for the pre-operative evaluation of patients with spinal metastases comprising six variables: the Karnofsky performance status, the number of extraspinal bone metastases, the number of metastases in the vertebral body, the presence of metastases in

major organs, the site of the primary cancer, and presence of spinal cord palsy (4). The presence of malignant neural compression requires special and rapid clinical attention to include regional radiotherapy and/or surgery in addition to systemic and bisphosphonates therapy, in order to avoid permanent paralysis, sensory loss, and/or sphincter dysfunction (5). As illustrated in the current case study, a valuable contribution of the CT data of PET/CT is the fact that it facilitates the identification of vertebral collapse and the presence of extension of the tumor mass into the epidural space (6, 7).

## Take-home message

- Fused PET/CT data allow for risk stratification of metastatic skeletal lesions.
- Destruction of the posterior aspect of the vertebral body by the tumor impinging on the thecal sac are findings that should be specifically looked for when reporting a PET/CT scan in a patient with metastatic spread to the vertebrae, and should be clearly addressed in the report, if found.

## References

1. Kennedy JA, Israel O, Frenkel A, Bar-Shalom R, Azhari H. Improved image fusion in PET/CT using hybrid image reconstruction and Super-Resolution. *Int J Biomed Imaging*. **2007**;2007: 46846.

2. Hirsh V. Skeletal disease contributes substantially to morbidity and mortality in patients with lung cancer. *Clin Lung Cancer*. 2009; **10**(4):223–229.

3. Taoka T, Mayr NA, Lee HJ *et al.* Factors influencing visualization of vertebral metastases on MR imaging versus bone scintigraphy. *Am J Roentgenol* 2001; **176**(6):1525–30.

4. Tokuhashi Y, Matsuzaki H, Toriyama S, Kawano H, Ohsaka S. Scoring system for the preoperative evaluation of metastatic spine tumor prognosis. *Spine* 1990;**15**:1110–13.

5. Loblaw A, Perry J, Chambers A, Laperriere NJ. Systematic review of the diagnosis and management

of malignant extradural spinal cord compression: the Cancer Care Ontario Practice Guidelines Initiative's Neuro-Oncology Disease Site Group. *J Clin Oncol* 2005;**23**(9):2028–37.

6. Metser U, Lerman H, Blank A *et al.* Malignant involvement of the spine: assessment by 18F-Fluorodeoxyglucose PET/CT. *J Nucl Med* 2004;**45**:279–84.

7. Guermazi A, Brice P, de Kerviler EE *et al.* Extranodal Hodgkin disease: spectrum of disease. *Radiographics* 2001;**21**:161–79.

A 56-year-old female was referred for FDG-PET/CT imaging 8 years after chemo-radiotherapy to treat an infiltrative ductal carcinoma of her left breast, due to rising serum marker levels while on hormonal therapy with tamoxifen, a non-steroidal estrogen antagonist.

## Acquisition and processing parameters

Baseline and follow-up FDG-PET/CT studies were performed after fasting for a period of 4 hours with blood sugar levels of 87 mg/dL in the initial study and 96 mg/dL in the follow-up study. A dose of 555 MBq (15 mCi) of FDG was injected for each of the

studies and oral contrast was given. After 70 min distribution time in the initial study and 90 min in the follow-up study, reduced-dose CT acquisitions were performed with the patient in the supine position with her arms up followed by the PET acquisition. The unenhanced CT and PET acquisition protocols and reconstruction parameters were as described in Case 1 (1).

## Findings

Figure 15.5 represents the initial study and Figure 15.6 the follow-up study after therapy. Each figure is composed of four panels: unenhanced transaxial CT (top left), PET (top right),

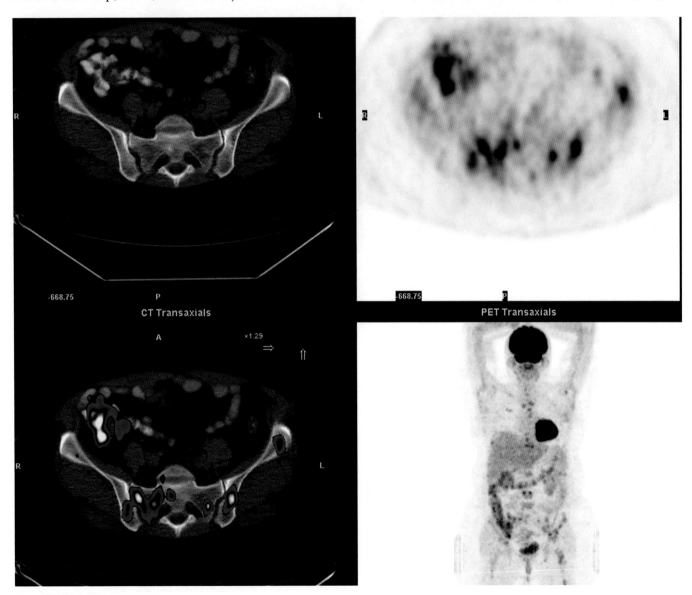

**Figure 15.5** Baseline FDG-PET/CT.

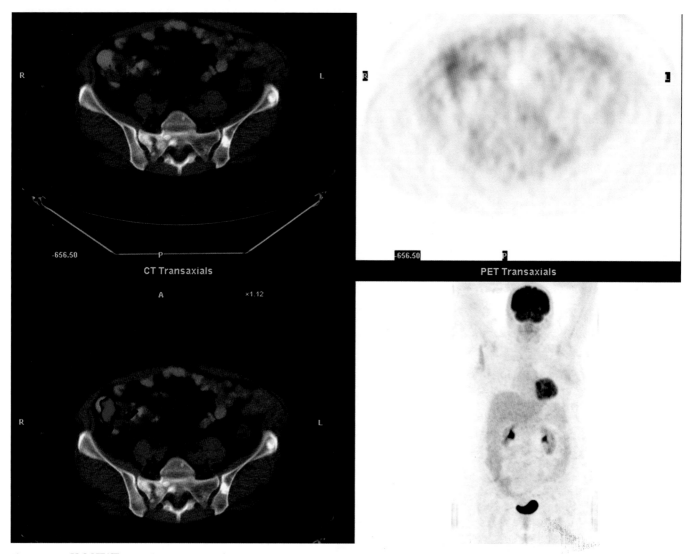

CT Transaxials

A         ×1.12

PET Transaxials

**Figure 15.6** FDG-PET/CT to monitor response to therapy.

PET/CT (bottom left), and MIP. On Figure 15.5 multiple bone lesions are detected on the MIP, and their intensity of FDG uptake is well visualized in the axial plane images. These scintigraphic abnormalities appear to be marrow-based with no clear cortical lesions observed on CT images. Based on these findings, treatment was altered to Letrozole, an aromatase inhibitor, combined with bisphosphonates therapy. Repeat FDG-PET/CT (Figure 15.6) was performed 8 months after the initial study for monitoring response to therapy. After treatment no FDG uptake is seen, while on the CT there are multiple "new" sclerotic lesions in the sacrum and left iliac bone.

## Diagnosis and clinical follow-up

The first PET/CT study performed due to rising tumor serum markers identified extensive marrow-based metastatic spread characterized by increased FDG uptake and normal-appearing bone on CT. Therefore hormonal therapy was altered and treatment with bisphosphonates was initiated. On FDG-PET/

CT after treatment FDG uptake disappeared while "new" sclerotic lesions were detected on CT. These latter changes represent repair and not disease progression. Normalization of the scintigraphic data indicates response and may suggest that the metastatic spread is no longer active. Currently, a year away from the second PET/CT study, the patient is receiving hormonal and bisphosphonates therapy and based on clinical and laboratory parameters she has no evidence for active metastatic disease.

## Discussion and teaching points

This case illustrates the high sensitivity of FDG for detection of early bone metastases prior to their identification on CT in a patient with breast cancer. After successful treatment, tracer uptake disappeared while morphological abnormalities, delayed in appearance on CT, persisted.

In patients with breast cancer, the risk for bone metastases increases with stage, reaching over 70% in advanced disease (2–6). Bone metastases from breast cancer may be lytic, sclerotic, or mixed in their radiographic appearance. Lytic lesions are predominant but 15–20% of patients have osteoblastic metastases. The superiority of FDG compared with BS in detection of metastatic skeletal spread is related to its high sensitivity to detect marrow-based early disease and lytic lesions overlooked on BS (7, 8). However, FDG-PET has been reported to have a somewhat limited sensitivity in depicting blastic metastases (8–10). The availability of corresponding CT images in the integrated PET/CT technology improves the ability of this single study to detect blastic metastases even if they are not showing increased uptake. For this matter, the high sensitivity of FDG-PET for detecting marrow and lytic lesions and the high sensitivity of CT in detecting blastic lesions are complementary (11).

There are a variety of treatment strategies for patients with bone metastases from breast cancer. These include bisphosphonates, antitumor hormonal and cytotoxic systemic drugs, and radiotherapy (12). Bisphosphonates bind to the surface of the bone, and are taken up by and induce apoptosis of osteoclasts during osteolysis, thus reducing their viability and function, and subsequently decrease the abnormally high levels of bone resorption characteristic of malignant skeletal involvement. In patients with bone metastases, the goal of bisphosphonate therapy is to prevent the onset and recurrence of skeletal-related events and to palliate bone pain (13).

Du et al. have assessed using sequential FDG-PET/CT examinations the temporal changes induced by treatment in the appearance of bone metastases in 25 patients with breast cancer. After treatment, the majority (80.5%) of lytic metastases became FDG-negative and blastic on CT, while other relatively large lesions (19.5%), remained FDG avid. Of the FDG-avid blastic metastases, 52% became negative, while in the others, uptake of FDG did not change and the lesions increased in size on CT (14). It appears that while uptake of FDG reflects tumor activity of bone metastases independent of the morphologic appearance on CT, radiographic changes may remain abnormal even when disease is no longer active, as they may represent also the repair process itself. This study also suggested that persistent positive FDG findings correlated with poorer prognosis. Tateishi et al. reviewed FDG-PET/CT studies performed before and after therapy in 102 patients with metastatic breast cancer. An increase in density on CT images after therapy correlated significantly with a decrease in uptake of FDG, expressed by changes in SUV in metastases with a positive response to therapy. A decrease in SUV of $\geq 8.5\%$ was a good predictor of long-term favorable response whereas a decrease in density and increase in SUV were associated with increased risk of disease progression (15).

## Take-home message

- Increased FDG-uptake may be seen in early bone metastases prior to the detection of cortical changes on CT.
- After successful therapy, mainly with bisphosphonates, sclerotic changes related to repair may be detected on CT, but FDG-PET becomes negative.

## References

1. Kennedy JA, Israel O, Frenkel A, Bar-Shalom R, Azhari H. Improved image fusion in PET/CT using hybrid image reconstruction and Super-Resolution. *Int J Biomed Imaging* **2007**;2007:46846.

2. Hamaoka T, Madewell JE, Podoloff DA, Hortobagyi GN, Ueno NT. Bone imaging in metastatic breast cancer. *J Clin Oncol* 2004;22(14):2942–53.

3. Yeh KA, Fortunato L, Ridge JA et al. Routine bone scanning in patients with T1 and T2 breast cancer: a waste of money. *Ann Surg Oncol* 1995;2:319–24.

4. Schirrmeister H, Kuhn T, Guhlmann A et al. Fluorine-18 2-deoxy-2-fluoro-D-glucose PET in the preoperative staging of breast cancer: comparison with the standard staging procedures. *Eur J Nucl Med* 2001;28:351–8.

5. Maffioli L, Florimonte L, Pagani L, Butti I, Roca I. Breast cancer: diagnostic and therapeutic options. *Eur J Nucl Med Mol Imaging* 2004;31:S143–8.

6. Ben-Haim S, Israel O. Breast cancer: role of SPECT and PET in imaging bone metastases. *Semin Nucl Med* 2009; **39**(6):408–15.

7. Lonneux M, Borbath I, Berliere M, Kirkove C, Pauwels S. The place of whole-body PET FDG for the diagnosis of distant recurrence of breast cancer. *Clin Positron Imag* 2000;3:45–9.

8. Abe K, Sasaki M, Kuwabara Y et al. Comparison of 18FDG-PET with 99mTc-HMDP scintigraphy for the detection of bone metastases in patients with breast cancer. *Ann Nucl Med* 2005;19:573–9.

9. Cook GJ, Houston S, Rubens R et al. Detection of bone metastases in breast cancer by 18FDG PET: differing metabolic activity in osteoblastic and osteolytic lesions. *J Clin Oncol* 1998;16:3375–9.

10. Nakai T, Okuyama, Kubota T et al. Pitfalls of FDG-PET for the diagnosis of osteoblastic bone metastases in patients with breast cancer. *Eur J Nucl Med Mol Imag* 2005;32:1253–8.

11. Even-Sapir E. Imaging of malignant bone involvement by morphologic, scintigraphic, and hybrid modalities. *J Nucl Med* 2005;**46**:1356–67.

12. Kohno N. Treatment of breast cancer with bone metastasis: bisphosphonate treatment – current and future. *Int J Clin Oncol* 2008;13(1):18–23.

13. Costa L, Major PP. Effect of bisphosphonates on pain and quality of life in patients with bone metastases. *Nature Rev Clin Oncol* 2009;6:163–74.

14. Du Y, Cullum I, Illidge TM, Ell PJ. Fusion of metabolic function and morphology: sequential [18F] fluorodeoxyglucose positron-emission tomography/computed tomography studies yield new insights into the natural history of bone metastases in breast cancer. *J Clin Oncol* 2007; 25(23):3440–7.

15. Tateishi U, Gamez C, Dawood S et al. Bone metastases in patients with metastatic breast cancer: morphologic and metabolic monitoring of response to systemic therapy with integrated PET/CT. *Radiology* **2008**; 47:189–96.

A 58-year-old female with multiple myeloma (MM) after chemotherapy, bone marrow transplantation, and right hip surgery due to a pathological fracture. Patient was referred for an FDG-PET/CT to assess activity and extent of disease.

## Acquisition and processing parameters

After a fasting period of 6 hours blood sugar was 100 mg/dL. A dose of 555 MBq (15 mCi) FDG was injected and oral contrast was given. After 60 minutes of distribution time, reduced-dose CT acquisition was performed with the patient in the supine position with her arms up followed by PET. The unenhanced CT and PET acquisition protocols and reconstruction parameters were as described in Case 1 (1).

## Findings

Figure 15.7 is composed of four panels: unenhanced coronal CT (left), PET (second from left), PET/CT (third from left), and MIP (right). Focal increased FDG uptake is seen in the spleen and within muscles along both thighs. Uptake is more prominent in a mass in the left adductor muscle; consistent with sites of extra-medullary active MM. Focal increased tracer uptake is also detected in an intra-medullary MM deposit in the midshaft of the left femur (red marker).

## Diagnosis and clinical follow-up

The patient was diagnosed with intra- and extra-medullary sites of active multiple myeloma. Guided by the FDG-PET/CT findings, biopsy of the left adductor magnus muscle was performed, which demonstrated the presence of infiltration by myeloma cells.

## Discussion and teaching points

Myelomatous involvement initiates in the marrow followed by bone destruction later during the course of disease. Marrow involvement cannot be evaluated using conventional radiography, which demonstrates the appearance of lytic lesions only when 30–50% of the bone mineral density is already lost (2). Assessment of non-invasive modalities which may identify

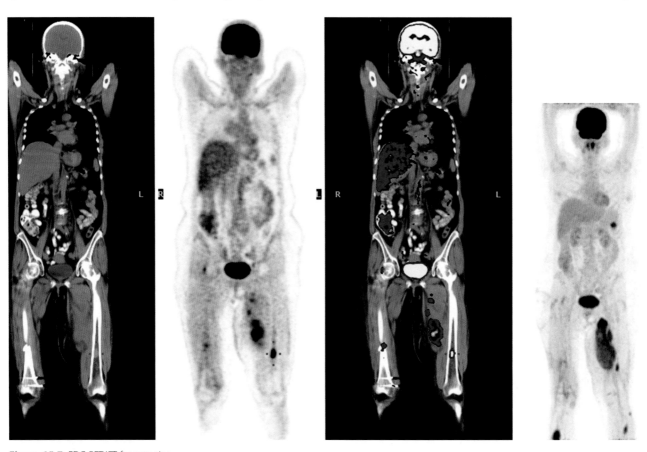

**Figure 15.7** FDG-PET/CT for restaging.

early marrow involvement in patients with MM, including magnetic resonance imaging (MRI) and FDG imaging, is now evolving. On MRI loss of fatty bone marrow components and their replacement by pathologic cells can be evaluated. FDG-PET imaging allows detection of focal sites of abnormal tracer uptake consistent with early disease confined to the marrow. Performance of FDG-PET/CT at the time of initial diagnosis has been reported to result in upstaging of disease and thus more aggressive therapy (3).

Monoclonal gammopathy of undetermined significance (MGUS) is defined by the presence of serum monoclonal (M) protein < 3 g/dL or bone marrow plasma cells < 10%. Smoldering disease is defined by serum M protein ≥ 3 g/dL or bone marrow plasma cells ≥ 10%. In both clinical settings anemia, hypocalcemia, lytic bone lesions, or renal failure are absent (4). Durie et al. assessed the role of FDG-PET in 66 patients with MM and MGUS. A positive FDG-PET reliably indicates the presence of active MM while a negative study strongly suggested the diagnosis of MGUS (5). In a series of 43 patients Shirrmeister et al. reported a sensitivity of 93% for detection of osteolytic MM by FDG-PET (6). The use of integrated PET/CT was suggested as a beneficial screening modality for MM with

uptake of FDG and bone destruction on CT indicative of active disease (7, 8). In a report by Nanni et al. on 28 patients with MM, FDG-PET/CT and MRI of the spine were shown to have a complementary role. While the former modality detected more lesions, all located outside the field of view of MRI, the latter modality was found superior to FDG-PET/CT to diagnose an infiltrative pattern in the spine (9).

FDG-PET/CT is also of value for monitoring response to therapy. FDG uptake decreases rapidly after effective therapy while a persistent positive study correlates with earlier relapse (7). Detection of extramedullary sites of disease has been associated with poor prognosis (5). An advantage of FDG-PET is its ability to detect skeletal as well as unexpected extramedullary involvement as illustrated in the present case (5, 6).

## Take-home message

- In patients with multiple myeloma, FDG-PET/CT allows identification of active disease even when confined to the bone marrow, prior to any cortical destruction.
- FDG-PET/CT allows for identification of unexpected extramedullary sites of disease.

## References

1. Kennedy JA, Israel O, Frenkel A, Bar-Shalom R, Azhari H. Improved image fusion in PET/CT using hybrid image reconstruction and Super-Resolution. *Int J Biomed Imaging* **2007**;2007:46846.

2. Lütje S, de Rooy JW, Croockewit S et al. Role of radiography, MRI and FDG-PET/CT in diagnosing, staging and therapeutical evaluation of patients with multiple myeloma. *Ann Hematol* 2009; **88**(12):1161–8.

3. Bredella MA, Steinbach L, Caputo G. Value of FDG PET in the assessment of patients with multiple myeloma. *Am Roentgen Ray Soc* 2204;**184**:1199–204.

4. International Myeloma Working Group. Criteria for the classification of monoclonal gammopathies, multiple myeloma and related disorders: a report of the International Myeloma Working Group. *Br J Haematol* 2003;**121**:749–57.

5. Durie BG, Waxman AD, D'Agnolo A, Williams CM. Whole-body 18F-FDG PET identifies high-risk myeloma. *J Nucl Med* 2002;**43**: 1457–63.

6. Schirrmeister H, Bommer M, Buck A et al. Initial results in the assessment of multiple myeloma using F-18 FDG PET. *Eur J Nucl Med Mol Imag* 2002;**29**:361–6.

7. Durie BG. The role of anatomic and functional staging in myeloma: description of Durie/Salmon plus staging system. *Eur J Cancer* 2006;**42**:1539–43.

8. Antoch G, Vogt FM, Freudenberg LS et al. Whole-body dual-modality PET/CT and whole-body MRI for tumour staging in oncology. *J Am Med Assoc* 2003;**290**: 3199–206.

9. Nanni C, Zamagni E, Farsad M et al. Role of (18)F-FDG PET/CT in the assessment of bone involvement in newly diagnosed multiple myeloma: preliminary results. *Eur J Nucl Med Mol Imag* 2006;**33**:1–7.

A 23-year-old male presented with a 6-month history of painful swelling in the lower aspect of the left chest wall. Biopsy diagnosed Ewing sarcoma. FDG-PET/CT was obtained for initial staging.

## Acquisition and processing parameters

After fasting for a period of 4 hours, fasting blood sugar was 88 mg/dL. A dose of 499.5 MBq (13.5 mCi) of FDG was injected and oral contrast was given. After 90 min of uptake time, a reduced-dose CT acquisition was performed with the patient in the supine position with his arms up followed by PET emission images. The unenhanced CT and PET acquisition protocols and reconstruction parameters were as described in Case 1 (1).

## Findings

Figure 15.8 is composed of four panels: unenhanced transaxial CT (top left), PET (top right), PET/CT (bottom left), and MIP.

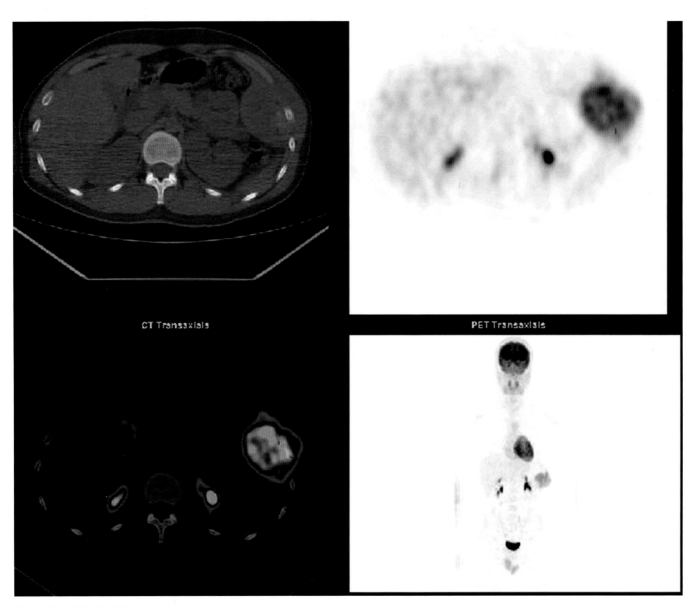

CT Transaxials

PET Transaxials

**Figure 15.8** FDG-PET/CT for initial staging.

On PET heterogeneous increased uptake of FDG is detected in the anterior aspect of the left chest wall corresponding to an 8 cm mass on CT, involving the anterolateral aspects of the 8th and 9th left ribs, and extending to surrounding soft tissues with calcifications (red marker). No other sites of disease were identified, as seen on the MIP image.

## Diagnosis and clinical follow-up

Primary Ewing sarcoma involving the bone and adjacent soft tissues with no evidence for disseminated metastases. The patient was referred for surgical resection of the primary tumor followed by chemotherapy.

## Discussion and teaching points

FDG-PET/CT is not used as a routine imaging modality in patients with primary bone malignancy. Benign bone lesions and low-grade primary malignant tumors may show overlapping intensity of FDG uptake. Therefore, this imaging modality cannot replace the need for tissue sampling in order to characterize these lesions as malignant or benign. Moreover, MRI is the modality of choice for the assessment of local tumor invasion (2).

Lung is the most common organ for metastatic spread of sarcoma and CT is more sensitive than FDG-PET for detection of small lung lesions. However, FDG-PET/CT is clinically useful in patients with primary bone malignancy, because of its ability for whole-body anatomo-metabolic assessment of metastatic spread (3, 4). As shown in the first case we discussed, FDG-PET/CT is highly sensitive for detection of skeletal metastases.

Skeletal involvement of osteosarcoma occurs in 10–20% of patients and is the second most common metastatic site after the lung and pleura. FDG-PET has been found to be a sensitive screening technique to detect bone metastases from Ewing sarcoma even when confined to the marrow (5). In pediatric patients, for instance, FDG-PET can detect skip metastases in cases with equivocal MRI findings due to the presence of physiologic red blood marrow in the long bones (6). FDG-PET/CT has been reported by Arush et al. to be useful and complementary to other imaging modalities for the detection of recurrent pediatric sarcomas, especially at the primary site (7). In a prospective multicenter study, Völker et al. evaluated the role of FDG-PET in 46 pediatric sarcoma patients and reported the important additional information provided by this test, and the relevant impact on therapy planning (8).

FDG-PET seems to be successful in monitoring response to neoadjuvant chemotherapy in patients with primary bone malignancy by identifying poor responders early during therapy (9). In a recent paper by Benz et al., changes in FDG-SUVmax at the end of neoadjuvant treatment identified histopathologic responders and non-responders in adult patients with primary bone sarcoma (10).

## Take-home message

- FDG-PET/CT allows detection of primary bone malignancy and is of value in a whole-body search for metastases.
- FDG-PET/CT provides important additional information that impacts therapy planning.

## References

1. Kennedy JA, Israel O, Frenkel A, Bar-Shalom R, Azhari H. Improved image fusion in PET/CT using hybrid image reconstruction and Super-Resolution. *Int J Biomed Imaging* 2007;**2007**:46846.

2. Schleiermacher G, Peter M, Oberlin O et al. Increased risk of systemic relapses associated with bone marrow micrometastasis and circulating tumor cells in localized Ewing tumor. *J Clin Oncol* 2003;**21**:85–9.

3. Ben Arush MW, Bar Shalom R, Postovsky S et al. Assessing the use of FDG-PET in the detection of regional and metastatic nodes in alveolar rhabdomyosarcoma of extremities. *J Pediatr Hematol Oncol* 2006; **28**(7):440–5.

4. Benz MR, Tchekmedyian N, Eilber FC et al. Utilization of positron emission tomography in the management of patients with sarcoma. *Curr Opin Oncol* 2009;**21**(4):345–51.

5. Daldrup-Link HE, Franzius C, Link TM et al. Whole-body MR imaging for detection of bone metastases in children and young adults: comparison with skeletal scintigraphy and FDG PET. *Am J Roentgenol* 2001;**177**:229–36.

6. Wuisman P, Enneking WF. Prognosis of patients who have osteosarcoma with skip metastasis. *J Bone Joint Surg Am* 1990;**72**:60–8.

7. Arush MW, Israel O, Postovsky S et al. Positron emission tomography/computed tomography with 18fluoro-deoxyglucose in the detection of local recurrence and distant metastases of pediatric sarcoma. *Pediatr Blood Cancer* 2007;**49**(7):901–5.

8. Völker T, Denecke T, Steffen I et al. Positron emission tomography for staging of pediatric sarcoma patients: results of a prospective multicenter trial. *J Clin Oncol* 2007;**25**(34):5435–41.

9. Hawkins DS, Schuetze SM, Butrynski JE et al. [18F]Fluorodeoxyglucose positron emission tomography predicts outcome for Ewing sarcoma family of tumors. *J Clin Oncol* 2005;**23**:8828–34.

10. Benz MR, Czernin J, Tap WD et al. FDG-PET/CT imaging predicts histopathologic treatment responses after neoadjuvant therapy in adult primary bone sarcomas. *Sarcoma* 2010; **2010**:143540.

A 65-year-old male with malignancy of unknown primary site with metastases to the liver. Biopsy confirmed a neuroendocrine origin. The patient was referred for a [68]Ga-somatostatin-PET/CT study to characterize the tumoral expression of somatostatin receptors and the extent of disease.

## Acquisition and processing parameters

A dose of 166.4 MBq (4.5 mCi) of [68]Ga-DOTA-NOC was injected intravenously, and the study was performed after 60 min of uptake time. The unenhanced CT acquisition protocol included 140 kVp, 80 mA, 0.8 s per CT rotation, pitch of 6 and a table speed of 22.5 mm/s. PET acquisition included 5 bed positions, 4 minutes each over the head and neck, chest, abdomen, pelvis and proximal femurs. Transaxial images (35 per field of view) were reconstructed as 128 × 128 pixel images having a pixel size of 4 mm × 4 mm and a slice thickness of 4.25 mm. The axial FOV was 14.5 cm. An ordered subsets expectation maximization (OSEM) algorithm using 2 iterations and 28 subsets was used for reconstructing the 2-D whole-body data from the PET projections (1).

## Findings

Figure 15.9 is composed of four panels: unenhanced transaxial CT (top left), PET (top right), PET/CT (bottom left), and MIP. Multiple sites of increased [68]Ga-DOTA-NOC uptake in the liver are shown on the MIP image, representing bilobar metastatic spread of a tumor overexpressing somatostatin receptors. In addition, [68]Ga-DOTA-NOC-PET identified focal uptake in the rectum and left pelvic lymph nodes (MIP image) suggestive of a primary rectal tumor with lymph nodes metastases. Transaxial CT, PET, and fused images at the level of the left midthorax demonstrate the presence of increased tracer uptake in the left scapula, localized to the marrow component of the bone which appears hyperdense on CT, consistent with a marrow-based metastasis (red marker).

## Diagnosis and clinical follow-up

The patient had a metastatic neuroendocrine tumor (NET) overexpressing somatostatin receptors. In addition to the known metastatic spread to the liver, [68]Ga-DOTA-NOC PET/CT showed that the primary lesion was in the rectum, a finding further validated by biopsy. Previously unknown metastases in pelvic lymph nodes and bone were also identified. The patient was referred for treatment with [177]Lu-labelled somatostatin.

## Discussion and teaching points

This case illustrates early metastatic spread confined to the bone marrow identified by the abnormal accumulation of [68]Ga-DOTA-NOC on PET preceding the presence of a cortical abnormality on CT.

In NET over-expressing somatostatin receptors, scintigraphy with radiolabeled-somatostatin has been reported to be more sensitive and specific for detection of tumor sites compared with morphological imaging modalities such as CT. Imaging with labeled somatostatin allows characterization of tumor receptor expression in individual patients. Metastatic tumors over-expressing the receptor can be treated with radio-immunotherapy using somatostatin labeled with beta-emitting radionuclides such as [80]Y or [177]Lu. Before therapy, scintigraphy aims at assessing the extent of disease, thus differentiating between localized disease where surgery can be considered, and disseminated disease. After therapy, scintigraphy is used to monitor response to treatment and for restaging in cases of clinically suspected recurrence. Until recently, scintigraphy was performed using somatostatin-analogs labeled with gamma-emitting radioisotopes, mainly [111]In (Octreoscan) (2,3). PET is now increasingly used to study patients with NET using new tracers of somatostatin labeled with [68]Ga. The tracer is composed of somatostatin and a [68]Ga-DOTA peptide such as TOC, TATE, or NOC. Recent papers have described the superiority of [68]Ga-labeled somatostatin PET imaging compared with Octreoscan. [68]Ga-DOTA-NOC, the tracer used in the illustrated case, is characterized by affinity to somatostatin receptors subtypes 2, 3, and 5 (4–6).

Detection of bone metastases is of clinical relevance in patients with NET as the presence of extrahepatic sites of disease has been previously associated with poor prognosis, and characterizes a subgroup of patients in whom an aggressive treatment approach is indicated (7). Several publications have reported on the superiority of [68]Ga-DOTA peptide PET over other imaging modalities including CT and bone scintigraphy for the detection of skeletal metastases in patients with NET (8, 9).

In a recent study by Ambrosini et al., the sensitivity, specificity, and accuracy of [68]Ga-DOTA-NOC-PET/CT and CT alone for the evaluation of bone metastases were retrospectively assessed in 223 patients with NET. On a patient-based analysis PET showed a higher sensitivity compared with CT (100% vs. 80%), specificity (100% vs. 98%), positive predictive value (100% vs. 92%), and negative predictive value (100% vs. 95%). PET detected more lesions than CT (246 vs. 194). In nine patients with skeletal metastatic spread detected on PET,

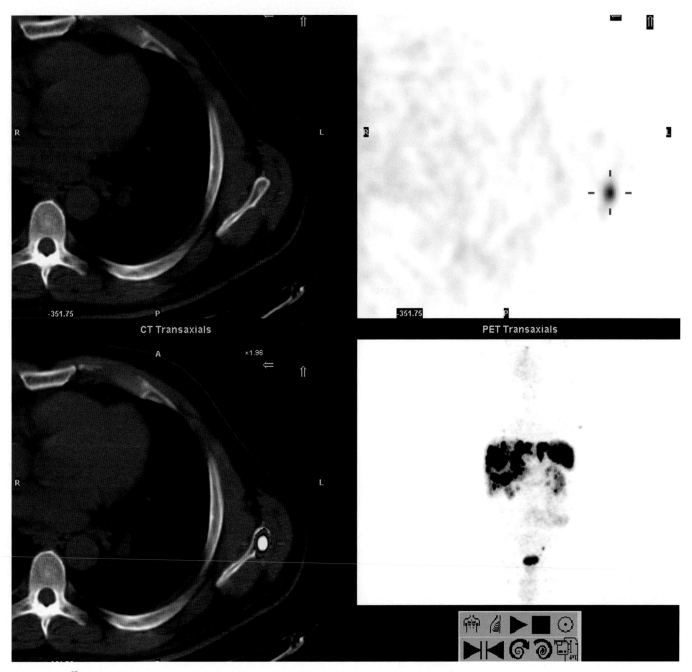

**Figure 15.9** ⁶⁸Ga-DOTA-NOC–somatostatin-PET/CT for staging.

CT was false-negative. ⁶⁸Ga-somatostatin PET upstaged the disease in four patients, and the positive functional scintigraphic lesions altered the clinical management by excluding surgery in two patients, while three patients were referred for radioimmunotherapy (10).

## Take-home message

- PET imaging with ⁶⁸Ga-DOTA peptide-somatostatin allows for the detection of soft tissue and early skeletal malignant involvement in patients with neuroendocrine tumors overexpressing somatostatin receptors.

## References

1. Kennedy JA, Israel O, Frenkel A, Bar-Shalom R, Azhari H. Improved image fusion in PET/CT using hybrid image reconstruction and Super-Resolution. *Int J Biomed Imaging* **2007**; 2007:46846.

2. Bombardieri E, Coliva A, Maccauro M *et al.* Imaging of neuroendocrine tumors with gamma-emitting radiopharmaceuticals. *Q J Nucl Med Mol Imaging* 2010; 54(1):3–15.

3. Wong KK, Cahill JM, Frey KA, Avram AM. Incremental value of 111-in pentetreotide SPECT/CT fusion imaging of neuroendocrine tumors. *Acad Radiol* 2010;**17**(3):291–7.

4. Gabriel M, Decristoforo C, Kendler D et al. 68Ga-DOTA-Tyr3-octreotide PET in neuroendocrine tumors: comparison with somatostatin receptor scintigraphy and CT. *J Nucl Med* 2007;**48**(4):508–18.

5. Buchmann I, Henze M, Engelbrecht S et al. Comparison of (68)Ga-DOTATOC PET and (111)In-DTPAOC (Octreoscan) SPECT in patients with neuroendocrine tumors. *Eur J Nucl Med Mol Imaging* 2007;**34**(10):1617–26.

6. Antunes P, Ginj M, Zhang H et al. Are radiogallium-labelled DOTA-conjugated somatostatin analogues superior to those labelled with other radiometals? *Eur J Nucl Med Mol Imaging* 2007;**34**(7):982–93.

7. Panzuto F, Nasoni S, Falconi M et al. Prognostic factors and survival in endocrine tumor patients: comparison between gastrointestinal and pancreatic localization. *Endocr Relat Cancer* 2005;**12**:1083–92.

8. Putzer D, Gabriel M, Henninger B et al. Bone metastases in patients with neuroendocrine tumor: 68Ga-DOTA-Tyr3-octreotide PET in comparison to CT and bone scintigraphy. *J Nucl Med* 2009;**50**(8):1214–21.

9. Ambrosini V, Tomassetti P, Castellucci P et al. Comparison between 68Ga-DOTA-NOC and 18F-DOPA PET for the detection of gastro-entero-pancreatic and lung neuro-endocrine tumors. *Eur J Nucl Med Mol Imaging* 2008;**35**(8):1431–8.

10. Ambrosini V, Nanni C, Zompatori M et al. 68Ga-DOTA-NOC PET/CT in comparison with CT for the detection of bone metastasis in patients with neuroendocrine tumors. *Eur J Nucl Med Mol Imaging* 2010;**37**:722–7.

A 53-year-old male after prostatectomy for prostate cancer with a Gleason score of 8 was referred for [11]C-choline PET/CT due to elevated PSA levels of 15 ng/mL and normal bone scan and CT.

## Acquisition and processing parameters

A dose of 370 MBq (10 mCi) of [11]C-choline was administered intravenously. The patient was instructed to void prior to scanning and the study was initiated 5 min after injection. Reduced-dose CT acquisition was performed with the patient in the supine position with his arms up. Imaging started at the level of the upper femurs and pelvis up to the abdomen, chest, and head and neck. The unenhanced CT acquisition protocol included 140 kVp, 80 mA, 0.8 s per CT rotation; pitch of 6 and a table speed of 22.5 mm/s. PET acquisition included 7 bed positions for duration of 5 min each. Transaxial images (35 per FOV) were reconstructed as $128 \times 128$ pixel images having a pixel size of 4 mm × 4 mm and a slice thickness of 4.25 mm. The axial FOV was 14.5 cm. An ordered-subsets expectation maximization (OSEM) iterative algorithm using 2 iterations and 28 subsets was employed to reconstruct the 2-D whole-body data from the PET projections (1).

## Findings

Figure 15.10 is composed of four panels: unenhanced coronal CT (left), PET (second from left), PET-CT (third from left), and MIP (right). Increased uptake of [11]C-choline is observed in the intramedullary region of the right proximal femur at the level of the lesser trochanter corresponding to sclerotic changes on CT (red marker).

## Diagnosis and clinical follow-up

The presence of skeletal metastasis in the right femur was validated by biopsy. The patient was referred for radiotherapy.

## Discussion and teaching points

Prostate cancer is the most common malignancy in men. Clinical nomograms based on prostate-specific-antigen (PSA) levels, Gleason score at biopsy, and clinical stage, have been generated for risk stratification and prediction of the probability of local recurrence or distant metastatic spread, in order to categorize patients as having low-risk or high-risk cancer (2–4). The use of clinical nomograms has refined the selection of high-risk patients in whom assessment of malignant bone involvement should be performed at diagnosis prior to

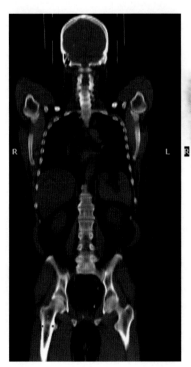
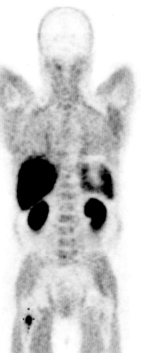
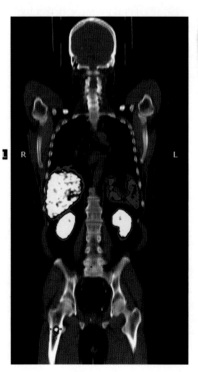
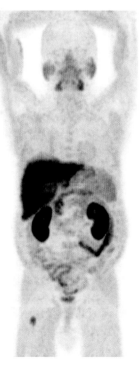

**Figure 15.10** [11]C-Choline-PET/CT.

treatment (5, 6). Later in the course of the disease patients may experience biochemical progression, local recurrence, or metastatic spread. The most frequent sites of metastases are lymph nodes and bone.

The majority of patients, almost 90%, who die of prostate cancer harbor metastatic spread to bone. Restaging is indicated in cases of rising PSA or alkaline phosphatase levels and/or new complaints of bone pain. In patients receiving bone-specific treatment, imaging aims at evaluating the efficacy of therapy intended to reduce future bone-associated morbidity (3).

For decades, bone scintigraphy (BS) has been the most widely used method to evaluate skeletal metastases from prostate cancer. However, more recent reports have debated whether BS is as effective for detection of skeletal metastases, and for monitoring response to therapy as previously perceived (5–7).

The role of PET in patients with prostate cancer has been the scope of many studies. On earlier reports, FDG, the most commonly used PET tracer, seemed to be of limited value in this group of patients due to generally low accumulation in prostate cancer cells (8). It is now thought that FDG-PET in prostate cancer should not be automatically dismissed but rather performed in selected groups of patients. In aggressive tumors with high Gleason scores and in patients with advanced stage-disease FDG-PET may be beneficial in identifying disease progression and monitoring response to therapy including discriminating active from quiescent osseous lesions (9, 10).

Other PET tracers have also been evaluated for imaging patients with prostate cancer including $^{18}$F-fluoride, a bone-seeking agent highly sensitive for detection of bone pathology, 16β-[$^{18}$F]fluoro-5α-dihydrotestosterone (FDHT), a tracer detecting the androgen receptor expression, $^{11}$C-acetate, with uptake based on fatty acid synthesis, and $^{11}$C- and $^{18}$F-choline, which are radiolabeled phospholipids (10) (see Chapter 1). Choline is a precursor for the biosynthesis of phosphatidylcholine and other phospholipids, which are major components of the cell membrane (11). Moreover, overexpression of choline kinase has been found in human-derived prostate cancer cell lines (12).

Many studies have addressed the role of radiolabeled choline-PET for detection of bone metastases in patients with prostate cancer during staging and restaging (13–16). In a recent manuscript by Beheshti et al. the role of $^{18}$F-choline-PET/CT was prospectively assessed for the pre-operative staging of patients with prostate cancer and with intermediate or high risk of extracapsular disease. The test was highly sensitive for detection of early bone metastases. $^{18}$F-choline avid lesions on PET/CT led to a change in therapy in 15% of all patients, and in 20% of the high-risk group (17). The appearance of skeletal metastases on labeled choline-PET/CT is characterized by dynamic changes. Initial involvement confined to the marrow presents as a positive PET and negative CT, followed by a positive PET and positive CT pattern due to the appearance of cortical lesions, mainly of osteoblastic type. After successful treatment, lesions show dense sclerotic changes on CT and no increased uptake thus becoming PET negative CT positive (18).

A major role of labeled choline-PET/CT is for restaging of patients with rising serum PSA levels as in the present case. $^{11}$C-choline-PET was found to be sensitive to detect local and distant recurrences even with mildly increased PSA levels (19). Cimitan et al. examined 100 such patients with $^{18}$F-choline-PET/CT. Increased uptake in bone metastases was identified in 21% of the patients (13).

## Take-home message

- PET imaging with $^{11}$C-choline allows for the early detection of metastatic skeletal spread in patients with prostate cancer and suspected recurrence.

## References

1. Kennedy JA, Israel O, Frenkel A, Bar-Shalom R, Azhari H. Improved image fusion in PET/CT using hybrid image reconstruction and Super-Resolution. Int J Biomed Imaging 2007;2007:46846.

2. Hricak H, Schoder H, Pucar D et al. Advances in imaging in the postoperative patient with a rising prostate-specific antigen level. Semin Oncol 2003; 30:616–34.

3. Han M, Partin AW, Zahurak M et al. Biochemical (prostate specific antigen) recurrence probability following radical prostatectomy for clinically localized prostate cancer. J Urol 2003;169:517–23.

4. Schoder H, Larson SM. Positron emission tomography for prostate, bladder, and renal cancer. Semin Nucl Med 2004;34:274–92.

5. Sabbatini P, Larson SM, Kremer A. Prognostic significance of extent of disease in bone in patients with androgen-independent prostate cancer. J Clin Oncol 1999;17:948–57.

6. Rigaud J, Tiguert R, Le Normand L. Prognostic value of bone scan in patients with metastatic prostate cancer treated initially with androgen deprivation therapy. J Urol 2002; 168:1423–6.

7. Even-Sapir E, Metser U, Mishani E et al. The detection of bone metastases in patients with high-risk prostate cancer: 99mTc-MDP planar bone scintigraphy, single- and multi-field-of-view SPECT, 18F-fluoride PET, and 18F-fluoride PET/CT. J Nucl Med 2006;47(2):287–97.

8. Effert PJ, Bares R, Handt S et al. Metabolic imaging of untreated prostate cancer by positron emission tomography with 18fluorine-labeled deoxyglucose. J Urol 1996;155:994–8.

9. Seltzer MA, Barbaric Z, Belldegrun A et al. Comparison of helical computerized tomography, positron emission tomography and monoclonal antibody scans for evaluation of lymph node metastases in patients with prostate specific antigen relapse after treatment for localized prostate cancer, J Urol 1999;162:1322–8.

10. Beheshti M, Langsteger W, Fogelman I. Prostate cancer: role of SPECT and PET in imaging bone metastases. *Semin Nucl Med* 2009;**39**(6):396–407.

11. Breeuwsma AJ, Pruim J, Jongen MM *et al.* In vivo uptake of [11C]choline does not correlate with cell proliferation in human prostate cancer. *Eur J Nucl Med Mol Imaging* 2005;**32**:668–73.

12. Zheng QH, Gardner TA Raikwar S *et al.* [11C]choline as a PET biomarker for assessment of prostate cancer tumor models. *Bioorg Med Chem.* 2004;**12**:2887–2893.

13. Cimitan M, Bortolus R, Morassut S *et al.* [(18)F]fluorocholine PET/CT imaging for the detection of recurrent prostate cancer at PSA relapse: experience in 100 consecutive patients. *Eur J Nucl Med Mol Imaging* 2006;**33**:1387–98.

14. Husarik DB, Miralbel R, Dubs M *et al.* Evaluation of [(18)F]-choline PET/CT for staging and restaging of prostate cancer. *Eur J Nucl Med Mol Imaging* 2008;**35**:253–63.

15. Langsteger W, Beheshti M, Nader M *et al.* Evaluation of lymph node and bone metastases with fluorocholine (FCH) PET-CT in the follow up of prostate cancer patients, *Eur J Nucl Med Mol Imaging* 2006; **33**(suppl 2):208–9.

16. Langsteger W, Beheshti M, Loidl W *et al.* Fluorocholine (FCH) PET – CT in preoperative staging of prostate cancer. *Eur J Nucl Med Mol Imaging* 2006; **33**(suppl 2):207–8.

17. Beheshti M, Imamovic L, Broinger G *et al.* 18F choline PET/CT in the preoperative staging of prostate cancer in patients with intermediate or high risk of extracapsular disease: a prospective study of 130 patients. *Radiology* 2010;**254**(3): 925–33.

18. Beheshti M, Vali R, Waldenberger P *et al.* The use of F-18 choline PET in the assessment of bone metastases in prostate cancer: correlation with morphological changes on CT. *Mol Imaging Biol* 2009; **11**(6):446–54.

19. Boukaram C, Hannoun-Levi JM. Management of prostate cancer recurrence after definitive radiation therapy. *Cancer Treat Rev* 2010; **36**(2):91–100.

# 16

# Pediatric oncology

Laura A. Drubach, Frederick D. Grant, and S. Ted Treves

## Introduction

Cancer is the fourth leading cause of death in the pediatric population with boys having a higher death rate than girls (1). Even though only 2% of the total number of cancers occurs in children it accounts for 10% of all childhood deaths in the USA and is second only to accidents (1, 2).

The most common cancers in the pediatric population are leukemia, lymphomas, and central nervous system tumors (3). Together these cancers account for 63% of all cases presenting each year. Other common cancers that present in childhood are neuroblastoma, Wilms' tumor, and rhabdomyosarcoma (3). These tumors most commonly occur in younger children while osteosarcoma, Ewing's sarcoma, and Hodgkin's disease tend to present in children older than 10 years of age (3).

The treatment of children with cancer is in the great majority performed in pediatric cancer treatment centers that are members of the Children's Oncology Group, the single pediatric cooperative clinical trials group that resulted from the recent unification of four pediatric cooperative groups, the Children's Cancer Group, the Pediatric Oncology Group, the National Wilms Tumor Study Group, and the Intergroup Rhabdomyosarcoma Study Group (2). This guarantees access to state-of-the-art treatment protocols and diagnostic investigations.

High suspicion in detecting cancer in children is needed since the majority of these tumors present insidiously and with very few initial signs and symptoms. PET/CT is a valuable assessment tool for children with cancer that provides information that is not apparent on conventional imaging. The clinically acceptable application of FDG-PET in pediatric oncology has

been rising and now FDG-PET plays a clear and important role in the evaluation of many pediatric tumors.

FDG-PET is sensitive in the detection of the primary tumor and metastasis. The intensity of FDG uptake has in addition been shown to correlate with tumor grade and has assisted in establishing prognosis. FDG-PET is frequently used in the assessment of tumor response to chemotherapy and radiation therapy. In addition FDG-PET has been proven to be useful for the determination of the exact location of viable tumor within a particular mass, thus facilitating tumor biopsy. For more details on this please refer to Chapter 20.

Well-accepted indications for use of FDG-PET in pediatric cancers are the evaluation of lymphomas, soft tissue tumors, and bone sarcomas, although this list continues to expand (4). In lymphoma FDG-PET finds additional areas of tumor involvement as compared with CT alone (5, 6). FDG-PET has also been shown to be a reliable source for evaluation of grade of malignancy in brain tumors (7). The intensity of radiotracer uptake correlates with the grading of sarcomas and assists in establishing prognosis (8). In addition, FDG-PET is frequently used in the assessment of tumor response after chemotherapy and/or radiation therapy in patients with sarcomas (9). FDG-PET is also useful to determine the exact viable tumor location within a particular mass with the goal to facilitate tumor biopsy and to minimize sampling errors.

The indications for FDG-PET in the evaluation of pediatric tumors continues to grow as more studies are performed in this age group and as more knowledge emerges in the coming years.

## References

1. Ries LAG, Smith MA, Gurney JG et al. (Eds). *Cancer Incidence and Survival among Children and Adolescents: United States SEER Program 1975–1995.* Bethesda, MD: National Cancer Institute, SEER Program, 1999.

2. Ross JA, Severson RK, Pollock BH, Robison LL. Childhood cancer in the United States. A geographical analysis of cases from the Pediatric Cooperative Clinical Trials groups. *Cancer* 1996;77:201–7.

3. Kufe DW, Pollock RE, Weichselbaum R et al. Pediatric oncology: principles and

practice. In GH Reaman (Ed.), *Cancer Medicine.* Hamilton, ON: BC Decker Inc., 2003.

4. McCarville MB. PET-CT imaging in pediatric oncology. *Cancer Imaging* 2009;9:35–43.

5. Moog F, Bangerter M, Diederichs CG et al. Lymphoma: role of whole-body

2-deoxy-2-[F-18]fluoro-D-glucose (FDG) PET in nodal staging. *Radiology* 1997;**203**:795–800.

6. Moog F, Bangerter M, Diederichs CG *et al*. Extranodal malignant lymphoma: detection with FDG PET versus CT. *Radiology* 1998;**206**:475–81.

7. Hoffman JM, Hanson MW, Friedman HS *et al*. FDG-PET in pediatric posterior fossa brain tumors. *J Comput Assist Tomogr* 1992;**16**:62–8.

8. Benz MR, Tchekmedyian N, Eilber FC *et al*. Utilization of positron emission tomography in the management of patients with sarcoma. *Curr Opin Oncol* 2009;**21**:345–51.

9. Hawkins DS, Schuetze SM, Butrynski JE *et al*. [18F]Fluorodeoxyglucose positron emission tomography predicts outcome for Ewing sarcoma family of tumors. *J Clin Oncol* 2005;**23**:8828–34.

An 11-year-old girl with a 6-month history of left knee pain. X-ray and MRI performed at presentation showed a left knee lesion suspicious for osteosarcoma. Biopsy of the lesion confirmed high-grade osteosarcoma. An FDG-PET scan was performed at presentation and after the patient underwent chemotherapy and surgical resection of the tumor with allograft reconstruction.

## Acquisition and processing parameters

After fasting for a period of 4 hours, the patient was injected intravenously with 5 mCi of FDG on a weight-based calculation (150 μCi/kg, with a maximum of 10 mCi and a minimum of 500 μCi) and an uptake phase of 60 min was allowed prior to imaging. Her glucose level at the time of radiotracer administration was 88 mg/dL.

The patient was instructed to avoid heavy exercise and caffeine for at least 12 hours prior to the study. The administration of radiopharmaceutical was performed after the patient was in a room at 75 °F (~24 °C) temperature for at least 30 min in an attempt to diminish brown fat uptake.

The PET scan was obtained in 2-D mode with 8 min per bed position. The acquisition included 3 min for the transmission and 5 min for the emission scan.

## Findings

The initial PET scan (Figure 16.1) shows intense FDG uptake in the region of the left distal femur (arrow) at the site where the lesion was seen on X-ray. Expected physiologic uptake is seen in the genitourinary and gastrointestinal tracts. No metastases were seen. The area of increased uptake in the distal lower leg corresponded clinically to a site of skin inflammation.

The follow-up PET scan (Figure 16.2) was performed after the patient underwent chemotherapy and resection of the tumor with allograft reconstruction. The study shows no abnormal uptake at the site where the initial lesion was seen, consistent with surgical resection. The allograft shows less uptake than the surrounding tissues, which is consistent with the typical appearance of an allograft. There is a linear area of uptake just proximal to the allograft (arrow) consistent with uptake at the surgical site. Uptake in the thymus is secondary to thymic rebound due to chemotherapy. No metastases are seen.

## Discussion and teaching points

Osteosarcoma is the most common primary malignant bone tumor in children and is characterized by the production of osteoid and immature bone by the tumor cells. The highest incidence is between ages 12 and 25 years and the most common location of occurrence is the metaphysis of the long bones. The distal femur is the most common location with 75% of cases presenting in this site.

Osteosarcoma is associated with several genetic conditions, such as retinoblastoma, Werner syndromes, Li-Fraumeni syndrome, and Rothmund–Thomson syndrome. The typical symptoms at presentation are localized pain and swelling without other systemic symptoms.

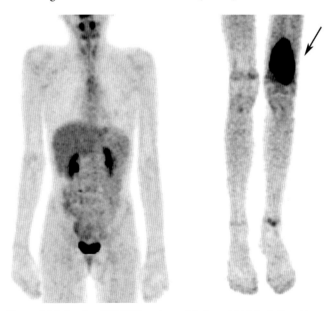

**Figure 16.1** Baseline FDG-PET from base of skull to mid thighs (left) and lower extremities (right).

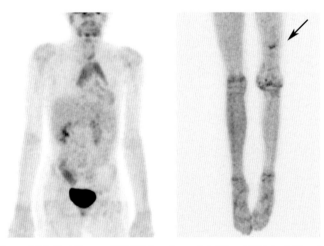

**Figure 16.2** Post-therapy FDG-PET from base of skull to mid thighs (left) and lower extremities (right).

The initial work up includes X-ray that characteristically shows a permeative infiltrating process of the bone with or without an associated soft tissue mass. The local extension of the tumor is generally evaluated with MRI.

FDG-PET is used at presentation for the evaluation of metastases and for evaluation of uptake by the primary tumor. FDG-PET is highly sensitive for the detection of the primary tumor showing typically very intense uptake such as in this patient (1). The detection of metastasis at initial staging is an important prognostic factor associated with worse outcome. FDG-PET is a sensitive tool for the evaluation of metastasis and serves as a tool in the assessment of prognosis.

The response of the tumor to chemotherapy is another important prognostic factor. FDG-PET is used in this setting for the evaluation of response to chemotherapy. The intensity of tumor FDG uptake correlates positively with the histologic response to chemotherapy. An SUV of less than 2.5 has been described to correlate with a good response (2).

The progression of metastasis while receiving chemotherapy is a sign of non-operability and FDG-PET is a sensitive tool for detection of metastasis (2, 3).

One drawback of dedicated FDG-PET is that it has been found to be not as sensitive as CT in the evaluation of small metastases to the lung. This shortcoming could be overcome by the use of FDG-PET/CT (4), which has been shown to increase the sensitivity of detection of small lung metastases.

## Take-home message

- FDG-PET is highly sensitive for the detection of the primary osteosarcoma showing very intense uptake at presentation.
- FDG-PET plays a role in restaging patients with osteosarcoma and in the detection of metastasis while receiving chemotherapy.
- Dedicated FDG-PET was found to not be as sensitive as CT in the evaluation of small metastases to the lung. This shortcoming of FDG-PET could be overcome by the use of FDG-PET/CT.

## References

1. Charest M, Hickeson M, Lisbona R et al. FDG PET/CT imaging in primary osseous and soft tissue sarcomas: a retrospective review of 212 cases. *Eur J Nucl Med Mol Imaging* 2009;**36**:1944–51.

2. Hamada K, Tomita Y, Inoue A et al. Evaluation of chemotherapy response in osteosarcoma with FDG-PET. *Ann Nucl Med* 2009;**23**:89–95.

3. Costelloe CM, Macapinlac HA, Madewell JE et al. 18F-FDG PET/CT as an indicator of progression-free and

overall survival in osteosarcoma. *J Nucl Med* 2009;**50**:340–7.

4. Benz MR, Tchekmedyian N, Eilber FC et al. Utilization of positron emission tomography in the management of patients with sarcoma. *Curr Opin Oncol* 2009;**21**:345–51.

A 6-year-old boy with a complaint of intermittent right knee pain for 1 year. X-ray and MRI performed at presentation showed a lesion in the right upper femur. The patient underwent a biopsy of the lesion that confirmed the diagnosis of Ewing's sarcoma. He was started on chemotherapy treatment. He also received granulocyte colony-stimulating factor (GCSF) during treatment.

## Acquisition and processing parameters

After fasting for a period of 4 hours, the patient was injected intravenously with 3.66 mCi of FDG on a weight-based dose (150 µCi/kg with a maximum of 10 mCi and a minimum of 500 µCi) with an uptake phase of 60 min allowed prior to imaging. The blood glucose at the time of administration was 90 mg/dL.

The patient was instructed to avoid heavy exercise and to avoid caffeine for 12 hours prior to the study. The administration of radiopharmaceutical was performed after the patient was in a room at 75 °F (~24 °C) temperature for at least 30 min in an attempt to diminish brown fat uptake.

The FDG-PET scan was obtained in 2-D mode with 8 min per bed position. The acquisition included 3 min for the transmission and 5 min for the emission scan.

## Findings

FDG-PET scan performed at presentation (Figure 16.3) shows intense radiotracer uptake in the proximal right femur. No metastatic disease was present. There is normal genitourinary and gastrointestinal uptake. Fused FDG-PET and MRI images (Figure 16.4C) show that the area of increased uptake corresponded to a soft tissue mass and the bone (arrow).

The patient underwent five cycles of chemotherapy and a repeat FDG-PET scan was performed to evaluate tumor response to therapy. The follow-up FDG-PET (Figure 16.5) shows resolution of the abnormal uptake in the right proximal femur seen in the prior study. There is now uptake in the bone marrow that is consistent with bone marrow stimulation secondary to GCSF administration. In addition there is mild linear uptake in the esophagus that may represent an inflammatory process such as esophagitis. No metastases are seen.

## Diagnosis and clinical follow-up

The patient underwent biopsy of the lesion which confirmed the diagnosis of Ewing's sarcoma. He received chemotherapy and is doing well.

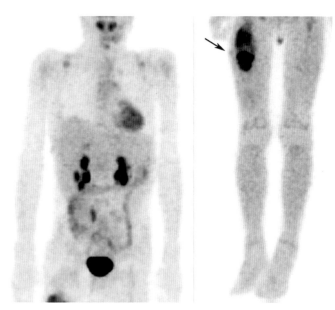

**Figure 16.3** MIP FDG-PET from base of skull to mid thigh (left) and lower extremities (right).

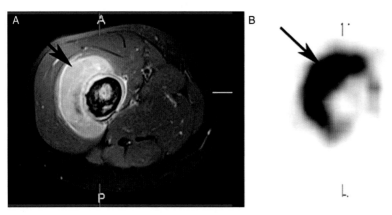
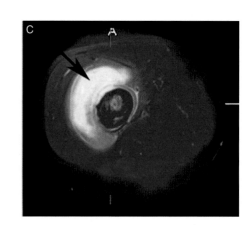

**Figure 16.4** (A) Axial MRI; (B) FDG-PET; (C) fused FDG-PET/MRI images of the proximal right thigh.

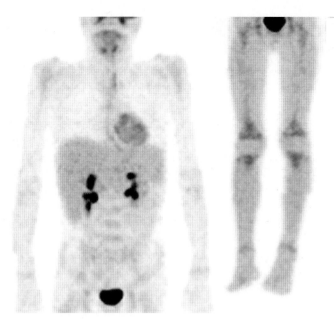

**Figure 16.5** MIP FDG-PET from base of skull to mid thigh (left) and lower extremities (right).

## Discussion and teaching points

Ewing's sarcoma is the second most common primary bone tumor in the pediatric population (after osteosarcoma). This is a tumor of neuroectodermal origin that can present in the bone or soft tissue.

The highest incidence is between ages 5 and 30 years. The most common bones involved by Ewing's sarcoma are the long bones of the upper and lower extremities, pelvis and less frequently the ribs, vertebral bodies, hands, and feet. This tumor usually presents with longstanding localized pain with or without a soft tissue mass.

FDG-PET plays a role in the initial staging and follow-up of patients with Ewing's sarcoma typically showing very intense uptake by the tumor and in metastatic sites. It is not unusual to see sites of lower uptake within the tumor representing necrosis. A study comparing bone scintigraphy with FDG-PET for the detection of metastasis from Ewing tumors found that FDG-PET was superior to bone scintigraphy in this regard (1).

The intensity of FDG uptake correlates with histologic response to chemotherapy, with SUV less than 2.5 being predictive of good response independent of initial disease stage (2).

A drawback of FDG-PET imaging in the evaluation of Ewing's sarcoma is that the sensitivity of FDG-PET for detecting small lung lesions, either at initial staging or during follow-up, is lower than CT. This can be improved if FDG-PET/CT is used (3). FDG-PET/CT was found to be more sensitive than FDG-PET alone, but not CT alone, for the detection of metastases to the lungs. However, the specificity of FDG-PET/CT for the characterization of pulmonary metastases with a diameter $> 0.5$ cm and lymph node metastases with a diameter of $< 1$ cm was significantly increased over that of CT alone (4).

## Take-home message

- FDG-PET has been found to be superior to bone scintigraphy in the detection of bone metastases from Ewing tumors.
- FDG-PET imaging of Ewing's sarcoma correlates with histologic response to neoadjuvant chemotherapy.

## References

1. Dutour A, Decouvelaere AV, Monteil J et al. 18F-FDG PET SUVmax correlates with osteosarcoma histologic response to neoadjuvant chemotherapy: preclinical evaluation in an orthotopic rat model. *J Nucl Med* 2009;**50**:1533–40.

2. Hawkins DS, Schuetze SM, Butrynski JE et al. [18F]Fluorodeoxyglucose positron emission tomography predicts outcome for Ewing sarcoma family of tumors. *J Clin Oncol* 2005;**23**:8828–34.

3. Gerth HU, Juergens KU, Dirksen U et al. Significant benefit of multimodal imaging: PET/CT compared with PET alone in staging and follow-up of patients with Ewing tumors. *J Nucl Med* 2007;**48**:1932–9.

4. Kleis M, Daldrup-Link H, Matthay K et al. Diagnostic value of PET/CT for the staging and restaging of pediatric tumors. *Eur J Nucl Med Mol Imaging* 2009;**36**:23–36.

A 10-year-old boy who was initially diagnosed with neuroblastoma at age 5, when he presented with a left adrenal mass and diffuse bone metastasis. The patient was initially treated with chemotherapy and bone marrow transplantation. After a long period of stability the patient presents with back pain. FDG-PET was performed as part of the evaluation and restaging.

## Acquisition and processing parameters

After fasting for a period of 4 hours, the patient was injected intravenously with 5 mCi of FDG (150 µCi/kg with a maximum of 10 mCi and a minimum of 500 µCi) and an uptake phase of 60 min was allowed prior to imaging. The blood glucose was 98 mg/dL. The patient was instructed to avoid heavy exercise and caffeine for 12 hours prior to the study. The administration of radiopharmaceutical was performed after the patient was in a room at 75 °F (~24 °C) temperature for at least 30 minutes in an attempt to diminish brown fat uptake. The FDG-PET scan was obtained in 2-D mode with 8 min per bed position. The acquisition included 3 min for the transmission and 5 min for the emission scan.

## Findings

The FDG-PET scan shows an area of abnormal uptake just anterior to the seventh thoracic vertebral body (Figure 16.7, arrows).

This area of abnormal uptake is likely to represent tumor recurrence. Bilateral FDG uptake in the cervical regions corresponds to brown fat uptake. Due to the proximity to the spine, an MRI was performed to evaluate for spinal canal involvement. The sagittal view of the thoracic spine MRI (T1 post gadolinium) (Figure 16.7) shows an enhancing mass centered at the T7 vertebral body (arrow) in the same location where the abnormality was seen on FDG-PET.

## Diagnosis and clinical follow-up

Biopsy of the mass revealed neuroblastoma. The patient received chemotherapy with good results.

## Discussion and teaching points

Neuroblastoma is the most common solid tumor in children. It is a tumor with a wide range of degree of malignancy, with some tumors undergoing spontaneous regression and others presenting with widely disseminated disease.

In the USA there are approximately 650 new cases every year, with the most common location being the adrenal glands.

The initial work-up for staging of neuroblastoma includes bone scintigraphy to evaluate for skeletal metastasis, and

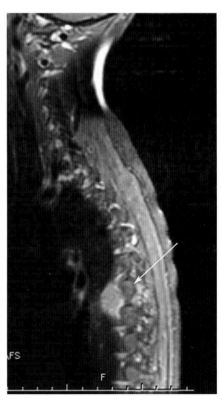

**Figure 16.7** Sagittal spinal MRI.

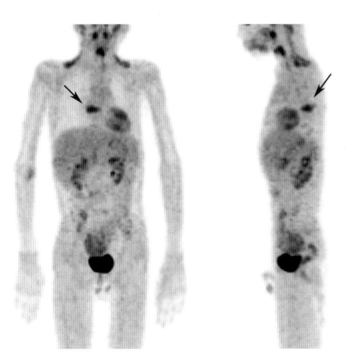

**Figure 16.6** MIP-Coronal (left) and sagittal (right) FDG-PET.

iodine-123 metaiodobenzylguanidine ([123]I-MIBG) imaging. [123]I-MIBG scintigraphy is a very sensitive method for evaluation of the primary tumor and the detection of metastases (1).

Although not routinely used in this setting, FDG-PET is also a sensitive method for detection of the primary tumor and for the detection of metastases with few specific indications. [123]I-MIBG imaging was found to be significantly more sensitive for individual lesion detection in relapsed neuroblastoma than FDG-PET, however, FDG-PET can sometimes play a complementary role, particularly in soft tissue lesions. Complete response by FDG-PET metabolic evaluation was found to not always correlate with complete response by [123]I-MIBG uptake (2).

FDG-PET was found to be superior to [123]I-MIBG in depicting stage I and II neuroblastoma, but [123]I-MIBG may be needed to exclude higher-stage disease. FDG-PET also can provide important information for patients with tumors that weakly accumulate [123]I-MIBG. [123]I-MIBG was found to be superior in the evaluation of stage IV neuroblastoma, especially during initial chemotherapy, primarily because of the better detection of bone or marrow metastases (3).

One area where FDG-PET is of great importance is in the evaluation of neuroblastomas that are [123]I-MIBG negative (4, 5).

## Take-home message

- FDG-PET is useful for the evaluation of [123]I-MIBG negative neuroblastomas.
- FDG-PET is superior in stage I and II neuroblastoma.

## References

1. Vik TA, Pfluger T, Kadota R et al. (123)I-mIBG scintigraphy in patients with known or suspected neuroblastoma: results from a prospective multicenter trial. *Pediatr Blood Cancer* 2009;**52**:784–90.

2. Taggart DR, Han MM, Quach A et al. Comparison of iodine-123 metaiodobenzylguanidine (MIBG) scan and [18F]fluorodeoxyglucose positron emission tomography to evaluate response after iodine-131 MIBG therapy for relapsed neuroblastoma. *J Clin Oncol* 2009;**27**:5343–9.

3. Sharp SE, Shulkin BL, Gelfand MJ, Salisbury S, Furman WL. 123I-MIBG scintigraphy and 18F-FDG PET in neuroblastoma. *J Nucl Med* 2009;**50**:1237–43.

4. Nguyen NC, Bhatla D, Osman MM. 123I-MIBG Scintigraphy and 18F-FDG PET in neuroblastoma. *J Nucl Med* 2010;**51**:330–1.

5. Mc Dowell H, Losty P, Barnes N, Kokai G. Utility of FDG-PET/CT in the follow-up of neuroblastoma which became MIBG-negative. *Pediatr Blood Cancer* 2009;**52**:552.

An 11-year-old boy with a 5-month history of weight loss, decreased appetite, fever, and night sweats. Physical exam was positive for generalized cervical adenopathy. Chest X-ray showed a mediastinal mass. A biopsy of the cervical nodes revealed Hodgkin's lymphoma.

## Acquisition and processing parameters

After fasting for a period of 4 hours, the patient was injected intravenously with 9 mCi of FDG (weight equivalent dose of 150 μCi/kg with a maximum of 10 mCi and a minimum of 500 μCi) with an uptake phase of 60 min allowed prior to imaging. The blood glucose was 104 mg/dL at the time of radiotracer administration. The patient was instructed to avoid heavy exercise and caffeine for 12 hours prior to the study. The administration of radiopharmaceutical was performed after the patient was in a room at 75 °F (~24 °C) temperature for at least 30 min in an attempt to diminish brown fat uptake. The FDG-PET scan was obtained in 2-D mode with 8 min per bed position. The acquisition included 3 min for the transmission and 5 min for the emission scan.

## Findings

The FDG-PET images (Figure 16.8) acquired as part of the initial staging evaluation shows a large lobulated area of

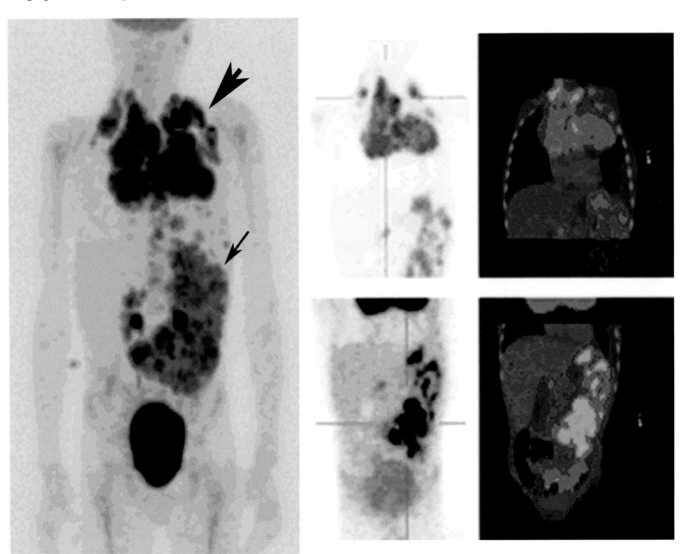

**Figure 16.8** Initial staging FDG-PET and fused FDG-PET/CT images.

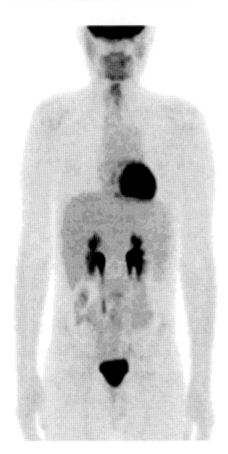

**Figure 16.9** Post-chemotherapy FDG-MIP.

## Discussion and teaching points

Hodgkin's lymphoma in the pediatric age group occurs predominantly during adolescence, with the nodular sclerosis type being the most common in this age group. It has typically an insidious onset with monthly history of fever, night sweats, and weight loss.

FDG-PET and CT are the preferred imaging methods for staging Hodgkin's disease. Multiple investigators have found that the information obtained on FDG-PET changes the patient's stage (1). In addition, FDG-PET is more sensitive than CT for the detection of distant metastases (2).

Confirmed involvement of the spleen changes the staging in Hodgkin's disease. Tumor involvement of the spleen can be facilitated by the use of FDG-PET (3). The sensitivity of CT for detection of splenic involvement is lower than that of FDG-PET in the setting of lymphoma (4).

A frequently seen problem is that residual masses may remain visible on CT after termination of chemotherapy. This does not always signify that there is still viable tumor present. The identification of remaining viable tumor tissue is difficult to assess with anatomic imaging only. FDG-PET provides an advantage over anatomic imaging in that it detects viable tissue, as it interrogates the biologic behavior of the lesion without relaying on tumor size and shape. Relapse was found to occur in 100% of patients that had FDG uptake on FDG-PET at the site of a residual mass detected on CT (5). The detection of viable tumor by FDG-PET after the end of treatment has higher predictive value for relapse than classical CT scan imaging.

increased FDG uptake that corresponds to the CT soft tissue mass (thick arrow). In addition, there is abnormal uptake in supraclavicular, prevascular, paratracheal and hilar adenopathy. There is also a massively enlarged spleen with abnormal uptake that is consistent with splenic tumor involvement (thin arrow). There is extensive retroperitoneal adenopathy that is also FDG avid.

## Diagnosis and clinical follow-up

A lymph node biopsy confirmed Hodgkin's lymphoma. The patient was placed on chemotherapy, with complete response to treatment as confirmed by FDG-PET after therapy (Figure 16.9).

## Take-home message

- The addition of FDG-PET imaging can change the staging of Hodgkin's lymphoma.
- FDG-PET has been shown to increase the detection of metastases when compared with CT alone.
- Detection of tumor involvement of the spleen can be facilitated by FDG-PET imaging.

## References

1. Hoh CK, Glaspy J, Rosen P *et al.* Whole-body FDG-PET imaging for staging of Hodgkin's disease and lymphoma. *J Nucl Med* 1997;**38**:343–8.

2. Schaefer NG, Hany TF, Taverna C *et al.* Non-Hodgkin lymphoma and Hodgkin disease: coregistered FDG PET and CT at staging and restaging – do we need contrast-enhanced CT? *Radiology* 2004;**232**:823–9.

3. Moog F, Bangerter M, Diederichs CG *et al.* Extranodal malignant lymphoma: detection with FDG PET versus CT. *Radiology* 1998;**206**:475–81.

4. de Jong PA, van Ufford HM, Baarslag HJ *et al.* CT and 18F-FDG PET for noninvasive detection of splenic involvement in patients with malignant lymphoma. *Am J Roentgenol* 2009;**192**:745–53.

5. Jerusalem G, Beguin Y, Fassotte MF *et al.* Whole-body positron emission tomography using 18F-fluorodeoxyglucose for posttreatment evaluation in Hodgkin's disease and non-Hodgkin's lymphoma has higher diagnostic and prognostic value than classical computed tomography scan imaging. *Blood* 1999;**94**:429–33.

A 16-year-old boy with a 3-week history of early morning headaches, nausea, and vomiting over the last month. The patient also developed double vision and right ear pressure that worsen at night. MRI of the brain showed a bi-thalamic mass (Figure 16.10B). Due to the high risk location of the tumor biopsy was not attempted. The presumed diagnosis of astrocytoma was entertained and the patient was started on therapy.

## Acquisition and processing parameters

After fasting for a period of 4 hours, the patient was injected intravenously with 10 mCi FDG (150 µCi/kg with a maximum of 10 mCi and a minimum of 500 µCi) and an uptake phase of 30 min was allowed in a quiet and dimly lit environment prior to imaging. The patient's glucose at the time of administration was 108 mg/dL. The patient was positioned in a head holder and the FDG-PET scan was obtained in 3-D mode with a 5-min transmission using Ge-68 as a source and a 10-min emission scan.

## Findings and differential diagnosis

The MRI (T2 flair AX) (Figure 16.10B) clearly demonstrates the bi-thalamic mass. The FDG-PET (Figure 16.10A) shows that the bi-thalamic mass has negligible FDG uptake in the region where the tumor was detected on MRI (Figure 16.10C: fused MRI-FDG-PET). This would be consistent with a low-grade tumor. For comparison also shown is another patient with a posterior fossa mass, proven to be lymphoma, which shows increased uptake of FDG (Figure 16.11, arrows).

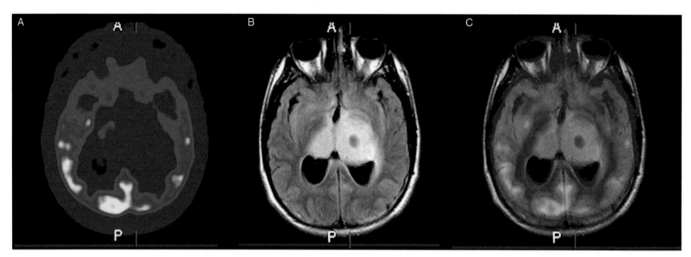

**Figure 16.10** (A) Axial FDG-PET; (B) MRI; (C) fused FDG-PET/MRI slices.

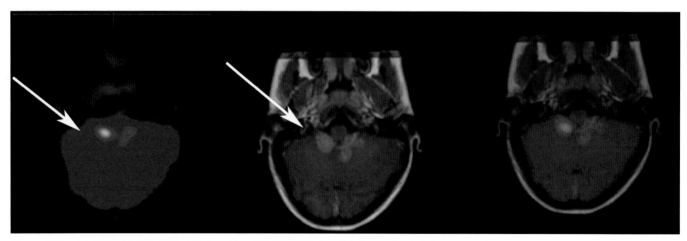

**Figure 16.11** Axial FDG-PET (left), MRI (middle), and fused FDG-PET/MRI slices (right) at the level of the posterior fossa.

## Diagnosis and clinical follow-up

Correlation of all studies determined that the patient has astrocytoma. The patient underwent radiation therapy.

## Discussion and teaching points

Primary brain tumors are the second most common malignancy in children and adolescents, after leukemia, and the most common solid organ tumors.

In young children the most common site of involvement is in the posterior fossa, with medulloblastoma and cerebellar astrocytoma being the most common tumors in this location.

In older children and adolescents supratentorial tumors are more common. Supratentorial tumors include astrocytomas, glioblastomas, and ependymomas.

Currently FDG-PET is not routinely used at all centers as part of the work-up for brain tumors, but it can provide useful information. FDG-PET is very useful to differentiate recurrent tumor from changes due to radiotherapy, especially when fusion and registration with MR imaging is used (1). FDG-PET scans can differentiate malignant lesions with a high metabolic rate from lesions with a low metabolic rate (2). FDG-PET brain imaging has been shown to assist in determining the location within the tumor with the highest activity to assist with biopsy localization (2).

One difficulty of CNS tumor imaging with FDG-PET is that it has limited ability to distinguish uptake in primary CNS tumors from the normally high background gray matter brain activity – especially for small lesions and for low-grade lesions that typically would have low-grade uptake similar to that of white matter (2). In order to overcome some of these limitations other PET probes that have been used for the evaluation of brain tumors are: $^{11}$C-L methylmethionine, $^{18}$F-fluorothymidine, $^{18}$F-fluoromisonidazole, $^{18}$F-fluoroethyl-L-tyrosine, and $^{18}$F-FDOPA (see Chapters 2 and 5).

## Take-home message

- FDG-PET imaging has been shown to assist in determining the location of highest metabolic activity within the tumor for biopsy guidance.
- FDG-PET is very useful to differentiate recurrent tumor from changes due to radiotherapy, especially when fusion and registration with MR imaging is used.
- Multiple other PET agents (not FDA-approved yet) are available in certain centers for evaluation of brain tumors.

## References

1. Hustinx R, Pourdehnad M, Kaschten B, Alavi A. PET imaging for differentiating recurrent brain tumor from radiation necrosis. *Radiol Clin North Am* 2005;**43**:35–47.

2. Hagge RJ, Wong TZ, Coleman RE. Positron emission tomography: brain tumors and lung cancer. *Radiol Clin North Am* 2001;**39**:871–81.

A 13-year-old girl presenting with chest pain, cough, and dyspnea. A chest CT showed multiple pulmonary nodules. The patient was found to have a thyroid nodule on physical exam. Biopsy of the nodule showed papillary thyroid carcinoma. She underwent a FDG-PET scan as part of restaging after a course of chemotherapy treatment.

## Acquisition and processing parameters

After fasting for a period of 4 hours, the patient was injected intravenously with 9 mCi of FDG (weight equivalent dose of 150 μCi/kg with a maximum of 10 mCi and a minimum of 500 μCi) and an uptake phase of 60 min was allowed prior to imaging. The blood glucose was 104 mg/dL at the time of administration. The patient was instructed to avoid heavy exercise and to avoid caffeine for 12 hours prior to the study. The administration of radiopharmaceutical was performed after the patient was in a room at 75 °F (∼24 °C) temperature for at least 30 min in an attempt to diminish brown fat uptake. The FDG-PET scan was obtained in 2-D mode with 8 minutes

per bed position (3 min for transmission and 5 min for the emission scan).

## Findings

Coronal and axial FDG-PET images of the chest show multiple areas of abnormal FDG avidity within the chest (Figure 16.12) (arrow) that correlate with the abnormal nodules seen on the corresponding CT (Figure 16.13). This pattern is consistent with metabolically active lung metastases.

## Diagnosis and clinical follow-up

Biopsy showed papillary thyroid cancer, and the patient underwent chemotherapy treatment.

## Discussion and teaching points

For decades, radioiodine has been the standard agent for diagnostic imaging and radiotherapy of differentiated thyroid 1carcinoma. Well-differentiated thyroid cancer is less iodine-avid

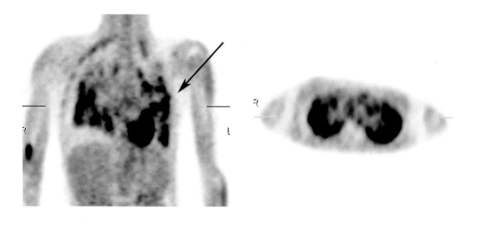

Figure 16.12 Coronal (left) and axial (right) FDG-PET images of the chest.

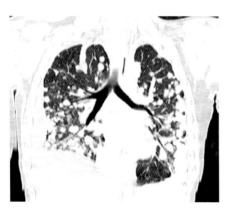
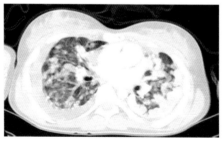

Figure 16.13 Coronal (left) and axial (right) CT images of the chest.

than normal thyroid tissue, but typically demonstrates sufficient radioiodine uptake to be detected with a radioiodine scan. Thyroid cancer also can be detected with FDG-PET, although there can be a reciprocal relationship between radioiodine uptake and FDG avidity. In the same patient, some sites of disease can be detected by both radioiodine and FDG-PET, while other lesions will show discordant uptake of one tracer, either radioiodine or FDG, but not the other (1, 2). Some investigators have demonstrated that well-differentiated metastases tend to be iodine-avid, while more aggressive and less differentiated lesions tend to show FDG, but not iodine uptake (1, 2). FDG-PET can be particularly helpful in patients with evidence of disease (such as an elevated serum thyroglobulin level or radiographic evidence of pulmonary metastases), but an unrevealing iodine scan (3, 4). In these patients, FDG-PET is more than 80% sensitive for finding sites of occult disease (5). However, even the combination of both a radioiodine whole-body scan and an FDG-PET study will not detect all sites of metastatic disease, as spread to small cervical lymph nodes may not be detected with either radiopharmaceutical (6).

When using FDG-PET to identify metastatic thyroid cancer, higher serum thyroglobulin levels are associated with improved sensitivity (4, 7) and co-registered FDG-PET/CT improves specificity and anatomic localization (8). Empiric radioiodine therapy may be of benefit when differentiated thyroid cancer is not iodine-avid, but shows FDG uptake. However, empiric radioiodine therapy lacks efficacy in patients with evidence of persistent disease (such as an elevated serum thyroglobulin level), but a negative radioiodine scan and negative FDG-PET (9).

## Take-home message

- FDG-PET is beneficial in patients with high serum thyroglobulin, but with an unrevealing iodine scan.
- Well-differentiated metastases from thyroid cancer tend to be iodine-avid, while more aggressive and less differentiated lesions tend to show FDG, but not iodine uptake.

## References

1. Feine U, Lietzenmayer R, Hanke JP et al. Fluorine-18-FDG and iodine-131-iodide uptake in thyroid cancer. *J Nucl Med* 1996;**37**:1468–72.

2. Grunwald F, Schomburg A, Bender H et al. Fluorine-18 fluorodeoxyglucose positron emission tomography in the follow-up of differentiated thyroid cancer. *Eur J Nucl Med* 1996;**23**:312–19.

3. Hooft L, Hoekstra OS, Deville W et al. Diagnostic accuracy of 18F-fluorodeoxyglucose positron emission tomography in the follow-up of papillary or follicular thyroid cancer. *J Clin Endocrinol Metab* 2001;**86**:3779–86.

4. Wang W, Macapinlac H, Larson SM et al. [18F]-2-fluoro-2-deoxy-D-glucose positron emission tomography localizes residual thyroid cancer in patients with negative diagnostic (131)I whole body scans and elevated serum thyroglobulin levels. *J Clin Endocrinol Metab* 1999;**84**:2291–302.

5. Dietlein M, Scheidhauer K, Voth E, Theissen P, Schicha H. Fluorine-18 fluorodeoxyglucose positron emission tomography and iodine-131 whole-body scintigraphy in the follow-up of differentiated thyroid cancer. *Eur J Nucl Med* 1997;**24**:1342–8.

6. Robbins RJ, Larson SM. The value of positron emission tomography (PET) in the management of patients with thyroid cancer. *Best Pract Res Clin Endocrinol Metab* 2008;**22**:1047–59.

7. Shammas A, Degirmenci B, Mountz JM et al. 18F-FDG PET/CT in patients with suspected recurrent or metastatic well-differentiated thyroid cancer. *J Nucl Med* 2007;**48**:221–6.

8. Freudenberg LS, Frilling A, Kuhl H et al. Dual-modality FDG-PET/CT in follow-up of patients with recurrent iodine-negative differentiated thyroid cancer. *Eur Radiol* 2007;**17**:3139–47.

9. Kim EY, Kim WG, Kim WB et al. Clinical outcomes of persistent radioiodine uptake in the neck shown by diagnostic whole body scan in patients with differentiated thyroid carcinoma after initial surgery and remnant ablation. *Clin Endocrinol (Oxf)* 2010; **73**:257–63.

A 16-year-old boy with a 4-month history of slowly growing masses and swelling of the left leg. The masses were not painful. Just prior to presentation to the hospital the patient also noted swelling of the left inguinal region. FDG-PET was performed at the time of presentation for staging.

## Acquisition and processing parameters

After fasting for a period of 4 hours, the patient was injected intravenously with 14 mCi of FDG and an uptake phase of 60 min was allowed prior to imaging. The patient was instructed to avoid heavy exercise and to avoid caffeine for 12 hours prior to the study. The administration of radiopharmaceutical was performed after the patient was in a room at 75 °F (~24 °C) temperature for at least 30 minutes to diminish brown fat uptake. The FDG-PET scan was obtained in 2-D mode with 8 min per bed position (each bed position consisted of 3 min for transmission and 5 min for emission scanning).

## Findings

The lower extremities MIP images show three large areas of increased FDG uptake (Figure 16.14) (arrows) localized in the popliteal region of the left leg and the other two just inferiorly. These areas corresponded to the masses palpable on physical exam. The lower extremities and the whole-body images also show increased uptake in the left inguinal region. The corresponding CT of the pelvis shows that the abnormal FDG-PET uptake in the inguinal region corresponds to abnormal adenopathy (Figure 16.15) (arrow). There are no other areas of abnormal uptake in the chest or abdomen. The increased uptake in the right hand corresponds to the injection site.

## Diagnosis and clinical follow-up

Biopsy of the mass was consistent with rhabdomyosarcoma. The patient underwent chemotherapy treatment and is now doing well.

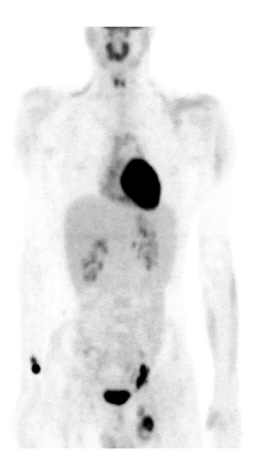
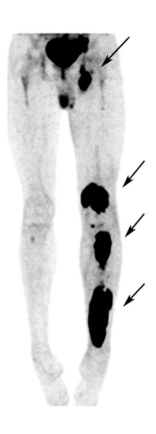

**Figure 16.14** MIP FDG-PET from base of skull to mid thigh (left) and lower extremities (right).

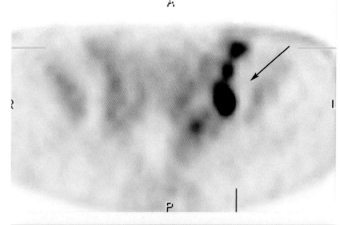

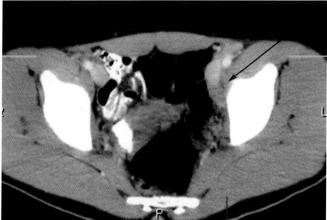

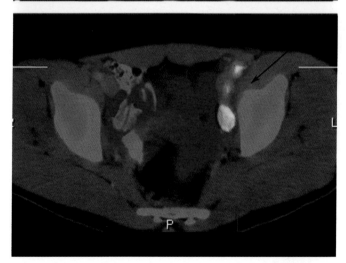

**Figure 16.15** Axial FDG-PET (top), CT (middle), and fused FDG-PET/CT (bottom) at the level of the pelvis.

## Discussion and teaching points

Rhabdomyosarcoma is one of the most common soft tissue sarcomas in children. The clinical symptoms at presentation depend on the location of the tumor. The most common sites are the head and neck and genitourinary system, but it can occur in any other location of the body. This tumor is very common in young children with 70% of the rhabdomyosarcomas diagnosed in patients younger than 10 years. It has a peak incidence between 1 and 5 years of age.

The initial imaging staging of patients with rhabdomyosarcoma calls for evaluation with CT and/or MRI. FDG-PET is often part of the initial radiologic evaluation as well. The overall staging accuracy of FDG-PET/CT has been found to be significantly higher than that of conventional imaging alone in patients with rhabdomyosarcoma (1), and it has been suggested that FDG-PET be included as part of the initial staging of all patients with rhabdomyosarcoma (2).

The local recurrence of tumor occasionally can be difficult to assess with conventional imaging alone, especially if the patient underwent resection of the primary tumor and post-surgical changes are present. FDG-PET/CT was found to be useful and complementary to other conventional imaging modalities for the detection of recurrent pediatric sarcomas, especially at the primary site (3, 4).

The changes in tumor FDG uptake correlates significantly with the histopathologic response of the tumor and the survival of patients with sarcoma (5), and it was found to be useful in the evaluation of chemotherapy and radiation therapy response (4). FDG-PET is also valuable for the evaluation of rhabdomyosarcoma of the alveolar type which is characterized by a worse prognosis (6).

## Take-home message

- FDG-PET imaging is emerging as an important imaging modality in the management of patients with sarcoma. Its applications include tumor grading, staging, and therapeutic monitoring.

# References

1. Tateishi U, Hosono A, Makimoto A *et al.* Comparative study of FDG PET/CT and conventional imaging in the staging of rhabdomyosarcoma. *Ann Nucl Med* 2009;**23**:155–61.

2. Klem ML, Grewal RK, Wexler LH *et al.* PET for staging in rhabdomyosarcoma: an evaluation of PET as an adjunct to current staging tools. *J Pediatr Hematol Oncol* 2007;**29**:9–14.

3. Arush MW, Israel O, Postovsky S *et al.* Positron emission tomography/ computed tomography with 18fluoro-deoxyglucose in the detection of local recurrence and distant metastases of pediatric sarcoma. *Pediatr Blood Cancer* 2007;**49**:901–5.

4. McCarville MB, Christie R, Daw NC, Spunt SL, Kaste SC. PET/CT in the evaluation of childhood sarcomas. *Am J Roentgenol* 2005;**184**: 1293–304.

5. Benz MR, Tchekmedyian N, Eilber FC *et al.* Utilization of positron emission tomography in the management of patients with sarcoma. *Curr Opin Oncol* 2009;**21**:345–51.

6. Ben Arush MW, Bar Shalom R, Postovsky S *et al.* Assessing the use of FDG-PET in the detection of regional and metastatic nodes in alveolar rhabdomyosarcoma of extremities. *J Pediatr Hematol Oncol* 2006; **28**:440–5.

# Malignancy of unknown origin

### Hubert H. Chuang, Denis J. Gradinscak, and Homer A. Macapinlac

## Introduction

Malignancy of unknown origin, also referred to as occult primary or cancer with unknown primary (CUP), presents a diagnostic and therapeutic challenge. Approximately 10–15% of patients present with metastatic disease without an obvious primary tumor, and in many cases a primary tumor is not found even at autopsy (1). These include the paraneoplastic syndromes, where a patient presents with the humoral effects of an occult primary. In the absence of a known primary tissue of origin, the therapy is empiric and the outcome is generally poor. However, there are several favorable presentations that should be considered, and there are advances in personalized therapy that may improve outcomes. The role of FDG-PET/CT in cancer with an unknown primary is still being defined, but it is likely to play an increased role not only in the initial evaluation of these patients, but also in the assessment of response and in the direction of subsequent therapy.

Patients with an occult primary frequently present with general symptoms such as anorexia, weight loss, and fatigue, or with a localizing finding, such as lymphadenopathy, pathologic fracture, or a large fluid collection. The tumors in these patients are heterogeneous in histological appearance, but are characterized by their aggressiveness, propensity for early dissemination, and atypical metastatic pattern. The existence of metastatic disease at presentation is associated with a poor prognosis, and with a median survival of less than a year (2, 3). However, patients with only loco-regional disease have a better prognosis (4).

The inability to identify a primary tumor is often a source of anxiety, and may leave both the patient and the clinician feeling that the evaluation is inadequate (5). In addition to the psychological benefits, identification of a primary tumor may also lead to more effective therapy or allow access to clinical trials. However, a prolonged search may lead to increased costs to the healthcare system, and identifying an occult primary may take years in patients with a paraneoplastic syndrome (6, 7).

The initial diagnostic approach focuses on identifying a primary tumor and determining the extent of disease. A thorough clinical exam and basic laboratory work may provide some clues. CT scan of the chest, abdomen, and pelvis is usually performed. Additional studies are suggested by the clinical presentation and imaging findings (8–10). Serum alpha-fetoprotein (AFP), human chorionic gonadotropin (HCG), and prostate specific antigen (PSA) may be checked in men; however, evaluation of other serum tumor markers is not recommended as they are often not specific to a particular tumor type, although they are sensitive indicators of disease burden with a known tumor. In women with isolated axillary nodal disease, breast imaging is recommended. Clinical signs and symptoms are used to guide endoscopic evaluation. Histology and immunohistochemistry also offer clues as to the tissue of origin.

In general, tumors are classified as carcinomas (epithelial origin), sarcomas (connective tissue origin), melanomas, and lymphomas; germ cell tumors are rare and resemble carcinomas. A first-line immunohistochemical panel may be applied to help classify the tissue type, for example using an epithelial marker (e.g., pan-cytokeratin AE1/3), a melanocytic marker (e.g., S100), and a lymphoid marker (e.g., CLA). A sarcoma marker (e.g., vimentin) may not be included in this panel, because sarcomas are rare and their morphology is often distinctive. These markers typically have high sensitivity for the histological subtype, but have lower specificity. Identification of a non-epithelial tissue type will result in altered management, and improved outcomes are associated with some tissues such as lymphoma and germ cell tumors.

When the cells are of epithelial origin, a specific organ of origin is often not possible to be ascertained based on histology alone, but may be made in conjunction with clinical and imaging findings. Cytokeratins are the principal markers of adenocarcinomas, and staining for CK7, widely expressed on simple glandular epithelium, and for CK20, found on gastrointestinal epithelium, is commonly used for initial characterization and to direct additional immunohistochemical stains.

Additional markers help further narrow possible origins. For example, thyroid transcription factor 1 (TTF1) is commonly used to help identify primary lung tumors as it is expressed in 70–90% of non-mucinous lung adenocarcinomas;

*A Case-Based Approach to PET/CT in Oncology*, ed. Victor H. Gerbaudo. Published by Cambridge University Press.
© Cambridge University Press 2012.

however, it is also found on virtually all thyroid cancers and more than 50% of poorly differentiated neuroendocrine tumors. Estrogen or progesterone receptors are commonly found in breast, ovarian, and endometrial carcinomas, but also in a small number of lung, prostate, colon, and gastric adenocarcinomas. Serum carcinoembryonic antigen (CEA) is commonly used to follow patients with known colonic carcinomas, but immunohistochemical staining for CEA is also common in pancreatic, upper gastrointestinal tumors and hepatocellular carcinomas, and less frequently in lung, breast, and ovarian tumors. Caudal type homeobox transcription factor-2 (CDX2) is a highly sensitive and specific marker for gastrointestinal carcinomas; however, its staining is variable, tending to be stronger in the lower gastrointestinal tract and weaker in gastroesophageal and pancreaticobiliary tumors. AFP, although useful as a serum marker for hepatocellular carcinoma, stains only 20–30% of these tumors. RCC is a highly specific antibody for renal cell carcinomas, although its sensitivity has been reported at between 55–85%. The plethora of different markers and combinations of staining patterns can be overwhelming; a recent review by Oien (11) provides further details, but is not a substitute for an experienced pathologist.

When the patient cannot be steered to a particular treatment pathway based upon tumor origin, therapy is empiric. Adenocarcinomas and poorly differentiated carcinomas represent the majority of these cases (80–90%) (11). Phase II studies have demonstrated efficacy of cisplatin-based and gemcitabine-based regimens. Poorly or undifferentiated tumors may be more responsive to cisplatin-based therapy. Cisplatin-based therapy is also used in patients with disseminated squamous cell carcinomas. Recent phase III studies have shown that combining cisplatin and 5-fluorouracil with either docetaxel or paclitaxel results in improved outcomes (3, 8).

Neuroendocrine tumors are uncommon but have a better prognosis than other cancers of unknown primary. Well-differentiated neuroendocrine tumors are treated similarly to metastatic carcinoid tumors, and may be candidates for octreotide therapy when unresectable. Poorly differentiated or small cell neuroendocrine tumors are treated similarly to small cell lung cancer, and a recent study using combination paclitaxel, carboplatin, and etoposide reported responses in more than 50% of the patients (12).

Recent efforts have incorporated advances in molecular biology into treatment strategies. Varadhachary and Raber (13) used gene expression profiles to assign a tissue of origin in 63 of 104 patients (61%). Although patients with lung and pancreatic profiles did poorly, patients who received colon cancer-specific therapy had a better outcome compared with empiric therapy. Molecular characterization of tumors may allow selection of patient-specific therapy and lead to an improved outcome.

The favorable clinical presentations represent only 10–20% of patients with an unknown primary (4, 10). These include women with adenocarcinoma in isolated axillary lymph nodes (suggesting breast cancer), women with peritoneal adenocarcinoma (suggesting ovarian or primary peritoneal), men with blastic bone metastases and increased prostate-specific antigen (PSA) (suggesting prostate cancer), young men with a mediastinal or retroperitoneal mass and elevated alpha fetoprotein (AFP) or the beta subunit of human chorionic gonadotropin (beta-hCG) (suggesting extragonadal germ cell tumor), cervical squamous cell carcinomas (suggesting a head and neck primary) or inguinal lymph nodes (suggesting genital or anorectal primary), neuroendocrine carcinomas, and any patient with limited extent of disease. Imaging studies in these cases are important to confirm limited disease without distant metastases.

FDG-PET has had a large impact in clinical oncology practice as it frequently detects disease missed by conventional radiologic evaluation; it predicts response to therapy, and can be used to assess residual abnormalities after therapy. Its application is rapidly expanding, and the use of hybrid imaging such as FDG-PET/CT is rapidly becoming the standard. Both the National Comprehensive Cancer Network (NCCN) and the European Society of Medical Oncology (ESMO) currently acknowledge that FDG-PET/CT imaging may be helpful in the evaluation of carcinoma with an unknown primary, particularly when presenting with cervical metastases or suspected limited extent of disease (8, 9). However, they note a lack of prospective studies evaluating its utility compared with established diagnostic evaluation strategies.

A number of retrospective studies have reported on the utility of FDG-PET or FDG-PET/CT in identifying a primary tumor site. In 2006, a meta-analysis showed that FDG-PET found a primary tumor in 41% of patients with negative conventional workup (14). Another meta-analysis by Kwee and Kwee (15) reported that FDG-PET/CT identified a primary tumor in 37% of patients. Dong et al. (16) also reviewed the literature and found similar detection rates between FDG-PET and FDG-PET/CT, at 29% and 31%, respectively.

One of the difficulties in evaluating the effectiveness of FDG-PET in patients with an unknown primary is the lack of uniform conventional work-up before FDG-PET imaging. Current NCCN guidelines suggest CT scan of the chest, abdomen, and pelvis as part of the evaluation of patients presenting with biopsy-proven metastatic malignancy. Of the ten studies reviewed by Seve et al., only two had whole-body CT as part of the conventional work-up. In these, FDG-PET identified a primary in 17% of patients, including all of the tumors detected by CT, confirming its greater sensitivity.

Identification of a primary tumor in FDG-PET was associated with improved outcome in a study by Mantaka et al. (17); however, of the eight patients where a primary tumor was not identified, only one received therapy, calling into question the significance of identifying a primary tumor. In contrast, Kole et al. (18) reported no survival benefit when the primary tumor site was identified by FDG-PET. Other studies also suggest that when a treatable malignancy is not present, identification of a primary tumor does not alter the prognosis (19, 20).

Limited disease is considered to be a favorable prognostic finding, and FDG-PET is useful in identifying unrecognized distant metastases. Seve *et al.* reported FDG-PET detection of previously unrecognized metastases in 37% of patients. A similar rate of 27% for the detection of previously unrecognized metastases was reported in a meta-analysis by Rusthoven *et al.* for studies with cervical lymph node metastases and an unknown primary (21). Overall, FDG-PET findings led to a change in management in 20–35% of patients with an unknown primary, by directing specific chemotherapy, modifying radiation therapy fields, or allowing surgical resection with curative intent.

The next generation of positron emitting radiotracers is currently under development and clinical evaluation. Tracers binding to specific sites, such as the estrogen or somatostatin receptors, may indicate the appropriateness of specific therapy, and markers for cell proliferation or apoptosis may prove more reliable in predicting tumor response to treatment. These agents will allow the in vivo assessment of therapy and allow further tailoring of patient-specific therapy.

In summary, imaging studies play an important role in evaluation of patients with occult primary tumors. Although there are limited data and few well-controlled studies comparing different modalities, published work suggests that FDG-PET frequently identifies an occult primary tumor, even after negative conventional evaluation, including CT scans. Moreover, the ability of FDG-PET to identify metastatic disease and to predict tumor responses can play an important role in selecting the initial treatment strategy and subsequent management decisions. Development of new FDG-PET tracers may allow further characterization of tumors and direct personalized treatments. The cases that follow will highlight the developing role of FDG-PET/CT in the management of patients with malignancy of unknown origin.

# References

1. Pentheroudakis G, Golfinopoulos V, Pavlidis N. Switching benchmarks in cancer of unknown primary: from autopsy to microarray. *Eur J Cancer* 2007;**43**:2026–36.

2. Pavlidis N, Briasoulis E, Hainsworth J, Greco FA. Diagnostic and therapeutic management of cancer of an unknown primary. *Eur J Cancer* 2003;**39**:1990–2005.

3. Greco FA. Therapy of adenocarcinoma of unknown primary: are we making progress? *J Natl Compr Canc Netw* 2008;**6**:1061–7.

4. Fizazi K. Treatment of patients with specific subsets of carcinoma of an unknown primary site. *Ann Oncol* 2006;**17**(Suppl 10):177–80.

5. Abbruzzese JL, Abbruzzese MC, Lenzi R, Hess KR, Raber MN. Analysis of a diagnostic strategy for patients with suspected tumors of unknown origin. *J Clin Oncol* 1995;**13**:2094–103.

6. Vedeler CA, Antoine JC, Giometto B et al. Management of paraneoplastic neurological syndromes: report of an EFNS Task Force. *Eur J Neurol* 2006;**13**:682–90.

7. Voltz R. Paraneoplastic neurological syndromes: an update on diagnosis, pathogenesis, and therapy. *Lancet Neurol* 2002;**1**:294–305.

8. Ettinger DS, Agulnik M, Cristea M et al. Occult primary. *J Natl Compr Canc Netw* 2008;**6**:1026–60.

9. Briasoulis E, Pavlidis N, Felip E. Cancers of unknown primary site: ESMO clinical recommendations for diagnosis, treatment and follow-up. *Ann Oncol* 2009;**20**(Suppl 4): 154–5.

10. Hainsworth JD, Fizazi K. Treatment for patients with unknown primary cancer and favorable prognostic factors. *Semin Oncol* 2009;**36**:44–51.

11. Oien KA. Pathologic evaluation of unknown primary cancer. *Semin Oncol* 2009;**36**:8–37.

12. Hainsworth JD, Spigel DR, Litchy S, Greco FA. Phase II trial of paclitaxel, carboplatin, and etoposide in advanced poorly differentiated neuroendocrine carcinoma: a Minnie Pearl Cancer Research Network Study. *J Clin Oncol* 2006;**24**:3548–54.

13. Varadhachary GR, Raber MN. Gene expression profiling in cancers of unknown primary. *J Clin Oncol* 2009;**27**:e85–6; author reply e87–8.

14. Seve P, Billotey C, Broussolle C, Dumontet C, Mackey JR. The role of 2-deoxy-2-[F-18]fluoro-D-glucose positron emission tomography in disseminated carcinoma of unknown primary site. *Cancer* 2007;**109**:292–9.

15. Kwee TC, Kwee RM. Combined FDG-PET/CT for the detection of unknown primary tumors: systematic review and meta-analysis. *Eur Radiol* 2009;**19**:731–44.

16. Dong MJ, Zhao K, Lin XT et al. Role of fluorodeoxyglucose-PET versus fluorodeoxyglucose-PET/computed tomography in detection of unknown primary tumor: a meta-analysis of the literature. *Nucl Med Commun* 2008; **29**:791–802.

17. Mantaka P, Baum RP, Hertel A et al. PET with 2-[F-18]-fluoro-2-deoxy-D-glucose (FDG) in patients with cancer of unknown primary (CUP): influence on patients' diagnostic and therapeutic management. *Cancer Biother Radiopharm* 2003;**18**:47–58.

18. Kole AC, Nieweg OE, Pruim J et al. Detection of unknown occult primary tumors using positron emission tomography. *Cancer* 1998;**82**:1160–6.

19. Stewart JF, Tattersall MH, Woods RL, Fox RM. Unknown primary adenocarcinoma: incidence of overinvestigation and natural history. *Br Med J* 1979;**1**:1530–3.

20. Abbruzzese JL, Abbruzzese MC, Hess KR et al. Unknown primary carcinoma: natural history and prognostic factors in 657 consecutive patients. *J Clin Oncol* 1994;**12**:1272–80.

21. Rusthoven KE, Koshy M, Paulino AC. The role of fluorodeoxyglucose positron emission tomography in cervical lymph node metastases from an unknown primary tumor. *Cancer* 2004;**101**:2641–9.

A 69-year-old male with poorly differentiated carcinoma in left cervical nodes. CT scan of the head and neck did not reveal a primary tumor site, and history, physical exam, and laboratory results were unremarkable. Endoscopic evaluation under anesthesia was planned, but had not been performed at the time of the staging FDG-PET study.

## Acquisition and processing parameters

The day before the study, the patient was called and instructed on a high protein, low carbohydrate, and low sugar meal, and to take nothing by mouth, except water, for at least 6 hours before the appointment. Upon arrival, a peripheral intravenous catheter was placed, and 9.3 mCi of FDG was administered intravenously; the catheter was removed after injection, and the entire setup was counted to determine the residual FDG. Fingerstick glucose level was 91 mg/dL at the time of injection. He was instructed to rest quietly in a room, with a warm blanket and the lights dimmed. After a 90-min uptake period, the patient was encouraged to void before imaging on a combined PET/CT scanner. Unenhanced CT from the thoracic inlet to the mid thighs was obtained first, with the patient in the supine position and arms above the head, and without any specific breath-holding instructions. CT scan parameters were 120 kVp, 300 mA, 0.5 s rotation speed, 1.375 pitch, with a reconstructed slice thickness of 3.75 mm. The CT data were reconstructed using a soft algorithm and a $512 \times 512$ matrix, with a transaxial field of view of 50 cm. PET emission images were then acquired over the same body region, starting superiorly and moving inferiorly, in 3-D mode, for 3 min per bed position and 47 image planes per bed position with a 7-slice overlap between them, and a 15.4 cm longitudinal field of view. PET data were reconstructed using an ordered-subset expectation maximization iterative algorithm (20 subsets and 2 iterations).

Subsequently, the patient was instructed to lower his arms to the side of the body, and non-contrast CT and PET emission images were obtained from the vertex of the head to the thoracic inlet. The acquisition parameters were the same as for the previously acquired whole-body images.

## Findings and differential diagnosis

MIP image of the head and neck shows hypermetabolism in multiple left cervical lymph nodes (Figure 17.1A), as also shown in the axial fusion image (Figure 17.1B). There is subtle soft tissue fullness in the left fossa of Rosenmuller (Figure 17.1C) with focal hypermetabolism on fusion images (Figure 17.1D), suggesting a primary tumor site.

## Diagnosis and clinical follow-up

Nasopharyngoscopy did not identify any mucosal abnormalities; however, biopsies at the fossa of Rosenmuller revealed a non-keratinizing nasopharyngeal carcinoma WHO grade II/III. He went on to have chemoradiation therapy, with 70 Gy to the area of gross disease followed by consolidation chemotherapy with 5-fluorouracil and cisplatin. His post-therapy course was complicated by xerostomia (dry mouth), mucositis, and lymphedema of the anterior neck and lower face.

## Discussion and teaching points

Primary tumors of the head and neck frequently present with metastatic disease involving cervical nodes. A primary site is often found in the palatine tonsil, base of tongue, or nasopharynx; however, in 3–7% of cases a primary tumor is not identified (1, 2). These patients commonly undergo unilateral comprehensive neck dissection followed by comprehensive irradiation of the neck and mucosal surfaces (1). Generally, patients who present with cervical nodal metastases and an occult primary in the head and neck represent a favorable subset of patients with an unknown primary; however, the extent of nodal disease greatly affects the prognosis, and comprehensive irradiation leads to frequent complications, including xerostomia, mucositis, skin damage, dysphagia, and stricture. Identification of a primary tumor site allows targeted radiation therapy, potentially sparing the patient unnecessary morbidity.

The role of FDG-PET in identifying an occult primary is perhaps best described for patients presenting with cervical metastases. A meta-analysis by Rusthoven *et al.* reported identification of a primary tumor in 25% of patients after a negative conventional work-up (3). Other previously unrecognized metastases were also identified in 39 patients (27%), with distant metastases in 12 cases (11%). In a prospective study, Johansen *et al.* studied 64 patients with metastatic disease in cervical nodes and a negative conventional evaluation, and reported that FDG-PET identified a primary tumor in 29% of patients after conventional evaluation, and resulted in changes in therapy in 25% of patients (4). This included reduction in radiation treatment volume in 10 cases (17%), and detection of disseminated metastases or a distant primary site in the other five cases (9%). Roh *et al.* compared the accuracy of FDG-PET/CT against contrast-enhanced CT scans in 44 patients presenting with cervical nodal metastases, and found that FDG-PET/CT had higher sensitivity, identifying 14/16 primary sites (88%) versus 7/16 (44%), with similar specificity of 82% vs. 89% (5).

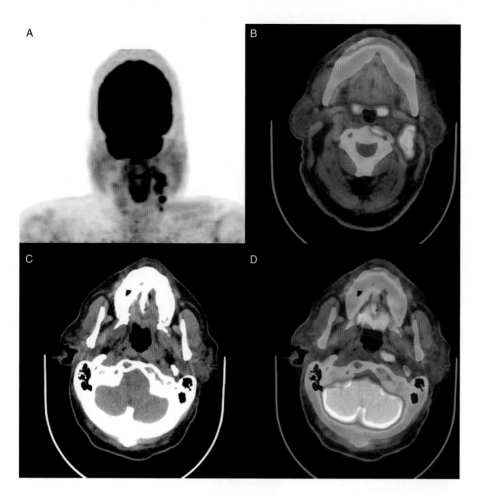

**Figure 17.1** (A) MIP image of the head and neck; (B) fused FDG-PET/CT of the neck; (C) axial CT; (D) fused FDG-PET/CT at the level of the fossa of Rosenmuller.

In this case, an occult primary in the head and neck was suspected; however, conventional work-up was unrevealing, and there were no suspicious mucosal lesions on endoscopic evaluation. However, based upon the FDG-PET/CT findings, biopsies of the fossa of Rosenmuller revealed the primary tumor, which was likely deep to the mucosal surface. These findings allowed relative sparing of other mucosal surfaces during radiation therapy, perhaps saving this patient from worse complications.

## Take-home message

- FDG-PET/CT frequently identifies an occult primary tumor site in the head and neck, even after a negative conventional evaluation.
- FDG-PET/CT frequently alters patient management, by identifying a primary tumor outside the head and neck or distant metastases, or by allowing targeted radiation therapy.

## References

1. Galer CE, Kies MS. Evaluation and management of the unknown primary carcinoma of the head and neck. *J Natl Compr Canc Netw* 2008;**6**:1068–75.

2. Miller FR, Karnad AB, Eng T *et al.* Management of the unknown primary carcinoma: long-term follow-up on a negative PET scan and negative panendoscopy. *Head Neck* 2008;**30**:28–34.

3. Rusthoven KE, Koshy M, Paulino AC. The role of fluorodeoxyglucose positron emission tomography in cervical lymph node metastases from an unknown primary tumor. *Cancer* 2004;**101**:2641–9.

4. Johansen J, Buus S, Loft A *et al.* Prospective study of 18FDG-PET in the detection and management of patients with lymph node metastases to the neck from an unknown primary tumor. Results from the DAHANCA-13 study. *Head Neck* 2008;**30**:471–8.

5. Roh JL, Kim JS, Lee JH *et al.* Utility of combined (18)F-fluorodeoxyglucose-positron emission tomography and computed tomography in patients with cervical metastases from unknown primary tumors. *Oral Oncol* 2009;**45**:218–24.

A 56-year-old male with a 2-month history of fatigue and anorexia, who presented with a left neck mass. Biopsy revealed poorly differentiated squamous cell carcinoma. Fiberoptic inspection of the head and neck was unrevealing. A FDG-PET/CT study was ordered for staging.

## Acquisition and processing parameters

After fasting for least 6 hours, 16.6 mCi of FDG was administered intravenously. He was instructed to rest quietly in a room, with a warm blanket and dimmed lights. After an 80-min uptake period, the patient was encouraged to void before imaging on a combined PET/CT scanner. He was placed in the supine position and imaged without any specific breath-holding instructions. The unenhanced CT scan was performed first, from skull vertex to mid thighs, using the following acquisition parameters:

140 kVp, 120 mA, 0.5 s rotation speed, 1.375 pitch, with a reconstructed slice thickness of 3.75 mm. The CT images were used to generate the transmission maps for attenuation correction of the PET acquisitions and for diagnostic purposes.

Immediately after the CT scan, and without changing the patient's position, the PET emission scan was acquired over the same body area, starting superiorly and moving inferiorly, in 2-D mode for 3 min per bed position. PET data were reconstructed using an ordered-subset expectation maximization iterative algorithm (30 subsets and 2 iterations).

## Findings and differential diagnosis

MIP images show extensive hypermetabolism, not only in the left neck, but also involving the abdomen (Figure 17.2A). Fusion images suggest a primary distal esophageal tumor

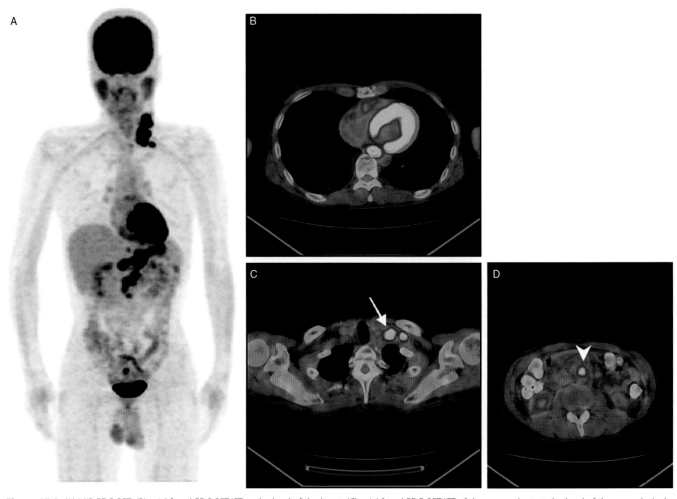

**Figure 17.2** (A) MIP FDG-PET; (B) axial fused FDG-PET/CT at the level of the heart; (C) axial fused FDG-PET/CT of the upper chest at the level of the supraclavicular regions; (D) axial fused FDG-PET/CT at the level of the abdomen.

(Figure 17.2B) in addition to non-regional nodal involvement, including left supraclavicular (Figure 17.2C, arrow) and retroperitoneal nodes (Figure 17.2D, arrow head).

## Diagnosis and clinical follow-up

Subsequent upper endoscopy and biopsy revealed a poorly differentiated squamous cell carcinoma in the mid-esophagus. The presence of cervical and distal retroperitoneal nodes made him ineligible for surgery. His disease was initially stable, after starting carboplatin, paclitaxel, and capecitabine with palliative radiation (45 Gy) to the left neck mass; however, he had subsequent progression and rapid decline, and was referred for hospice care.

## Discussion and teaching points

The initial presentation of this patient is typical for occult malignancy, with several months of weight loss, fatigue, and malaise preceding diagnosis. He was originally referred to an ENT specialist, and considered to have an occult primary in the head and neck with N2b disease. However, in this case, the cervical nodes represented distant metastases with a primary tumor outside the head and neck. In the National Oncologic PET Registry, PET imaging was found to alter management in 36.5% of cases (1); similar frequencies have also been reported for patients with carcinoma of unknown primary (2, 3).

In the absence of symptoms or findings suggesting disease beyond the head and neck, evaluation of the rest of the body is often cursory. However, spread to left supraclavicular nodes by visceral organ tumors is a well-known phenomenon, described in 1848 by Virchow and in 1889 by Troisier. In one large series, supraclavicular nodal involvement was reported in only 2.8% of 4,365 patients with thoracic or abdominal cancers (4). However, another study in 1956 suggested the incidence of involvement is much greater when carefully examined for, being present in 37% of patients with "tumor death" (5), suggesting that metastases to left supraclavicular or lower cervical nodes via the thoracic duct is fairly common but may be difficult to palpate.

Whole-body FDG-PET is a convenient way to assess the extent of disease in one procedure, and in this case identified a primary tumor outside the head and neck, in addition to substantial retroperitoneal disease. This led to a dramatic change in management. Chemotherapy became the primary treatment modality, and radiation therapy was used in a palliative role. PET was also useful in recognizing the lack of response to therapy, and the subsequent decision for hospice care.

## Take-home message

- Thoracic and abdominal malignancies frequently metastasize to left supraclavicular and cervical nodes.
- Whole body FDG-PET/CT is a convenient way to quickly identify non-regional tumor involvement.

## References

1. Hillner BE, Siegel BA, Liu D *et al.* Impact of positron emission tomography/computed tomography and positron emission tomography (PET) alone on expected management of patients with cancer: initial results from the National Oncologic PET Registry. *J Clin Oncol* 2008;**26**:2155–61.

2. Rusthoven KE, Koshy M, Paulino AC. The role of fluorodeoxyglucose positron emission tomography in cervical lymph node metastases from an unknown primary tumor. *Cancer* 2004;**101**:2641–9.

3. Seve P, Billotey C, Broussolle C, Dumontet C, Mackey JR. The role of 2-deoxy-2-[F-18]fluoro-D-glucose positron emission tomography in disseminated carcinoma of unknown primary site. *Cancer* 2007;**109**:292–9.

4. Viacava EP, Pack GT. Significance of supraclavicular signal node in patients with abdominal and thoracic cancer. A study of one hundred and twenty-two cases. *Arch Surg* 1944;**48**:109–19.

5. Young JM. The thoracic duct in malignant disease. *Am J Pathol* 1956;**32**:253–69.

A 65-year-old female with progressive ataxia over 4 months, and now requiring a wheelchair. Imaging of the head did not reveal any focal abnormality; however, her work-up was notable for anti-Yo antibodies, consistent with a paraneoplastic syndrome. FDG-PET/CT was requested for identification of an occult primary neoplasm.

## Acquisition and processing parameters

The patient was instructed to take nothing by mouth, except water, for at least 6 hours before the appointment. Upon arrival, the height and weight were checked, and the patient was interviewed. A peripheral intravenous catheter was placed, and 20 mCi of FDG was administered intravenously along with 250 cc normal saline. Fingerstick glucose level was 98 mg/dL at time of injection. She was instructed to rest quietly in a room.

After a 50-min uptake period, the patient was encouraged to void before imaging on a combined PET/CT scanner. She was imaged in the supine position, with arms above the head and without any specific breath-holding instructions. The unenhanced CT scan was performed first, from orbits to mid thighs, using the following acquisition parameters: 120 kVp, 200 mA, 0.5 s rotation speed, 0.984 pitch, with a reconstructed slice thickness of 3.75 mm. The CT images were used to generate the transmission maps for attenuation correction of the PET emission data and for diagnostic purposes. Immediately after the CT scan, and without changing the patient's position, the PET emission scan was acquired over the same region, starting superiorly and moving inferiorly, in 2-D mode for 4 min per bed position. PET data were reconstructed using an ordered-subset expectation maximization iterative algorithm (21 subsets, 2 iterations).

## Findings and differential diagnosis

The MIP image shows hypermetabolic foci in the left chest and axilla (Figure 17.3). A left breast mass is seen on the CT image (Figure 17.4A) corresponding to a hypermetabolic focus shown on the fusion image (Figure 17.4B), consistent with occult breast cancer. Enlarged left axillary nodes (Figure 17.5A) are also hypermetabolic (Figure 17.5B, arrow) and consistent with regional nodal involvement.

## Diagnosis and clinical follow-up

Biopsy revealed invasive ductal carcinoma in the left breast. The patient underwent a modified radical left mastectomy. The tumor was less than 2 cm in size (T1), estrogen (ER) and progesterone receptor (PR) negative, with more than 10 lymph nodes were involved (N3).

## Discussion and teaching points

Paraneoplastic syndromes are characterized by an indirect biologic effect by a tumor. These can be hormone-mediated, such as vasopressin-mediated syndrome of inappropriate antidiuretic hormone secretion (SIADH) in lung cancer, or associated with antibodies, such as anti-acetylcholine receptor antibody mediated myasthenia gravis in thymoma. Paraneoplastic syndromes affecting the nervous system are relatively rare, and there are several well-defined presentations associated with specific auto-antibodies (1). These patients usually present with neurologic symptoms and an occult primary tumor. The initial search for an occult malignancy may be negative, and experts suggest repeat imaging, as a tumor may be identified a year or more after presentation (2).

Progressive cerebellar ataxia is associated with anti-Yo antibodies, directed against Purkinje cells. It is associated with breast and ovarian cancers, but has also been reported with Hodgkin's lymphoma, uterine, gastric, and lung cancers (2, 3). These patients are often severely incapacitated and become bedridden within a few months of presentation. Identification and treatment of the tumor is the best chance for stabilization

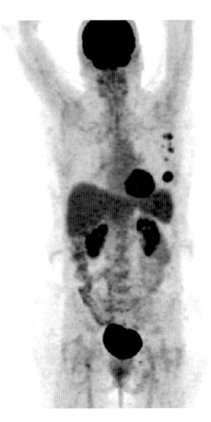

**Figure 17.3** FDG-MIP.

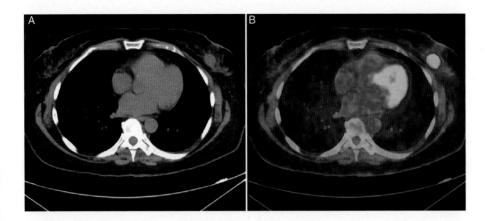

**Figure 17.4** (A) Axial CT; (B) Fused FDG-PET/CT of the chest.

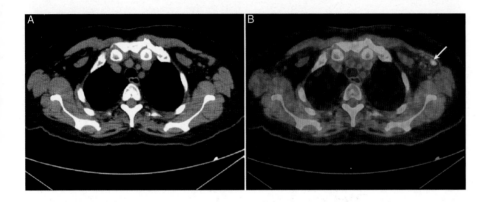

**Figure 17.5** (A) axial CT; (B) fused FDG-PET/CT of the upper chest including the axillae.

of the symptoms; however, the symptoms may persist even after treatment of the primary tumor (4).

FDG-PET/CT allows for evaluation of the whole body in one procedure, and provides important information about loco-regional and distant spread of tumor. A recent study reported that FDG-PET identified an occult primary in two of four patients with an antibody-positive paraneoplastic neurologic syndrome, but only four of 46 patients with clinically suspected paraneoplastic syndrome without an associated antibody (5). Similarly, Hadjivassiliou *et al.* reported that FDG-PET identified a primary tumor in seven of 37 (19%) of patients with antibody-positive paraneoplastic neurologic syndromes but in only two of 43 (5%) of patients without an associated antibody (6). These studies suggest that FDG-PET is more effective in evaluating patients with an antibody-positive paraneoplastic syndrome. Several studies also report that FDG-PET identifies an occult primary in patients with an antibody-associated paraneoplastic syndrome, even after a negative conventional work-up including CT scans (7, 8).

In this case, the patient presented with rapidly progressing cerebellar ataxia. Evaluation did not reveal a lesion within the central nervous system to explain the clinical presentation, and the presence of anti-Yo antibodies suggested an occult malignancy in a paraneoplastic syndrome. Based on the PET findings, the patient underwent surgical resection and was started on adjuvant therapy.

## Take-home message

- Paraneoplastic syndromes are characterized by an indirect biologic effect from an occult malignancy. Paraneoplastic neurologic syndromes are usually antibody mediated; the clinical manifestations precede identification of the occult tumor by more than a year. Identification and treatment of the occult tumor is the best hope for clinical stabilization.

- Whole-body FDG-PET/CT allows rapid identification of an occult malignancy in paraneoplastic syndromes. FDG-PET/CT detects primary tumors not found on conventional work-up.

## References

1. Darnell RB, Posner JB. Paraneoplastic syndromes involving the nervous system. *New Engl J Med* 2003;**349**:1543–54.

2. Vedeler CA, Antoine JC, Giometto B *et al.* Management of paraneoplastic neurological syndromes: report of an EFNS Task Force. *Eur J Neurol* 2006;**13**:682–90.

3. Noorani A, Sadiq Z, Minakaran N et al. Paraneoplastic cerebellar degeneration as a presentation of breast cancer – a case report and review of the literature. *Int Semin Surg Oncol* 2008;**5**:8.

4. Shams'ili S, Grefkens J, de Leeuw B *et al*. Paraneoplastic cerebellar degeneration associated with antineuronal antibodies: analysis of 50 patients. *Brain* 2003; **126**:1409–18.

5. Bannas P, Weber C, Derlin T *et al*. (18) F-FDG-PET/CT in the diagnosis of paraneoplastic neurological syndromes: a retrospective analysis. *Eur Radiol* 2010;**20**(4): 923–30.

6. Hadjivassiliou M, Alder SJ, Van Beek EJ *et al*. PET scan in clinically suspected paraneoplastic neurological syndromes: a 6-year prospective study in a regional neuroscience unit. *Acta Neurol Scand* 2009; **119**:186–93.

7. Linke R, Schroeder M, Helmberger T, Voltz R. Antibody-positive paraneoplastic neurologic syndromes: value of CT and PET for tumor diagnosis. *Neurology* 2004;**63**:282–6.

8. Younes-Mhenni S, Janier MF, Cinotti L *et al*. FDG-PET improves tumour detection in patients with paraneoplastic neurological syndromes. *Brain* 2004;**127**:2331–8.

A 69-year-old female with newly diagnosed squamous cell carcinoma of the supraglottic larynx. CT scan showed involvement of the thyroid cartilage and bilateral cervical nodal involvement, consistent with T4N2c disease. An FDG-PET scan was requested to evaluate for distant metastatic disease.

## Acquisition and processing parameters

The patient was instructed to take nothing by mouth, except water, for at least 6 hours before the appointment. A peripheral intravenous catheter was placed, and 19.4 mCi of FDG was administered intravenously. Fingerstick glucose level was 92 mg/dL at time of injection. She was allowed to rest quietly in a room, with a warm blanket and the lights dimmed. After a 100-min uptake period, the patient was encouraged to void before imaging on a combined PET/CT scanner. She was placed in a supine position, with arms above the head and without any specific breath-holding instructions. The unenhanced CT scan was performed first, from the orbits to mid thighs, using the following acquisition parameters: 120 kVp, 300 mA, 0.5 s rotation speed, 1.375 pitch, with a reconstructed slice thickness of 3.75 mm. The CT images were used to generate the transmission maps for attenuation correction of the PET acquisitions and for diagnostic purposes.

Immediately after the CT scan, and without changing the patient's position, the PET emission images were acquired over the same region, starting superiorly and moving inferiorly, in 2-D mode for 3 min per bed position. PET data were reconstructed using an ordered-subset expectation maximization iterative algorithm (20 subsets, 2 iterations).

## Findings and differential diagnosis

MIP images show multiple suspicious foci in the neck and chest (Figure 17.6). CT and fusion images show a right laryngeal mass and contralateral cervical nodal involvement (Figure 17.7A, 17.7B). A spiculated left upper lobe nodule is also FDG avid (Figure 17.8A, 17.8B). In addition, increased activity is seen in hilar and axillary lymph nodes (Figure 17.9A, 17.9B, respectively). These findings may be consistent with thoracic metastases from a primary laryngeal tumor, with an unrelated primary lung neoplasm with nodal metastases, and with reactive or metastatic axillary nodes.

## Diagnosis and clinical follow-up

Biopsy of the left upper lobe nodule revealed a poorly differentiated squamous cell carcinoma, and subsequent endobronchial ultrasound and biopsy revealed metastatic carcinoma involving the left hilar nodes without mediastinal nodal involvement. This was considered to be a separate lung primary. Biopsy of axillary nodes did not identify malignancy; however, a left breast mass was seen on mammography, and biopsy revealed invasive ductal carcinoma.

After induction chemotherapy with Taxol and carboplatin, the patient went on to have surgery, with involvement of three surgical teams. Final diagnosis revealed three synchronous primaries: a T4N2c squamous cell carcinoma of the larynx, a T1N1 squamous cell carcinoma of the left upper lobe of the lung, and a T1N0 invasive ductal carcinoma of the left breast. She received adjuvant chemoradiation with cisplatin and 57–70 Gy of radiation to the neck, before starting Arimidex (Anastrozole) as adjuvant therapy for her breast cancer.

## Discussion and teaching points

Patients with malignancies of the head and neck share many of the same risks for lung and other cancers, and may have synchronous cancers at presentation or subsequently develop a second or third malignancy. Large studies have reported the identification of an unrelated malignancy in 1–5% of FDG-PET studies (1–3). These include lung, thyroid, colorectal, breast, esophageal, uterus or ovary, and other head and neck tumors.

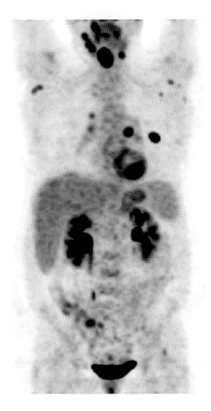

**Figure 17.6** FDG MIP image.

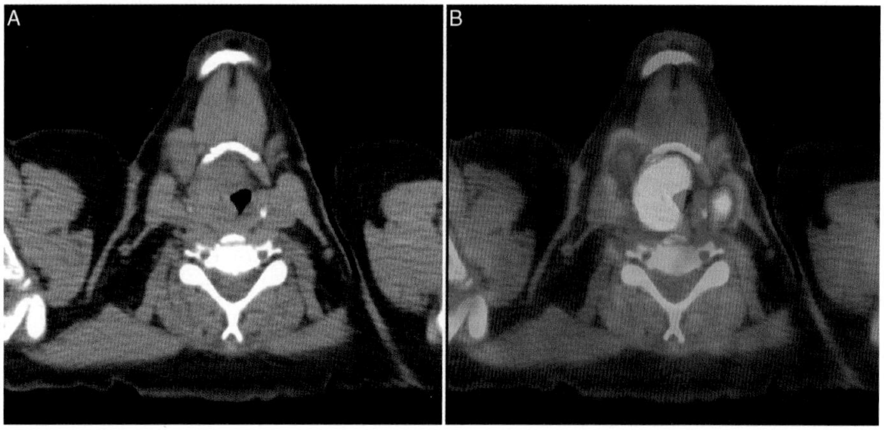

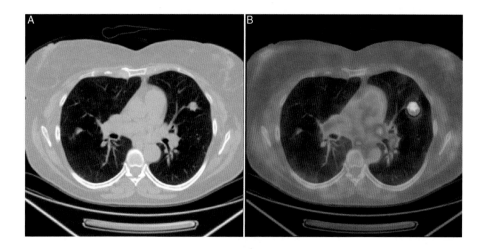

**Figure 17.7** (A) axial CT; (B) fused FDG-PET/CT of the neck.

**Figure 17.8** (A) axial CT; (B) fused FDG-PET/CT of the upper chest.

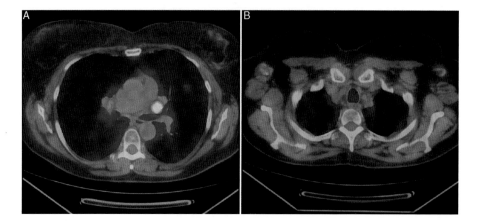

**Figure 17.9** Axial fused FDG-PET/CT images of the chest: (A) hilar regions; (B) upper chest and axillae.

In this case, an unrelated primary lung cancer was identified on FDG-PET, and although the axillary nodal activity was a false-positive finding, further evaluation led to the identification of another unrelated tumor in the breast. The presence of surgically treatable, synchronous tumors in the lung and the breast influenced the decision to undergo laryngectomy and neck dissection rather than chemoradiation therapy.

## Take-home message

- A second malignancy is found incidentally on 1–5% of FDG-PET/CT studies.

# References

1. Agress H, Jr., Cooper BZ. Detection of clinically unexpected malignant and premalignant tumors with whole-body FDG PET: histopathologic comparison. *Radiology* 2004;**230**:417–22.

2. Choi JY, Lee KS, Kwon OJ *et al.* Improved detection of second primary cancer using integrated [18F] fluorodeoxyglucose positron emission tomography and computed tomography for initial tumor staging. *J Clin Oncol* 2005;**23**:7654–9.

3. Ishimori T, Patel PV, Wahl RL. Detection of unexpected additional primary malignancies with PET/CT. *J Nucl Med* 2005;**46**:752–7.

A 65-year-old male, with metastatic carcinoma involving mediastinal nodes, with presumed lung primary, referred for staging evaluation.

## Acquisition and processing parameters

The patient was called and instructed to take nothing by mouth, except water, for at least 6 hours before the appointment. Upon arrival, a peripheral intravenous catheter was placed, and 9.8 mCi of FDG was administered intravenously. Fingerstick glucose level was 100 mg/dL at the time of injection. He was instructed to rest quietly in a room, with a warm blanket and the lights dimmed. After a 100-min uptake period, the patient was encouraged to void before imaging on a combined PET/CT scanner. He was imaged in the supine position, with arms above the head and without any specific breath-holding instructions. The unenhanced CT scan was performed first, from orbits to mid thighs, using the following acquisition parameters: 120 kVp, 296 mA, 0.5 s rotation speed, 1.375 pitch, with a reconstructed slice thickness of 3.75 mm. The CT images were used to generate the transmission maps for attenuation correction of the PET acquisitions and for diagnostic purposes.

Immediately after the CT scan, and without changing the patient's position, the PET emission scan was acquired over the same region, starting superiorly and moving inferiorly, in 3-D mode for 3 min per bed position with a 7 slice overlap between bed positions. PET data were reconstructed using an ordered-subset expectation maximization iterative algorithm (20 subsets and 2 iterations).

## Findings and differential diagnosis

A rounded left lower lobe nodule is not FDG avid (Figure 17.10A, 17.10B). Fusion images show no uptake in the right hilar (Figure 17.11A) or other mediastinal regions, despite the enlarged lymph nodes seen on contrast CT (Figure 17.11B).

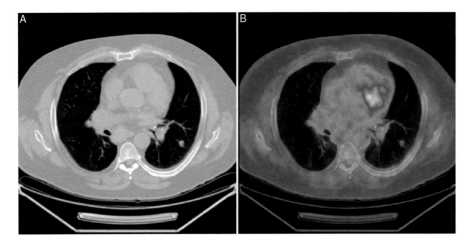

**Figure 17.10** (A) axial CT; (B) fused FDG-PET/CT of the chest.

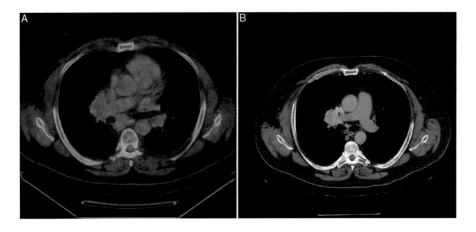

**Figure 17.11** (A) axial fused FDG-PET/CT; (B) axial contrast enhanced CT of the chest.

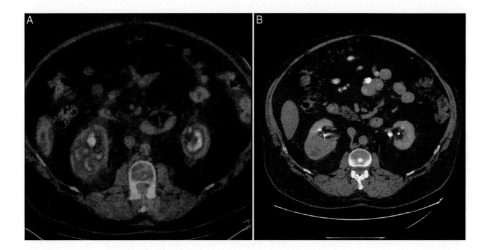

**Figure 17.12** (A) Fused FDG-PET/CT; (B) axial contrast enhanced CT of the abdomen.

A right renal mass, also not FDG avid, is seen in the fusion images (Figure 17.12A). The differential diagnoses include metastatic renal cell carcinoma, versus unusual non-small cell lung cancer with non-regional and distant metastases, versus unrelated renal mass with a non-avid thoracic tumor.

## Diagnosis and clinical follow-up

Tissue from fine-needle aspirates of the mediastinal nodes was originally reported as non-small cell carcinoma. Additional immunohistochemistry stains were positive for vimentin and CD10, consistent with sarcoma or renal cell carcinoma. Subsequent contrast-enhanced CT scan confirmed a right renal mass (Figure 17.12B), and right nephrectomy revealed a 6 cm clear cell renal cell carcinoma, with extension into the renal vein (T3b).

## Discussion and teaching points

The FDG avidity of a tissue also contributes to its characterization. Although non-avid tissues are usually considered benign, it is important to remember that not all malignant tumors are positive on FDG-PET. These can loosely be categorized by mechanism: low cellular density (e.g., mucinous or lipomatous tumors and bronchioloalveolar carcinomas), relatively slow proliferation/metabolic rate (e.g., thyroid and prostate cancers), rapid clearance of FDG (e.g., well-differentiated hepatocellular carcinomas which have high glucose-6-phosphatase (1)), and regional high background activity (e.g., bladder and brain tumors). Renal cell carcinomas (RCC) are variable in presentation on FDG-PET, with a lower sensitivity for slowly growing RCC (2, 3). The variable uptake and superimposed renal excretion of FDG makes identification of primary renal cell carcinomas challenging (2, 4, 5).

In this case, the patient presented with metastatic carcinoma involving mediastinal nodes, thought to originate from a primary lung site. However, these sites were not FDG avid, bringing into question the presumed diagnosis of lung cancer. The interpreting physician also identified a non-avid renal mass on non-contrast CT images, suggesting a possible primary tumor site, and prompting re-evaluation of pathology samples. Only limited tissue was available for immunohistochemistry, but the staining pattern was consistent with renal cell carcinoma. Subsequent imaging and surgery confirmed the presence of a renal neoplasm. The early recognition of a possible renal primary tumor facilitated additional evaluation, subsequent diagnosis, and the initiation of appropriate therapy in this patient. Restaging studies, after therapy with the receptor tyrosine kinase inhibitor, sunitinib, showed a positive response, with decreased size of mediastinal nodes and of the left lower lobe nodule.

## Take-home message

- The FDG avidity of a lesion can be used to characterize it. It is important to remember that not all malignant tumors are FDG avid.
- When confronted by a non-avid tumor, the CT component of the study is important in identifying other sites of disease.

## References

1. Gallagher BM, Fowler JS, Gutterson NI et al. Metabolic trapping as a principle of oradiopharmaceutical design: some factors responsible for the biodistribution of [18F] 2-deoxy-2-fluoro-D-glucose. *J Nucl Med* 1978;**19**:1154–61.

2. Bihl H, Lang O, Schleicher J et al. Metastatic renal cell carcinoma (mRCC). Is there a role of F-18-FDG-PET? *Clin Positron Imaging* 1999;**2**:340.

3. Ramdave S, Thomas GW, Berlangieri SU et al. Clinical role of F-18 fluorodeoxyglucose positron emission tomography for detection and management of renal cell carcinoma. *J Urol* 2001;**166**:825–30.

4. Ak I, Can C. F-18 FDG PET in detecting renal cell carcinoma. *Acta Radiol* 2005;**46**:895–9.

5. Lin SP, Bierhals AJ, Lewis JS, Jr. Best cases from the AFIP: metastatic renal cell carcinoma. *Radiographics* 2007;**27**:1801–7.

A 47-year-old male with biopsy-proven metastatic carcinoid to the liver. Multiphase contrast-enhanced CT of the abdomen and pelvis showed two hypervascular metastases in the liver and a mass near the pancreatic body/root of mesentery. A $^{68}$Ga-DOTA-TATE PET/CT was performed to localize the primary and for initial staging.

## Acquisition and processing parameters

After fasting for a period of 4 hours, and pre-hydration with water, the patient was injected with 5.4 mCi of $^{68}$Ga-DOTA-TATE, and an uptake period of 45 min was allowed prior to imaging. Iodine-based oral contrast (Ioscan) was administered at 50% dilution at 60 min, 30 min and 0 min before the scan. The patient was asked to void prior to scanning. Images were obtained from proximal thigh to the vertex of the skull with the patient lying supine with arms placed above his head. CT was performed with the following parameters: CT EffmAs 80 (CareDose), 80 kVp, 18.0 mm feed per rotation, and 3 mm slice reconstructions. Immediately following the CT acquisition, without changing the patient's position, the emission scan was acquired from thigh to skull, to minimize misregistration in the pelvis due to bladder distension during scanning, for a total of 7 bed positions of 4 min each. PET data were reconstructed using OSEM (3 subsets and 4 iterations).

## Findings and differential diagnosis

MIP image from $^{68}$Ga-DOTA-TATE PET shows normal activity in the spleen greater than the liver, with renal excretion (Figure 17.13A). There is focal activity in the liver, consistent with known hepatic metastasis (Figure 17.13A, 17.13B, arrow heads). CT images show subtle thickening of the jejunal wall with enlarged adjacent mesenteric nodes (Figure 17.14A). In addition to activity within mesenteric nodal disease, fusion images also show focal uptake in the adjacent proximal small

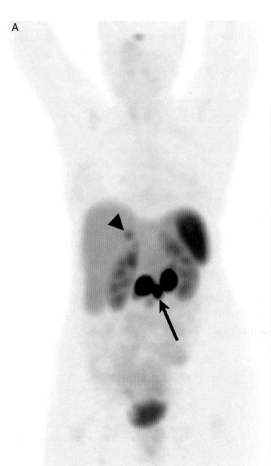
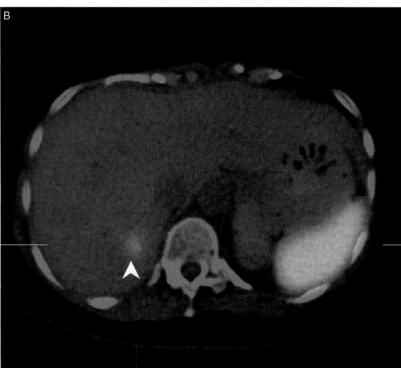

**Figure 17.13** (A) $^{68}$Ga-DOTA-TATE MIP image; (B) axial fused $^{68}$Ga-DOTA-TATE PET/CT.

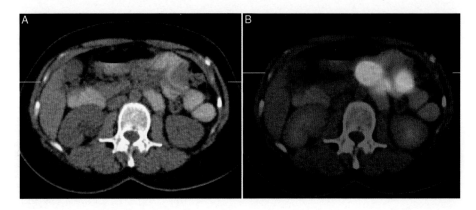

**Figure 17.14** (A) axial CT; (B) fused [68]Ga-DOTA-TATE PET/CT.

bowel (Figure 17.14B, Figure 17.13A, arrow). The differential diagnoses are primary carcinoid of the small bowel, versus metastatic pancreatic carcinoid, versus unknown primary neuroendocrine tumor with metastases.

## Diagnosis and clinical follow-up

The patient underwent partial resection of the small bowel and the mesenteric metastases, with concomitant partial hepatectomy. Pathology revealed primary neuroendocrine tumor of the jejunum, with mesenteric nodal and hepatic metastases.

## Discussion and teaching points

Gastroenteropancreatic neuroendocrine tumors (GEP NET) are a heterogeneous group of tumors deriving from endocrine cells; they are classified according to location or embryologic origin (foregut, midgut, and hindgut) (1, 2). Incidence is 1–4/100,000 per annum, of which approximately 50% are carcinoid tumors (3). Carcinoids of the foregut, including the jejunum, are uncommon, accounting for less than 10% of all carcinoids.

Somatostatin receptors (SR) are overexpressed at the cell membrane of a large variety of NET. Of the five subtypes, SR2 is predominant in NETs and exhibits greatest affinity for the available somatostatin analogs (4). Indium111-DTPA-octreotide is the principal analog in SR scintigraphy, and is the investigation of choice over conventional anatomical imaging because of the capability for whole-body imaging without additional radiation burden to the patient. Somatostatin receptor binding can also be used to evaluate patients for octreotide or radiopeptide therapy (1). FDG-PET has a limited role in staging of GEP NETs as most tumors in this group are slow growing and well differentiated with poor uptake of FDG. FDG-PET utility is limited primarily to assessment of poorly differentiated NETs (5). There appears to be a "flip-flop pattern" where FDG-positive lesions are SR-negative and vice-versa (6).

Several [68]Ga-labelled somatostatin analogs have been developed and are in clinical use outside the USA (7). A small number of reports suggest the [68]Ga-DOTA-peptides have high sensitivity and specificity for neuroendocrine tumors. Gabriel *et al.* studied 84 patients with neuroendocrine tumors, and reported 97% sensitivity and 92% specificity using PET/CT with [68]Ga-DOTA-peptide, compared with 52% and 92% for SPECT/CT with SRS, or 61% and 71% for contrast-enhanced CT (8). Kayani *et al.* also reported high sensitivity of [68]Ga-DOTA-peptide PET/CT, with detection in 31 of 38 patients (82%) compared with detection in 25 of 38 patients (66%) by FDG-PET/CT (9). A study by Prasad *et al.* reported detection of a primary tumor site using [68]Ga-DOTA-peptide PET/CT in 35 of 59 (59%) patients with metastatic neuroendocrine tumor and an unknown primary (10).

[68]Ga-DOTA-TATE PET was particularly useful in this case because it identified the bowel primary not detected on conventional anatomical imaging and correctly localized the mass anterior to the pancreas as a mesenteric nodal metastasis, which was confirmed at surgery. Whilst multiphase CT is excellent for identifying and characterizing liver lesions as metastases, it is not as good for identifying bowel primaries in NET. Moreover, although this patient's metastases were resectable, he would also be a candidate for somatostatin-based therapy.

## Take-home message

- [68]Ga-DOTA-TATE is a PET agent that binds to somatostatin receptors.
- Detection of neuroendocrine tumors (NETs) by [68]Ga-DOTA-peptide PET may be superior to other imaging techniques, including somatostatin receptor scintigraphy (SRS), contrast CT, and FDG-PET.

## References

1. Oberg K, Jelic S. Neuroendocrine gastroenteropancreatic tumors: ESMO clinical recommendations for diagnosis, treatment and follow-up. *Ann Oncol* 2008;**19**(Suppl 2): ii104–5.

2. Modlin IM, Kidd M, Latich I, Zikusoka MN, Shapiro MD. Current status of gastrointestinal carcinoids. *Gastroenterology* 2005; **128**:1717–51.

3. Modlin IM, Lye KD, Kidd M. A 5-decade analysis of 13,715 carcinoid tumors. *Cancer* 2003;**97**:934–59.

4. Rufini V, Calcagni ML, Baum RP. Imaging of neuroendocrine tumors. *Semin Nucl Med* 2006; **36**:228–47.

5. Adams S, Baum R, Rink T *et al.* Limited value of fluorine-18 fluorodeoxyglucose positron emission tomography for the imaging of neuroendocrine tumours. *Eur J Nucl Med* 1998;**25**:79–83.

6. Sundin A, Garske U, Orlefors H. Nuclear imaging of neuroendocrine tumours. *Best Pract Res Clin Endocrinol Metab* 2007;**21**:69–85.

7. Meyer GJ, Macke H, Schuhmacher J, Knapp WH, Hofmann M. 68Ga-labelled DOTA-derivatised peptide ligands. *Eur J Nucl Med Mol Imaging* 2004;**31**:1097–104.

8. Gabriel M, Decristoforo C, Kendler D *et al.* 68Ga-DOTA-Tyr3-octreotide PET in neuroendocrine tumors: comparison with somatostatin receptor scintigraphy and CT. *J Nucl Med* 2007;**48**:508–18.

9. Kayani I, Bomanji JB, Groves A *et al.* Functional imaging of neuroendocrine tumors with combined PET/CT using 68Ga-DOTATATE (DOTA-DPhe1, Tyr3-octreotate) and 18F-FDG. *Cancer* 2008;**112**:2447–55.

10. Prasad V, Ambrosini V, Hommann M *et al.* Detection of unknown primary neuroendocrine tumours (CUP-NET) using (68)Ga-DOTA-NOC receptor PET/CT. *Eur J Nucl Med Mol Imaging* 2010;**37**:67–77.

A 73-year-old male, with poorly differentiated carcinoma in the right pelvis, found after the patient complained of right lower abdominal pain. Immunohistochemsitry was positive for epithelial markers (cytokeratin and CAM5.2) and a squamous cell marker (p63); the staining pattern suggested urothelial carcinoma or squamous carcinoma. FDG-PET was acquired for staging.

## Acquisition and processing parameters

The patient was instructed to take nothing by mouth, except water, for at least 6 hours before the appointment. Upon arrival, the height and weight were checked and the patient was encouraged to void before the injection. A peripheral intravenous catheter was placed, and 18.6 mCi FDG was administered intravenously. He was instructed to rest quietly in a room, with a warm blanket and the lights dimmed.

After an uptake period of 65 min, the patient was encouraged to void before imaging on a combined PET/CT scanner. He was imaged in the supine position, with arms above the head and without any specific breath-holding instructions. The unenhanced CT scan was performed first, from orbits to mid thighs, using the following acquisition parameters: 120 kVp, 293 mA, 0.5 s rotation speed, 1.375 pitch, with a reconstructed slice thickness of 3.75 mm. The CT images were used to generate the transmission maps for attenuation correction of the PET acquisitions and for diagnostic purposes.

Immediately after the CT scan, and without changing the patient's position, the PET emission scan was acquired over the same region, starting superiorly and moving inferiorly, in 2-D mode for 3 min per bed position. PET data were reconstructed using an ordered-subset expectation maximization iterative algorithm (30 subsets and 2 iterations).

## Findings and differential diagnosis

Fusion images show a partially necrotic, lobulated, hypermetabolic focus in the right pelvis (Figure 17.15B). As shown on the MIP image, no other hypermetabolic foci are identified to suggest a primary tumor or other sites of disease (Figure 17.15A).

## Diagnosis, clinical follow-up, and further imaging to monitor response to therapy

The patient was diagnosed with cancer of unknown primary (CUP), and started on gemcitabine and cisplatin, as this would also cover bladder cancer. After two cycles, a restaging FDG-PET/CT scan showed interval progression, with enlargement of the pelvic mass and evidence of new right hydronephrosis and hydroureter (Figure 17.16A, 17.16B). The chemotherapy regimen was changed to Taxol, and restaging after 6 weeks also showed interval progression, with increasing size and persistent hypermetabolism. The patient was referred for definitive radiation therapy, with 50 Gy, boosted to 63 Gy along the pelvic sidewall. Restaging FDG-PET/CT (Figure 17.17A, 17.17B) showed minimal metabolic activity in the necrotic pelvis mass, similar to background, and no distant metastases. The mass decreased slightly in size, but remains without suspicious metabolic activity almost 2 years later. The patient is considered to be in remission.

A
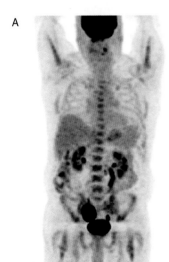

B
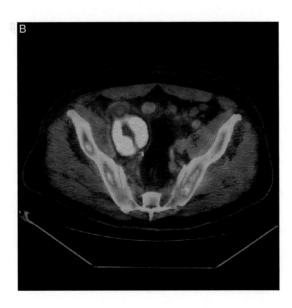

**Figure 17.15** Initial staging FDG-PET/CT.

A
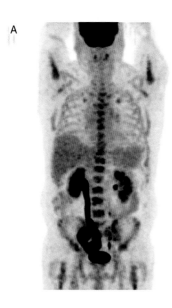
B
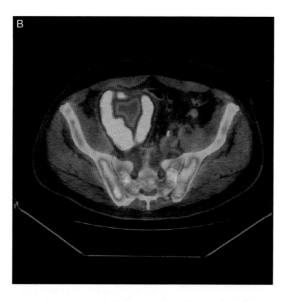

**Figure 17.16** FDG-PET/CT after two cycles of gemcitabine and cisplatin.

A
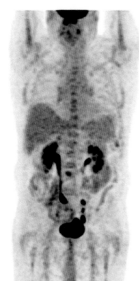
B
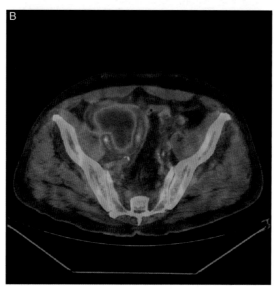

**Figure 17.17** Restaging FDG-PET/CT after definitive radiation therapy.

## Discussion and teaching points

When there is limited extent of disease, definitive local therapy may result in an improved outcome. In this case, there was clinical suspicion for more extensive disease than was detected on staging evaluation, and therefore empiric systemic therapy was used initially. Unfortunately, there was progression on two different chemotherapy regimens; however, despite local growth of the tumor in the pelvis, no distant metastases were revealed on restaging studies, suggesting the pelvic tumor as the only site of involvement. There are several theories for why a primary tumor is not found, including the embryologic migration error and the cancer stem cell theory (1).

FDG-PET is frequently used for post-therapy response assessment, and decreased activity has been reported to predict response to therapy in many different cancers, including esophageal, breast, and lung cancers (2–4).

FDG-PET evaluation has been incorporated into response assessment criteria for lymphoma (5), and also proposed as part of response criteria for solid tumors (6, 7). Perhaps even more intriguing, the early FDG-PET scan has been proposed to predict higher risk of treatment failure, and as an indicator to change to aggressive therapy in these individuals (8, 9), and this has become an active research topic in lymphoma.

In this case, FDG-PET was used to direct therapy. Although the staging exam suggested limited extent of disease, systemic therapy was used initially. Restaging FDG-PET studies showed that despite local progression after different chemotherapy regimens, there were no distant sites of tumor. The patient received definitive radiation therapy, with successful metabolic response and is considered in remission despite a persistent residual anatomic abnormality.

## Take-home message

- FDG-PET/CT may evaluate treatment response and direct subsequent therapy.

- Metabolic responses may precede anatomic changes, and FDG-PET may also be used to evaluate soft tissue abnormalities that remain after therapy.

## References

1. Greco FA, Hainsworth JD. Introduction: unknown primary cancer. *Semin Oncol* 2009;**36**:6–7.

2. Lordick F, Ott K, Krause BJ *et al.* PET to assess early metabolic response and to guide treatment of adenocarcinoma of the oesophagogastric junction: the MUNICON phase II trial. *Lancet Oncol* 2007;**8**:797–805.

3. Wahl RL, Zasadny K, Helvie M *et al.* Metabolic monitoring of breast cancer chemohormonotherapy using positron emission tomography: initial evaluation. *J Clin Oncol* 1993;**11**:2101–11.

4. Patz EF, Jr., Connolly J, Herndon J. Prognostic value of thoracic FDG PET imaging after treatment for non-small cell lung cancer. *Am J Roentgenol* 2000;**174**:769–74.

5. Cheson BD, Pfistner B, Juweid ME *et al.* Revised response criteria for malignant lymphoma. *J Clin Oncol* 2007;**25**:579–86.

6. Young H, Baum R, Cremerius U *et al.* Measurement of clinical and subclinical tumour response using [18F]-fluorodeoxyglucose and positron emission tomography: review and 1999 EORTC recommendations. European Organization for Research and Treatment of Cancer (EORTC) PET Study Group. *Eur J Cancer* 1999;**35**:1773–82.

7. Wahl RL, Jacene H, Kasamon Y, Lodge MA. From RECIST to PERCIST: evolving considerations for PET response criteria in solid tumors. *J Nucl Med* 2009;**50**(Suppl 1): 122S–50S.

8. Kasamon YL, Jones RJ, Wahl RL. Integrating PET and PET/CT into the risk-adapted therapy of lymphoma. *J Nucl Med* 2007;**48**(Suppl 1): 19S–27S.

9. Kasamon YL, Wahl RL, Ziessman HA *et al.* Phase II study of risk-adapted therapy of newly diagnosed, aggressive non-Hodgkin lymphoma based on midtreatment FDG-PET scanning. *Biol Blood Marrow Transplant* 2009;**15**:242–8.

# 18 Sarcoma

Katherine A. Zukotynski and Chun K. Kim

Sarcomas are solid malignant tumors arising from mesenchymal tissue with distinct clinical and pathological features. They constitute a diverse group of tumors with more than 50 different histological subtypes divided into two broad categories: sarcomas of soft tissues (including fat, muscles, nerves, blood vessels, and other connective tissues) and sarcomas of bones (1, 2). Several classification schemes for sarcoma exist. In general, classification is based on histology with tumors subdivided according to the presumed tissue of origin.

Sarcomas can occur anywhere in the body and at all ages in both men and women. The age of incidence depends, at least in part, on the type as well as the subtype. For example, osteosarcomas tend to develop in young adults while chondrosarcomas are more common in older patients. Sarcomas found within certain organs may be difficult to differentiate from other malignancies; therefore, the true incidence of sarcomas is likely underestimated (3). Collectively, sarcomas are believed to account for approximately 1% of all adult malignancies and 15% of all pediatric malignancies (1). While soft tissue sarcomas are overall more frequent in middle-aged and older adults than in children and young adults, some subtypes such as rhabdomyosarcoma and synovial sarcoma are more common in young patients. Indeed soft tissue sarcomas account for a large proportion of pediatric malignancies, i.e., 7–10%. The incidence of primary bone tumors is approximately one-fifth that of soft tissue sarcomas. However, primary bone tumors also represent a significant percentage of malignancies in patients under the age of 20. Sarcomas are an important cause of death in the 14–29 years age group (4). Even in adults, the number of years of life lost is substantial despite the very low incidence of the disease, because people are often affected during the prime of their life (3).

While the risk factors and etiology of most soft tissue sarcomas remain unknown, it is thought to be an association with hereditary syndromes, prior viral infection, occupational chemicals and/or radiotherapy for another cancer. Genetic aberrations associated with the disease also contribute significantly to the malignant potential of these tumors and can have an impact on prognosis, management, and survival.

Symptoms related to the sarcoma can be substantially different depending on the site of disease. The clinical course of sarcoma patients is variable. In patients with soft tissue sarcomas, the 5-year metastasis-free rate was found to be more dependent on the **histologic grade** rather than on the histologic type. While there were no statistically significant differences in the 5-year metastasis-free rate among tumors of different histologic type (but of the same grade), there were statistically significant differences in the 5-year metastasis-free rate amongst grade 1, grade 2, and grade 3 groups of combined soft tissue sarcomas, i.e., 91%, 71%, and 44%, respectively (5). The overall survival in patients with a soft tissue sarcoma is approximately 50% at 5 years, and the key determinant of survival is the control of both local recurrence as well as distant dissemination. The clinical presentation, course, and prognosis of patients with osteosarcoma, Ewing sarcoma, gastrointestinal stromal tumor (GIST), malignant peripheral nerve sheath tumor (MPNST) and synovial sarcoma will be discussed in the clinical cases that follow.

## Clinical management of patients with sarcoma

Effective management of patients with sarcoma requires accurate diagnosis and staging. In addition to the TNM stage, the histological grade (G) is taken into account to determine the sarcoma stage, which is different from staging the majority of other cancers. The histologic grade is based on tissue characteristics such as cellularity, differentiation, and mitotic rate, and may predict biologic behavior. The histologic grade is commonly evaluated using the FNCLCC (The Federation Nationale des Centre de Lutte Contre le Cancer) (1, 5). Typically, sarcomas are large heterogeneous masses with multiple components of differing biological characteristics and therefore, a tissue biopsy is essential for histologic grading. For TNM staging in patients with sarcoma, the T stage includes the **location** (depth) of the tumor in addition to the **size** of the tumor. Indeed, in patients with N0M0 disease, sarcoma size is a more important prognostic factor than the depth, and the histologic grade is a more important prognostic factor than the T stage (size and depth).

*A Case-Based Approach to PET/CT in Oncology*, ed. Victor H. Gerbaudo. Published by Cambridge University Press.
© Cambridge University Press 2012.

Management of patients with sarcoma is challenging because of the broad spectrum of disease with variable responses to surgery, radiation, and chemotherapy. Although increasing insight into the molecular pathways has recently led to the development of targeted therapies, in general, the mainstay of curative therapy is complete surgical resection. Even in the presence of metastatic disease, surgical resection of both the primary tumor and metastases may improve survival. Although sarcomas are relatively resistant to radiation, adjuvant radiation may be helpful for local control in certain cases. Multi-agent chemotherapy is often helpful, although the efficacy varies depending on the sarcoma subtype. One difficulty is that response following therapy may be difficult to assess by conventional response evaluation criteria in solid tumors (RECIST). $^{18}$F-fluorodeoxyglucose (FDG) positron emission tomography (PET) has shown promising results in this regard. The remainder of this chapter will primarily review the clinical utility of FDG-PET for diagnosis, staging, and assessment of treatment response and for follow-up in patients with sarcomas.

## Sarcoma staging with anatomic imaging

Conventional radiography is generally the first-line diagnostic modality to image sarcomas. It is useful for initial detection and characterization of skeletal sarcomas, but less valuable for evaluation of soft tissue sarcoma due to its poor contrast resolution.

Additional characterization of sarcomas beyond plain radiography is better achieved by magnetic resonance imaging (MRI) compared with computed tomography (CT). Advantages of MRI over CT include its exquisite contrast resolution, i.e., the capability to show soft tissue and blood vessels in greater detail, the higher sensitivity for the detection of marrow abnormalities, and the absence of ionizing radiation. With regards to sarcoma patients, MRI may be used to detect, characterize, and evaluate the extent of malignancy, and is considered to be the imaging modality of choice for locoregional staging of musculoskeletal masses. Although MRI is not as useful for the characterization of skeletal sarcomas, it is still the best modality for the evaluation of bone marrow involvement. MRI is also used to monitor tumor response to neoadjuvant therapy. However, the image acquisition time is significantly longer than for CT, which can be particularly problematic for claustrophobic patients, pediatric patients (who often require sedation), and seriously ill patients. Furthermore, gadolinium-induced nephrogenic systemic fibrosis is a grim complication in patients with renal insufficiency and may limit the use of MRI in this setting. Also, MRI may be contraindicated in patients with implanted metal devices.

CT can be particularly useful for sarcoma staging, particularly for imaging osseous lesions or when MRI is contraindicated. With regards to the evaluation of skeletal lesions, CT provides excellent cortical detail and shows the type and presence of cortical bone destruction. It also allows for the assessment of the presence and patterns of matrix mineralization. Mineralization as well as varying densities in soft tissue sarcoma also can be evaluated with CT. Other indications include characterization of adjacent tissues and assessment of fracture risk. CT angiography may be used to evaluate tumor size, extent, and vascularity. CT of the chest is a valuable tool for M staging as it is the most sensitive technique for detecting lung metastases (6). While CT is less expensive than MRI or PET, its main disadvantages include exposure to ionizing radiation and the need for intravenous contrast that may be associated with a risk of allergic reaction and/or contrast nephropathy.

Anatomic imaging, although essential for TNM staging, does not assess histology. Certain imaging features, such as the presence of necrosis, may suggest more aggressive disease, however, tissue sampling is needed to define histologic grade. Unfortunately, biopsies may be dictated by surgical convenience and miss the most aggressive portion of the tumor. Misinterpretation of the histologic grade due to sampling error can lead to inappropriate patient management, which may be catastrophic for the patient.

## Utility of FDG-PET in sarcoma

The main advantages of FDG-PET compared with conventional anatomic imaging modalities include the large field of view, consisting of imaging of the whole body and extremities, as well as the capability to evaluate tumor metabolic activity. Therefore, FDG-PET and conventional imaging are complementary for identifying sites of distant metastases. FDG-PET also identifies the most biologically aggressive portion of a tumor and may predict overall biologic behavior.

The intensity of FDG uptake on PET is typically described semi-quantitatively using the maximum standardized uptake value (SUVmax), peak SUV, or average SUV (SUVavg). These values have their respective advantages and disadvantages. The average SUV should not be used for the evaluation of sarcomas, however, particularly in the case of primary tumor grading, because it will often be erroneously low due to the heterogeneity of the tumor.

## Differential diagnosis and grading

The usefulness of FDG-PET for differentiating between benign lesions and sarcomas as well as for non-invasive grading of sarcomas has been assessed by numerous investigators. The intensity of FDG uptake by sarcomas generally correlates with tumor grade as well as markers of cell proliferation such as cellularity, mitotic activity, Ki-67 labeling index and p53 overexpression (7–10). A meta-analysis of seven studies with 157 primary soft tissue lesions published in 2003 (11) showed that the sensitivity and specificity of FDG-PET for diagnosing malignant versus benign lesions was 79% and 77% using SUV $\geq$ 2.0, and 60% and 86% using SUV $\geq$ 3.0 as the criteria, respectively. Upon correlation of SUV with tumor grade, an SUV higher than 2.0 was seen in 59/66 (89.4%) intermediate/high-grade malignant lesions, 8/24 (33.3%) low-grade malignant lesions, and 13/68 (19.1%) benign lesions. An SUV above 3.0 was seen in 45/66 (68.2%) intermediate/high-grade malignant lesions, 3/24 (12.5%) low-grade malignant lesions, and 8/68 (11.8%) benign lesions, respectively. With either cut-off, there was no statistically significant difference between the low-grade malignant lesions and the benign lesions, whereas intermediate/high-grade malignant lesions differed significantly from both other groups. It was concluded that FDG-PET may be helpful in tumor grading but offers inadequate discrimination between low-grade tumors and benign lesions. Another meta-analysis from mixed types of sarcomas published in 2004 found similar results, i.e., statistically significant difference in FDG avidity between high-grade sarcomas and low-grade sarcomas, but not between low-grade sarcomas and benign tumors. It has also been reported that certain benign diseases such as giant cell tumors are associated with FDG uptake that may be as high as or even higher than that of high-grade sarcomas (12–15).

A recent report describes the correlation of FDG uptake with grade not only within the group of sarcomas as a whole but also within individual sarcoma subtypes, using the French 3-tier grading system (low, intermediate, and high) and a proposed 2-tier system (low and high). While FDG uptake increases with grade for most sarcoma subtypes, there was a considerable overlap in FDG uptake between tumors of different grades as shown by earlier studies of mixed sarcomas. Some subtypes showed relatively higher FDG uptake, e.g., malignant peripheral nerve sheath tumors (MPNST) and "not otherwise specified" (NOS), or lower uptake, e.g., desmoid, GIST, and primitive neuroectodermal tumor, than other subtypes. However, individual sarcoma subtypes could not be discriminated on the basis of FDG uptake alone due to a significant overlap.

In summary, FDG uptake in sarcomas is generally higher than in benign lesions. Also, FDG uptake generally correlates with the tumor grade. However, there is considerable overlap in intensity of FDG uptake between grades as well as between subtypes, limiting the ability of FDG to differentiate, especially between low-grade sarcomas and benign lesions. Therefore, tissue sampling is still needed for both diagnosis and histologic grading.

## Detection/monitoring of malignant transformation

While the differentiation between sarcomas and benign lesions cannot be made solely on the basis of FDG uptake, FDG-PET can be useful in specific clinical settings, such as, for example, the detection of or monitoring of malignant transformation. Individuals with neurofibromatosis 1 (NF1) have 8–12% lifetime risk of developing malignant peripheral nerve sheath tumors (MPNSTs) (15, 16). Differentiating between benign and malignant tumors has important prognostic and therapeutic implications, but can be difficult, especially in individuals who have multiple benign tumors. The sensitivity and specificity of FDG-PET for the identification of malignant

change has been reported to be 97% and 87%, respectively, in a series of 69 patients with NF1 (17), and 89% and 95%, respectively, in another series of 105 patients (18). The utility of FDG-PET for the diagnosis of malignant transformation has also been published in patients with fibrous dysplasia and giant cell tumors (19, 20).

## Guidance of biopsy

As already emphasized, the histologic grade of a sarcoma is a more important prognostic indicator than the T stage. Further, the overall tumor behavior is dictated by the most biologically aggressive component. However, sarcomas are notoriously heterogeneous tumors, and improper tissue sampling can potentially result in an incorrect or inconclusive diagnosis. Even if tissue sampling is diagnostic of malignancy, the histologic grade may be incorrect, resulting in improper treatment and a higher risk for disease progression or recurrence. The most biologically aggressive portion of the tumor is thought to have the highest FDG uptake (20). Therefore, FDG-PET can be used to guide biopsy to the most metabolically active tumor site, and can provide a more accurate determination of tumor histology (see Chapter 20).

In a series of 20 patients in whom the results of initial biopsy guided by FDG-PET were compared with those from subsequently performed complete surgical resection of the mass, the biopsy site suggested by PET was found to be representative of the most malignant site of the whole mass histology (20).

FDG-PET can be particularly helpful for guiding biopsy in patients with NF1 because determining the specific lesion out of several benign lesions that is undergoing malignant transformation is often challenging using anatomic imaging alone. Also, correctly sampling the portion of the tumor that has undergone malignant transformation within a large benign neurofibroma can be difficult; the value of PET in such a case has been reported (20).

In summary, effective biopsy guidance in sarcoma patients is essential: (1) to avoid incorrect diagnosis, (2) for correct histologic grading, and (3) for correct identification of malignant transformation. In this role, FDG-PET has been found to be invaluable.

## N and M staging

The capacity of FDG-PET to image the whole body and to interrogate tumor metabolic activity is helpful to identify distant metastatic sites. In a prospective multicenter study of 46 pediatric patients with sarcomas including osteosarcoma, rhabdomyosarcoma, and the Ewing sarcoma family of tumors, PET was found to be superior to conventional imaging for the detection of lymph node involvement (21). The sensitivity of PET and conventional imaging was 95% and 25%, respectively, on a lesion basis, and 88% and 62%, respectively, on a patient basis.

The lung is typically the first site of distant metastases in patients with sarcoma. High-resolution chest CT is the most sensitive imaging modality for the detection of pulmonary metastases and is indispensable in this regard. The sensitivity of FDG-PET is reported to be low – as low as 25% (22, 23), because the pulmonary lesions are often too small to be reliably characterized. Despite this low sensitivity, FDG-PET may have added value, i.e., higher specificity. For example, in the presence of high FDG uptake at other sites of disease, the absence of significant uptake in a large lung nodule makes a metastatic lesion unlikely. The low sensitivity of PET for the detection of lung metastases has been partially overcome by the use of hybrid PET/CT imaging, which may improve the ability to detect lung metastases.

For the identification of skeletal metastases, PET is more sensitive than conventional imaging including $^{99m}$Tc-MDP-bone scintigraphy, with a sensitivity of 89% vs. 57%, respectively (23). Another group of investigators also found FDG-PET to be more sensitive (100% vs. 68%) and more specific (96% vs. 87%) than bone scintigraphy in patients with Ewing's sarcoma, however, FDG-PET had lower sensitivity compared with bone scintigraphy in patients with osteosarcoma (24). Of note, PET images in this study were reconstructed by filtered back-projection, and not attenuation-corrected. Today, the quality of PET is considerably superior, and in addition, CT images are often obtained immediately before the PET acquisition using hybrid PET/CT scanners. In certain circumstances MRI may be more accurate than FDG-PET for identifying skeletal metastases. A retrospective study of 33 patients with myxoid liposarcoma showed that MRI was superior to FDG-PET for the early detection of spinal metastases (24). Although hybrid PET/MR scanners have recently been introduced into clinical practice, their utility is still under investigation. Alternatively, co-registration of PET with MRI, though more difficult than co-registration with CT, may be performed (25).

In summary, FDG-PET, CT, and MRI are all valuable imaging tools that are often complementary for the assessment of metastatic disease in patients with sarcoma.

## Monitoring therapeutic response

Sarcoma histopathologic response to neoadjuvant chemotherapy is primarily assessed based on the degree of tumor necrosis present in the surgically resected tumor. For example, the response of osteosarcomas to treatment is categorized as a good response when ≥ 95% tumor necrosis is present in the specimen, a partial response when ≥ 90% and < 95% tumor necrosis is present in the specimen, and a lack of response when < 90% tumor necrosis is present in the specimen (26). The early prediction of the degree of tumor necrosis in response to neoadjuvant chemotherapy is essential, especially in non- or poor responders because inefficient but toxic and expensive therapy can be stopped, and more importantly, because poor responders may benefit from altering the therapeutic regimen. Waiting for weeks to months to complete neoadjuvant chemotherapy without identifying poor

responders may potentially result in the loss of opportunity for cure or improved outcome.

While core biopsy and/or anatomical imaging obtained during treatment may be useful for assessing early therapy response in some malignancies, neither is reliable in sarcoma patients. Pre-existing necrosis and therapy-induced necrosis cannot be differentiated based on a small sample, because necrosis is often present in a sarcoma even before therapy begins. Furthermore, tissue heterogeneity itself can introduce sampling error. Also, anatomical imaging is not useful in sarcoma patients because malignancies of connective tissue may not significantly change anatomically despite good response to therapy, or at least may not change for a considerable period of time following the completion of therapy. For these reasons, the need for a dependable, non-invasive means to provide an accurate prediction of the histologic response of the sarcoma to neoadjuvant therapy is especially high.

Results in the literature suggest that FDG-PET predicts and accurately assesses histologic treatment response through a decrease in intensity of FDG uptake on follow-up imaging compared with baseline tumor activity (27–33). The percent decrease in FDG uptake suggested as an optimal cut-off value separating good and poor responders ranges from 25% to 60% amongst articles. This variation is likely due to multiple factors. For example, the number of cycles of chemotherapy given before the repeat PET scan varies amongst the reports in the literature. The subtype and/or grade of the sarcoma are also variable. The intensity of FDG uptake was measured using a tumor-to-background ratio by some investigators while others used the SUV. In case of SUV, some investigators used the SUVmax measured from a single pixel while others have used the peak SUV measured from a small fixed size ROI placed in the region of highest FDG uptake. Furthermore, attenuation correction was generally not performed before 2000, while more recent studies have used attenuation-corrected images. Despite the variation in the optimal cut-off value of parameters representing FDG uptake used to separate good and poor responders, most investigators agree that FDG-PET is an accurate and valuable non-invasive tool for predicting histologic response. The response criteria recommended by the European Organization for Research and Treatment of Cancer are: **partial metabolic response** is classified as a reduction of a minimum of 15–25% in tumor SUV after one cycle of chemotherapy, and > 25% after more than one cycle, and **complete metabolic response** implies complete resolution of FDG uptake within the tumor volume so that it is indistinguishable from surrounding normal tissue (34). However, it should be remembered that these criteria were derived from studies on other malignancies and therefore may not necessarily apply to the evaluation of sarcoma response. At any rate, careful standardization of patient preparation and imaging technique is required to avoid fluctuations in FDG uptake due to other causes.

## Assessment of prognosis

Metabolic response evaluated by FDG-PET following treatment has also been shown to be a strong predictor of outcome in patients with soft tissue and bone sarcomas (35–37). In a study of patients with the Ewing sarcoma family of tumors receiving neoadjuvant chemotherapy (27), post-treatment SUVmax of < 2.5 was found to be a significant predictor of progression-free survival, while a ≥ 50% decline in the SUVmax was not. On the other hand, another study of patients with high-grade sarcomas (pleomorphic undifferentiated sarcoma/malignant fibrous histiocytoma, synovial sarcoma, and leiomyosarcoma accounting for 76% of the cases), showed that a ≥ 40% decline in the SUVmax after chemotherapy was a significant predictor for lower risk of recurrence and death after complete resection and adjuvant radiotherapy (33). The discrepancy in results between these reports may be related to the different subtypes and histologic grades of sarcomas of their patient cohort, as well as to differences in study design. Regardless of small variations in the indices evaluated and in the results, changes in FDG uptake after treatment appear to be a useful prognostic indicator. For example, imatinib mesylate (Gleevec), a tyrosine kinase inhibitor, has been successfully used to treat gastrointestinal stromal tumor (GIST), and good treatment response assessed by FDG-PET was associated with a longer progression-free survival (92% vs. 12% at 1 year) (34).

Several groups of investigators have found that the degree of FDG uptake by sarcoma at baseline alone is an independent predictor (independent of histologic grade) of overall survival and disease-free survival (38–40). Again, the methods, e.g., SUV vs. tumor-to-background ratio, SUVmax vs. SUVavg, used for risk stratification varied amongst the reports, but there was a good overall correlation between the level of FDG intensity and survival. In one study, tumor heterogeneity assessed using an FDG image heterogeneity analysis was shown to be a strong independent predictor of patient outcome (41). In this study, SUVmax was a significant predictor of overall survival and disease-free survival in univariate analysis, but not in multivariate analysis. The histologic grade and tumor heterogeneity were the only two independent predictors for overall survival, while the tumor heterogeneity was the only independent predictor of disease-free survival.

In summary, three independent indices derived from FDG-PET have been reported to be helpful for prognostication in sarcoma patients. These include: (1) metabolic response on post-treatment PET, (2) the intensity of tumor FDG uptake on pre-treatment PET, and (3) tumor heterogeneity on pre-treatment PET. While tumor heterogeneity has been shown in one study to be the best predictor, it has not been evaluated by many groups of investigators, and further research is needed for validation.

## Evaluation of recurrence

FDG-PET and PET/CT appear to have high sensitivity and moderate specificity for the assessment of local and distant sarcoma recurrence (42–47). However, low to intermediate levels of tracer uptake may remain at the site of treated disease due to inflammation. In order to accurately distinguish tumor recurrence from post-intervention inflammation, knowledge of the intensity of tumor metabolic uptake at baseline coupled with the results of other studies is essential.

## Other PET tracers for the evaluation of sarcoma

There are PET radiopharmaceuticals other than FDG that have been used to target oncogenic processes in patients with sarcomas. $3'$-deoxy-$3'$-$^{18}$F-fluorothymidine (FLT) uptake reflects cell proliferation (48). In a prospective trial, FLT-PET accurately detected all soft tissue and bone sarcomas and the intensity of tracer uptake correlated with tumor grade (48, 49). $^{18}$F-fluoromisonidazole (FMISO) has been used to assess tumor tissue hypoxia in sarcoma lesions (50, 51). Hypoxia may result from upregulation of stress-reactive proteins, unregulated tumor growth, and neovascularization. Initial work with FMISO suggests that sarcomas have regional hypoxia and that areas of hypoxia do not necessarily correlate with areas of increased metabolism (51). Ultimately, it is hoped that new PET radiopharmaceuticals will improve imaging and direct targeted therapy.

## Summary

To date, large prospective trials of FDG-PET in patients with specific individual sarcoma histology are limited. Nevertheless, the accumulated data have clearly shown that FDG-PET is a valuable imaging modality that provides complementary information to anatomic imaging. The role of FDG-PET in patients with sarcoma may be summarized as follows:

- The role of FDG-PET in distinguishing malignant from benign processes based on imaging alone is limited.
- MRI and/or CT are superior to PET in the evaluation of the tumor size and depth location (T stage). However, histologic grade (G stage) is more important than T stage in sarcoma patients, and the G stage of a sarcoma can be correlated with the intensity of tumor FDG uptake. However, FDG-PET alone cannot be used for G staging and ultimately tissue sampling is required.
- FDG-PET is valuable for effectively guiding biopsy of sarcomas such that an accurate diagnosis and histologic grade can be determined both in patients with proven malignancy, and in those with suspected malignant transformation.
- FDG-PET is helpful for N and M staging. Specifically, FDG-PET appears to be a sensitive and specific modality in the evaluation of bone metastases. Although FDG-PET is not sensitive for the detection of lung metastases, it increases the specificity for larger nodules found on CT.
- FDG-PET is helpful for monitoring therapy response in sarcoma patients, since anatomic imaging and core biopsy is unreliable in this group of patients.

- FDG-PET results are a strong predictor of patient outcome.
- FDG-PET is reported to be highly sensitive and reasonably specific for the detection of recurrent sarcoma.

- It is expected that increasing uses of hybrid PET/CT scanners and new PET tracers will result in improved management of patients with sarcoma.

# References

1. Demetri GD, Antonia S, Benjamin RS et al.; National Comprehensive Cancer Network Soft Tissue Sarcoma Panel. Soft tissue sarcoma. *J Natl Compr Canc Netw.* 2010;**8**(6):630–74.

2. National Cancer Institute Fact Sheet (http://www.cancer.gov/cancertopics/factsheet/Sites-Types/soft-tissue-sarcoma).

3. National Cancer Institute: a snapshot of sarcoma (http://www.cancer.gov/aboutnci/servingpeople/snapshots/sarcoma.pdf).

4. Grimer R, Judson I, Peake D, Seddon B. Guidelines for the management of soft tissue sarcomas. *Sarcoma* 2010;2010:506182.

5. Coindre J-M, Terrier P, Gouillou L et al. Predictive value of grade for metastasis development in the main histologic types of adult soft tissue sarcomas: a study of 1240 patients from the French Federation of Cancer Centers Sarcoma Group. *Cancer* 2001;**91**:1914–26.

6. Fadul D, Fayad L. Advanced modalities for the imaging of sarcoma. *Surg Clin N Am* 2008;**88**:521–37.

7. Adler LP, Blair HF, Makley JT et al. Noninvasive grading of musculoskeletal tumors using PET. *J Nucl Med* 1991;**32**:1508–12.

8. Eary JF, Conrad EU, Bruckner JD et al. Quantitative [F-18]fluorodeoxyglucose positron emission tomography in pretreatment and grading of sarcoma. *Clin Cancer Res* 1998;**4**:1215–20.

9. Folpe AL, Lyles RH, Sprouse JT et al. (F-18) fluorodeoxyglucose positron emission tomography as a predictor of pathologic grade and other prognostic variables in bone and soft tissue sarcoma. *Clin Cancer Res* 2000;**6**:1279–87.

10. Schulte M, Brecht-Krauss D, Heymer B et al. Grading of tumors and tumor like lesions of bone: evaluation by FDG PET. *J Nucl Med* 2000;**41**:1695–701.

11. Ioannidis JP, Lau J. 18F-FDG PET for the diagnosis and grading of soft-tissue sarcoma: a meta-analysis. *J Nucl Med* 2003;**44**:717–24.

12. Feldman F, van Heertum R, Saxena C et al. 18FDG-PET applications for cartilage neoplasms. *Skeletal Radiol* 2005;**34**(7):367–74.

13. Aoki J, Watanabe H, Shinozaki T et al. FDG PET of primary benign and malignant bone tumors: standardized uptake value in 52 lesions. *Radiology* 2001;**219**:774–7.

14. Ducatman BS, Scheithauer BW, Piepgras DG et al. Malignant peripheral nerve sheath tumors. A clinicopathologic study of 120 cases. *Cancer* 1986;**57**:2006–21.

15. McGaughran JM, Harris DI, Donnai D et al. A clinical study of type 1 neurofibromatosis in north west England. *J Med Genet* 1999;**36**:197–203.

16. Warbey VS, Ferner RE, Dunn JT, Calonje E, O'Doherty MJ. [18F]FDG PET/CT in the diagnosis of malignant peripheral nerve sheath tumours in neurofibromatosis type-1. *Eur J Nucl Med Mol Imaging* 2009;**36**(5):751–7.

17. Ferner RE, Golding JF, Smith M et al. [18F]2-fluoro-2-deoxy-D-glucose positron emission tomography (FDG PET) as a diagnostic tool for neurofibromatosis 1 (NF1) associated malignant peripheral nerve sheath tumours (MPNSTs): a long-term clinical study. *Ann Oncol* 2008;**19**:390–4.

18. Berrebi O, Steiner C, Keller A, Rougemont AL, Ratib O. F-18 fluorodeoxyglucose (FDG) PET in the diagnosis of malignant transformation of fibrous dysplasia in the pelvic bones. *Clin Nucl Med* 2008;**33**(7):469–71.

19. Makis W, Hickeson M. Spindle cell sarcoma degeneration of giant cell tumor of the knee, imaged with F-18 FDG PET-CT and Tc-99m MDP Bone Scan. *Clin Nucl Med* 2010;**35**:112–15.

20. Hain SF, O'Foherty MJ, Bingham J, Chinyama C, Smith MA. Can FDG PET be used to successfully direct preoperative biopsy of soft tissue tumors? *Nucl Med Commun* 2003;**24**(11):1130–43.

21. Volker T, Denecke T, Steffen I et al. Positron emission tomography for staging of pediatric sarcoma patients: results of a prospective multicenter trial. *J Clin Oncol* 2007;**25**:5435–41.

22. Franzius C, Daldrup-Link HE, Sciuk J et al. FDG-PET for detection of pulmonary metastases from malignant primary bone tumors: Comparison with spiral CT. *Ann Oncol* 2001;**12**:479–86.

23. Franzius C, Sciuk J, Daldrup-Link HE et al. FDG-PET for detection of osseous metastases from malignant primary bone tumours: comparison with bone scintigraphy. *Eur J Nucl Med* 2000;**27**:1305–11.

24. Schwab JH, Boland PJ, Antonescu C et al. Spinal metastases from myxoid liposarcoma warrant screening with magnetic resonance imaging. *Cancer* 2007;**110**:1815–22.

25. Somer EJR, Marsden PK, Banatar NA et al. PET-MR image fusion in soft tissue sarcoma: accuracy, reliability and practicality of interactive point-based and automated mutual information techniques. *Eur J Nucl Med* 2003;**30**:54–62.

26. Huvos AG, Rosen G, Marcove RC. Primary osteogenic sarcoma: pathologic aspects in 20 patients after treatment with chemotherapy en bloc resection, prosthetic bone replacement. *Arch Pathol Lab Med* 1977;**101**(1):14–18.

27. Hawkins DS, Schuetze SM, Butrynski JE et al. [F-18] Fluorodeoxyglucose positron emission tomography predicts outcome for Ewing's sarcoma family of tumors. *J Clin Oncol* 2005;**23**(34):8828–34.

28. Evilevitch V, Weber WA, Tap WD et al. Reduction of glucose metabolic activity is more accurate than change in size at predicting histopathologic response to neoadjuvant therapy in high-grade soft-tissue sarcomas. *Clin Cancer Res* 2008;**14**:715–20.

29. Benz MR, Allen-Auerbach MS, Eilber FC et al. Combined assessment of metabolic and volumetric changes for assessment of tumor response in

patients with soft-tissue sarcomas. *J Nucl Med* 2008;**49**:1579–84.

30. Hawkins DS, Rajendran JG, Conrad EU 3rd *et al.* Evaluation of chemotherapy response in pediatric bone sarcomas by [F-18]-fluorodeoxy-D-glucose positron emission tomography. *Cancer* 2002;**94**:3277–84.

31. Benz MR, Czernin J, Allen-Auerbach MS *et al.* FDG-PET/CT imaging predicts histopathologic treatment responses after the initial cycle of neoadjuvant chemotherapy in high grade soft tissue sarcomas. *Clin Cancer Res* 2009;**15**:2856–63.

32. Schulte M, Brecht-Krauss D, Werner M *et al.* Evaluation of neoadjuvant therapy response of osteogenic sarcoma using FDG PET. *J Nucl Med* 1999;**40**:1637–43.

33. Schuetze SM, Rubin BP, Vernon C *et al.* Use of positron emission tomography in localized extremity soft tissue sarcoma treated with neoadjuvant chemotherapy. *Cancer* 2005;**103**:339–48.

34. Stroobants S, Goeminne J, Seegers M *et al.* 18FDG-Positron emission tomography for the early prediction of response in advanced soft tissue sarcoma treated with imatinib mesylate (Glivec). *Eur J Cancer* 2003;**39** (14):2012–20.

35. Young H, Baum R, Cremerius U *et al.* Measurement of clinical and subclinical tumor response using [F-18]-fluorodeoxyglucose and positron emission tomography: review and 1999 EORTC recommendations. *Eur J Cancer* 1999;**35**(13):1773–82.

36. Costelloe CM, Macapinlac HA, Madewell JE *et al.* 18F-FDG PET/CT as an indicator of progression-free and overall survival in osteosarcoma. *J Nucl Med* 2009;**50**(3):340–7.

37. Eary JF, O'Sullivan F, Powitan Y *et al.* Sarcoma tumor FDG uptake measured by PET and patient outcome: a retrospective analysis. *Eur J Nucl Med* 2002;**29**(9):1149–54.

38. Schwarzbach MH, Hinz U, Dimitrakopoulou-Strauss A *et al.* Prognostic significance of preoperative [18-F] fluorodeoxyglucose (FDG) positron emission tomography (PET) imaging in patients with resectable soft tissue sarcomas. *Ann Surg* 2005;**241**:286–94.

39. Lisle JW, Eary JF, O'Sullivan J, Conrad EU. Risk assessment based on FDGPET imaging in patients with synovial sarcoma. *Clin Orthop Relat Res* 2009;**467**(6):1605–11.

40. Brenner W, Friedrich RE, Gawad KA *et al.* Prognostic relevance of FDG PET in patients with neurofibromatosis type-1 and malignant peripheral nerve sheath tumours. *Eur J Nucl Med Mol Imaging* 2006;**33**:428–32.

41. Eary JF, O'Sullivan F, O'Sullivan J, Conrad EU. Spatial heterogeneity in sarcoma 18F-FDG uptake as a predictor of patient outcome. *J Nucl Med* 2008;**49**:1973–9.

42. Franzius C, Daldrup-Link HE, Wagner-Bohn A *et al.* FDG-PET for detection of recurrences from malignant primary bone tumors: comparison with conventional imaging. *Ann Oncol* 2002;**13**(1):157–60.

43. Johnson GR, Zhuang H, Khan J *et al.* Roles of positron emission tomography with fluorine-18-deoxyglucose in the detection of local recurrent and distant metastatic sarcoma. *Clin Nucl Med* 2003;**28**:815–20.

44. Kole AC, Nieweg OE, van Ginkel RJ *et al.* Detection of local recurrence of soft-tissue sarcoma with positron emission tomography using [18F] fluorodeoxyglucose. *Ann Surg Oncol* 1997;**4**:57–63.

45. Schwarzbach MH, Dimitrakopoulou-Strauss A, Willeke F *et al.* Clinical value of [18-F] fluorodeoxyglucose positron emission tomography imaging in soft tissue sarcomas. *Ann Surg* 2000;**231**:380–6.

46. Arush MW, Israel O, Postovsky S *et al.* Positron emission tomography/computed tomography with 18fluoro-deoxyglucose in the detection of local recurrence and distant metastases of pediatric sarcoma. *Pediatr Blood Cancer* 2007;**49**:901–5.

47. Park JY, Kim EN, Kim DY *et al.* Role of PET or PET/CT in the posttherapy surveillance of uterine sarcoma. *Gynecol Oncol* 2008;**109**:255–62.

48. Shields AF, Grierson JR, Dohmen BM *et al.* Imaging proliferation in vivo with [F-18]FLT and positron emission tomography. *Nat Med* 1998;**4**:1334–6.

49. Buck AK, Herrmann K, Buschenfelde CM *et al.* Imaging bone and soft tissue tumors with the proliferation marker [18F]fluorodeoxythymidine. *Clin Cancer Res* 2008;**14**: 2970–7.

50. Rasey JS, Koh WJ, Evans ML *et al.* Quantifying regional hypoxia in human tumors with positron emission tomography of [F-18] fluoromisonidazole: a pre-therapy study of 37 patients. *Int J Radiat Oncol Biol Phys* 1996;**36**:417–28.

51. Rajendran JG, Wilson DC, Conrad EU et al. [18-F] FMISO and [18-F] FDG PET imaging in soft tissue sarcomas: correlation and hypoxia, metabolism and VEGF expression. *Eur J Nucl Med Mol Imaging* 2003;**30**(5):695–704.

# Osteosarcoma

A 68-year-old female who presented to her local hospital with longstanding back pain that had recently become more severe. Initial plain films disclosed an abnormality of the left pelvis. Subsequent evaluation with an MRI of the pelvis revealed a $12 \times 7 \times 9$ cm mass involving both the left iliac bone and adjacent soft tissue. Chest CT identified pulmonary metastases. FDG-PET/CT was performed for further evaluation of the mass and to assess for additional sites of metabolically active disease.

## Acquisition and processing parameters

In our nuclear medicine department, we ask patients to fast for at least 4–6 hours before FDG-PET/CT. The patient's blood glucose level is checked prior to the FDG injection because an elevated blood glucose level may result in an altered biodistribution of radiotracer. The standard FDG dose for an adult oncology patient is approximately 740 megabequerel (20 mCi) for a 2-D acquisition and 444 megabequerel (12 mCi) for a 3-D acquisition. After an uptake period of 60 min, CT is performed from the skull base through the upper/mid thighs without breath-hold, for attenuation correction of PET and anatomic correlation, but not for primary interpretation, as it is not of standard diagnostic quality. We do not routinely use IV or oral contrast. This study was acquired using a 16-slice PET/CT scanner. For the CT portion of the study the parameters were as follows: $16 \times 1.25$ mm detector configuration, 3.75 mm slice reconstruction thickness with ordered subset expectation maximization (OSEM), 3.27 mm slice interval, 90 mA, 140 kVp, and 50 cm scan field of view. Immediately following the CT scan, the PET portion of the study was performed over the same anatomic range. Images were acquired for 3–5 min per bed position. Longer times are used in larger patients, or to compensate for lower counts, e.g., relatively lower injected activity, or more delayed imaging. PET parameters were $128 \times 128$ matrix, and reconstruction algorithm using OSEM with 2 iterations and 21 subsets. Both attenuation-corrected and non-attenuation-corrected images are generated and displayed.

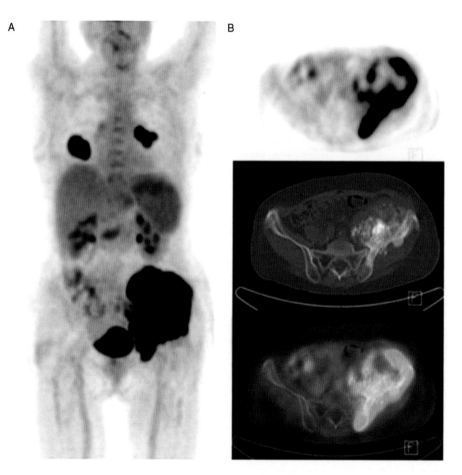

A   B

**Figure 18.1** (A) MIP standard-body FDG-PET. (B) Cross-sectional FDG-PET, CT, and fused FDG-PET/CT images of the pelvis centered on the FDG-avid mass.

Please note: the acquisition protocols and processing parameters employed for Cases 2–5 are essentially identical to those presented above.

## Findings and differential diagnosis

The FDG-PET/CT images show a large intensely FDG-avid lesion arising from the left iliac bone with a significant extra-osseous soft tissue component that demonstrates heterogeneous tracer uptake. The SUVmax of the most intense region of the iliac lesion is 13. In addition, there are intensely FDG-avid pulmonary nodules in both lungs. Metabolic activity elsewhere within the gastrointestinal and genitourinary tracts is physiologic.

The findings are highly suspicious for malignancy and metastatic osteosarcoma would be the most likely diagnosis with this appearance on FDG-PET/CT.

## Diagnosis and clinical follow-up

Pathology confirmed osteosarcoma of the left iliac bone arising in the setting of Paget's disease with pulmonary metastases. Standard pre-operative chemotherapy with curative intent was not possible in this case and palliative chemotherapy was initiated.

## Discussion and teaching points

### Malignant bone tumors

Malignant bone tumors, although uncommon, are a major contributor to morbidity and mortality particularly in children and young adults. They typically originate from the periosteum, osseous cortex, medullary cavity, or joint surfaces. Outcome depends on the histologic type and tumor grade, the disease stage, and the use of appropriate therapy. For most bone tumors, successful treatment requires a combination of chemotherapy and local control with surgery or radiotherapy. Clinical management and prognosis depends on the disease stage at diagnosis and the assessment of response to therapy. FDG-PET can play an important role in guiding biopsy, staging, assessing response to therapy, and evaluating recurrence. The advantages include the large field of view, consisting of the whole body and extremities, as well as the capability to evaluate tumor biology.

### Osteosarcoma

Osteosarcomas are the most common primary bone tumors of children and young adults and are primarily aggressive tumors of the extremities that occur in the long bone metaphyses. The peak incidence is between the ages of 5–25 years (1). A second peak in incidence occurs in older adults due to secondary osteosarcomas, usually at sites of prior bone pathology such as Paget's disease, chondromas, or fibrous dysplasia.

Classified according to the FNCLCC grading system for sarcomas, there are several histologic subtypes such as: chondroblastic, fibroblastic, osteoblastic, parosteal, telangiectatic, small cell, periosteal, high-grade surface type, and secondary osteosarcoma. Prior retinoblastoma or radiation is associated with an increased risk of osteosarcoma.

The clinical presentation of patients with an osteosarcoma is variable and may be a result of trauma, pain, or the presence of an osseous-based mass. More than 50% of patients with osteosarcoma have metastases at the time of diagnosis or shortly thereafter. It is estimated that 15–20% of patients present with pulmonary metastases, the most common site of metastatic disease (2). Osseous metastases are seen in approximately 10–20% of patients with metastatic disease, while metastases to the lymph nodes and brain are rare (3).

The prognosis of patients with an osteosarcoma depends on staging and clinical management. Osteosarcomas are resistant to radiotherapy and surgery is the mainstay of local control. Inadequate local control is associated with recurrence and poor outcome. Neoadjuvant chemotherapy may facilitate limb-sparing procedures. Multi-agent chemotherapy is helpful and, overall, the 5-year survival using a combination of multi-agent chemotherapy and local control is estimated to be over 65% (4). The treatment of recurrent disease and/or metastases is also important for survival.

## FDG-PET in osteosarcoma staging and diagnosis

FDG-PET has been used for staging patients with osteosarcoma. The site of the primary malignancy is often heterogeneous with peripheral tracer uptake and relative central photopenia (5). In general, the intensity of tracer uptake is higher than in most other sarcomas (6) and may be associated with histologic grade and prognosis (7). FDG-PET may be helpful to identify osseous skip lesions as well as other sites of metastatic disease.

Although early reports suggested that FDG-PET had a similar accuracy as single detector CT for the detection of lung metastases, subsequent studies have shown that spiral CT is significantly more sensitive (8).

In a study of 32 patients with osteosarcoma published in 2000, comparing FDG-PET with planar $^{99m}$Tc-MDP-bone scintigraphy for the detection of bone disease, all of the osseous metastatic lesions in five patients were detected with $^{99m}$Tc-MDP-bone scintigraphy and none were identified by FDG-PET (7). The authors concluded that FDG-PET could not replace $^{99m}$Tc-MDP-bone scintigraphy for the detection of osseous metastases, since osteosarcoma metastases to bone are often sclerotic (osteoblastic). In contrast, a study published in 2007 reported a 90% sensitivity for FDG-PET compared with 81% for $^{99m}$Tc-MDP-bone scintigraphy in identifying osseous metastases (6). While the PET images in the former study were reconstructed using filtered back projection and were uncorrected for attenuation, the PET images presented in the latter article were likely reconstructed with an iterative algorithm and were attenuation corrected. These differences should be taken into consideration in the interpretation of the respective results. At any rate, when the images from all modalities were combined for the analysis, the sensitivity was 100%.

In summary, although the role of FDG-PET in osteosarcoma patients remains to be further refined, it can complement routine anatomic imaging, assess tumor biology and help guide effective biopsy, which is ultimately needed for diagnosis. Staging patients with osteosarcoma includes: MRI for local staging and high-resolution chest CT to evaluate for pulmonary metastases; FDG-PET can increase the specificity of pulmonary nodules found on CT. While FDG-PET and $^{99m}$Tc-MDP-bone scintigraphy may both be used to identify skeletal disease, further research is needed to refine the comparative utility of these two modalities.

## FDG-PET in osteosarcoma for assessing therapy response

Several studies have shown that a decrease of 30–40% in tumor-to-background FDG-uptake ratio after neoadjuvant chemotherapy correlates with a favorable histological response (9, 10). Other studies have reported that a decrease in FDG uptake may correlate with tumor necrosis, but these studies had false-positive findings from benign processes such as inflammation (11, 12). In addition, the SUVmax on post-therapy-pre-surgical studies has been proposed as a predictor of histopathologic response to neoadjuvant chemotherapy (12). In summary, pre-operative FDG-PET prior to and following neoadjuvant chemotherapy may provide an estimate of disease extent and predict histological response.

## FDG-PET in osteosarcoma for assessing recurrence

There is a small body of literature evaluating FDG-PET for the assessment of recurrent osteosarcoma. It is important to note that FDG uptake may be seen at the site of limb amputation for many months following surgery (13) and that uptake due to inflammation may obscure recurrent disease (14). In a study of six patients with primary malignant bone tumors, all sites of local recurrence were detected with FDG-PET, although there was one false-positive study (15). The performance of MRI and FDG-PET for the detection of local disease recurrence was compared (16). Although MRI appeared to be more sensitive, it was adversely affected by implant artifact. Further, FDG-PET found 13 additional sites of metastatic recurrent disease that were not in the field of view of the MRI. In summary, FDG-PET may complement anatomic imaging for the detection of recurrent disease and has the advantage of a large field of view.

### Take-home message

- Osteosarcomas are the most common primary bone tumor of children with a second peak in older adults usually at sites of bone pathology such as Paget's disease, chondromas, or fibrous dysplasia.
- The most common site of osteosarcoma metastasis is the lungs.
- An important advantage of FDG-PET is the ability to interrogate disease by the way of whole-body imaging.

## References

1. Ries LAG, Smith MA, Gurney JG et al. (eds). *Cancer Incidence and Survival among Children and Adolescents: United States SEER Program 1975–1995*. NIH Pub. No. 99–4649. Bethesda, MD: National Cancer Institute, SEER Program, 1999.

2. Eary J. Sarcomas. In RL Wahl (Ed.), *Principles and Practice of PET and PET/CT*, 2nd edn. Philadelphia, PA: Lippincott Williams & Wilkins, 2010, pp. 392–401.

3. Brenner W, Bohuslavizki KH, Eary JF. PET imaging of osteosarcoma. *J Nucl Med* 2003;44:930–42.

4. Bakhshi S, Radhakrishnan V. Prognostic markers in osteosarcoma. *Exp Rev Anticancer Ther* 2010;10(2):271–87.

5. Eary JF, Conrad EU, Bruckner JD et al. Quantitative [F-18] fluorodeoxyglucose positron emission tomography in pretreatment and grading of sarcoma. *Clin Cancer Res* 1998;4:1215–20.

6. Volker T, Denecke T, Steffen I et al. Positron emission tomography for staging of pediatric sarcoma patients: results of a prospective multicenter trial. *J Clin Oncol* 2007;25:5435–41.

7. Franzius C, Sciuk J, Daldrup-Link HE, Jurgens H, Schober O. FDG-PET for detection of osseous metastases from malignant primary bone tumours: comparison with bone scintigraphy. *Eur J Nucl Med* 2000;27:1305–11.

8. Franzius C, Daldrup-Link HE, Sciuk J et al. FDG-PET for detection of pulmonary metastases from malignant primary bone tumors: comparison with spiral CT. *Ann Oncol* 2001;12:479–86.

9. Schulte M, Brecht-Krauss D, Werner M et al. Evaluation of neoadjuvant therapy response of osteogenic sarcoma using FDG PET. *J Nucl Med* 1999;40:1637–43.

10. Ye Z, Zhu J, Tian M et al. Response of osteogenic sarcoma to neoadjuvant therapy: evaluated by 18F-FDG-PET. *Ann Nucl Med* 2008;22:475–80.

11. Jones DN, McCowage GB, Sostman HD et al. Monitoring of neoadjuvant therapy response of soft-tissue and musculoskeletal sarcoma using fluorine-18-FDG PET. *J Nucl Med* 1996;37:1438–44.

12. Hawkins DS, Conrad EU III, Butrynski JE, Schuetze SM, Eary JF. [F-18]-fluorodeoxy-D-glucose positron emission tomography response is associated with outcome for extremity osteosarcoma in children and young adults. *Cancer* 2009;115:3519–25.

13. Jadvar H, Gamie S, Ramanna L, Conti PS. Musculoskeletal system. *Semin Nucl Med* 2004;34:254–61.

14. Hain SF, O'Doherty MJ, Lucas JD, Smith MA. 18F-FDG PET in the evaluation of stumps following amputation for soft tissue sarcoma. *Nucl Med Comm* 1999;20:490.

15. Franzius C, Daldrup-Link HE, Wagner-Bohn A et al. FDG-PET for detection of recurrences from malignant primary bone tumors: comparison with conventional imaging. *Ann Oncol* 2002;13:157–60.

16. Lucas JD, O'Doherty MJ, Cronin BF et al. Prospective evaluation of soft tissues masses and sarcomas using fluorodeoxyglucose positron emission tomography. *Br J Surg* 1999;86:550–6.

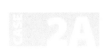

A 66-year-old male with metastatic gastrointestinal tumor (GIST) who was followed for several years with FDG-PET/CT to assess response to therapy: at the time of the FDG-PET/CT in 2008, the patient was post-surgery and had been on imatinib mesylate (Gleevec) for 2 years. The FDG-PET/CT performed in 2009 was done following cryoablation of a hepatic lesion and replacement of imatinib mesylate with sunitinib. This study showed significant disease progression. Despite additional changes to the chemotherapy regimen continued disease progression was seen on the FDG-PET/CT in 2010.

## Findings and differential diagnosis

The FDG-PET/CT done in 2008 shows a metabolically active lesion in the dome of the right hepatic lobe. Additional hepatic and splenic lesions identified on a prior diagnostic CT were not FDG avid. FDG uptake in the left inguinal region was favored to be due to inflammation (Figure 18.2A, white arrow) and there was physiologic distribution of tracer elsewhere in the body. The FDG-PET/CT done in 2009 was performed following cryoablation of the hepatic lesion identified in 2008 as well as modification of the chemotherapy regimen. While the cryoablated lesion is no longer seen, there are new FDG-avid hepatic metastases as well as a new FDG-avid osseous lesion in the region of the left 6th rib (Figure 18.2B, black arrow). The FDG-PET/CT done in 2010 shows disease progression with interval increase in size, number, and intensity of FDG-avid lesions in the liver and bone (Figure 18.2C).

This was a case of known metastatic GIST, although several other malignancies could also have this appearance on FDG-PET. Indeed, due to the absence of characteristic features and the rarity of the disease, the diagnosis of GIST is infrequently made on initial imaging. Occasionally identification of a rounded, well-defined exophytic mass originating from the stomach may suggest the diagnosis.

## Diagnosis and clinical follow-up

Initial pathology confirmed a GIST arising from the stomach. At presentation only the stomach was involved and gastric resection was performed. The patient was subsequently started on imatinib mesylate chemotherapy. Unfortunately, follow-up FDG-PET/CT in 2008 revealed recurrent metastatic disease in the liver and the patient underwent cryoablation of the liver lesion followed by sunitinib chemotherapy. Despite this therapy, significant interval disease progression was identified on the subsequent FDG-PET/CT study. The chemotherapy regimen was changed; however, the disease was not controlled.

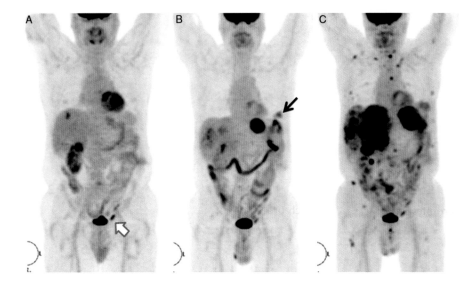

**Figure 18.2** (A) MIP whole-body FDG-PET in 2008 post-surgery and 2 years of imatinib mesylate. (B) MIP whole-body FDG-PET in 2009 post-cryoablation of hepatic lesion and sunitinib. (C) MIP whole-body FDG-PET in 2010 after additional chemotherapy regimens.

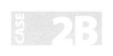

# Gastrointestinal stromal tumor

An 82-year-old male with a GIST arising from the distal esophagus and several enlarged mediastinal lymph nodes identified on diagnostic CT. FDG-PET/CT was performed for initial staging (Figure 18.3A), and at follow-up after treatment with imatinib mesylate (Figure 18.3B).

## Findings and differential diagnosis

The initial FDG-PET/CT study (Figure 18.3A) showed intense FDG uptake at the site of the known GIST involving the distal esophagus, but no abnormal uptake in the enlarged mediastinal lymph nodes (images not shown), suggesting these were of a benign etiology. Intense tracer accumulation in a horseshoe kidney was incidentally noted and there was no tracer accumulation in the distended urinary bladder. Indeed, the patient was found to have an enlarged prostate gland and bladder outlet obstruction at the time of this study.

The follow-up FDG-PET/CT study (Figure 18.3B) performed to evaluate tumor response to imatinib mesylate treatment showed virtually complete resolution of the FDG avidity in the GIST while there was little interval change in size of the mass. Also noted on CT was no significant interval change in size of the mediastinal lymph nodes (images not shown).

## Diagnosis and clinical follow-up

Pathology confirmed a GIST arising from the esophagus. At presentation only the esophagus was involved. Follow-up post-therapy revealed resolution of metabolically active disease.

## Discussion and teaching points

GISTs are relatively uncommon tumors that account for approximately 3% of all gastrointestinal (GI) neoplasms. Although FDG-PET is not used for initial diagnosis, it is very helpful for monitoring response to therapy.

GISTs were initially thought to be of smooth muscle origin. However, further evaluation has led to the hypothesis that these tumors originate from the interstitial cells of Cajal located in the myenteric plexus of the gastrointestinal tract (GI), which are responsible for coordinating GI motility (1, 2). The rate of occurrence in both men and women is similar, although the incidence in men may be slightly higher. The most common site of involvement is the stomach, followed by the small intestine, and rectum. Other locations that are not

uncommonly involved by the malignancy include the colon, mesentery, omentum, esophagus, and diaphragm (1). CT and MRI can be used to identify the location and size of the primary tumor, and can assess for the presence or absence of metastatic disease. The most common site for metastases is the liver (3).

Recently, there has been widespread scientific interest in GIST, because the principal pathogenic defect has been identified and specific molecular inhibitors have been developed. Indeed, GISTs are thought to represent a spectrum of neoplastic diseases ranging from benign to malignant, depending, at least in part, on tumor size, mitotic activity and anatomic site of origin (4). Malignancy is associated with mutations in the KIT gene, which promote activation of tyrosine kinase and ultimately result in mitosis and tumorigenesis (5, 6). Imatinib mesylate (Gleevec) is a tyrosine kinase inhibitor that has been used to successfully treat patients with GIST (7). For patients who are or who develop resistance to imatinib mesylate therapy, other tyrosine kinase inhibitors may be used.

FDG-PET can detect metabolic response to therapy and may be more effective than anatomic imaging in this respect (8, 9). For example, a study combining FDG-PET and CT found that FDG-PET and CT viewed side-by-side correctly identified response in 95% of patients after 1 month, as opposed to 85% for FDG-PET alone, and 44% for CT alone (8). Furthermore, a decrease in tumor metabolism on PET is thought to be highly predictive of patient outcome. Finally, a significant number of patients develop secondary resistance to imatinib mesylate within 2 years of treatment. It is believed that this results from new KIT mutations in existing tumor cells. FDG-PET can be used to detect tumors that have become resistant to therapy by their increased FDG uptake.

## Take-home message

- GISTs originate from the interstitial cells of Cajal located in the myenteric plexus of the GI tract.
- GISTs are associated with mutations in the KIT gene, which promote activation of tyrosine kinase. Tyrosine kinase inhibitors such as imatinib mesylate (Gleevec) have been used to treat patients with GIST.
- FDG-PET is more effective than anatomic imaging for monitoring therapy response, and has prognostic value.

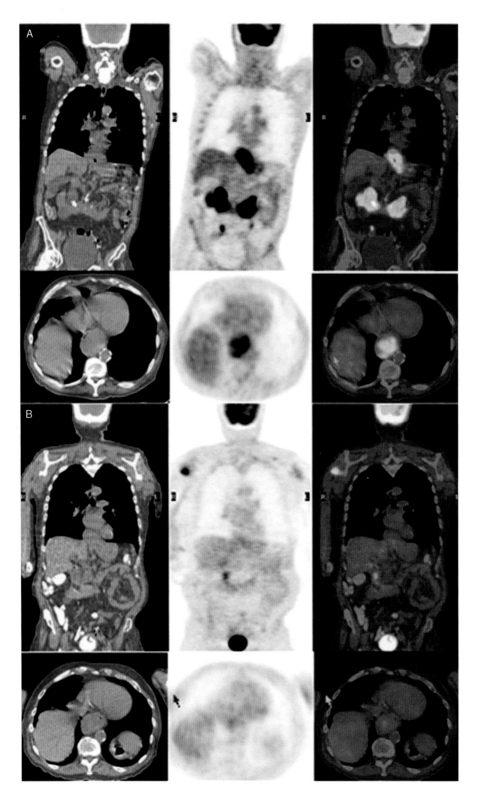

**Figure 18.3** (A) Coronal (top row) and axial (bottom row), CT, FDG-PET, and fused images of the site of disease at staging. (B) Coronal (top row) and axial (bottom row), CT, FDG-PET, and fused images of the site of prior disease post-imatinib mesylate therapy.

# References

1. DeMatteo RP, Lewis JJ, Leung D *et al.* Two hundred gastrointestinal stromal tumors: recurrence patterns and prognostic factors for survival. *Ann Surg* 2000;**231**(1):51–8.

2. Kindblom LG, Remotti HE, Aldenborg F *et al.* Gastrointestinal pacemaker cell tumor (GIPACT): gastrointestinal stromal tumors show phenotypic characteristics of the interstitial cells of Cajal. *Am J Pathol* 1998;**152**(5):1259–69.

3. Lau S, Tam KF, Kam CK *et al.* Imaging of gastrointestinal stromal tumour (GIST). *Clin Radiol* 2004;**59**(6):487–98.

4. DeMatteo RP. The GIST of targeted cancer therapy: a tumor (gastrointestinal stromal tumor), a mutated gene (c-kit), and a molecular inhibitor (STI571). *Ann Surg Oncol* 2002;**9**(9):831–9.

5. Hirota S, Isozaki K, Moriyama Y *et al.* Gain-of-function mutations of c-kit in human gastrointestinal stromal tumors. *Science* 1998; 279(5350):577–80.

6. Eary J. Sarcomas. In RL Wahl(Ed.), *Principles and Practice of PET and PET/ CT*, 2nd edn. Philadelphia, PA: Lippincott Williams & Wilkins, 2010, pp. 392–401.

7. Demetri GD, von Mehren M, Blanke CD *et al.* Efficacy and safety of imatinib mesylate in advanced gastrointestinal stromal tumors. *New Engl J Med* 2002;**347**(7):472–80.

8. Antoch G, Kanja J, Bauer S *et al.* Comparison of PET, CT, and dual-modality PET/CT imaging for monitoring of imatinib (STI571) therapy in patients with gastrointestinal stromal tumors. *J Nucl Med* 2004;**45** (3):357–65.

9. Choi H, Charnsangavej C, de Castro Faria S *et al.* CT evaluation of the response of gastrointestinal stromal tumors after imatinib mesylate treatment: a quantitative analysis correlated with FDG PET findings. *Am J Roentgenol* 2004; **183**(6):1619–28.

# FDG-PET for surveillance and biopsy guidance in patients with neurofibromatosis type I

A 30-year-old female with a history of neurofibromatosis type I and multiple neurofibromas throughout the body, presenting with left knee pain. FDG-PET was ordered to evaluate for malignant transformation of the known neurofibromas and to guide effective biopsy of suspicious lesions, as clinically warranted.

## Findings and differential diagnosis

CT shows a large soft tissue mass with mixed densities posterior to the left femur. FDG uptake within this mass is also heterogeneous with portions of the tumor showing moderate uptake (SUVmax 6) while other sites of the tumor are not significantly FDG avid. There is also low-level FDG uptake in a soft tissue nodule posterior to the right femur (Figure 18.4).

The portions showing moderate FDG avidity were felt to be suspicious for malignant transformation, i.e., MPNST. Core biopsy of the left thigh mass was guided by the PET findings. The mildly FDG-avid soft tissue nodule in the right femur was felt to represent a neurofibroma.

## Diagnosis and clinical follow-up

Pathology confirmed MPNST in the left leg lesion and the patient was scheduled for left leg amputation. The right leg lesion and the lesions in the rest of the body were to be followed with imaging.

## Discussion and teaching points

Patients with neurofibromatosis type 1 (NF1) are thought to have increased risk of developing an MPNST (1, 2). An MPNST is an aggressive soft tissue sarcoma with an associated risk of mortality.

Detecting transformation of a benign neurofibroma into an MPNST is difficult. Clinical symptoms such as increasing neurofibroma size, neurological symptoms and/or pain are suspicious but not definitive for malignant transformation. CT and MRI are effective to characterize the anatomic extent of a tumor but are unable to distinguish benign from malignant lesions. Furthermore, tumors may be heterogeneous, containing both benign and malignant components. The literature suggests that FDG-PET and FDG-PET/CT may be used to detect and monitor malignant transformation in patients with NF1(3–5). In particular, a study by Ferner *et al.* (3) evaluated the accuracy of FDG-PET in detecting malignant transformation in 105 NF1 patients with 116 lesions. MPNST was diagnosed with a sensitivity and specificity of 89% and 95%, respectively. The authors concluded that symptomatic neurofibromas with an SUVmax of 3.5 g/mL or more should be resected, whereas symptomatic lesions with an SUVmax between 2.5 and 3.5 g/mL should be closely monitored with follow-up FDG-PET imaging. Other studies have also shown significantly higher FDG uptake associated with MPNSTs compared with benign neurofibromas (6, 7).

## Take-home message

- Patients with NF1 are thought to be at increased risk of developing an MPNST.
- Detecting transformation of a benign neurofibroma into an MPNST is difficult using anatomic imaging alone.
- FDG-PET/CT may be used to monitor patients with NF1 since significantly higher FDG uptake is associated with MPNSTs when compared with neurofibromas.
- FDG-PET/CT can be helpful in identifying the most adequate biopsy site within the tumor.

A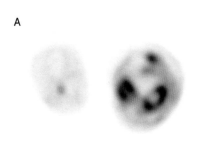

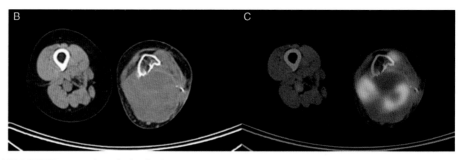

**Figure 18.4** Axial (A) FDG-PET, (B) CT, and (C) fused FDG-PET/CT images through the thighs.

# References

1. Ducatman BS, Scheithauer BW, Piepgras DG *et al.* Malignant peripheral nerve sheath tumors. A clinicopathologic study of 120 cases. *Cancer* 1986;**57**:2006–21.

2. McGaughran JM, Harris DI, Donnai D *et al.* A clinical study of type 1 neurofibromatosis in north west England. *J Med Genet* 1999;**36**:197–203.

3. Ferner RE, Golding JF, Smith M *et al.* [18F]2-fluoro-2-deoxy-D-glucose positron emission tomography (FDG PET) as a diagnostic tool for neurofibromatosis 1 (NF1) associated malignant peripheral nerve sheath tumours (MPNSTs): a long-term clinical study. *Ann Oncol* 2008;**19**:390–4.

4. Ferner RE, Lucas JD, O'Doherty MJ *et al.* Evaluation of (18) fluorodeoxyglucose positron emission tomography ((18)FDG PET) in the detection of malignant peripheral nerve sheath tumours arising from within plexiform neurofibromas in neurofibromatosis 1. *J Neurol Neurosurg Psychiatry* 2000;**68**:353–7.

5. Warbey VS, Ferner RE, Dunn JT *et al.* [(18)F]FDG PET/CT in the diagnosis of malignant peripheral nerve sheath tumours in neurofibromatosis type-1. *Eur J Nucl Med Mol Imaging* 2009;**36**:751–7.

6. Bredella MA, Torriani M, Hornicek F *et al.* Value of PET in the assessment of patients with neurofibromatosis type 1. *Am J Roentgenol* 2007;**189**:928–35.

7. Cardona S, Schwarzbach M, Hinz U *et al.* Evaluation of F18-deoxyglucose positron emission tomography (FDG-PET) to assess the nature of neurogenic tumours. *Eur J Surg Oncol* 2003;**29**:536–41.

A 23-year-old male with metastatic Ewing sarcoma who presented with back pain, leg pain, headache, and fatigue. Initial CT of the chest, abdomen, and pelvis demonstrated widespread disease including osseous involvement and several pulmonary nodules. FDG-PET/CT was ordered for further evaluation of metabolic avidity of known disease prior to chemotherapy.

## Findings and differential diagnosis

The FDG-PET/CT in October 2009 prior to chemotherapy shows widespread FDG-avid disease including FDG-avid osseous lesions and pulmonary nodules (Figure 18.5A). The FDG-PET/CT in March 2010 immediately following chemotherapy shows significant interval decrease in FDG-avid disease with near-complete resolution of FDG-avid pulmonary and osseous lesions (Figure 18.5B). Only minimal residual uptake was identified in the soft tissue and marrow at the site of disease in the left thigh. Unfortunately, the follow-up study in August 2010 showed new intensely FDG-avid pulmonary nodules and a new FDG-avid sclerotic lesion in the left iliac bone highly suggestive of recurrent metastasis (Figure 18.5C). The low-level FDG uptake in the mid left thigh was also slightly more FDG-avid.

This was a case of known metastatic Ewing's sarcoma, although other malignancies could also have this appearance on PET. The intense tracer uptake in the left mid thigh as well as the numerous other sites of osseous disease and pulmonary nodules are highly suspicious for a primary osseous sarcoma such as Ewing's sarcoma.

## Diagnosis and clinical follow-up

Pathology confirmed metastatic Ewing's sarcoma originating from the left femur.

## Discussion and teaching points

The Ewing's sarcoma family of tumors (ESFT) is a complex group of aggressive tumors arising from primordial mesenchymal stem cells of the bone marrow and includes Ewing's sarcoma, extraosseous Ewing's sarcoma, Askin tumor (chest wall primary tumor), and primitive neuroectodermal tumor. Based on the Surveillance, Epidemiology, and End Results (SEER) data, the incidence of the ESFT is estimated to be 3 per 1,000,000 per year (1). In particular, Ewing's sarcoma is thought to be the second most commonly diagnosed primary bone tumor of children and young adults. The majority of patients are adolescents (1). Ewing's sarcoma can occur throughout the body but is typically found in the extremities

and pelvis. There are no known risk factors for the disease but there may be a link with a family history of cancer. Several factors suggest improved prognosis, such as limited stage (2) and small volume disease (3).

The clinical presentation of patients with Ewing's sarcoma is variable and depends on the disease extent and location. In some cases, the disease may be present for several years before coming to clinical attention while in other cases it may present early with pain or with an osseous-based mass. It is estimated that 20–30% of patients have metastatic disease at the time of diagnosis, often involving the lungs and bones.

Depending on the clinical presentation, the initial evaluation of patients with Ewing's sarcoma often includes radiographs followed by MRI for local staging. Chest CT is performed to evaluate for lung metastases. Bone scintigraphy and bone marrow biopsy may be helpful to identify distant bone disease, although some centers advocate the use of spine MRI as a sensitive and less invasive alternative approach to assessing bone marrow involvement (4). The utility of FDG-PET for the evaluation of the primary site of disease is limited, but it can be helpful for the identification of other sites of soft tissue disease as well as bone metastases (5). In general, diagnostic CT is superior to FDG-PET for the detection of pulmonary nodules (6). However, FDG-PET is more sensitive than either MRI or planar $^{99m}$Tc-MDP bone scintigraphy (7, 8) for the identification of osseous metastases. The high sensitivity of FDG-PET for osseous disease is likely related to the fact that FDG-PET investigates malignant cells while planar bone scintigraphy assesses the osteoblastic reaction to the malignant cells. In addition, Ewing's sarcoma metastases often involve bone marrow and are lytic, which decreases the sensitivity of bone scintigraphy.

FDG-PET/CT has superior sensitivity and specificity to FDG-PET alone for the detection and localization of sites of disease (9). Also, SPECT bone scintigraphy and $^{18}$F-NaF-PET are more sensitive than planar bone scintigraphy for the detection of osseous disease. Further investigation is needed to determine the precise role of FDG-PET/CT, SPECT bone scintigraphy, and $^{18}$F-NaF-PET in patients with Ewing's sarcoma.

Therapy for patients with Ewing's sarcoma has changed over the past few years. Currently, the combination of local control and multi-agent chemotherapy has improved the 5-year survival to 60–70% in patients with localized disease of the extremities. However, patients with distant metastases continue to have poor survival.

There is relatively scarce literature on the value of FDG-PET for the evaluation of patients with Ewing's sarcoma

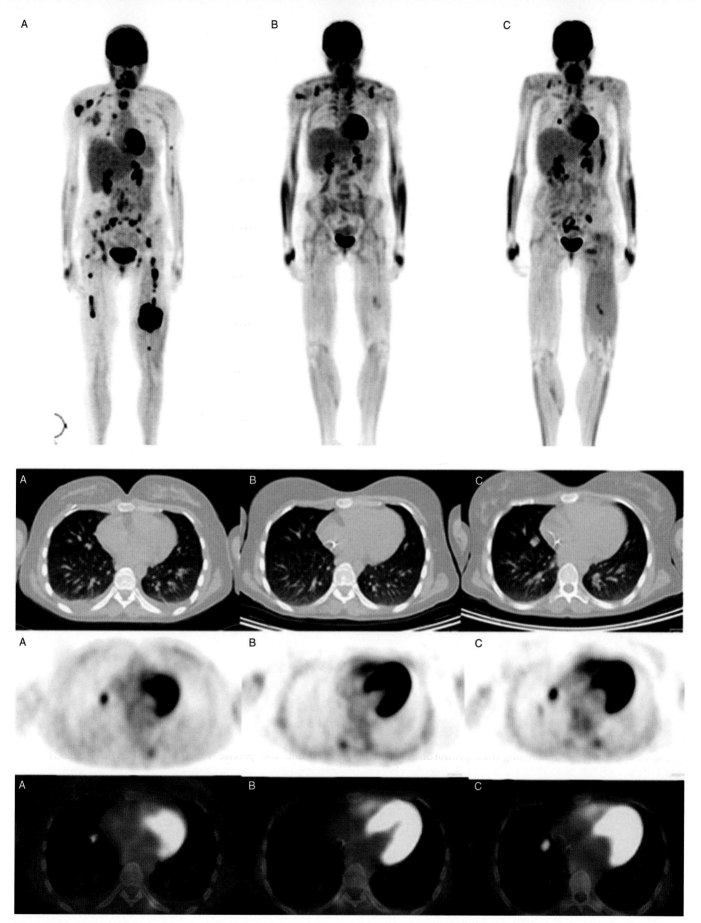

**Figure 18.5** (A) MIP whole-body PET and axial CT, PET. and fused images of the lungs in October 2009 prior to chemotherapy. (B) MIP whole-body PET and axial CT, PET, and fused images of the lungs in March 2010 after chemotherapy. (C) MIP whole-body PET and axial CT, PET, and fused images of the lungs in August 2010 at the time of follow-up.

pre- and post-therapy. MRI is routinely used to evaluate the response of local disease to therapy. Preliminary results suggest, however, that pre- and post-therapy FDG-PET can show response to treatment (10), may be used to predict progression-free survival (11) and is useful to detect sites of recurrent disease (12).

## Take-home message

- Ewing's sarcoma belongs to the Ewing's sarcoma family of tumors, a complex group of aggressive tumors arising from primordial mesenchymal stem cells.

- MRI is performed for local staging and chest CT, bone scintigraphy, bone marrow biopsy, and/or spine MRI may be helpful for the assessment of distant disease.
- The utility of FDG-PET for the evaluation of localized disease is limited, but it can be helpful to guide biopsy, and identify soft tissue and bone metastases.
- Preliminary studies suggest FDG-PET can be used to predict progression-free survival and to identify sites of recurrent disease.

## References

1. http://www.cancer.gov/cancertopics/pdq/treatment/ewings/healthprofessional#Section_153 [accessed November 25 2010].

2. Coterill SJ, Ahrens S, Paulussen M et al. Prognostic factors in Ewing's tumor of bone: analysis of 975 patients from the European intergroup cooperative Ewing's sarcoma study group. *J Clin Oncol* 2000;**18**:3108–14.

3. Paulussen M, Ahrens S, Dunst J et al. Localized Ewing tumor of the bone: final results of the cooperative Ewing's sarcoma study CESS 86. *J Clin Oncol* 2001;**19**:1818–29.

4. Mentzel H-J, Kentouche K, Sauner D et al. Comparison of whole-body STIR-MRI and 99mTc-methylene-diphosphonate scintigraphy in children with suspected multifocal bone lesions. *Eur Radiol* 2004;**14**:2297–302.

5. Völker T, Denecke T, Steffen I et al. Positron emission tomography for staging pediatric sarcoma patients: results of a prospective multicenter trial. *J Clin Oncol* 2007;**25**:5435–41.

6. Franzius C, Daldrup-Link HE, Sciuk J et al. FDG-PET for detection of pulmonary metastases from malignant primary bone tumors: comparison with spiral CT. *Ann Oncol* 2001;**12**:479–86.

7. Daldrup-Link HE, Franzius C, Link TM et al. Whole-body MR imaging for detection of bone metastases in children and young adults: comparison with skeletal scintigraphy and FDG PET. *Am J Radiol* 2001;**177**: 229–36.

8. Franzius C, Sciuk J, Daldrup-Link HE et al. FDG-PET for detection of osseous metastases from malignant primary bone tumours: comparison with bone scintigraphy. *Eur J Nucl Med* 2000;**27**:1305–11.

9. Gerth HU, Juergens KU, Dirksen U et al. Significant benefit of multi-modal imaging: PET/CT compared with PET alone in staging and follow-up of patients with Ewing tumors. *J Nucl Med* 2007;**48**(12):1932–9.

10. Furth C, Amthauer H, Denecke T et al. Impact of whole-body MRI and FDG-PET on staging and assessment of therapy response in a patient with Ewing sarcoma. *Pediatr Blood Cancer* 2006;**47**:607–11.

11. Hawkins DS, Rajendran JG, Conrad EU 3rd et al. Evaluation of chemotherapy response in pediatric bone sarcomas by [F-18]-fluorodeoxy-D-glucose positron emission tomography. *Cancer* 2002;**94**:3277–84.

12. Arush MW, Israel O, Postovsky S et al. Positron emission tomography/computed tomography with 18Fluoro-deoxyglucose in the detection of local recurrence and distant metastases of pediatric sarcoma. *Pediatr Blood Cancer* 2007;**49**:901–5.

A 38-year-old female with a history of left pleural synovial sarcoma, post-surgical resection of the tumor and chemotherapy 1 year ago. FDG-PET/CT was ordered for the evaluation of possible recurrent disease and distant metastatic disease.

## Findings and differential diagnosis

FDG-PET/CT shows extensive changes in the left hemithorax including metabolically active pleural-based disease that was suspicious for recurrent malignancy (Figure 18.6). The sites of intense tracer uptake could be used to guide biopsy to the most histologically aggressive portion of disease (see Chapter 20). Of note, the radiological appearance of pleuropulmonary synovial sarcoma is similar to that of other diseases of the lung and pleura such as primary and metastatic lung cancer and malignant mesothelioma.

## Diagnosis and clinical follow-up

Pathology confirmed recurrent synovial sarcoma and therapy was initiated.

## Discussion and teaching points

Synovial sarcomas are uncommon soft tissue tumors that are thought to arise *de novo* from mesenchymal tissue (1). Malignancy most frequently involves the para-articular extremities of young adults, although other sites of disease may include the head and neck, chest, abdomen, and paravertebral region. The typical clinical presentation of a patient with a synovial sarcoma is of a painful slow-growing palpable mass; however, the clinical presentation may vary depending on the site of the disease and the involvement of adjacent structures. Larger volume disease at diagnosis is thought to be associated with a worse prognosis. It is estimated that 25% of patients have metastases at presentation, most commonly to the lungs (1).

Pleuropulmonary synovial sarcoma is a subtype of synovial sarcoma that may arise in the chest wall, pleura, heart, mediastinum, or lungs (2). The typical clinical presentation includes a cough, chest pain, or dyspnea.

Often radiographs are obtained at the time of presentation and may reveal a well-defined lobulated soft tissue mass. In most cases of pleuropulmonary synovial sarcoma, the mass is pleural-based. In a minority of cases, the disease may involve more than 50% of the hemithorax (2). MRI is the modality of choice for local staging (3) while chest CT is helpful to assess for pulmonary metastases. MRI or bone scintigraphy may be helpful for the evaluation of distant sites of osseous disease. FDG-PET can show increased uptake at sites of metabolically active disease (2). Since extrathoracic synovial sarcoma with pulmonary metastases is more common than pleuropulmonary synovial sarcoma, whole-body FDG-PET/CT is particularly helpful to exclude extrathoracic sites of disease.

The primary management for patients with pleuropulmonary synovial sarcoma is surgery, with post-operative radiation to improve local control and multi-regimen chemotherapy in certain cases (2–3). MRI is typically done following therapy to evaluate for local recurrence while follow-up chest radiographs or CT are routinely performed to monitor for metastases. There are limited preliminary results in the literature suggesting that pre-therapy FDG-PET may be helpful to predict progression-free survival (4).

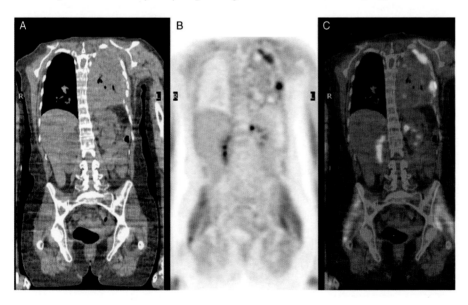

**Figure 18.6** Coronal (A) CT, (B) FDG-PET, and (C) fused FDG-PET/CT centered on the left hemithorax disease.

## Take-home message

- Pleuropulmonary synovial sarcoma is a subtype of synovial sarcoma.
- Surgery is the cornerstone of therapy, although post-operative radiation and multi-regimen chemotherapy may be helpful.

- FDG-PET can be useful in detection of recurrence and guiding biopsy.

## References

1. O'Sullivan PJ, Harris AC, Munk PL. Radiological features of synovial cell sarcoma: pictorial review. *Br J Radiol* 2008;81: 346–56.

2. Frazier A, Franks TJ, Pugatch RD, Galvin JR. From the archives of the AFIP: pleuropulmonary synovial sarcoma. *Radiographics* 2006;**26**:923–40.

3. Mirzoyan M, Muslimani A, Setrakian S, Swedeh M, Daw HA. Primary pleuropulmonary synovial sarcoma. *Clin Lung Cancer* 2008;9:257–61.

4. Lisle J, Eary JF, O'Sullivan J, Conrad EU. Risk assessment based on FDG-PET imaging in patients with synovial sarcoma. *Clin Orthop Relat Res* 2009;**467**:1605–11.

# 19

# Methodological aspects of therapeutic response evaluation with FDG-PET

Saiyada N. F. Rizvi, Ronald Boellaard, Sigrid Stroobants, and Otto S. Hoekstra

Predicting and evaluating response to therapy may become one of the most important indications for FDG-PET in oncology. The FDG-PET result could serve as a surrogate for actual patient outcomes in clinical practice and in drug development. The FDG-PET end result can be qualitative or, increasingly often, quantitative.

In this context, three methodological aspects of a totally different nature are of crucial importance: getting the right numbers out of the scan (standardization, validation of simplified quantitative measures), validating the biological relevance of the tracer signal (changes), and developing and validating the response criteria. In this chapter, examples of each of these domains (physics, biology, and epidemiology) will be discussed. To some extent, the cases have been modified from actual practice for didactical reasons.

*A Case-Based Approach to PET/CT in Oncology*, ed. Victor H. Gerbaudo. Published by Cambridge University Press.
© Cambridge University Press 2012.

A 62-year-old female with locally advanced cancer of the left breast was treated with experimental neoadjuvant chemotherapy. No data have been published on FDG-PET and this new therapeutic agent. A secondary aim of the study is to explore the use of FDG-PET to evaluate the response to this therapy.

## Acquisition and processing parameters and findings

Dynamic FDG-PET scans were obtained at baseline and after one cycle of therapy. The PET scanner (ECAT EXACT HR+; Siemens/CTI, Knoxville) used provides an axial field of view of 15.5 cm and produces 63 transaxial slices with a slice thickness of 2.5 mm. The patient fasted for at least 6 hours prior to the imaging sessions. The patient was scanned in the supine position with arms at her sides. The patient was positioned in such a way that the dominant lesions were in the center of the field of view. The distance between the suprasternal notch and the upper field of view (laser beam alignment) was recorded and used on subsequent scans. First, a 10-min transmission scan was acquired using three rotating $^{68}$Ge rod sources; this was followed by intravenous injection of a bolus of approximately 10 mCi of FDG, simultaneously starting a dynamic emission scan in 2-D mode. Data acquisition ($6 \times 5$, $6 \times 10$, $3 \times 20$, $5 \times 30$, $5 \times 60$, $8 \times 150$, $6 \times 300$ s frames) was identical for the baseline and post-therapy scans. Emission data were corrected for decay, dead time, scatter, random coincidences, and measured photon attenuation. Scans were reconstructed into $128 \times 128$ matrices using both filtered backprojection (FBP) with a 0.5 Hanning filter and ordered subsets expectation maximization (OSEM, 2 iterations with 16 subsets), followed by post-smoothing with a 0.5 Hanning filter. The resulting transaxial spatial resolution for both reconstruction methods was ~7 mm full-width at half-maximum at the center of the field of view. VOIs were defined on summed images of the last three frames (i.e., 45–60 min post-injection) as follows: VOIs were generated automatically using a region growing method, which only included pixels greater than a preset threshold, 75% of the maximum value within a lesion. SUV was corrected for lean body mass and for plasma glucose. SUVs were calculated using the average counts within the threshold-defined VOI, in the OSEM reconstructed images ($2 \times 16$).

In this patient, the $SUV_{75}$ of the primary tumor decreased by 50% after one cycle of chemotherapy.

## Discussion and teaching points

*Question*: Is the decrease of the metabolic rate of glucose ($MR_{glu}$) consumption also 50%?

*Answer*: This is not necessarily so.

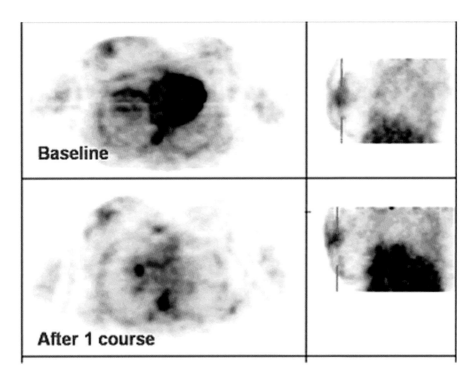

**Figure 19.1** Representative axial (left) and sagittal slices of FDG-PET scan obtained at baseline and after one course of therapy.

In response-monitoring studies with FDG-PET, one assumes that the level of tracer uptake is somehow proportional to tumor "activity," i.e., that a reduction in uptake following therapy reflects lower tumor "activity" and vice versa. The most commonly used method is a very simple semiquantitative method: the standardized uptake value (SUV). This method is attractive for clinical studies as it requires only a single (static) scan, usually acquired 60 min after intravenous injection of FDG, and no blood sampling. SUV is then calculated as tumor uptake, normalized to injected dose and a factor that takes into account the total distribution space of FDG. The main disadvantage, however, is the inherent assumption that plasma clearance is always the same. If plasma clearance of FDG changes as a result of therapy (i.e., due to changing uptake in other tissues), the relationship between uptake at a certain time and injected dose will also change (1). This cannot be accounted for in the SUV calculation and, consequently, comparison of pre- and post-therapy scans might be misleading.

The currently available evidence shows no substantial effects of classic cytotoxic drugs on the kinetics of FDG, at least not in settings in which therapy is administered for short periods, ample time is allowed between courses to allow for recovery, and FDG-PET scanning is performed after such a recovery period (i.e., just prior to the next course). At present, new drugs are being introduced which are administered continuously. Under these conditions it cannot be assumed that there will be no effects on the kinetics of FDG at the time of repeat scans during therapy. Therefore, it has been recommended to validate the use of SUV in cases of investigational drug classes, and to start with dynamic studies to explore whether SUV is a valid alternative for metabolic rate of glucose (2).

## Take-home message

- With appropriate normalizations, SUV is closely related to metabolic rate of glucose ($MR_{glu}$).
- This is also true for use during cytotoxic therapy.
- Drugs altering pharmacokinetics of FDG may affect the association with $MR_{glu}$.
- Validating the use of SUV to monitor response to therapy with new investigational drug classes is essential.

## References

1. Doot RK, Dunnwald LK, Schubert EK *et al*. Dynamic and static approaches to quantifying 18F-FDG uptake for measuring cancer response to therapy, including the effect of granulocyte CSF. *J Nucl Med* 2007;**48**(6):920–5.

2. Shankar LK, Hoffman JM, Bacharach S *et al*. Consensus recommendations for the use of 18F-FDG PET as an indicator of therapeutic response in patients in National Cancer Institute Trials. *J Nucl Med* 2006;**47**(6):1059–66.

A 50-year-old male presenting with an adenocarcinoma of the esophagus, clinically staged as T3N1M0.

## Acquisition and processing parameters

A staging PET scan was obtained using an HR+ scanner, 60 min after injection of 10 mCi of FDG. The scan was obtained in 2-D mode. The scanner was calibrated according to the NEDPAS protocol (1).

The scan showed increased FDG uptake in the known esophageal cancer with an SUVmax of 8.0 (Figure 19.2).

Thereafter, the patient was referred to a hospital recruiting patients for a clinical trial evaluating the predictive value of FDG-PET early during neoadjuvant chemoradiotherapy.

This scan was also acquired with an HR+ PET scanner, also calibrated using the NEDPAS protocol, and the acquisition also started 60 min after injection of 10 mCi of FDG, in 2-D mode (Figure 19.3).

## Findings, discussion, and teaching points

On the scan obtained during therapy there is still intense uptake in the primary tumor, with a SUVmax of 9.9. The response to therapy was classified as "progressive disease" since the FDG uptake in the primary tumor had increased by 24% (2).

However, after reading the report and reviewing the images, the attending physician asks why the images of the second scan are so "noisy."

*Question*: Is he right, and if so, what is the likely explanation? Can this affect the response classification assigned to this case?

*Answer*: The clinician was right. It seems that different reconstruction parameters have been used during the processing of these scans. In fact, the initial FDG-PET scan proved to have been reconstructed with OSEM 1 iteration, 8 subsets, and the second with 2 iterations, 16 subsets. In fact, reconstruction of the first scan with the same parameters as the second one

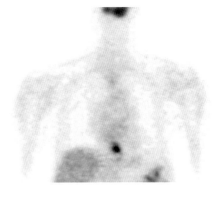

**Figure 19.2** Coronal slice of FDG-PET at presentation.

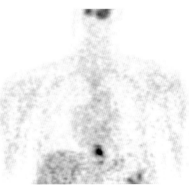

**Figure 19.3** Coronal slice of the FDG-PET scan obtained during therapy.

revealed that the tumor SUVmax in the first scan was also 9.9. (3–5).

## Take-home message

- Standardized uptake values depend on acquisition, reconstruction, and region of interest (ROI) definition parameters.
- In multicenter studies as well as in daily clinical practice, such parameters need to be controlled.

## References

1. Boellaard R, Oyen WJ, Hoekstra CJ et al. The Netherlands protocol for standardisation and quantification of FDG whole body PET studies in multi-centre trials. *Eur J Nucl Med Mol Imaging* 2008;**35**(12):2320–33.

2. Young H, Baum R, Cremerius U et al. Measurement of clinical and subclinical tumour response using [18F]-fluorodeoxyglucose and positron emission tomography: review and 1999 EORTC recommendations. European Organization for Research and Treatment of Cancer (EORTC) PET Study Group. *Eur J Cancer* 1999; **35**(13):1773–82.

3. Boellaard R, Krak NC, Hoekstra OS, Lammertsma AA. Effects of noise, image resolution, and ROI definition on the accuracy of standard uptake values: a simulation study. *J Nucl Med* 2004;**45**(9):1519–27.

4. Westerterp M, Pruim J, Oyen W et al. Quantification of FDG PET studies using standardised uptake values in multi-centre trials: effects of image reconstruction, resolution and ROI definition parameters. *Eur J Nucl Med Mol Imaging* 2007;**34**(3):392–404.

5. Boellaard R, O'Doherty MJ, Weber WA et al. FDG PET and PET/CT: EANM procedure guidelines for tumour PET imaging: version 1.0. *Eur J Nucl Med Mol Imaging* 2010;**37**(1):181–200.

A patient presented with locally advanced (stage IIIA-N2) non-small cell lung cancer (NSCLC, adenocarcinoma).

## Acquisition and processing parameters

FDG-PET scans of the chest before induction chemotherapy were obtained 55 min after injection of FDG. Images were reconstructed to yield a post-reconstruction resolution of about 7 mm FWHM.

## Findings, discussion, and teaching points

In Figure 19.4 the two images on the left show the baseline pre-induction chemotherapy (pre-IC) contrast-enhanced CT scan, and the attenuation-corrected FDG-PET scan, showing intense uptake in the primary tumor of the left upper lobe lesion on CT. The lesion SUVmax was 9.

The patient was treated with three cycles of platinum-based induction chemotherapy. After completion, the patient was referred for PET (CT and PET images on the right of Figure 19.4: post-IC), which was acquired using exactly the same parameters as during the first scan. The post-IC CT revealed partial lesion remission, but FDG-PET still showed intense uptake in the primary tumor, with an SUVmax of 5.

The attending physician has read a research article expanding on the impressive survival stratification of the SUV post-IC (Figure 19.5) (8), and suggests to you that his patient (with a tumor SUV of 5) is in the poor prognostic group.

*Question*: Is he right?

*Answer*: This is impossible to answer without knowledge of the FDG-PET methodology applied in the published study. One needs to know specific details on the time between tracer injection and the scan, the region of interest definition, scanner calibration, and image reconstruction parameters.

The importance of standardizing the interval between FDG injection and scan acquisition is demonstrated in Figure 19.6. In this case the measured activity in the primary tumor (obtained in another NSCLC patient who underwent a dynamic FDG-PET scan) increases by more than 20% between 55 and 90 min after injection.

The latter was the time delay after injection used by the authors cited by the attending physician.

## Take-home message

- Generalizability of SUV thresholds is limited due to methodological heterogeneity in the PET literature.
- This is especially true for absolute SUV levels, less so for relative changes (provided that baseline and follow-up scans have been performed similarly).

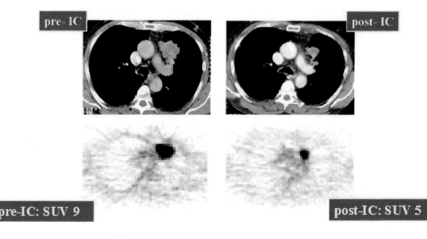

pre- IC

post- IC

pre-IC: SUV 9

post-IC: SUV 5

**Figure 19.4** Left: Pre-therapy axial CT (top) and FDG-PET (bottom). Right: Post-therapy axial CT (top) and FDG-PET (bottom).

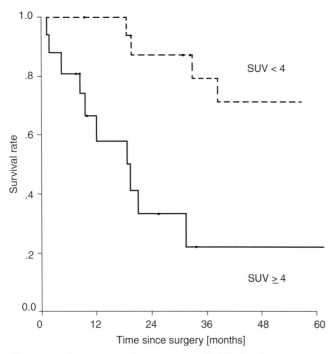

**Figure 19.5** Prognostic stratification upon residual FDG uptake in the primary tumor after induction chemotherapy.

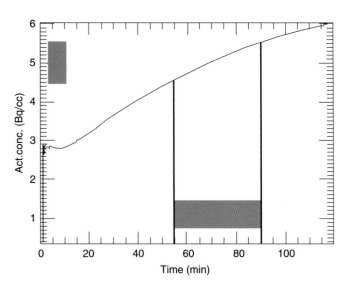

**Figure 19.6** Time-activity curve of NSCLC (random patient).

# Reference

1. Hellwig D, Graeter TP, Ukena D *et al.* Value of F-18-fluorodeoxyglucose positron emission tomography after induction therapy of locally advanced bronchogenic carcinoma. *J Thorac Cardiovasc Surg* 2004;**128**(6):892–9.

You are participating in a phase II clinical trial evaluating a new drug.

Figure 19.7 shows a coronal slice of the patient prior to therapy. The image reveals liver metastases with central necrosis and a viable rim.

The second scan obtained post-therapy with the new drug shows resolution of the earlier abnormalities (Figure 19.8)

*Question*: does this finding have predictive impact?

*Answer*: Even without any quantification, it is quite clear that the FDG signal has dramatically changed due to this therapy.

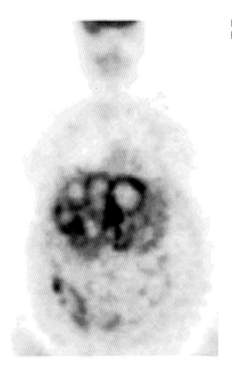

**Figure 19.7** Coronal FDG-PET at baseline.

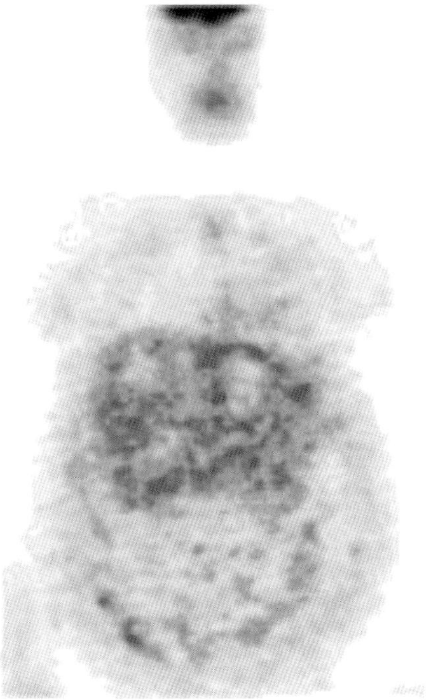

**Figure 19.8** Coronal FDG-PET after therapy.

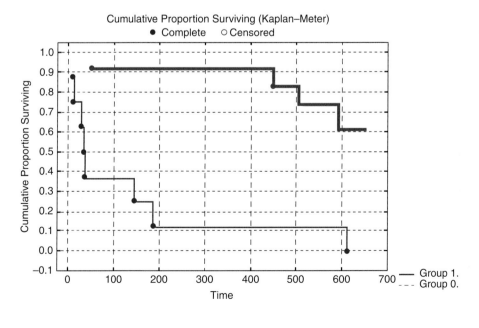

**Figure 19.9** Survival analysis of patients with GIST tumors treated with imatinib, stratified by FDG response. With permission from S Stroobants, J Goeminne, M Seegers *et al*. 18FDG-Positron emission tomography for the early prediction of response in advanced soft tissue sarcoma treated with imatinib mesylate (Glivec). *Eur J Cancer* 2003;**39**(14):2012–20.

However, in order to qualify as a suitable biomarker of response, the association between FDG-PET response patterns and patient outcome needs to be established. In this particular case of gastro-intestinal stromal cell tumor (GIST) treated with imatinib, studies have confirmed the suitability of FDG-PET in this context (1): patients with this type of PET response (blue) do much better than the ones with unchanged uptake (red) (Figure 19.9).

## Take-home message

- With classic cytotoxic chemotherapy, FDG is an appropriate read-out of response.
- For newer, "targeted" agents, this predictive value remains to be validated.

## Reference

1. Stroobants S, Goeminne J, Seegers M *et al.* 18FDG-Positron emission tomography for the early prediction of response in advanced soft tissue sarcoma treated with imatinib mesylate (Glivec). *Eur J Cancer* 2003;**39**(14):2012–20.

A patient with non-Hodgkin's lymphoma of the diffuse large cell type was referred for response evaluation after completed CHOP chemotherapy.

The baseline FDG-PET scan was acquired at another hospital. The report of that scan stated that there were multiple intense foci of FDG uptake in enlarged nodes in the right axillary region, as well as multiple skeletal, and especially vertebral, lesions.

Figure 19.10 represents a coronal slice of the post-therapy scan showing clearly enhanced uptake on the right side of a mid-lumbar vertebra. You read the scan as persistent uptake and report that this is suspicious of persistent lymphoma.

*Question*: The hematologist asks whether they should perform a biopsy to confirm the suspicion. Is this the most logical step?

*Answer*: The hematologist is correct that FDG-PET positive findings do not replace a biopsy (1); however, the issue is whether your interpretation is correct without having reviewed the baseline scan.

A few days later, you receive the images of the baseline FDG-PET scan (Figure 19.11).

When reviewing the baseline study, you realize that it is obvious that the "abnormality" on the post-therapy FDG-PET scan reflected normal bone marrow activity, considering that the baseline scan revealed enhanced activity on the left side of this lumbar vertebra, rather than on its right side.

## Take-home message

- Baseline FDG-PET scans are mandatory in malignant lymphoma subtypes that may not be FDG avid (1, 2).
- FDG-PET response criteria in lymphoma require comparison with baseline imaging, but since the added value of FDG-PET in staging is limited, the baseline CT scan can also be used.
- There are some indications that observer variation may improve upon the use of baseline FDG-PET scans (3).

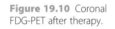

Figure 19.10 Coronal FDG-PET after therapy.

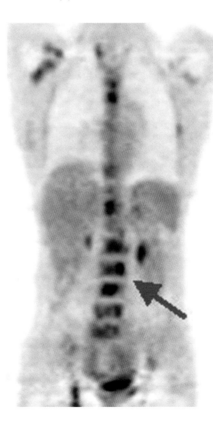

Figure 19.11 Coronal slice at the same level as the post-therapy scan.

# References

1. Cheson BD, Pfistner B, Juweid ME *et al.* Revised response criteria for malignant lymphoma. *J Clin Oncol* 2007;**25**(5):579–86.

2. Juweid ME, Stroobants S, Hoekstra OS *et al.* Use of positron emission tomography for response assessment of lymphoma: consensus of the Imaging Subcommittee of International Harmonization Project in Lymphoma. *J Clin Oncol* 2007;**25**(5):571–8.

3. Quarles van Ufford H, Hoekstra OS, de Haas M *et al.* On the added value of baseline FDG-PET in malignant lymphoma. *Mol Imaging Biol* 2010;**12**(2):225–32.

A 60-year-old female patient has diffuse large cell non-Hodgkin's lymphoma (NHL) with pre-therapy findings in the neck and mediastinum. Upon completion of CHOP therapy the patient is referred for response evaluation with FDG-PET. CT has revealed a complete remission.

## Acquisition and processing parameters and findings

Figure 19.12 shows contiguous 1 cm non-attenuation corrected coronal slices, obtained with an HR+ PET scanner, 60 min after 10 mCi of FDG. The scan is unremarkable, except for an intense focus of FDG uptake in the periphery of the upper lobe of the right lung (p32-p34).

## Discussion and teaching points

You are one of the central reviewers of an observational trial which evaluates the predictive value of FDG-PET in this context. You are provided with this scan only.

*Question*: How do you classify the response?

*Answer*: The original NHL localizations in the neck and mediastinum are normal. The initial report did not indicate the presence of pulmonary lesions. If that is correct, and the intrapulmonary lesion has emerged during therapy, it should be considered inflammatory until proven otherwise (1). With respect to her lymphoma, the patient is very likely to be in complete remission. In this case, the final diagnosis of the pulmonary lesion was coccidiodiomycosis.

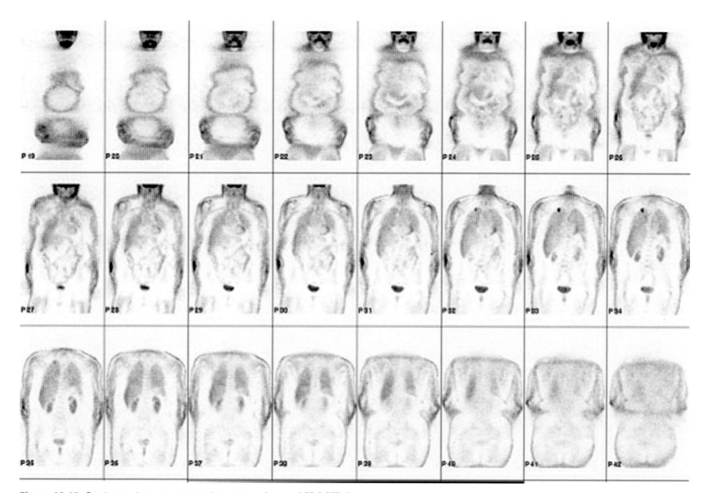

**Figure 19.12** Contiguous 1 cm non-attenuation corrected coronal FDG-PET slices.

497

## Take-home message

- In case of resolution of former lymphoma sites, any new lesion is non-malignant until proven otherwise.

- During chemotherapy, pulmonary infections are common and may be opportunistic.

## Reference

1. Juweid ME, Stroobants S, Hoekstra OS *et al.* Use of positron emission tomography for response assessment of lymphoma: consensus of the Imaging Subcommittee of International Harmonization Project in Lymphoma. *J Clin Oncol* 2007; 25(5):571–8.

A 50-year-old male was treated with platinum-based chemoradiotherapy for locally advanced non-small cell lung cancer (IIIA-N2). The patient underwent dynamic FDG-PET imaging before and after the therapy was completed.

## Acquisition and processing parameters

A 10- to 15-min transmission scan was acquired to correct for photon attenuation followed by a bolus injection of 10 mCi of FDG in 5 mL of saline at a rate of 0.8 mL/s, after which the line was flushed with 42 mL of saline (2.0 mL/s). Simultaneously with the injection of FDG, a dynamic 2-D emission scan was started with a total duration of 60 min with variable frame length (6 × 5, 6 × 10, 3 × 20, 5 × 30, 5 × 60, 8 × 150, and 6 × 300 seconds). All dynamic scan data were corrected for dead time, decay, scatter, randoms, and photon attenuation and were reconstructed with a 128 × 128 matrix using filtered back projection (FBP) with a Hanning filter (cut-off, 0.5 cycles/pixel). This resulted in a transaxial spatial resolution of around 7-mm full width at half maximum. In addition, three venous blood samples were drawn at 35, 45, and 55 min after FDG injection as quality control for the image-derived input function and for plasma glucose measurement.

## Findings, discussion, and teaching points

The metabolic rate of glucose in the primary tumor after therapy was 0.08 μmol/mL/min. This is well below the 0.13 μmol/mL/min threshold of residual FDG uptake after therapy reported by Hoekstra *et al.* (1) in similar patients during induction chemotherapy (Figure 19.13).

*Question*: Does this finding imply that this patient is likely to have a 60% probability of surviving 3 years?

*Answer*: No, for two different reasons:

1. The therapeutic regimen of the primary study involved induction chemotherapy, and not chemoradiation. The whole idea behind following the metabolic behavior of the primary tumor builds on the hypothesis that this will reflect the efficacy of the therapy on the cancer process, i.e., not only on the primary tumor but also on the clinically occult distant metastases that will ultimately kill most patients. Adding a local therapy (radiotherapy) to systemic therapy does not automatically imply that the association

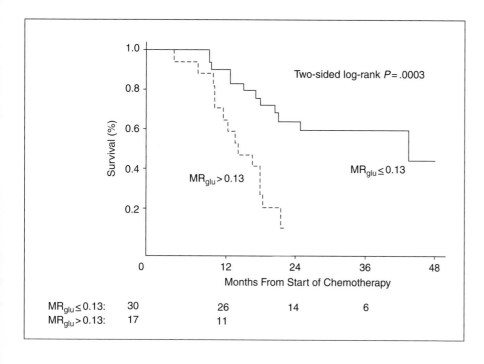

**Figure 19.13** Survival by absolute value of residual metabolic rate of glucose (MR_glu) after induction chemotherapy. With permission from CJ Hoekstra, SG Stroobants, EF Smit *et al.* Prognostic relevance of response evaluation using [18F]-2-fluoro-2-deoxy-d-glucose positron emission tomography in patients with locally advanced non-small-cell lung cancer. *J Clin Oncol* 2005;**23** (33):8362–70.

of the FDG biomarker and survival is maintained. This needs to be re-established.

2. The 0.13 µmol/mL/min threshold was data-driven and needs external validation. In the same study the authors prospectively validated an earlier proposed 50% change threshold (2), but residual FDG uptake was a better predictor.

## Take-home message

- Data-driven thresholds of response require external validation.
- Validity of imaging biomarkers of response may be intervention dependent.

## References

1. Hoekstra CJ, Stroobants SG, Smit EF *et al.* Prognostic relevance of response evaluation using [18F]-2-fluoro-2-deoxy-d-glucose positron emission tomography in patients with locally advanced non-small-cell lung cancer. *J Clin Oncol* 2005; **23**(33):8362–70.

2. Vansteenkiste JF, Stroobants SG, De Leyn PR, Dupont PJ, Verbeken EK. Potential use of FDG-PET scan after induction chemotherapy in surgically staged IIIa-N2 non-small-cell lung cancer: a prospective pilot study. The Leuven Lung Cancer Group. *Ann Oncol* 1998;**9**(11):1193–8.

# Chapter 20

# FDG-PET/CT-guided interventional procedures in oncologic diagnosis

Servet Tatli, Victor H. Gerbaudo, and Stuart Silverman

The unique ability of FDG-PET/CT imaging to investigate the biologic behavior of tumors by providing metabolic information has revolutionized the management of oncological diseases. In addition to its contribution to the diagnosis, staging, restaging, and monitoring of cancer therapy, FDG-PET/CT has been shown by our group as a useful technique to guide various interventional procedures (1). FDG-PET/CT has been used to plan biopsies (2, 3), surgery (4), and radiotherapy (5–9), and was recently added to the armamentarium of interventional radiologists as a guiding tool for biopsies and percutaneous ablations (1, 10).

Despite recent advances in medicine, particularly in imaging, definite diagnoses of a vast majority of cancers still rely on histopathological diagnosis. **Percutaneous image-guided biopsies** have become an invaluable tool in the care of patients with cancer. Biopsy with fine needles, or large needles in some cases, can be obtained with a percutaneous approach under cross-sectional imaging guidance. However, commonly used cross-sectional imaging modalities such as ultrasound (US), CT, and MRI provide largely anatomical and morphological information that sometimes may not be adequate enough to select the appropriate mass or a part of a mass to biopsy. Besides helping to select the metabolically active viable tumor tissue in order to improve pathological yield and to minimize sampling errors, the metabolic information provided by FDG-PET/CT allows for the visualization of a metabolically active mass without morphologic correlate on other cross-sectional imaging modalities while targeting the tumor during biopsy.

Minimally invasive image-guided **percutaneous tumor ablation** is now being used to treat patients with a variety of cancers, including those that are focal, small in size and limited in number, and particularly those patients who are not candidates for surgery (11–13). Although work is preliminary, FDG-PET/CT can be used to guide tumor ablations (1). The concept is similar to how PET/CT used to guide biopsy; FDG-PET/CT can be used to target and ablate the metabolically active tumors and the metabolically active portions of the tumor. As with any image-guided ablation FDG-PET/CT can contribute to assuring that the ablation is complete and not harmful to adjacent organs (1, 10).

FDG-PET/CT imaging can be utilized to guide percutaneously an intervention in three ways: (1) prior PET/CT images can be reviewed and an intervention can be planned and executed under another cross-sectional imaging modality (CT or MRI) with the aid of the metabolic information provided by the previously acquired FDG-PET/CT; (2) using special computer software, prior FDG-PET/CT images demonstrating metabolically active tumor in the area of interest are registered and fused with the images of the cross-sectional imaging modality being used for the interventional procedure; and (3) the intervention can be performed in the nuclear medicine suite directly under FDG-PET/CT scan guidance.

In this chapter, we will demonstrate and discuss different cases in which FDG-PET/CT images were utilized to guide different stages of intervention.

## References

1. Tatli S, Gerbaudo VH, Mamede M *et al.* Abdominal masses sampled at PET/CT-guided percutaneous biopsy: initial experience with registration of prior PET/CT images. *Radiology* 2010;**256**(1):305–11.

2. Hain SF, Curran KM, Beggs AD *et al.* FDG-PET as a "metabolic biopsy" tool in thoracic lesions with indeterminate biopsy. *Eur J Nucl Med* 2001;**28**(9):1336–40.

3. Mallarajapatna GJ, Kallur KG, Ramanna NK, Susheela SP, Ramachandra PG. PET/CT-guided percutaneous biopsy of isolated intramuscular metastases from postcricoid cancer. *J Nucl Med Technol* 2009;**37**(4):220–2.

4. Cohn DE, Hall NC, Povoski SP *et al.* Novel perioperative imaging with 18F-FDG PET/CT and intraoperative 18F-FDG detection using a handheld gamma probe in recurrent ovarian cancer. *Gyn Oncol* 2008;**110**(2):152–7.

5. Aerts HJ, van Baardwijk AA, Petit SF *et al.* Identification of residual metabolic-active areas within individual NSCLC tumours using a pre-radiotherapy (18)Fluorodeoxyglucose-PET-CT scan. *Radiother Oncol* 2009;**91**(3):386–92.

6. Roels S, Slagmolen P, Nuyts J *et al.* Biological image-guided radiotherapy in rectal cancer: challenges and pitfalls. *Int J Radiat Oncol Biol Phys* 2009;**75**(3):782–90.

7. Abramyuk A, Tokalov S, Zöphel K *et al.* Is pre-therapeutical FDG-PET/CT capable to detect high risk tumor subvolumes responsible for local failure in non-small cell lung cancer? *Radiother Oncol* 2009;**91**(3):399–404.

8. Ford EC, Herman J, Yorke E, Wahl RL. 18F-FDG PET/CT for image-guided and intensity-modulated radiotherapy. *J Nucl Med* 2009;**50**(10):1655–65.

9. Vila A, Sánchez-Reyes A, Conill C *et al.* Comparison of positron emission tomography (PET) and computed tomography (CT) for better target volume definition in radiation therapy planning. *Clin Transl Oncol* 2010;**12**(5):367–73.

10. Schoellnast H, Larson SM, Nehmeh SA *et al.* Radiofrequency ablation of non-small-cell carcinoma of the lung under real-time FDG PET CT guidance. *Cardiovasc Intervent Radiol* 2011; **34**(Suppl 2):182–5.

11. Silverman SG, Tuncali K, Morrison PR. MR Imaging-guided percutaneous tumor ablation. *Acad Radiol* 2005; **12**(9):1100–9.

12. Shankar S, van Sonnenberg E, Silverman SG, Tuncali K. Interventional radiology procedures in the liver. Biopsy, drainage, and ablation. *Clin Liver Dis* 2002; **6**(1):91–118.

13. Uppot RN, Silverman SG, Zagoria RJ *et al.* Imaging-guided percutaneous ablation of renal cell carcinoma: a primer of how we do it. *Am J Roentgenol* 2009; **192**(6):1558–70.

CT-guided biopsy using prior FDG-PET/CT images to select a metabolically active mass to biopsy in a 49-year-old male with progressive metastatic gastrointestinal stromal tumor detected on a recent FDG-PET/CT scan.

## FDG-PET/CT acquisition and processing parameters

Patient was fasted for at least 6 hours before the IV injection of 20 mCi of FDG. FDG-PET/CT scans were acquired after 60–90 min post-injection of FDG using a PET/CT scanner (Discovery ST, General Electric, Milwaukee, WI). The CT scans were performed with the patient in the supine position from the head to the proximal thighs for attenuation correction and anatomic co-registration without oral or IV contrast material, and with the following imaging parameters of 140 kVp, 90–120 mA, 1.25 collimation. Images were reconstructed to 3.75 mm section thickness using a 512 × 512 matrix, with a filtered backprojection algorithm. Immediately after the CT scan, FDG-PET scans were obtained for the same volume as the CT scans in 2-D mode for 4 min acquisitions, for 6–7 bed positions. FDG-PET images were reconstructed using a 128 × 128 matrix with an iterative ordered subsets expectation maximization (OSEM) algorithm (2 iterations, 30 subsets), yielding a volume of 47 sections with a voxel size of 3.25 × 3.25 × 3.25 mm³.

Maximum standardized uptake values were generated for each lesion corrected for body weight [$SUVmax = (tissue\ activity\ concentration) \times (body\ weight)/(administered\ activity)$]. Maximal lesional SUVs were measured as the maximum point on the axial image with highest activity.

## Interventional procedure

In this case, the FDG-PET/CT images were used for procedure planning in order to target a peripancreatic mass. By using 18-gauge large needles, tissue samples were obtained under US guidance (Figure 20.1D) using a transhepatic approach to a 6 cm mass lesser sac mass showing mild FDG avidity (arrowheads in Figures 20.1A–C). Note a non-FDG-avid 5 cm mass between the anterior chest wall and liver, which was not selected for biopsy (arrow in Figures 20.1A–C).

## Diagnosis and clinical follow-up

Pathology revealed metastasis from patient's known gastrointestinal stromal tumor.

## Discussion and teaching points

In this case, because of the FDG-PET/CT scan findings; the peripancreatic mass was biopsied rather than the photopenic mass anterior to the liver. The peripancreatic mass was mildly FDG avid (activity equal to liver), whereas the mass anterior to the liver demonstrated lack of metabolic activity. Although easier and possibly safer, biopsy of the metabolically inactive mass would have most likely yielded a non-diagnostic biopsy result.

In patients with multiple tumors, selection of an appropriate site for biopsy can potentially increase the yield. FDG-PET/CT provides a metabolic map of the tumor mass, and FDG avidity may represent the presence of active tumor cells in it. When a prior FDG-PET/CT scan is available, it may be helpful to consider not only visibility and/or accessibility of the mass but also metabolic activity of the tumor when planning a biopsy procedure and selecting a mass to biopsy.

## Take-home message

- In the presence of multiple tumors, FDG-PET/CT may be helpful in selecting which mass to biopsy.

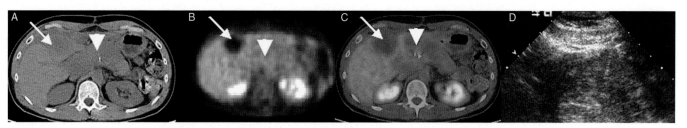

**Figure 20.1** (A) axial CT; (B) FDG-PET; (C) fused FDG-PET/CT; (D) ultrasound image.

- While planning a biopsy procedure and selecting a mass to biopsy, an interventional radiologist should consider not only visibility and/or accessibility of the mass but also metabolic activity of the tumor whenever the FDG-PET/CT scan is available (1).

## Reference

1. Tatli S, Gerbaudo VH, Mamede M *et al.* Abdominal masses sampled at PET/CT-guided percutaneous biopsy: initial experience with registration of prior PET/CT images. *Radiology* 2010; **256**(1):305–11.

A 51-year-old male with recurrent gastrointestinal stromal tumor that progressed despite treatment with a tyrosine kinase inhibitor. Whole-body FDG-PET/CT for restaging showed a large, partially FDG-avid mass in the mid abdomen (Figures 20.2A–C), and was referred for percutaneous biopsy before initiation of a different treatment protocol (Figure 20.2D).

## Interventional procedure technique

The prior PET/CT scan (Figures 20.2A–C) was reviewed and used to delineate regions of the large mass that was FDG-avid, and therefore most likely to contain viable tumor. Tissue samples were obtained using 18-gauge large needles under CT-guidance (Figure 20.2D).

## Diagnosis and clinical follow-up

Pathology revealed gastrointestinal stromal tumor.

## Discussion and teaching points

In this case, the abdominal mass was large and demonstrated a heterogeneous pattern of FDG uptake. Highly FDG-avid areas and non-avid areas were clearly delineated. High FDG uptake is usually consistent with viable malignant tissue, whereas non-FDG-avid areas most likely represent non-malignant tissue such as foci of necrosis or fibrosis. With the FDG-PET/CT findings, the biopsy route was planned and the most FDG-avid portion of the mass (Figures 20.2B, 20.2C) targeted (Figure 20.2D).

## Take-home message

- The information provided by FDG-PET/CT can be used to target the most metabolically active portion of a mass, and potentially improve the yield of the biopsy procedure.
- Targeting markedly FDG-avid foci during biopsy minimizes sampling errors, whereas obtaining tissue samples from non-FDG-avid areas may yield non-diagnostic results.

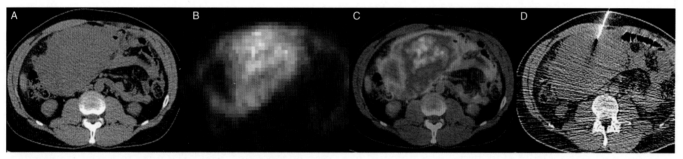

**Figure 20.2** (A) axial CT; (B) FDG-PET; (C) fused FDG-PET/CT; (D) CT guidance image.

## Reference

1. Tatli S, Gerbaudo VH, Mamede M *et al.* Abdominal masses sampled at PET/CT-guided percutaneous biopsy: initial experience with registration of prior PET/CT images. *Radiology* 2010; **256**(1):305–11.

A 73-year-old female with history of breast and lung cancers. Whole-body FDG-PET/CT scan showed an FDG-avid mass in the left lobe of the liver with no corresponding CT finding. The patient was referred to interventional radiology for biopsy.

## Interventional procedure technique

Fine-needle aspiration biopsy of the mass was performed under CT guidance. Since the mass was not visualized on unenhanced CT, prior FDG-PET/CT images were registered to the CT images obtained during the biopsy using special sofware that allowed the prior PET images to be fused with the CT images acquired during the biopsy procedure. The whole-body FDG-PET/CT images were transferred in DICOM format from the radiology network to a separate laptop computer. A FDG-PET/CT image dataset (typically 25 pairs of sections) that included the mass and surrounding anatomy was selected. The CT scanner is programmed to recognize the IP address of the laptop. Through a LAN connection, an intraprocedural planning CT scan (120 kVp, 120 mA, 5 mm section thickness) with a volume (typically 25 sections) that matches the selected FDG-PET/CT scan dataset was transferred to a laptop computer in DICOM format. A section containing the most FDG-avid portion of the mass was chosen from the PET images, and a matching section from the intraprocedural CT scan was selected. Four structures that were visible in both the FDG-PET/CT image and the planning CT image were identified and selected as landmarks. Based on these landmarks, the FDG-PET/CT and intraprocedural CT images were registered using Medical Image Processing Analysis and Visualization (MIPAV) software. This software is available on the Internet, and compatible with several platforms including Windows, MAC, UNIX, and LINUX. Interventional radiologists reviewed the registered images and placed an initial biopsy needle. A CT scan was repeated and registered to the FDG-PET/CT as described above. The needles

were re-positioned if the needle-tip was not in the most FDG-avid portion of the mass. Each registration was completed within 3–5 min. Figure 20.3 exemplifies in this case how the PET and CT images were initially registered by selecting four landmarks from each image; in (Figures 20.3A and 20.3B) posterior (1) and anterior border of the liver (2), anterior border of the spine (3), and posterior border of the left kidney (4), and then fused (Figure 20.3C). Axial CT image (Figure 20.3D) was obtained for needle-tip location confirmation. Registered image (Figure 20.3E) shows that one biopsy needle was within the FDG-avid mass (curved arrow) but the other was not (arrowhead).

## Diagnosis and clinical follow-up

Pathology revealed a metastasis from the patient's known primary breast adenocarcinoma.

## Discussion and teaching points

Previously acquired FDG-PET/CT images and registration software were used to biopsy a mass under CT scan guidance. The information provided by the FDG-PET/CT scan was used to target the FDG-avid mass (Figures 20.3A, 20.3C, 20.3E) that had no CT correlate (Figures 20.3B, 20.3D). Although anatomical landmarks and visual co-registration could have been used to place the needles in the expected location of the mass, accurate targeting would have been difficult, and the procedure may have been prolonged and radiation exposure to the patient and healthcare personnel may have been increased (1). In this case, preprocedural FDG-PET images registered to intraprocedural unenhanced CT images and displayed on a single screen helped target the mass.

If a mass is not well visualized with unenhanced CT, intravenous contrast material can be administered during a CT-guided biopsy. However, contrast enhancement of some

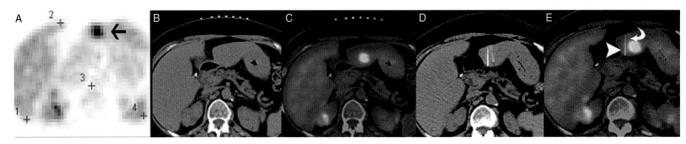

Figure 20.3 (A) axial FDG-PET; (B) axial CT; (C) fused FDG-PET/CT; (D) CT guidance image; (E) fused FDG-PET/CT guidance image. Printed with permission from *Radiology* 2010;**256**(1):305–11.

masses may not persist long enough to be useful during the entire biopsy procedure. Ultrasound or MRI guidance may also be used to biopsy masses that are not visible in unenhanced CT. However, some masses are not visible with US. MRI typically requires special, wide-bore, or open configuration scanners.

## Take-home message

- By using image registration software, prior FDG-PET/CT images can be registered to intraprocedural CT to aid in the targeting of malignant masses that are not visible with unenhanced CT alone.

## Reference

1. Tatli S, Gerbaudo VH, Mamede M *et al*. Abdominal masses sampled at PET/CT-guided percutaneous biopsy: initial experience with registration of prior PET/CT images. *Radiology* 2010; **256**(1):305–11.

A 79-year-old female with history of non-small lung cancer. Contrast-enhanced CT (Figure 20.4A) showed a new liver mass and the patient was referred for both a restaging FDG-PET/CT scan and a percutaneous biopsy of one of her liver masses.

## Interventional procedure technique

FDG-PET/CT and biopsy were both performed during the same session. Following the diagnostic FDG-PET/CT scan (acquired as described above), while the patient remained on the scanner table, FDG-PET/CT images were reviewed on the scanner monitor. The patient remained supine and a marker line grid was placed over the liver. After initiating IV conscious sedation medication, a CT scan (140 kVp, 40 mA, 3.75 mm section thickness) was obtained at one table position (~15 cm length) during quiet breathing. Then, an FDG scan (2-D mode, 3 min emission) was acquired during quiet breathing. CT and PET images were fused electronically using the scanner's software, and the fused images were reviewed to plan the interventional procedure.

The skin entry site was marked, prepped, and sterile drapes were applied. After local anesthesia with 2% of lidocaine, 22-gauge biopsy needles were placed into the FDG-avid mass with tandem technique using additional CT scans obtained with the same protocol above, and each fused with a previously obtained one-bed position planning PET scan. After the biopsy needles were placed into the mass, one-table position CT (Figure 20.4A) and PET (Figure 20.4B) scans were repeated with the same protocol used for the planning scan, and the positions of the needle-tips (Figure 20.4C) were confirmed on the fused PET/CT images (Figure 20.4D). After the needles were removed, a CT scan was performed to evaluate for bleeding or pneumothorax.

Following the biopsy procedure, the patient was observed for 2 hours.

## Diagnosis and clinical follow-up

Pathology revealed a metastasis from the patient's known non-small cell lung cancer.

## Discussion and teaching points

The patient was in need of a restaging FDG-PET/CT as well as a biopsy of the liver mass; we performed both studies in a single session, and biopsied the liver mass under FDG-PET/CT guidance. In addition to X-ray fluoroscopy, US, CT, and MRI, FDG-PET/CT can also be used to guide percutaneous interventions (1). Although, as presented in an earlier case, prior FDG-PET/CT images can be registered to the intraprocedural CT using special registration software, we opted to use the PET/CT scanner to guide the procedure in this case because this allowed for both the acquisition of the restaging FDG-PET/CT scan and the biopsy to be performed in the same visit. Another benefit of performing the biopsy during the same session as the FDG-PET/CT scan is that there are fewer misregistration artifacts that can occur as a result of a change in the patient's positioning between two scans. Although misregistration is not uncommon in FDG-PET/CT images, it is usually due to respiratory and cardiac motion, and is typically limited only to regions near the diaphragm. The added value of using FDG-PET/CT in this case to target and biopsy the mass was that the lesion was almost undetectable on CT. It is in cases like this where accurate lesion targeting is difficult without the metabolic information. By using fused anatomo-metabolic FDG-PET/CT images, planning and targeting of the mass was achieved without difficulty and an adequate biopsy specimen was obtained.

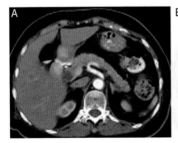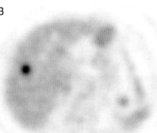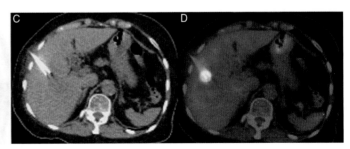

**Figure 20.4** (A) axial CT; (B) axial FDG-PET; (C) CT guidance image; (D) fused FDG-PET/CT guidance image.

## Take-home message

- Biopsy can be performed in a PET/CT scanner, and is particularly helpful when doing biopsies of FDG-avid masses that are not visible or poorly visible with unenhanced-CT.

- Biopsy in a PET/CT scan may allow a staging PET/CT and biopsy to be performed in the same session.

## Reference

1.   Tatli S, Gerbaudo VH, Feeley CM *et al.* PET/CT-guided percutaneous biopsy of abdominal masses: initial experience. *J Vasc Interv Radiol* 2011;**22**(4):507–14.

A 55-year-old male with metastatic colon cancer to the liver underwent a low anterior surgical resection of the primary tumor and recently completed chemotherapy. The liver lesion responded partially, and therefore was referred for percutaneous ablation. A staging PET/CT was also requested.

## Interventional procedure technique

A plan was made to perform a restaging FDG-PET/CT scan and biopsy in the same session. Following the FDG-PET/CT scan, while the patient remained on the scanner table, FDG-PET/CT images were reviewed on the scanner monitor and revealed that the liver lesion (Figure 20.5A, arrow) was not FDG avid (Figure 20.5B). However, a biopsy was performed to evaluate whether the mass contained neoplastic cells. The skin entry site was marked, prepped, and sterile drapes were applied. After local anesthesia with 2% of lidocaine, 25-gauge biopsy needles were placed into the mass with tandem technique using additional CT scans to confirm the positions of the needle-tips (Figure 20.5C). After the needles were removed, a CT scan was performed to evaluate for bleeding or pneumothorax. Following the biopsy procedure, the patient was observed for 2 hours.

## Diagnosis and clinical follow-up

Pathology revealed metastases from the patient's known colon cancer and the mass was treated with percutaneous CT-guided radiofrequency ablation (RF) on a subsequent visit.

## Discussion and teaching points

In this case, an FDG-PET/CT-guided biopsy was planned during the same session as the diagnostic whole-body PET/CT scan. However, when the mass was shown not to be FDG avid, biopsy was still undertaken, and indeed the diagnostic FDG-PET/CT scan was falsely negative. There are reasons for false-negative FDG-PET results. As with any imaging technique, the spatial resolution is limited and small (< 1 cm) malignant lesions may not be detected. Similarly, large masses that are mostly necrotic or contain fibrosis and only a few viable tumor cells may be falsely negative. Finally, cancers that contain a large amount of mucin may not be detectable (1, 2). In contrast, if a small mass or lymph node is FDG-avid compared with the surrounding background, the possibility of malignancy is high. In the illustrated case, although the liver mass was 1.7 cm, the lack of FDG avidity was probably related to the presence of only a small number of cancer cells within a partially treated lesion. It is believed that a cancerous lesion with fewer than $10^8$ cells will not be detected by today's state-of-the-art PET scanners, whether they are FDG avid or not (3). Another explanation for a false-negative FDG-PET result in this case is that the chemotherapy might have prevented FDG uptake by cancer cells via a phenomenon known as post-treatment stunning (3). Negative effect of recent therapy on the FDG uptake of malignant cells is a well-known fact, and FDG-PET/CT imaging is recommended to be performed at least 6–8 weeks after chemotherapy and 8–12 weeks after radiation therapy (3). In summary, therefore, negative PET findings do not necessarily indicate that the patient is disease-free, and biopsy can play an important role in determining the need for additional treatment, including ablation.

## Take-home message

- Cancerous masses (both small and large) may contain too small a number of viable tumor cells to be detected with FDG-PET.
- FDG-PET/CT's sensitivity decreases when adenocarcinoma cells have a high mucin content.
- Recent chemotherapy may prevent FDG uptake of residual tumor cells.
- Biopsy may be helpful in evaluating non-FDG-avid masses.

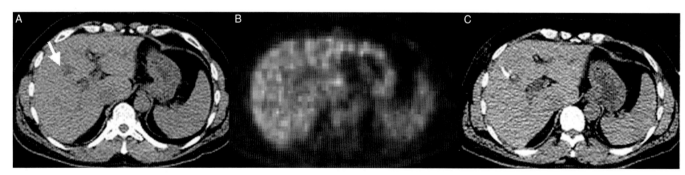

**Figure 20.5** (A) axial CT; (B) axial FDG-PET; (C) CT guidance image.

# References

1. von Schulthess GK, Steinert HC, Hany TF. Integrated PET/CT: current applications and future directions. *Radiology* 2006;**238**(2): 405–22.

2. Whiteford MH, Whiteford HM, Yee LF *et al.* Usefulness of FDG-PET scan in the assessment of suspected metastatic or recurrent adenocarcinoma of the colon and rectum. *Dis Colon Rectum* 2000;**43**(6):759–67.

3. Wahl RL, Jacene H, Kasamon Y, Lodge MA. From RECIST to PERCIST: evolving considerations for PET response criteria in solid tumors. *J Nucl Med* 2009; **50**(Suppl 1):122S–50S.

A 65-year-old female with adenocarcinoma of the colon treated with low anterior resection developed a new liver mass detected by MRI; findings suggested a metastasis. The patient was referred for a restaging FDG-PET/CT scan and percutaneous radiofrequency (RF) ablation. A plan was made to perform PET/CT and ablation in the same session.

## Interventional procedure technique

Following the diagnostic FDG-PET/CT scan, while the patient remained on the scanner table, images were reviewed on the scanner monitor. The patient remained supine and a grid was placed over the liver. After initiating IV conscious sedation, a CT scan (140 kVp, 40 mA, 3.75 mm section thickness) was obtained at one table position (~15 cm length) during quiet breathing. Then, a PET scan (2-D mode, 3 min emission) was performed during shallow breathing. CT and PET images were fused electronically using the scanner's built-in software, and the fused images were reviewed and the ablation was planned. The images revealed a highly FDG-avid liver mass with ill-defined margins on CT.

The skin entry site was marked, prepped, and sterile drapes were applied. After local anesthesia with 2% of lidocaine, a 22-gauge guiding needle was placed into the FDG-avid mass using additional CT scans obtained with the same protocol above, and each fused to the previously obtained one-bed position planning FDG-PET images. A clustered internally cooled RF device (Covidien, Mansfield, MA) was placed in the mass using a tandem technique. One-table position CT (Figure 20.6A) and FDG-PET (Figure 20.6B) scans were repeated using the same protocol used for the planning scan, and following confirmation of the position of the RF applicator on the fused FDG-PET/CT images (Figure 20.6C), RF energy was delivered for 12 minutes. After the applicator was removed, a CT scan was performed to evaluate for bleeding or pneumothorax. Following the ablation procedure, the patient was admitted for overnight observation.

## Diagnosis and clinical follow-up

MRI at 24 hours showed that the ablation volume encompassed the entire tumor. There was no residual tumor at follow-up MRI scan acquired 18 months later.

## Discussion and teaching points

Percutaneous RF ablation was performed under FDG-PET/CT guidance. PET/CT guidance helped visualize FDG-avid tumor with ill-defined margins on CT, and guide the placement of the ablation applicators (1). Proper positioning of ablation applicators is crucial to assure complete tumor treatment without injuring adjacent organs. While suboptimal probe placement could lead to under-treatment and residual viable tumor, ablation extending beyond the tumor carries the risk of damaging adjacent normal parenchyma as well as injuring adjacent organs.

As the ablation procedure progressed, tumor metabolic activity persisted and the tumor was FDG avid even after ablation. The persistence of FDG activity within the tumor throughout ablation helps during targeting and assures that the ablation applicators' positions remain appropriate. The lack of thermal effects on FDG activity within the tumor during FDG-PET/CT-guided RF ablation indicates that changes in FDG activity cannot be used to monitor ablation coverage or completeness at the time of the intervention (2).

## Take-home message

- FDG-PET/CT can be used to guide RF ablation procedures and is particularly helpful for guiding where to place RF applicators.

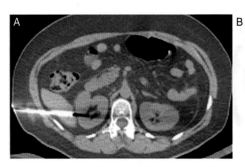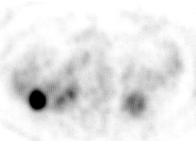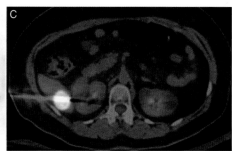

**Figure 20.6** (A) axial CT; (B) axial FDG-PET; (C) fused FDG-PET/CT guidance image.

- FDG activity persists throughout the ablation procedure as thermal effects do not result in dissipation of FDG uptake in tumors.
- The lack of thermal effects on FDG activity within the tumor during FDG-PET/CT-guided RFA, indicates that

changes in FDG activity cannot be used to monitor ablation coverage or completeness at the time of the intervention (1).

# References

1. Tatli S, Gerbaudo VH, Feeley CM *et al*. PET/CT-guided percutaneous biopsy of abdominal masses: initial experience. *J Vasc Interv Radiol* 2011; **22**(4):507–14.

2. Schoellnast H, Larson SM, Nehmeh SA *et al*. Radiofrequency ablation of non-small-cell carcinoma of the lung under real-time FDG PET CT guidance. *Cardiovasc Intervent Radiol* 2011;**34**(Suppl 2): 182–5.

A 53-year-old female with enlarging perihepatic metastasis from ovarian papillary cystadenocarcinoma. The patient was referred for restaging FDG-PET/CT and percutaneous ablation. A plan was made to perform the FDG-PET/CT and the ablation in the same session.

## Interventional procedure technique

Following the staging FDG-PET/CT scan, while the patient remained on the scanner table, FDG-PET/CT images were reviewed on the scanner monitor and revealed a partially FDG-avid perihepatic mass adjacent to the anterior chest wall, diaphragm, and the heart (Figure 20.7). The patient remained supine and a grid was placed over the liver. After initiating conscious sedation, a CT scan (140 kVp, 40 mA, 3.75 mm section thickness) was obtained at one table position (~15 cm length) during quiet breathing. Then, a FDG-PET scan (2-D mode, 3 min emission) was performed during quiet breathing. CT and PET images were fused electronically using the scanner's built-in software, and the procedure was planned based on the information observed in the fused images (Figure 20.7).

The skin entry site was marked, prepped, and sterile drapes were applied. After local anesthesia with 2% of lidocaine, a 22-gauge guiding needle was placed into the FDG-avid portion of the mass using additional CT scans obtained with the same protocol described above, and each fused to the previously obtained one-bed position planning PET images. A total of 5 ice-rod cryoablation applicators (Cryohit; Galil Medical, Yokneam, Israel) were placed within the mass using a tandem technique. One-table position CT and FDG-PET scans were repeated with the same protocol used for the planning CT scan, and the positions of the cryoablation applicators were confirmed by the fused FDG-PET/CT images for each application (Figure 20.8).

Two 15-min cycles of freezing separated by a 10-min passive thaw were delivered. Intermittent CT images were obtained and each was fused with the previously acquired PET scan to evaluate adequate coverage and adjacent organ involvement. After the applicator was removed, a CT scan was performed to evaluate for bleeding or pneumothorax. Following the ablation procedure, the patient was admitted for overnight observation.

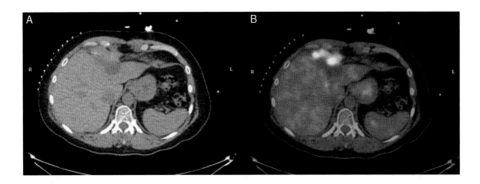

**Figure 20.7** (A) Ablation planning axial CT; (B) fused FDG-PET/CT images of the liver.

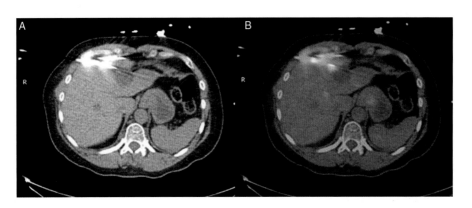

**Figure 20.8** (A) Axial CT; (B) fused FDG-PET/CT images of the liver demonstrating the position of the cryoablation applicators.

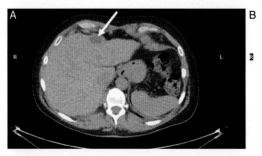 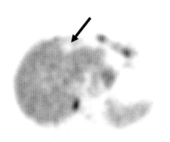 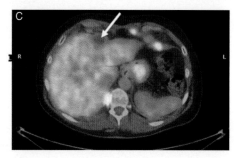

**Figure 20.9** (A) Axial CT; (B) FDG-PET; (C) fused FDG-PET/CT images of the liver 6 months after treatment.

## Diagnosis and clinical follow-up

MRI at 24 hours showed that the ablation volume encompassed the entire tumor. There was no residual tumor at follow-up MRI and PET/CT acquired 6 months later (Figure 20.9, arrows).

## Discussion and teaching points

Cryoablation was chosen to treat an ovarian carcinoma metastasis in this case because it was situated close to the heart. Using CT, the effects of freezing, manifested as an "iceball" can be visualized and the treatment monitored. This is an important advantage of cryoablation relative to RF ablation where the effects of heating are not as well delineated during imaging. This feature of cryoablation allows for monitoring the growth of the ice ball, which becomes particularly important while treating tumors located in close proximity to critical structures. If the iceball extends to the adjacent critical structure during freezing, the amount of cryogen gas may be decreased to prevent further growth to prevent injury. FDG-PET/CT added an additional important benefit in this case. The tumor was large and heterogeneous containing regions of non-FDG avidity. FDG-PET/CT guidance helped identify and ablate only metabolically active sites of tumor thus assuring further the safety of the procedure.

## Take-home message

- PET/CT can be used to guide percutaneous cryoablation.
- PET/CT guidance helps to ablate only the metabolically active portion of the mass and to prevent unnecessary extension of the ablation zone to critical structures.

## Reference

1. Tatli S, Gerbaudo VH, Feeley CM *et al.* PET/CT-guided percutaneous biopsy of abdominal masses: initial experience. *J Vasc Interv Radiol* 2011;**22**(4):507–14.

# Index